MEDICAL RADIOLOGY
Diagnostic Imaging

Editors:
A. L. Baert, Leuven
K. Sartor, Heidelberg

Springer
Berlin
Heidelberg
New York
Barcelona
Hong Kong
London
Milan
Paris
Tokyo

J. W. A. J. Reeders · P. C. Goodman (Eds.)

Radiology of AIDS

With Contributions by

J. Bedford · J. W. Berlin · M. R. Canninga-Van Dijk · A. Deville · E. K. Fishman
E. H. L. Gaensler · A. Geoffray · P. C. Goodman · R. M. Gore · L. B. Haramati · C. B. Hicks
A. J. Holz · K. M. Horton · H. J. Hulsebosch · E. R. Jenny-Avital · J. S. Klein · P. P. Maeder
J. R. Mathieson · A. J. Megibow · R. A. Meuli · F. H. Miller · E. H. Moore · G. M. Newmark
J. W. A. J. Reeders · G. S. Reiter · J. Sandhu · M. Spehl · J. Tehranzadeh · M. T. Tran
J. G. Van den Tweel · E. van Sonnenberg · M. L. Hansman Whiteman · V. Yaghmai · J. Yee

Foreword by
A. L. Baert

With 267 Figures in 453 Separate Illustrations, 33 in Color and 25 Tables

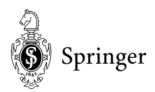
Springer

Jacques W. A. J. Reeders, MD, PhD
Consultant (Interventional) Radiologist
Department of Radiology
St. Elisabeth Hospital Willemstad
Breedestraat 193 (O)
Curaçao
Netherlands Antilles

Philip C. Goodman, MD
Department of Radiology
Duke University Medical Center
P.O. Box 3808
Durham, NC 22710
USA

Medical Radiology · Diagnostic Imaging and Radiation Oncology

Continuation of
Handbuch der medizinischen Radiologie
Encyclopedia of Medical Radiology

ISBN 3-540-66510-2   Springer-Verlag Berlin Heidelberg New York

Library of Congress Cataloging-in-Publication Data

Radiology of AIDS / (eds.) J.W.A.J. Reeders, P.C. Goodman ; foreword by A.L. Baert.
    p. ; cm. -- (Medical radiology)
    Includes bibliographical references and index.
    ISBN 3540665102 (alk. paper)
    1. AIDS (Disease)--Imaging. I. Reeders, Jacques W.A.J. II. Goodman, Philip C.
(Philip Charles), 1946- III. Series.
    [DNLM: 1. Acquired Immunodeficiency Syndrome--radiography. WC 503.1 R129 2001]
    RC607.A26 R232 2001
    616.97'920757--dc21   00-048254

Springer-Verlag Berlin Heidelberg New York
a member of BertelsmannSpringer Science+Business Media GmbH

http//www.springer.de
© Springer-Verlag Berlin Heidelberg 2001

Printed in Germany

Cover-Design and Typesetting: Verlagsservice Teichmann, 69256 Mauer

SPIN: 107 176 09   21/3130 – 5 4 3 2 1 0 – Printed on acid-free paper

To my mother,
the memory of Louis, my father,
and to my wife Nienke
and my children Loes and Puck

To the memory of Paul and Dorothy, my parents,
and to my wife Mary
and my children Whitney and Graydon

Foreword

Although astonishing progress has been achieved during recent years in the treatment of patients afflicted with AIDS, this disease is still spreading in much of the developing world, where economic resources are limited. Physicians working in these geographic areas increasingly face the dramatic and devastating consequences of this epidemic and will certainly benefit from the information imparted in this book. Indeed, it has now been well established that radiologic studies play a key role in the diagnosis and management of patients with HIV infection.

In the Western world the positive effects of new potent drugs are already discernible, resulting in decreased mortality from the illness. But as AIDS patients survive longer, the medical profession is confronted with changing radiologic findings related to longstanding AIDS.

This superb book provides a very comprehensive overview of our current knowledge about radiologic imaging features in AIDS. I would like to congratulate most sincerely the Editors for their tremendous field work, their enthusiasm, and their high level of expertise, which have resulted in the publication of this outstanding volume. To assist them in their task, they have recruited numerous leading specialists in the field. Meticulous editing has reduced the repetition that otherwise can easily occur in a multiauthored textbook. I am convinced that this comprehensive and richly illustrated work will be of great interest to all clinical disciplines involved in the management of AIDS patients.

I hope that this volume will have the same great success that other books in the Diagnostic Medical Radiology series have enjoyed. I would appreciate any constructive criticism that might be offered.

Leuven   ALBERT L. BAERT

Preface

The terrible AIDS epidemic that first gained notoriety in the medical literature in 1981 has only recently been alleviated somewhat in some countries by the introduction of highly active antiretroviral therapy (HAART). However, in other regions of the world where social and economic conditions are less favorable, AIDS continues to exact a heavy toll in human morbidity and mortality. Radiology has been an important discipline in diagnosing many of the diseases associated with AIDS and continues to be relied upon by clinical providers in order to offer the best care to their patients. Millions of those suffering with AIDS have benefited from an early or confirmatory diagnosis of disease of the brain, lungs, intra-abdominal organs, lymph nodes, musculoskeletal system, etc.

The value of imaging of AIDS is well established. Approximately one year ago the editors of this book met at the Radiological Society of North America (RSNA) meeting in Chicago, USA to discuss the value of an updated compendium of both down-to-earth and cutting-edge information regarding the imaging of AIDS. This book, *Radiology of AIDS*, is the culmination of our collaboration begun during that initial discussion. In preparing this book, we have enlisted the assistance of some of the leading experts in the field of AIDS diagnosis. Our intention was to provide a source of concise yet thorough, easily read, and amply illustrated material that would be useful to practicing clinicians and radiologists whether they reside in central Africa, western Europe, North America, or other parts of the globe where AIDS exists. We hope that the efforts of our contributors will be used to the benefit of those unfortunate individuals who suffer from this disease and that their care is facilitated by the information contained herein. Moreover, it is our fervent desire that the intensity of the continuing fight against the spread of this epidemic is maintained. It is already presumed that heterosexual contact is the most rapidly growing mode of transmission of HIV, and the spread of the virus continues. Given the latency period before symptoms appear, we must remain vigilant and remember that AIDS will be with us for years to come. A book about AIDS, in particular this book on the radiology of AIDS, should serve not only as a resource for diagnosis and treatment but also as a reminder that HIV remains a significant public health risk.

We would like to express our appreciation of the incredible efforts made by our contributing authors, whose dedication to the care of AIDS patients is so important. We would also like to thank our respective secretaries, Vera Mills and Carina Magloire-Juliana, for their diligent work in preparing the manuscripts, and Ursula Davis at Springer-Verlag, for her timely and persistent prodding. Without their efforts, this book would not have been produced.

Curaçao   J. W. A. J. REEDERS
Durham   P. C. GOODMAN

Contents

1 Introduction

JACQUES W. A. J. REEDERS

CONTENTS

1.1 History

Acquired immune deficiency syndrome (AIDS), the most severe clinical expression of immune suppression following infection with human immune deficiency virus (HIV), was first diagnosed as a clinical entity in 1981 (CDC 1986; GOTTLIEB et al. 1981; MASUR et al. 1981; SIEGAL et al.1981). At the Centers for Disease Control and Prevention (CDC) in Atlanta, Georgia, USA, the first indications of the impending AIDS epidemic became evident. Upon retrospective review of clinical cases and blood and tissue samples, the disease was found to have already existed at least as early as 1978 in the United States. The first report appeared in the *Morbidity and Mortality Weekly Report* of the CDC on 5 June 1981 (CDC 1981).

J.W.A.J. REEDERS, MD, PhD
Consultant Radiologist, Department of Radiology, St. Elisabeth Hospital Willemstad, Breedestraat 193 (O), Curaçao, Netherlands Antilles

It was at the beginning of the 1980s that the relatively few cases of homosexual male patients with unusual infections and tumors heralded the onset of one of the most devastating epidemics in medical history, an epidemic that has had a profound impact on all aspects of medical practice. Because the new disease was mainly seen in homosexuals with frequently changing sexual contacts, the name gay-related immune deficiency disease (GRID) was given.

After the initial reports of AIDS, the CDC set up a task force to detect the syndrome in the population and identify those at risk. Criteria for the definition of AIDS were drawn up based primarily on the diagnosis of opportunistic infections and rare tumors in individuals with no evidence of immune suppression. The CDC formulated the first case definition in 1981, and this definition has since been revised several times. Besides three additional clinical conditions, one laboratory parameter was included as an indicator for AIDS: the peripheral blood CD4 lymphocyte count (T cells in HIV-infected patients).

1.2 AIDS: a Retrovirus Infection

The course of HIV disease involves a latent period following initial infection. The likelihood of developing clinical AIDS is directly related to the duration of HIV infection. An estimated cumulative incidence of AIDS of 54% has been reported 11 years following seroconversion. During the period between seroconversion and the development of clinical AIDS, HIV-positive patients often demonstrate non-specific findings.

One can deduce that the human immune system does not (yet) have a satisfactory solution to suppressing or eliminating the infection. The cytotoxic T cell response and neutralizing antibodies, two important pillars on which the fight against other infections rests, do not appear to be capable of successfully combating an HIV infection. Two properties of the virus are partially responsible for this: the ability to remain latent in some cells and the ability to continually change those components at which the human immune response aims. Because the virus infection has direct effects on different compartments of the immune system, for many disorders it is difficult to indicate whether they are the cause or the result of disease progression (Goudsmit and Boucher 1998).

Intervention via administration of antiviral substances (zidovudine), neutralizing antibodies, and immune modulators (interferon, interleukins) can help to provide insights into the importance of the different processes in retarding or preventing progression of disease. Until a strategy has been developed which can eliminate host cells with (latent) provirus, it will remain impossible actually to cure the infection (Goudsmit and Boucher 1998).

Much research in the coming years will be aimed at developing methods to eliminate HIV and at developing an effective vaccine. Until this has been achieved, the medical profession can help AIDS patients by establishing diagnosis rapidly, so that adequate treatment can be initiated early on.

1.3
Epidemiology of HIV/AIDS

To develop public health care policies, and to plan and evaluate preventive measurements, predictions of the course of the AIDS epidemic are necessary. The first projections were based on extrapolation of the observed incidence of AIDS cases and predicted an exponential growth of the number of cases in the early years; this led to an overestimate of the expected number of cases. Now, more sophisticated mathematical models have been developed in which a variety of factors, depending on the region and the purpose for which a prediction is performed, can be incorporated. However, the predictions still have to be interpreted with caution, taking into account the assumptions and limitations of the mathematical model used. WHO estimated that by the year 2000, the global prevalence of HIV (including AIDS cases) would be 20 million and the cumulative number of HIV infections since the beginning of the epidemic would be 30–40 million. It was also predicted that by 2000 the number of children under 10 years orphaned due to AIDS would exceed 5 million (Bindels and Coutinho 1998).

1.4
CNS and Peripheral Nervous System Manifestations

Neurologic complications occur in at least 70% of all HIV-infected individuals, and in 10% of patients neurologic disease is the presenting manifestation of HIV infection. The stage of HIV infection is important in differential diagnosis. Some of these complications occur in early HIV infection: examples are HIV myopathy and inflammatory polyneuropathies. However, most complications occur during severe immunosuppression, when the CD4+ cell count is below $0.2\times10^9/1$ (normal is $>0.5\times10^9/1$) (Portegies and Enting 1998). Several clinical syndromes occur in HIV infection: meningitis, focal neurological symptoms, diffuse encephalopathy, dementia, myelopathy, and neuromuscular disorders. A specific diagnosis based on the clinical examination may be virtually impossible because of the overlap in clinical presentations. Ancillary investigation may not always distinguish between the different specific causes of disease. It is important to keep in mind that only a limited set of causes leads to a specific therapy. A rigorous search for these diagnoses by computed tomography (CT) or magnetic resonance imaging (MRI) is always necessary. Invasive diagnostic procedures, such as brain biopsy, should be reserved for patients in reasonable clinical condition. It is also important to realize that multiple neurologic complications may coexist, which further complicates the diagnosis (Portegies and Enting 1988).

1.4.1
Pulmonary Manifestations

Pneumocystis carinii pneumonia (PCP) and Kaposi's sarcoma were the harbingers of the AIDS epidemic almost 15 years ago. Since then, the spectrum of pulmonary disease affecting these individuals has become better understood. Although the majority of these conditions are infectious in nature, neoplastic and inflammatory diseases also occur with increased frequency among individuals infected with HIV.

The main infectious causes of pulmonary disease among HIV-infected individuals are *Pneumocystis carinii* , *Mycobacterium tuberculosis* , and pyogenic bacterial pneumonia secondary to *Streptococcus pneumoniae, Haemophilus influenzae,* or *Staphylococcus aureus* infection (Montaner and Phillips 1998). Less frequently a variety of fungi and viruses can give rise to pulmonary disease. Although initially a rare AIDS-related complication, aspergillosis has become the leading pulmonary mycosis in many centers.

Cytomegalovirus pneumonitis is uncommon. Although *Mycobacterium avium-intracellulare* (MAI) is a frequent late complication of AIDS, respiratory disease secondary to MAI is distinctly uncommon (WHITE and ZAMAN 1992; MONTANER and PHILLIPS 1998).

The main noninfectious causes of pulmonary disease among HIV-infected individuals are Kaposi's sarcoma, airways hyperreactivity (asthma), and emphysema (QUIEFFIN et al. 1991; MONTANER et al. 1993). Less frequently, lymphocytic interstitial pneumonitis, nonspecific interstitial pneumonitis, lymphoma, drug- or radiation-related pneumonitis, and pulmonary hypertension can be seen in these patients (MANI and SMITH 1994).

Not all lung diseases in patients with HIV infection or even AIDS are necessarily related to the HIV infection. Furthermore, the relative frequency of HIV-associated complications is continuously changing as new antiretrovirals and preventive therapies continue to alter the natural history of the disease. Despite this, PCP still remains the single most frequent AIDS index disease today (MONTANER and PHILLIPS 1998).

It has been generally accepted that specific patterns of pulmonary disease involvement in the AIDS patient, particularly at CT, can help suggest the likely diagnosis and guide further appropriate investigation (SIDER et al. 1993; HARTMAN et al. 1994).

1.4.2
Cardiovascular Manifestations

Cardiovascular system involvement, including pericardial effusion, ventricular dysfunction, endocarditis, cardiac tumors, and cardiac manifestations of various specific infections, is common in patients with HIV infection, particularly in those with advanced disease. Despite the high prevalence of cardiac involvement in AIDS, it is relatively uncommon for cardiovascular dysfunction to be responsible for the major symptoms of patients with AIDS or for hospital admission. Indeed, it has been estimated that less than 7% of HIV patients have symptomatic heart disease and that cardiac disease can be an expected cause of death in only 1%–6% of cases. Consequently, the chief value of familiarity with cardiac involvement in AIDS is perhaps that it enables common, but clinically unimportant disorders to be distinguished from those that are uncommon, but clinically very important.

Clinicians face patients with clinical syndromes of unknown etiology in whom it is important to establish the likely etiology, and patients with known infections in whom it is important to identify the organ systems involved (THOMPSON and KIESS 1998).

1.4.3
Luminal Gastrointestinal Tract Manifestations

Most patients with AIDS will exhibit gastrointestinal symptoms at some time during the course of their illness. In fact, clinical AIDS is often determined by identifying an opportunistic pathogen or neoplasm of the gastrointestinal (GI) tract. AIDS patients will often have multifocal abnormalities of the GI tract (WALL et al. 1986). GI symptoms in patients with AIDS are often nonspecific and so present diagnostic and management challenges. Radiology plays a key role in helping to make the diagnosis as well as in directing the management (WALL et al. 1998).

In an acute HIV infection, a mononucleosis-like illness can occur. This may include symptoms related to the GI tract, such as nausea and diarrhea. Usually this is self-limited and resolves spontaneously. Some patients complaint of pain on swallowing or, less commonly, dysphagia. Both endoscopy and double-contrast esophagograms may demonstrate giant (>2 cm), well-defined shallow ulceration of the esophagus with surrounding normal mucosa. Multiple lesions may occur, but solitary lesions are more frequent. Because biopsies, brushings, cultures, and histopathologic examination have failed to identify another causative organism, these lesions have been termed idiopathic esophageal ulcerations associated with HIV infection (FRAGER et al. 1994). Electron microscopy or biopsy specimens taken at ulcer margins have demonstrated retrovirus-like particles, supporting the diagnosis of HIV infection as the etiology (RABENECK et al. 1990). Corticosteroid treatment of the esophageal ulceration is effective, with 92% of patients having complete symptomatic response with prednisone, usually within a week (WILCOX and SCHWARTZ 1992). HIV-related esophageal ulcers also can occur later in the course of the disease, after recovery from the seroconversion illness (LEVINE et al. 1991). The lower GI tract may also be involved directly by HIV. This seroconversion illness often includes a sore throat, malaise, and myalgias. A maculopapular rash involves the upper trunk, arms, and face in 80% of patients. HIV has been isolated within the gut tissue in up to 50% of patients with AIDS (NELSON et al. 1988).

Idiopathic AIDS enteropathy is a chronic diarrheal illness without other identified infectious etiology. It is thought to be due to enteric HIV infection. Infection of the gut by HIV is associated with a decrease in the total number of intestinal T lymphocytes as well as a significant reversal of the normal mucosal helper/suppressor T cell ratio. HIV-infected mucosal cells demonstrate hypoproliferative changes with mucosal atrophy. Consequently, the structure and function of the gut are thought to be directly affected by the virus itself (WALL et al. 1998).

1.4.4
Hepatopancreaticobiliary Manifestations

Many patients with HIV infection undergo CT examination of the abdomen for evaluation of unexplained fever, abdominal pain, weight loss, palpable mass, organomegaly, or abnormal liver chemistries. The three most common sites of abnormal abdominal CT findings due to AIDS-related opportunistic infection or neoplasm are the lymph nodes, the liver, and the spleen. Often the radiologist can suggest a specific diagnosis or a short list of possible diagnoses on the basis of careful evaluation of abdominal CT findings. In many cases, diagnosis of the infection or neoplasm is made by analysis of blood, stool, or sputum specimens or bone marrow biopsy. However, in a significant percentage of cases, percutaneous fine-needle aspiration (FNAB) or core biopsy of an abdominal nodal or visceral lesion with sonographic or CT guidance may be the best or even the only means, other than open surgical biopsy, to establish the diagnosis (RADIN 1998).

Cooperation and communication between the radiology and cytology departments, together with the expertise of the radiology and cytology staff, will ensure excellent results.

1.4.5
Retroperitoneal Manifestations

In the early stages of HIV infection, retroperitoneal involvement is not frequent and is usually asymptomatic. Benign lymphadenopathy associated with numerous lymph nodes, normal or slightly enlarged, can be found during routine abdominal exploration with CT or ultrasound (US) examinations.

At the time of clinical presentation, patients with AIDS-related diseases of the retroperitoneum frequently have advanced disease involving multiple sites (e.g., nodes, digestive tract, liver, spleen, chest, or brain), but some diseases may be clinically silent and discovered only at autopsy (LAVAYSSIÈRE et al. 1998). US and CT are the modalities of choice for exploring the retroperitoneum, depending on the clinical presentation and status. FNAB under CT or US guidance is useful when it yields positive findings (e.g., non-Hodgkin's lymphoma or *Mycobacterium tuberculosis*). In practice, CT is the most useful method with the best cost-effectiveness ratio for the detection and study of the peritoneum in AIDS patients (LAVAYSSIÈRE et al. 1998).

1.4.6
Renal Manifestations

Parenchymal involvement of the solid abdominal organs has become increasingly common since AIDS was first described in 1981 (FRASSETTO et al. 1991). Renal complications are becoming more prevalent, owing to prolonged patient survival and an increased incidence of AIDS transmission in intravenous drug abusers (SCHACKER et al. 1996; MOORE and CHIASSON 1996). The kidneys in AIDS patients are subject to a wide variety of infectious, neoplastic, immunologic, vascular, and drug-related insults, which can produce a number of often confusing abnormalities on cross-sectional renal imaging studies (MILLER et al. 1993). Plain abdominal radiographs and intravenous urography do not play a major role in the evaluation of these complications (MILLER and GORE 1998).

Cross-sectional imaging is very useful in detecting and in some instances in characterizing the many infectious and neoplastic disorders that involve the kidney in AIDS patients. US has the advantages of lower cost and portability, and does not require intravenous contrast media that have the potential to be nephrotoxic. US may demonstrate striking abnormalities of HIV-associated nephropathy, while CT is normal or demonstrates only enlarged kidneys. In addition, diffuse echogenic foci may be noted in infections such as *Pneumocystis* and MAI, while CT scans remain unremarkable. CT and MRI may be required to demonstrate focal masses that are not well visualized on US. In addition, associated findings including lymphadenopathy, other organ involvement, and bowel pathology are often better appreciated on CT (MILLER and GORE 1998).

1.4.7
Musculoskeletal Manifestations

Since the recognition of HIV-associated disease 20 years ago, the profile of "typical" clinical musculoskeletal manifestations has changed. As supportive or suppressive therapy allows prolonged survival, we are seeing an expanding population manifesting the consequences of chronic immunosuppression and illness (MAGID 1998). Musculoskeletal imaging, like other medical fields, is confronted with an increasingly complex array of associated infections and inflammatory, arthritic, and neoplastic conditions. A high level of suspicion and an awareness of the non-specificity of the clinical and radiographic manifestations of many of these conditions may help in recognizing and diagnosing these abnormalities.

Most early musculoskeletal reports focused on the widespread resurgence of opportunistic infections and tumors which had been quite rare before HIV. More recent reports have explored the possible association between HIV and various inflammatory or arthritic manifestations.

Conventional radiography remains the gateway to diagnostic imaging. In an era of increasing economic limitations, it provides a readily available and economically feasible starting point for diagnostic assessment. It may suggest a diagnosis not yet considered, or confirm a clinical suspicion. Compared with imaging in other patients, imaging of suspected musculoskeletal disease in HIV patients is more different in quantity than in quality: both the clinical and the radiographic signs may be far more subtle than usual (MAGID 1998).

During the earliest part of the epidemic, CT was still relatively new and not routinely available; similarly, MRI did not become clinically available until halfway into the first decade of AIDS. Musculoskeletal scintigraphy became more sophisticated in the 1980s, as the development and availability of specially tagged cells or agents extended the scope and selectivity of available diagnostic tests.

In the face of increasingly complex and subtle clinical musculoskeletal problems, diagnostic imaging may play a major role in patient care and research (MAGID 1998).

1.5
Pediatric AIDS

In slightly more than a decade, HIV-1 infection and AIDS in children has evolved from a clinical syndrome meeting with skepticism as to its relationship to immunosuppressive disease in adults, to a well-characterized disease process, becoming the ninth leading cause of death in children and the seventh leading cause of death in adolescents in the United States. The number of reported cases of AIDS among children in the United States now exceeds 7,000 and it is estimated that there are 5–10 times more children with HIV-1 infection. This epidemic is more explosive in developing areas of the world. Over the same period, there have been dramatic advances in our understanding of human immunology and HIV-1, the causative agent of AIDS. New developments in radiologic techniques and additional experience with infected populations have advanced our understanding of the disease, enhanced diagnostic sensitivity and specificity, limited the need for invasive techniques, and improved our therapeutic approach to pediatric patients (GENIESER et al. 1998).

1.6
Dermatologic and Venereal Manifestations

Since the start of the HIV epidemic in the early 1980s, many dermatologic and venereal diseases have been described in association with HIV infection. The reasons for these associations were that well-known dermatologic and venereal diseases were seen with a higher frequency in HIV-infected patients, or that unusual expressions of these diseases were seen as a result of HIV-induced immunodeficiency. Moreover, otherwise rare dermatoses could be diagnosed in these patients, and even new skin and mucous membrane disease occurred. Gradually, what may be called HIV dermato-venereology has come into being.

Skin and mucous membrane involvement occurs in two phases of the HIV infection:
1. As part of the primary HIV infection;
2. In association with HIV-induced immune deficiency, or AIDS (HULSEBOSCH 1998)

1.7
Healthcare Workers in AIDS

Healthcare workers and surgical teams operating on HIV-infected patients run an unquestionable but probably low risk. The risk of HIV infection depends, in general, on three variables: (a) the prevalence of

HIV-infected patients to whom the healthcare workers are exposed, (b) the frequency of exposure (accidental injuries) to infected blood or body fluids, and (c) the risk of seroconversion after exposure. The risk of contracting HIV infection for a surgeon working during 30 years can be estimated at 0.6%–10%; for healthcare workers in general, the risk is lower.

The basis for the CDC recommendations is that healthcare workers should regard blood and other body fluids from all patients as potentially capable of transmitting blood-borne infection. Moreover, universal precautions should be observed. In this manner, healthcare workers can avoid unnecessary contamination or skin punctures/lacerations. This will greatly reduce the chance of transmission of HIV from the patient to the surgeon and his or her personnel. However, although none of the precautions will reduce the risk of contamination to zero, they will greatly decrease incidence. Nevertheless, in practice, these precautions are frequently partly ignored. Reasons for this common attitude could be inaccuracy, thought of invulnerability of the healthcare worker or surgical team, and/or inconvenience, e.g., loss of sensibility with double gloves (CONSTEN and VAN LANSCHOT 1998).

1.8
AIDS-Related Interventional Procedures

HIV/AIDS continues to exact a tremendous toll in both human and economic terms, having a devastating impact on those afflicted. It is almost a certainty that a radiologist will encounter an HIV-positive patient during the course of their routine practice. While the spectrum of radiologic abnormalities representing opportunistic infection and malignancy in the AIDS patient has received considerable attention over the past 20 years, the role of imaging (US/CT)-guided interventions in diagnosis and management of these patients has not been extensively detailed in the radiology literature.

Chapter 16 will review the use of interventional procedures in the HIV-infected individual.

1.9
Future Perspectives

Since the early 1990s many clinical trials have been conducted. Intense societal pressure and the urgency of the AIDS epidemic have also greatly reduced regulatory roadblocks to the approval of new and promising drugs and changed the position of regulators from extreme caution to active participation, resulting in a number of approvals of new antiviral compounds in record speed.

Many clinical trials are now cooperative efforts among pharmaceutical companies, academic investigators, governments regulators, and community participants.

Undoubtedly the HIV epidemic will continue to grow during this century. The harvest of new biomedical knowledge from expanded research efforts will hopefully continue. Progress will be incremental, and cures are not yet on the horizon. The knowledge gained may prolong useful lives and may change AIDS from a rapidly fatal disease to a controlled chronic illness.

References

Bindels PJE, Coutinho RA (1998) Surveillance and epidemiology of HIV/AIDS. In: Reeders JWAJ, Mathieson JR (eds) AIDS imaging; a practical clinical approach. Saunders, London, pp 20–36

CDC (1981) Kaposi's sarcoma and *Pneumocystis* pneumonia among homosexual men in New York City and California. MMWR 30:305–308

CDC (1986) Update: acquired immunodeficiency syndrome – United States. MMWR 35:17–21

Consten ECJ, van Lanschot JJB (1998) Surgery in AIDS. In: Reeders JWAJ, Mathieson JR (eds) AIDS imaging; a practical clinical approach. Saunders, London, pp 74–88

Frager D, Kotler DP, Baer J (1994) Idiopathic esophageal ulceration in the acquired immunodeficiency syndrome: radiology reappraisal in 10 patients. Abdom Imaging 19:2–5

Frassetto L, Schoenfeld PY, Humphreys MH (1991) Increasing incidence of human immunodeficiency virus-associated nephropathy at San Francisco General Hospital. Am J Kidney Dis 18:655–659

Genieser NB, Krasinski K, Roch KJ, Ambrosino MM (1998) Pediatric AIDS. In: Reeders JWAJ, Mathieson JR (eds) AIDS imaging; a practical clinical approach. Saunders, London, pp 260–280

Gottlieb MS, Schroff R, Schanker HM, et al. (1981) *Pneumocystis carinii* pneumonia and mucosal candidiasis in previously healthy homosexual men. N Engl J Med 305:1425–1431

Goudsmit J, Boucher CAB (1998) AIDS, a retrovirus infection in humans. In: Reeders JWAJ, Mathieson JR (eds) AIDS imaging; a practical clinical approach. Saunders, London, pp 8–14

Hartman TE, Primack SL, Müller NL, Staples CA (1994) Diagnosis of thoracic complications in AIDS: accuracy of CT. AJR 162:547–553

Hulsebosch HJ (1998) Dermatologic and venereal manifestations in AIDS. In: Reeders JWAJ, Mathieson JR (eds) AIDS imaging; a practical clinical approach. Saunders, London, pp 238–245

Laveyssièrre RL, Eliaszewicz M, Cabée AE, Trotot PM (1998) Imaging of the retroperitoneum. In: Reeders JWAJ, Mathieson JR (eds) AIDS imaging; a practical clinical approach. Saunders, London, pp 214–226

Levine MS, Loercher G, Katzka DA, et al. (1991) Giant, human immunodeficiency virus-related ulcers in the esophagus. Radiology 180:323–326

Magid D (1998) Musculoskeletal imaging in AIDS. In: Reeders JWAJ, Mathieson JR (eds) AIDS imaging; a practical clinical approach. Saunders, London, pp 246–259

Mani S, Smith GJ (1994) HIV and pulmonary hypertension: a review. South Med J 87:357–362

Masur H. Michelis MA, Greene JB, et al. (1981) An outbreak of community-acquired *Pneumocystis carinii* pneumonia. N Engl J Med 305:1431–1438

Miller FH, Gore RM (1998) Renal manifestations in AIDS. In: Reeders JWAJ, Mathieson JR (eds) AIDS imaging; a practical clinical approach. Saunders, London, pp 227–237

Miller FH, Parikh S, Gore RM, et al. (1993) Renal manifestations of AIDS. RadioGraphics 13:587–596.

Montaner JSG, Phillips P (1998) Clinical aspects of pulmonary complications in HIV/AIDS. In: Reeders JWAJ, Mathieson JR (eds) AIDS imaging; a practical clinical approach. Saunders, London, pp 131–140

Montaner JSSG, Guillemi SA, Januszewska M, et al. (1993) Unexpected lung lesions among patients with advanced HIV disease prior to PCP prophylaxis when using high resolution computed tomography. American Thoracic Society, San Francisco; 147:A1003

Moore RD, Chiasson RE (1996) Natural history of opportunistic disease in an HIV-infected urban clinical cohort. Am Intern Med 124:663–642

Nelson JA, Reynolds-Kohler C, Margaretten W, et al. (1988) HIV detected in bowel epithelium from patients with gastro-intestinal symptoms. Lancet 1:323–326

Portegies P, Enting RH (1998) Clinical neurology. In: Reeders JWAJ, Mathieson JR (eds) AIDS imaging; a practical clinical approach. Saunders, London, pp 91–97

Quieffin J, Hunter J, Schechter MT, et al. (1991) Aerosol pentamidine-induced bronchoconstriction. Chest 100:624–627

Rabeneck L, Popovic M, Gartner S, et al. (1990) Acute HIV infection presenting with painful swallowing and esophageal ulcers. JAMA 263:2318–2322

Radin DR (1998) Hepato-pancreato and biliary imaging in AIDS; computed tomography. In: Reeders JWAJ, Mathieson JR (eds) AIDS imaging; a practical clinical approach. Saunders, London, pp 203–213

Shacker T, Collier AC, Hughes J, et al. (1996) Clinical and epidemiologic features of primary HIV infection. Am Intern Med 125:257–269

Sider L, Gabriel H, Curry DR, Pham MS (1993) Pattern recognition of the pulmonary manifestations of AIDS on CT scans. RadioGraphics 13:771–784

Siegal FP, Lopez C. Hammer GS, et al. (1981) Severe acquired immunodeficiency in male homosexuals, manifested by chronic perianal ulcerative herpes simplex lesions. N Engl J Med 305:1439–1444

Thompson CR, Kiess MC (1998) Imaging of cardiac involvement in HIV disease. In: Reeders JWAJ, Mathieson JR (eds) AIDS imaging; a practical clinical approach. Saunders, London, pp 121–130

Wall SD, Ominsky S, Altman DT, et al. (1986) Multifocal abnormalities of the gastrointestinal tract in AIDS. AJR 146:1–5

Wall SD, Yee J, Reeders JWAJ (1998) Imaging of the lumenal gastrointestinal tract in AIDS. In: Reeders JWAJ, Mathieson JR (eds) AIDS imaging; a practical clinical approach. Saunders, London, pp 168–187

White DA, Zaman MK (1992) Pulmonary disease. Med Clin North Am 76:19–44

Wilcox CM, Schwartz DA (1992) A pilot study of corticosteroid therapy for idiopathic esophageal ulcerations associated with human immunodeficiency virus infection. Am J Med 93:131–134

2 HIV in America, 1981 to 2000: Therapeutic and Epidemiologic Considerations

GARY S. REITER and JOHN BEDFORD

CONTENTS

2.1 Introduction

The human immunodeficiency virus (HIV) epidemic in the United States has undergone dramatic therapeutic and demographic evolution in its first 19 years (CDC 1994). The immunodeficiency syndrome that first appeared to affect only homosexual men now touches all segments of American society. During the 1990s many cities in the northeast and south experienced rapid growth in the numbers of heterosexually infected men and women (CDC 1997). These trends were, and continue to be, exaggerated in people of color and communities of low socioeconomic status (CDC 1997). In dramatic contrast to early experience with AIDS, a large armamentarium of effective antiretroviral drugs has transformed HIV infection from a uniformly fatal illness to a chronic treatable illness (REITER 2000).

The earliest reports of what was to become the AIDS epidemic occurred in June of 1981. The U.S. Centers for Disease Control and Prevention (CDC) notified the medical world that *Pneumocystis carinii*

G.S. REITER, MD, FACP
Medical Director Holyoke Hospital, Director of River Valley HIV Services of Western Massachusetts, 575 Beech St., Holyoke, MA 01040, USA
J. BEDFORD, MD
Assistant Director, River Valley HIV Services of Western Massachusetts, 15 Hospital Drive, Suite 403, Holyoke, MA 01040, USA

pneumonia (PCP) and Kaposi's sarcoma (KS) were being seen in young homosexual men (GOTTLIEB et al. 1981a; FRIEDMAN-KIEN et al. 1981). In September of that year, the *Lancet* reported eight cases of KS arising over 2 years in young homosexual men in New York City (HYMES et al. 1981). Subsequent reports in the *New England Journal of Medicine* and elsewhere documented a loss of immune function with impaired cell-mediated immunity, lack of response to cutaneous recall antigens, and low levels of lymphocytes, especially T-helper cells, or CD4 cells (THOMSEN and JACOBSEN 1981; BRENNAN and DURACK 1981; GOTTLIEB et al. 1981b; SIEGAL et al. 1981).

The incidence of KS in the United States prior to 1981 was 0.02-0.06 per 100,000 population (OETTLE 1962; ROTHMAN 1962). Up until that time, KS affected predominantly older men of Jewish or Mediterranean origin, people in sub-Saharan Africa, or individuals who were severely malnourished or immunocompromised. Prior to 1981, PCP had also only been seen in individuals who were severely immunocompromised. What was occurring in these young homosexual men that allowed these opportunistic diseases to take hold in them?

The authors of the *Lancet* report were prescient in noting that, "All eight (patients) had a variety of sexually transmitted diseases...this unusual occurrence of KS in a population much exposed to sexually transmissible diseases suggests that such exposure may play a role in its pathogenesis" (HYMES et al. 1981). Not only was the immune deficit which allowed KS to take hold in these previously healthy men sexually transmitted, but KS itself has been subsequently linked to a sexually transmitted agent, known as human herpes virus 8 (HHV8) or Kaposi's sarcoma herpes virus (CHANG et al. 1994; AMBROZIAK et al. 1995; MOORE and CHANG 1995; SCHALLING et al. 1995; CHUCK et al. 1996).

By the fall of 1981, medical centers in San Francisco, New York, Los Angeles, Chicago, Philadelphia, and Miami were admitting several homosexual men daily with PCP. While many of these men, who were usually in the third and fourth decades of their lives, had been ill for months, some stated that they had been healthy until a few weeks prior to their presentation. PCP, when untreated, is an aggressive infection causing high fever, persistent dry cough, arterial oxygen desaturation, interstitial edema, pneumothorax, and death. Most of these initial victims of the epidemic died within days or weeks of hospital admission. In the winter of 1981, more articles began to appear in the medical literature documenting experience with a homosexual-associated immunodeficiency syndrome, briefly called gay-related immunodeficiency syndrome or GRIDS.

Caring for the early victims of HIV was both frightening and confusing. The initial sputum and bronchoscopic specimens and laboratory and radiographic studies were usually nondiagnostic. Cephalosporin antibiotics, which had undergone extensive development in the 1970s and 1980s, were not active against PCP. Many patients were empirically and unsuccessfully treated for *Legionella*. Finally, as clinical programs became aware of the CDC's reports of PCP, they began to have some success in treating the pneumonia with trimethoprim-sulfamethoxazole.

It was common in the summer of 1981 for impromptu case conferences to be arranged several times a week by the physicians caring for these young men. The professors of pulmonary medicine, dermatology, immunology, and infectious diseases would gather, present their most recent findings, and postulate the cause of this mysterious illness. Two principal hypotheses were favored to account for the immunodeficiency syndrome seen in these patients. One theory held that since most of these men had had many sexual encounters and contracted many communicable diseases, including cytomegalovirus (CMV), syphilis, gonorrhea, mononucleosis, herpes simplex, and hepatitis A and B, their immune systems had been overloaded. Fighting so many pathogens for so long had left their immune systems incompetent to respond successfully to usually nonvirulent, opportunistic agents such as *Candida albicans* or *Pneumocystis carinii*. Many investigators felt that repeated exposure to CMV, in particular, was responsible for creating a state of immunodeficiency. CMV mononucleosis had been shown in the past to cause temporary immunosuppression, with patterns of lymphocyte disturbance similar to those seen in the initial patients with AIDS (RINALDO et al. 1980).

Another theory held that many of these men had used numerous recreational drugs. At least one of these drugs, amyl nitrate, was thought to be potentially carcinogenic. It was felt that a carcinogen may have induced some mutation in the immune system,

rendering it incompetent. The exposure to a possible carcinogen could also account for the development of Kaposi's sarcoma in these individuals. Of course, many people subscribed to both of these theories.

Yet this illness was not multifactorial; it was not caused by immune system overload or recreational drugs, and it was not to be found only in homosexual men. This illness was proven to be an acquired immunodeficiency syndrome – AIDS, not GRIDS. It was caused by a virus that was simultaneously isolated in the United States and France (GALLO et al. 1984; BARRE-SINOUSSI et al. 1983; LEVY et al. 1984). The virus, which belonged to a family of lymphotrophic viruses, was initially called human T-cell lymphotrophic virus III (HTLVIII), and subsequently renamed human immunodeficiency virus 1 or HIV1.

2.2
The Changing Demographics of the Epidemic

Although the HIV epidemic in the United States was initially concentrated in homosexual Caucasian males, over time the scope of the disease expanded, encompassing many other demographic groups. The late 1980s saw the emergence of injection drug use as a major mode of HIV transmission, initially in the northeast and south, and subsequently in other regions of the country. This trend was followed by the spread of HIV in heterosexual and pediatric populations. Women now represent a growing percentage of infected individuals, with heterosexual contact the most common mode of transmission, followed by injection drug use. Between July 1998 and June 1999, one in three new cases of HIV occurred in women (CDC 1999).

HIV disproportionately affects communities of low socioeconomic status and people of color. As of June 1999, African Americans and Hispanics accounted for 55% of cumulative U.S. AIDS cases. Seventy-seven percent of women and 51% of men diagnosed with AIDS to date have been African American or Hispanic. This trend is persisting over time. Among women infected between July 1998 and June 1999, the CDC estimates that African American and Hispanic women accounted for 77% of new infections and 80% of new AIDS cases (CDC 1999). Meanwhile, African American and Hispanic men accounted for 58% of new infections among men during this same period.

The development of potent combination antiretroviral therapy in the mid 1990s led to steep declines in the incidence of AIDS and AIDS-related deaths. The incidence of AIDS in the United States dropped by 11% between 1997 and 1998. AIDS-related deaths decreased by 42% in 1997 and by 20% in 1998 (CDC 1999). One cohort of HIV patients, from the northeast, has shown no AIDS deaths over 3 years when treated with combination antiretroviral therapy (REITER et al. 2000a). Despite these dramatic overall advances in survival in the late 1990s, HIV-infected African American men were dying of AIDS four to five times more frequently than HIV-infected Caucasian men (CDC 2000). This discrepancy is due to differences in socioeconomic status and many other personal and social factors that decrease access to health care.

While the United States has experienced significant progress in helping people live with HIV, there has been less success in developing countries. It is estimated that 95% of HIV infections and AIDS-related deaths occur in the developing countries (PERRIENS 1999). Africa, in particular, is disproportionately affected. It accounts for approximately 70% of the world's HIV/AIDS cases while representing only 10% of the world's population (BUVE 2000). Presently, the southern and eastern parts of Africa are most heavily affected. In some African countries such as Botswana, Zimbabwe, Namibia, and Swaziland, more than a quarter of the adult population is HIV infected (PIOT and O'ROURKE 2000). At the XIII International AIDS Conference in Durban, South Africa, it was noted that 1,600 South Africans are infected daily with HIV, including a staggering 500 new perinatal infections daily. The epidemic is also explosive in the Caribbean. In Port-au-Prince, Haiti, 10% of the adult population is HIV infected. It is tragic that basic medical care is often out of reach for many people in the developing world. Antiretroviral therapy and the highly technical laboratory services necessary to support it are a distant hope for the vast majority of HIV-infected people in the world.

Heterosexual contact is the most common mode of HIV transmission in developing countries. Massive international cooperation will be necessary to stem the tide of HIV infection in these regions. Efforts should focus on prevention of sexual as well as perinatal transmission. While combination antiretroviral therapy is the standard of care for pregnant women in North America and Europe (GARCIA et al. 1999; MONFENSON et al. 1999), short courses of antiretroviral therapy, given during the last phase of pregnancy or during labor, have been shown to sig-

nificantly decrease the transmission of HIV from mother to child (OWOR et al. 2000; MOODLEY et al. 2000). Given the lack of available combination therapy in the developing world, further studies of simplified and short-course therapies are needed to decrease perinatal HIV transmission.

2.3
The Evolution of Antiretroviral Therapy

Treatment options for HIV-infected patients have expanded greatly since the first 6 years of the epidemic, when no HIV-specific therapy was available. Currently, several different classes of antiretroviral medication are effective in blocking HIV replication. The first medications to become available were the nucleoside reverse transcriptase inhibitors (NRTIs), led by AZT or zidovudine (see Table 2.1 for a list of commonly used medications, doses, and side-effects). Reverse transcriptase is the enzyme responsible for copying HIV's genetic material, RNA, into DNA. The DNA copy is then integrated into the host's nuclear DNA (Fig. 2.1). The NRTIs competitively inhibit this enzyme, and prevent the subsequent production of viral DNA.

The first study documenting the effectiveness of AZT therapy was published in 1987 in the *New England Journal of Medicine* by FISCHL et al. (1987). AZT's effect on survival was assessed in a double-blinded, placebo-controlled study, involving 282 AIDS patients. The study was terminated early after 24 weeks due to an excess of deaths in the placebo group. Of 20 patients who died during the study, 19 were in the placebo group while only one was in the AZT-treated group. Similar results by other researchers (VOLBERDING et al. 1990; VELLA et al. 1992) led to the approval of AZT by the U.S. Food and Drug Administration (FDA) for the treatment of AIDS patients. Other NRTIs were developed and approved over the next several years, including didanosine (DDI), zalcitabine (DDC), and stavudine (D4T).

The late 1980s and early 1990s were characterized by the treatment of HIV with reverse transcriptase inhibitors in sequential monotherapy. In time, clinicians came to realize the ineffectiveness of this practice. While monotherapy will lead to an initial fall in viral replication and a rise in the number of CD4 cells, reverse transcriptase inhibitors alone do not adequately suppress HIV viral replication. Sequential monotherapy promotes the development of viral resistance because the high rate of viral replication

Table 2.1. Medications commonly used in patients with AIDS, their doses, and their side-effects

Medication	Type of agent	Usual dosage	Side-effects
Zidovudine (AZT) (Retrovir)	NRTI	300 mg b.i.d.	Anemia, neutropenia, headache, fatigue
Didanosine (DDI) (Videx)	NRTI	125–200 mg b.i.d. or 250–400 mg q.d.[a]	Pancreatitis, peripheral neuropathy, nausea, diarrhea
Zalcitabine (DDC) (Hivid)	NRTI	0.75 mg t.i.d.	Peripheral neuropathy, stomatitis
Stavudine (D4T) (Zerit)	NRTI	30–40 mg b.i.d.	Peripheral neuropathy
Lamivudine (3TC) (Epivir)	NRTI	150 mg b.i.d. 300 mg q.d.[b]	Minimal side-effects
Abacavir (ABC) (Ziagen)	NRTI	300 mg b.i.d.	Hypersensitivity reaction
Nevirapine (Viramune)	NNRTI	200 mg q.d.+14 days then 200 mg b.i.d. or 400 mg q.d.	Rash, hepatitis
Delavirdine (Rescriptor)	NNRTI	400 mg t.i.d. 600 mg b.i.d.[c]	Rash
Efavirenz (Sustiva)	NNRTI	600 mg q.h.s.	Nightmares, dizziness, rash
Saquinavir (Fortovase)	PI	1200 mg b.i.d. with high fat meal or 400–600 mg with 100–200 mg ritonavir b.i.d.[d]	Elevated liver function tests, headache, nausea, diarrhea
Indinavir (Crixivan)	PI	800 mg@8h on empty stomach or with light meal or 800-1200 mg with 100–200 mg ritonavir b.i.d.[d]	Nephrolithiasis, abdominal pain, diarrhea, elevated LFTs, headache, dizziness, rash, altered taste, thrombocytopenia
Nelfinavir (Viracept)	PI	1250 mg b.i.d.	Diarrhea
Amprenavir (Agenerase)	PI	1200 mg b.i.d. or 600 mg with 100–200 mg ritonavir b.i.d.[d]	Nausea, headache, diarrhea
Ritonavir (Norvir)	PI	600 mg b.i.d.	Nausea, headache, diarrhea, circumoral paresthesias, elevated LFTs

NRTI, Nucleoside reverse transcriptase inhibitor; NNRTI, non-nucleoside reverse transcriptase inhibitor; PI, protease inhibitor
[a]Common dosage, not FDA approved, may not be as effective
[b]Common dosage, not FDA approved
[c]Under investigation
[d]Ritonavir raises C_{min} of concomitant protease inhibitor, which allows for simplified dosing and may overcome viral resistance

and HIV's tendency to mutate leads to viral resistance and therapeutic failure.

In the early 1990s, HIV clinicians began to have a better understanding of viral resistance and the factors contributing to its evolution. In January 1995 the Second Conference on Retroviruses in Washington D.C. heralded several new developments in the treatment of HIV that would revolutionize the field. The concept of combination therapy first arose at that time, concurrent with the introduction of a new NRTI, lamivudine. Lamivudine was found to have marked synergy with AZT. Viral resistance to AZT could be delayed and, in fact, reversed when the two drugs were used together. This realization helped to promote a paradigm shift with respect to the treatment of HIV, away from sequential monotherapy and towards combination therapy.

A new class of antiretroviral medications, the protease inhibitors, was also introduced at the Second Conference on Retroviruses in 1995. Protease inhibitors block the cleavage of large nonfunctional polypeptide products of HIV into smaller functional components essential for viral packaging (Fig. 2.1) Their inhibitory effect on viral replication was found to be more potent than that of any other available drugs. Protease inhibitors were then combined with reverse transcriptase inhibitors to form the first potent combination regimens used to treat HIV. Such regimens were found to dramatically decrease viral replication, halt disease progression, promote immune reconstitution, and allow many HIV-infected individuals to live essentially normal lives. Most of the opportunistic diseases that characterized the early years of the AIDS epidemic are unheard of in individuals on potent combination antiretroviral therapy.

Also in 1995 the practice of HIV viral load monitoring came into existence. This technology, which estimates the level of replicating virus in the bloodstream, was found by Dr. John Mellors and others to convey significant prognostic value with respect to HIV disease progression (MELLORS et al. 1996). Up until 1995, CD4 counts had been the primary laboratory parameter followed in HIV patients. While CD4

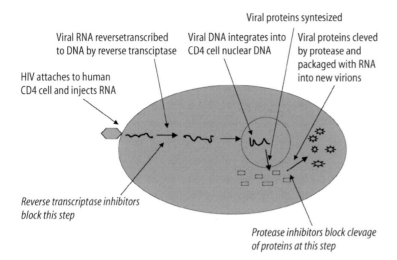

Viral proteins syntesized

Viral RNA reversetranscribed to DNA by reverse transciptase

Viral DNA integrates into CD4 cell nuclear DNA

Viral proteins cleved by protease and packaged with RNA into new virions

HIV attaches to human CD4 cell and injects RNA

Reverse transcriptase inhibitors block this step

Protease inhibitors block clevage of proteins at this step

Fig. 2.1. HIV life cycle

counts provide an estimate of the stage of disease progression and level of immune suppression, these values are not by themselves predictive of disease progression. Subsequent work by Mellors et al. showed that the likelihood of disease progression and death could be predicted by assessing both HIV viral load and CD4 count (MELLORS et al. 1997). In general, the higher the viral load and the lower the CD4 count, the higher the likelihood of progressing to AIDS or death.

In the late 1990s a third class of antiretroviral drugs, the non-nucleoside reverse transcriptase inhibitors (NNRTIs) became available. These medications act on the same enzyme that the NRTIs affect, but through a different mechanism. They inhibit reverse transcriptase by binding adjacent to its catalytic site, resulting in an allosteric change that renders the enzyme nonfunctional. The first drug in this class, nevirapine, was approved by the FDA in 1996, and subsequently, two other medications, delavirdine and efavirenz, have been approved as well. These medications have expanded the options available to clinicians when choosing a treatment regimen (Table 2.1).

At present, combination therapy with three or more antiretroviral medications is the accepted standard of care for HIV infection. The goal of therapy is to achieve maximal suppression of viral replication. A variety of possible combinations of the three classes of medications exist. The most commonly used regimens combine two or more NRTIs with either an NNRTI or a protease inhibitor. The effectiveness of this type of highly active antiretroviral therapy or HAART has been demonstrated in numerous studies (DEEKS et al. 1997; GULICK et al. 1997, 1999;

HAMMER et al. 1997). The earliest studies with triple therapy involved a protease inhibitor and two NRTIs. Therapy with indinavir, AZT, and lamivudine, when taken appropriately in antiretroviral naive patients, resulted in maximal viral suppression in up to 80% of patients at 52 weeks (GULICK et al. 1997). Later studies showed that regimens combining NRTIs with an NNRTI could also be very potent, particularly when efavirenz was used as the NNRTI (STASZEWSKI et al. 1999b). More recently, regimens employing the three NRTIs AZT, lamivudine, and abacavir have been shown to be very effective as well (STASZEWSKI et al. 1999a).

Many HIV clinicians are employing regimens with dual protease inhibitors, especially in patients with extensive treatment histories and evidence of antiretroviral resistance. These regimens are very potent and take advantage of pharmacokinetic interactions between the drugs which result in higher trough levels of medication. These changes in pharmacodynamics can allow for less frequent dosing, lower medication dosages, and often fewer side-effects, while achieving effective suppression of viral replication.

Recent advances in HIV therapeutics involve the use of viral resistance assays to guide therapy. Two different types of assay have been developed which analyze a sample of a patient's virus to characterize its susceptibility to the available antiretroviral medications. One type of assay, the genotypic resistance assay, involves sequence analysis of the viral genome. The results of this analysis are then compared with databases of known antiretroviral resistance conferring mutations in order to generate a resistance profile for that specific virus. The second type of assay is known as a phenotypic resistance assay. It is similar to the types of susceptibility assay used in standard microbiology laboratories with bacteria and fungi. Phenotypic assays assess the ability of a given HIV sample to replicate, in vitro, in the presence of varying concentrations of a panel of drugs. The concentration of drug required to inhibit replication by 50% (IC-50) is measured for each medication and compared with a standard. An increase of 2.5-fold or greater in the IC-50 is generally defined as demonstrating resistance. These data are collected for the available antiretroviral medications and used to construct a phenotypic resistance profile.

Results from genotypic and phenotypic assays do not always agree and are limited in their application. This is felt to be the result of a variety of factors, including the presence of small viral subpopulations in a patient's sample that may be analyzed by one assay but not another. In addition, both assays may miss subpopulations that may be present in the patient. These subpopulations may have resistance profiles different than those assayed and therefore undermine the effectiveness of the regimen chosen on the basis of the resistance assay. In addition, many patients who have been exposed to numerous drugs may have multiple subpopulations of virus.

Nevertheless, several recent studies have confirmed the value of viral resistance testing in guiding therapy. Two studies have demonstrated improved rates of viral suppression in patients who had genotypic resistance assays incorporated into the decision-making process when they were switched from a failing regimen to a new one (DURANT et al. 1999; BAXTER et al. 1999). On average, patients in these two studies who had undergone genotypic resistance testing had viral loads which were three times lower at 12–16 weeks of therapy than those in patients in whom the testing had not been performed. Similar results were found in a study randomizing patients failing therapy to either expert opinion only or expert opinion plus phenotypic resistance (DEMETER 2000). Resistance testing is becoming a routine aspect of HIV clinical care (DHHS 2000; CARPENTER et al. 2000).

2.4
Medication Adherence Is Key with Antiretroviral Therapy

The current group of antiretroviral medications must be adhered to 100% of the time in order to achieve maximal viral suppression and prevent the development of resistance. Two studies that matched viral suppression to degree of medication adherence have documented that missing as little as 5% or 10% of doses can lead to rapid loss of viral suppression (PATERSON et al. 1999; ARNSTEN et al. 2000). For most antiretroviral treatment regimens, missing 5% of doses is less than one missed dose a week. Another study documenting the key role of adherence, and the difficulty in maintaining it, compared directly observed therapy in a prison with community treatment in a clinical trial (FISCHL et al. 2000). Nearly 100% of the individuals on directly observed therapy achieved viral suppression, whereas only 68% of the individuals taking the medication on their own in the community did so.

Medication adherence is often viewed as a "patient-centered" issue. However, adherence is related to multiple interlocking factors including: the patient and his or her psychological and social characteristics; the mission, services, and general level of support at the clinical program where treatment is rendered; the expertise and interpersonal skills of the health care professional rendering treatment; and the unique characteristics of the antiretroviral regimen the patient is taking (REITER et al. 2000b). All of these elements need to be assessed and optimized to maximize an individual's medication adherence and chance of viral suppression.

2.5
New Challenges

The turn of the century has brought expanded treatment options for HIV patients, steep declines in mortality, and a marked decrease in the incidence of opportunistic infections (PALELLA et al. 1998), but it has not been without new challenges. HAART has the potential for numerous side-effects. Some patients tolerate their regimens better than others. Some of the side-effects, such as nausea and diarrhea, are readily treatable in many cases; others have been more troublesome. Some treated patients have developed metabolic complications and body composition changes, the mechanisms of which are not clearly understood, but may involve mitochondrial toxicity (SAINT-MARC et al. 1999). These changes include hyperlipidemia, insulin resistance, and alterations in body shape, characterized by central adiposity, dorsocervical fat pads, breast enlargement, and peripheral fat wasting. Patients may develop some or all of these changes. Initially it appeared that these abnormalities were related to protease inhibitors, but subsequent studies have implicated other medications as well, including the nucleoside analogues and non-nucleosides (Brinkman et al. 1999). The hyperlipidemia and insulin resistance are treatable with conventional medications used for these conditions in non-HIV patients (Reiter 2000), but the optimal treatment for the body habitus changes remains to be elucidated.

Another challenge involves the morbidity and mortality associated with hepatitis C in co-infected patients. HIV-infected patients with hepatitis C appear to be at higher risk of progression to end-stage liver disease than their non-HIV-infected counterparts (Thomas et al. 2000). The development of end-stage liver disease was found to occur more than twice as often in co-infected patients in a cohort followed prospectively at the Hemophilia Center of Philadelphia (Ragni 2000). Treatment with antiretroviral therapy, particularly protease inhibitors and non-nucleosides, may also result in hepatotoxicity in some co-infected patients, further complicating the care of these individuals (Sulkowski et al. 2000). It is not clear yet whether the optimal treatment strategy in these patients involves simultaneous or sequential therapy of hepatitis C and HIV.

2.6 Conclusion

The care of HIV patients is challenging in many ways. It involves much more than the prescription of antiretroviral therapy. HIV is a multidimensional illness. Patients may experience medication-related complications, opportunistic infections, cancers, wasting, and dementia as well as numerous psychosocial, existential, and spiritual stresses. Competent care of these patients demands clinicians who are experienced in treating HIV and committed to updating their knowledge of this rapidly changing disease. Patients benefit from a combined approach addressing the needs of the whole patient as well as those of the patient's family. The most successful clinical programs employ an interdisciplinary approach, including case managers, social workers, nutritionists, nurses, and psychologists, in addition to physicians. The integration of medical care with psychological and social support services for patients and their families maximizes the potential for successful treatment and promotes quality of life.

References

Ambroziak J, Blackbourn D, Herndier B, et al. (1995) Herpesvirus-like sequences in HIV-infected and uninfected Kaposi's sarcoma patients. Science 268:582–583

Arnsten J, Demas P, Gourevitch M, et al. (2000) Adherence and viral load in HIV-infected drug users: comparison of self-report and medication event monitors (MEMS). 7th Conference on Retroviruses and Opportunistic Infections, 30 January–2 February 2000, San Francisco, Calif., abstract 69

Barre-Sinoussi F, Chermann J, Rey P, et al. (1983) Isolation of a T-lymphotrophic retrovirus from a patient at risk for AIDS. Science 220:868–871

Baxter J, Mayers D, Wentworth D, et al. (1999) A pilot study of the short term effects of antiretroviral management based on plasma genotypic antiretroviral resistance testing (GART) in patients failing antiretroviral therapy. Sixth Conference on Retroviruses and Opportunistic Infections, February 1999, Chicago, Ill., abstract LB8

Brennan R, Durack D (1981) Gay compromise syndrome. Lancet 2:1338–1339

Brinkman K, Smeitink J, Romijn J, Reiss P (1999) Mitochondrial toxicity induced by nucleoside analogue reverse transcriptase inhibitors is a key factor in the pathogenesis of antiretroviral-therapy-related lipodystrophy. Lancet 354:1112–1115

Buvé A (2000) HIV/AIDS in Africa: Why so severe, why so heterogeneous? 7th Conference on Retroviruses and Opportunistic Infections, 30 January–2 February 2000, San Francisco, Calif., abstract S28

Carpenter CCJ, Cooper D, Fischl M, et al. (2000) Antiretroviral therapy in adults: updated recommendations of the International AIDS Society – USA Panel. JAMA 283:381–390

Centers for Disease Control and Prevention (1994) Update: trends in AIDS diagnosis and reporting under the expanded surveillance definition for adolescents and adults – United States, 1993. Morbidity Mortality Weekly Report 43:826–831

Centers for Disease Control and Prevention (1997) Update: trends in AIDS incidence– United States, 1996. Morbidity Mortality Weekly Report 46:861–867

Centers for Disease Control and Prevention (1999) U.S. HIV and AIDS cases reported through June 1999. Mid-Year Edition, vol 11, No. 1

Centers for Disease Control and Prevention (2000) U.S. HIV and AIDS cases reported through December 1999. Year-End Edition, vol 11, No. 2

Chang Y, Cesarman E, Pessin M, et al. (1994) Identification of herpes-like DNA sequences in AIDS-associated Kaposi's sarcoma. Science 266:165–169

Chuck S, Grant R, Katangole-Mbidde E, et al. (1996) Frequent presence of herpesviral-like DNA sequences in lesions of HIV-negative Kaposi's sarcoma. J Infect Dis 173:248–251

Deeks SG, Smith M, Holodniy M, Kahn J (1997) HIV-1 protease inhibitors. A review for clinicians. JAMA 277:145–153

Demeter L (2000) Drug resistance and the management of treatment failure. 7th Conference on Retroviruses and Opportunistic Infections, 30 January–2 February 2000, San Francisco, Calif., abstract S32

DHHS Panel on Clinical Practices for Treatment of HIV Infections (2000) Guidelines for use of antiretroviral agents in HIV-infected adults and adolescents. 28 January 2000 revision. Available at: http://havatis.org

Durant J, Clevenbergh P, Halfon P, et al. (1999) Drug resistance genotyping in HIV-1 therapy: the VIRADAPT randomized controlled trial. Lancet 353:2195–2199

Fischl MA, Richman D, Grieco M, et al. (1987) The efficacy of azidothymidine (AZT) in the treatment of patients with AIDS and AIDS-related complex: a double-blind, placebo controlled trial. N Engl J Med 371:185–191

Fischl M, Rodriguez A, Scerpella E, et al. (2000) The impact of directly observed treatment on virologic outcomes. 7th Conference on Retroviruses and Opportunistic Infections, 30 January–2 February 2000, San Francisco, Calif., abstract 71

Friedman-Kien A, Laubenstein L, Marmor M, et al. (1981) Kaposi's sarcoma and *Pneumocystis* pneumonia among homosexual men – New York City and California. Morbidity Mortality Weekly Report 30:305–383

Gallo R, Salahuddin S, Popovic M, et al. (1984) Frequent detection and isolation of cytopathic retroviruses (HTLVIII) from patients with AIDS and at risk for AIDS. Science 224:500–503

Garcia PM, Kalish LA, Pitt J, et al. (1999) Maternal levels of plasma human immunodeficiency virus type 1 RNA and the risk of perinatal transmission. Women and Infants Transmission Study Group. N Engl J Med 341:394–402

Gottlieb M, Schanker H, Fan P, et al. (1981a) *Pneumocystis* pneumonia– Los Angeles. Morbidity Mortality Weekly Report 30:250–252

Gottlieb M, Schroff R, Schanker H, et al. (1981b) *Pneumocystis carinii* pneumonia and mucosal candidiasis in previously healthy homosexual men – evidence of a new acquired cellular immunodeficiency. N Engl J Med 305:1425–1431

Gulick RM, Mellors J, Havlir D, et al. (1997) Treatment with indinavir, zidovudine, and lamivudine in adults with human immunodeficiency virus infection and prior antiretroviral therapy [see comments]. N Engl J Med 337:734–739

Gulick R, Mellors J, Havlir D, et al. (1999) Treatment with indinavir (IDV), zidovudine (ZDV) and lamivudine (3TC): three-year follow-up. 6th Conference on Retroviruses and Opportunistic Infections, Chicago, Ill., 388

Hammer SM, Squires K, Hughes M, et al. (1997) A controlled trial of two nucleoside analogues plus indinavir in persons with human immunodeficiency virus infection and CD4 cell counts of 200 per cubic millimeter or less. AIDS Clinical Trials Group 320 Study Team [see comments]. N Engl J Med 337:725–733

Hymes KB, Cheung T, Greene J, et al. (1981) Kaposi's sarcoma in homosexual men – a report of eight cases. Lancet 2:598–600

Levy J, Hoffman A, Dramer S, et al. (1984) Isolation of lymphocytopathic retroviruses from San Francisco patients with AIDS. Science 225:840–842

Mellors J, Rinaldo C, Grupta P, et al. (1996) Prognosis in HIV-1 infection predicted by the quantity of virus in plasma. Science 272:1167–1170

Mellors J, Munoz A, Giorgi J, et al. (1997) Plasma viral load and CD4+ lymphocytes as prognostic markers of HIV-1 infection. Ann Intern Med 126:946–954

Monfenson LM, Lambert J, Stiehm E, et al. (1999) Risk factors for perinatal transmission of human immunodeficiency virus type 1 in women treated with zidovudine. Pediatric AIDS Clinical Trials Group Study 185 Team. N Engl J Med 341:385–393

Moodley D, McIntyre J, for the SAINT Study Team (2000) Evaluation of safety and efficacy of two simple regimens for the prevention of mother to child transmission (MTCT) of HIV infection: nevirapine vs lamivudine and zidovudine used in a randomized clinical trial (the SAINT study). Program and abstracts of the XIII International AIDS Conference, 9–14 July 2000, Durban, South Africa, abstract TuOrB356

Moore P, Chang Y (1995) Detection of herpesvirus-like DNA sequences in Kaposi's sarcoma patients with and those without HIV infection. N Engl J Med 332:1181–1185

Oettle AG (1962) Geographical and racial differences in the frequency of Kaposi's sarcoma as evidence of environmental or genetic causes. Acta Un Int Cancer 18:330–363

Owor M, Deseyve M, Duefield C, et al. (2000) The one year safety and efficacy data of HIVNET 012 trial. Program and abstracts of the XIII International AIDS Conference, 9–14 July 2000, Durban, South Africa, abstract LbOr1

Palella FJ Jr, Delaney K, Moorman A, et al. (1998) Declining morbidity and mortality among patients with advanced human immunodeficiency virus infection. HIV Outpatient Study Investigators. N Engl J Med 338:853–860

Paterson D, Swindells S, Mohr J, et al. (1999) How much adherence is enough? A prospective study of adherence to protease inhibitor therapy using MEMS Caps. 6th Conference on Retrovirus and Opportunistic Infections, Chicago, Ill., 92

Perriens J (1999) AIDS – a global overview. Program and Abstracts of the Seventh European Conference on Clinical Aspects and Treatment of HIV-Infection, Lisbon, Portugal, 23–27 September 1999

Piot P, O'Rourke M (2000) AIDS in the developing world: an interview with Peter Piot. AIDS Clin Care 12:1–5

Ragni M (2000) Impact of HIV on progression to end-stage liver disease in HCV coinfected hemophiliacs. 7th Conference on Retroviruses and Opportunistic Infections, 30 January–2 February 2000, San Francisco, Calif., abstract 281

Reiter G (2000) Comprehensive clinical care in the era of potent combination therapy – managing HIV as a chronic illness. AIDS Clin Care 12:13–20

Reiter G, Wojtusik L, Wojnarowski C, et al. (2000a) Steep declines in mortality and no AIDS deaths in HAART treated patients. X111 International AIDS Conference, Durban, South Africa, 9–14 July 2000, abstract MoPeC2491

Reiter G, Stewart K, Wojtusik L, et al. (2000b) Elements of success in HIV clinical care. Top HIV Med 8:21–30

Rinaldo C, Carney W, Richter B, et al. (1980) Mechanisms of immunosuppression in cytomegaloviral mononucleosis. J Infect Dis 141:488–495

Rothman S (1962) Remarks on sex, age and racial distribution of Kaposi's sarcoma on possible pathogenetic factors. Acta Un Int Cancer 18:326–329

Saint-Marc T, Roizot-Martin I, Partisani M, et al. (1999) A syndrome of lipodystrophy in patients receiving stable nucleoside analogue therapy. Sixth Conference on Retroviruses and Opportunistic Infections, Chicago, Ill., abstract 653

Schalling M, Ekman M, Kaaya EE, Linde A, Biberfeld P (1995) A role for a new herpesvirus (KSAV) in different forms of Kaposi's sarcoma. Nature Med 1:707–708

Siegal F, Lopez C, Hammer G, et al. (1981) Severe acquired immunodeficiency in male homosexuals, manifested by chronic perianal ulcerative herpes simplex lesions. N Engl J Med 305:1439–1444

Staszewski S, Kaiser P, Gathe J, et al. (1999) Comparison of antiviral response with abacavir/combivir to indinavir/combivir in therapy-naive adults at 48 weeks (CNA3005). In: 39th Interscience Conference on Antimicrobial Agents and Chemotherapy, San Francisco, Calif., September 1999, abstract 505

Staszewski S, Morales-Ramirez J, Tashima K, et al. (1999) Efavirenz plus zidovudine and lamivudine, efavirenz plus indinavir, and indinavir plus zidovudine and lamivudine in the treatment of HIV-1 infection in adults. N Engl J Med 341:1865–1873

Sulkowski M, Thomas D, Chaisson R, et al. (2000) Hepatotoxicity associated with antiretroviral therapy in adults infected with human immunodeficiency virus and the role of hepatitis C or B virus infection. JAMA 283:74–80

Thomas D, Astemborski J, Rai R, et al. (2000) The natural history of hepatitis C virus infection. JAMA 284:450–456

Thomsen H, Jacobsen M (1981) Kaposi sarcoma among homosexual men in Europe. Lancet 2:688

Vella S, Giuliano M, Pezzotti P, et al. (1992) Survival of zidovudine-treated patients with AIDS compared with that of contemporary untreated patients. JAMA 267:1232–1236

Volberding PA, Lagakos S, Koch M, et al. (1990) Zidovudine in asymptomatic human immunodeficiency virus infection: a controlled trial in persons with fewer than 500 CD4-positive cells per cubic millimeter. N Engl J Med 322:941–949

3 The Clinical Spectrum of HIV Infection

Charles B. Hicks

CONTENTS

3.1
Introduction

Infection with the human immunodeficiency virus (HIV) initiates a process that begins with the primary HIV syndrome, is typically followed by an asymptomatic period that can last many years, and culminates with the variety of complications and manifestations that are collectively referred to as the acquired immune deficiency syndrome, or AIDS. The occurrence and pace of any or all of these elements of the so-called typical pattern of HIV infection varies significantly from patient to patient. In some instances, patients may progress from primary HIV infection to AIDS and death in 5 years or less. At the opposite end of the spectrum are well-documented cases of persons who have been HIV infected for greater than 20 years without any clinical symptoms or evidence of clinical progression. This latter group has been called "long-term nonprogressors." The introduction of more effective antiretroviral drugs in recent years has dramatically affected the course of disease for HIV-infected persons who receive treatment with highly active antiretroviral

C.B. Hicks, MD
Associate Clinical Professor of Medicine, Division of Infectious Diseases, Duke University Medical Center, Box 3360, Durham, NC 27710, USA

therapy (HAART). A more complete appreciation of the clinical spectrum of the infection and the impact of improved antiviral therapy on its manifestations facilitates the correct interpretation of radiographs in HIV-infected persons.

3.2
Pathophysiology of HIV Infection

The clinical manifestations of HIV infection are a consequence of an ongoing, active viral infection. Because most patients experience a relatively prolonged period of asymptomatic good health following initial infection, the intensity of the viral infection that is at work in HIV-infected persons is sometimes not fully appreciated. Indeed, when the first clinical cases of AIDS were described in 1981, the infectious nature of the underlying illness was not clear (Gottlieb et al. 1981; Masur et al. 1981). In an effort to elucidate the cause of this new condition, a case syndrome definition was developed by the Centers for Disease Control (CDC) in 1982, and the term acquired immune deficiency syndrome, or AIDS, entered the medical lexicon (CDC 1982). Once the human immunodeficiency virus (HIV) was identified and clearly established as the etiology of this infectious disorder, the distinction between HIV infection and AIDS became largely irrelevant. Despite this, the term AIDS is still widely used although it now properly only refers to the latest stages of immunologic suppression.

The process by which HIV infection causes progressive destruction of the human immune system is only partly understood (Fauci 1993). After HIV is acquired, it quickly invades cells of the immune system that have on their surfaces a molecule known as CD4 (for cluster designation 4) which serves as the receptor for the virus (Klatzmann et al. 1984). Inside these infected CD4+ cells, the virus replicates itself at a furious pace, producing numerous copies. This process leads to the death of the infected cell with release of the newly formed viruses. These progeny viruses in turn seek other CD4+ cells to invade and the sequence of cellular infection, viral replication, cell death, and release of new infectious viruses continues.

The viral replication process is initially unchecked by host defense mechanisms. Over a period of weeks to a few months (a period often referred to as primary HIV infection), most HIV-infected persons develop immune responses to the virus (COOPER et al. 1988). Unfortunately, these responses are only partially effective in controlling the amount of viral replication that continues. The degree of immunologic control that is established during this period in any particular patient can be inferred from measurements of viral concentrations in blood after the period of primary HIV infection. The measurement of virus concentration in blood, usually referred to as measuring viral load, has been shown to have considerable prognostic value and is vitally important to the clinical management of HIV-infected persons (MELLORS et al. 1996).

The primary target cells for HIV infection are CD4+ T lymphocytes, sometimes referred to as T helper cells. These cells play a crucial role in coordinating the complex interactions that are required for a properly functioning immune system. As their numbers decline, immune function becomes increasingly disordered. Thus the second factor that is important to understanding the manifestations of HIV infection in any individual patient is the CD4+ lymphocyte count. The two parameters viral load and CD4+ lymphocyte count are in general closely linked since the rate at which CD4+ lymphocytes are destroyed is directly proportional to the amount of ongoing viral replication as determined by the plasma viral load measurement. Thus, patients with high viral load measurements have more rapid destruction of CD4+ lymphocytes and usually have lower CD4 counts. As the number of CD4+ lymphocytes declines, the host becomes increasingly susceptible to a variety of complications that are a reflection of progressive loss of immune function (CROWE et al. 1991).

3.3
Natural History of HIV Infection

The clinical course of HIV infection begins with primary HIV infection (also referred to as the acute retroviral syndrome), goes into a period of asymptomatic clinical latency, evolves into early symptomatic disease, and finally becomes late-stage infection or true AIDS. Figure 3.1 graphically illustrates the "typical" course of HIV in an individual patient (FAUCI et al. 1996). Studies carried out before the availability of effective antiretroviral therapy provide information on the pace of progression in untreated patients. For example, in a cohort of homosexual men followed in San Francisco, the average time from documented infection with HIV to the

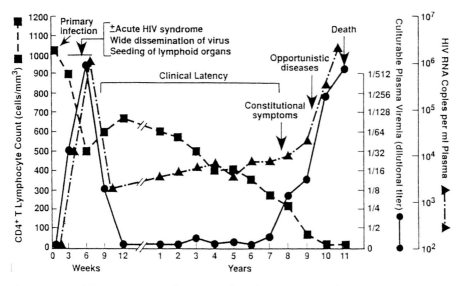

Fig. 3.1. Natural history of HIV infection in a hypothetical patient. This pattern assumes the patient did not receive antiretroviral therapy. The time frame for the various elements of HIV infection varies considerably from patient to patient. (From FAUCI 1996)

development of AIDS-defining conditions was 9.8 years (BACCHETTI and MOSS 1989). A compilation of data from other sources including persons infected sexually, by blood or blood product transfusions, or via injection drug use revealed time from infection to development of AIDS of between 7 and 10 years (ALCABES et al. 1993).

It is important to note that there is considerable variability among patients in the pace of the process, a fact that can be largely attributed to the differences in viral load that are seen from patient to patient. Patients with high viral load measurements progress more rapidly that those with lower viral loads. This fact explains the findings from an epidemiology analysis of a cohort of men who enrolled in a study of a hepatitis B vaccine (Rutherford et al. 1990). In this large group of 489 men for whom a time of acquisition of HIV could be reliably established, 13% progressed to AIDS within 5 years, 51% within 10 years, and 54% by the end of 11 years. After 11 years of follow-up, an additional 19% had symptomatic HIV infection but had not as yet developed an AIDS-defining condition, and 29% had a CD4+ lymphocyte count below 200 cells/mm^3. Thus a considerable majority of untreated HIV-infected persons progress to symptomatic, late-stage HIV infection over the course of 10 years or so.

3.3.1
Primary HIV Infection

The term primary HIV infection refers to the period following initial infection with the virus during which a clinically significant illness occurs in the majority of patients (QUINN 1997; KAHN and WALKER 1998). Following a typical incubation period of 2–4 weeks, patients develop signs and symptoms that may include fever, malaise, anorexia, rash, oral and/or genital ulcers, diffuse lymphadenopathy, myalgias, pharyngitis, and a variety of gastrointestinal and neurologic complaints. This presentation is often confused with infectious mononucleosis or other so-called viral syndromes, and a high index of suspicion is required to make the correct diagnosis. Testing for HIV infection in this setting can be quite difficult since almost all such patients have not developed a diagnostic antibody test at the time of presentation. It is not until the clinical illness subsides that the HIV antibody test typically becomes positive. Thus diagnosis of primary HIV infection usually requires a test for viral antigens (such as the p24 antigen test) or a viral amplification test (such as the polymerase

chain reaction or PCR). In most cases, primary HIV infection goes undetected and patients enter the period of asymptomatic clinical latency during which there is progressive loss of CD4+ lymphocytes due to repeated cycles of viral replication.

3.3.2
Clinical Latency and
Early Symptomatic HIV Disease

Following resolution of the primary HIV infection syndrome, there is usually a period of asymptomatic infection that precedes the development of HIV-associated symptoms and AIDS-defining conditions. As mentioned previously, this period is of variable length depending in large measure on the amount of chronic ongoing viral replication that is present (as measured by the HIV viral load). As the CD4+ lymphocyte count declines, the risk of symptomatic disease and opportunistic infections increases.

A variety of signs, symptoms, and conditions have been described in HIV-infected patients prior to the development of an AIDS-defining condition. One of the earliest such signs is persistent generalized lymphadenopathy which may begin during primary HIV infection and remain present thereafter (METROKA et al. 1983). This syndrome is defined as the presence of two or more extrainguinal sites of lymphadenopathy for a minimum of 3–6 months for which no other explanation can be found. It occurs in some 50%–70% of HIV-infected individuals and may be an early clue to the presence of HIV. Persistent generalized lymphadenopathy is caused by high levels of HIV infection of the CD4+ lymphocytes found in lymph nodes. In patients with advanced HIV infection, these enlarged nodes frequently involute as the CD4+ lymphocyte count falls to very low levels, and the process resolves spontaneously.

Other conditions noted in HIV-infected patients prior to the development of AIDS-defining opportunistic infections include nonspecific constitutional symptoms (fatigue, malaise, low-grade fever, night sweats, weight loss), intraoral conditions (candidiasis, oral hairy leukoplakia, gingivitis, aphthous ulcers), skin disorders [recurrent herpes simplex outbreaks, varicella zoster (shingles), molluscum contagiosum, warts], and renal dysfunction (HIV-associated nephropathy) (CHAISSON et al. 2000). The presence of any of these conditions in a person not known to be HIV infected should prompt consideration of the diagnosis and lead to appropriate testing.

3.3.3
Late-Stage HIV Infection (AIDS)

As the immune system becomes progressively more damaged by HIV, the risk of developing an opportunistic infection increases. Among the opportunistic infections that were routinely encountered in the early years of the HIV/AIDS pandemic were *Pneumocystis carinii* pneumonia, cerebral toxoplasmosis, disseminated *Mycobacterium avium-intracellulare* complex infection, cytomegalovirus infection (both retinitis and gastrointestinal infection), cryptococcal meningitis, and chronic *Cryptosporidium* diarrhea. The risk of developing any one of these AIDS-related opportunistic infections was found to be most closely related to the absolute CD4+ lymphocyte count (KOVACS and MASUR 2000). In the era before highly active antiretroviral therapy was available, patients whose CD4+ lymphocyte counts exceeded 200 cells/mm^3 were found to have little risk for the majority of HIV-associated opportunistic infections. This was best documented for the most commonly encountered opportunistic infection, *Pneumocystis carinii* pneumonia (PHAIR et al. 1990). Additional observations regarding the risk of various opportunistic infections relative to the degree of immunosuppression provided insights into the likelihood of any particular complication being seen as a function of the CD4+ lymphocyte count (Fig. 3.2).

Based on these findings, recommendations have been made to initiate prophylactic therapy with drugs active against particular pathogens when certain threshold CD4+ lymphocyte counts are reached. This strategy of initiating preventive therapy prior to developing an infection is termed primary prophylaxis. It is to be distinguished from the use of continuing therapy to prevent recurrence of an infection that has been successfully treated but may relapse if treatment is discontinued. The latter strategy is called secondary prophylaxis. An example of primary prophylaxis is the recommendation that preventive therapy for *Pneumocystis carinii* pneumonia be initiated for HIV-infected patients whose CD4+ lymphocyte count is less than 200 cells/mm^3. The recommendations for primary prophylaxis have been repeatedly updated as new information has become available (Table 3.1; Kovacs and MASUR 2000). The widespread acceptance and application of these recommendations led to decreases in the incidence of new opportunistic infections in HIV-infected patients receiving medical care even before the availability of more effective antiretroviral regimens.

3.4
Impact of Highly Active Antiretroviral Therapy

Although declines in the incidence of most opportunistic infections were noted before effective antiretroviral therapy was widely available, the major impact on HIV morbidity and mortality seen in the last few years is a consequence of highly active antiretroviral therapy (HAART) (PALELLA et al. 1998). In those areas of the world in which HAART is available, the natural history of HIV infection has been profoundly changed by the use of combinations of antiretroviral drugs that can suppress levels of viral replication to below the threshold of even the most sensitive available assays. These virologic responses are associated with significant immune reconstitution and increases in CD4+ lymphocyte counts,

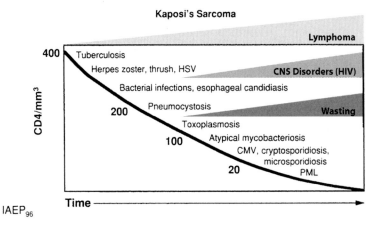

Fig. 3.2. Risk of various opportunistic infections in HIV-infected patients based on the CD4+ lymphocyte count. While there may be some variability in risk from patient to patient, the general patterns depicted here are sufficiently accurate that they form the basis for prophylactic strategies. (Adapted from the International AIDS Education Project 1996)

sometimes to normal levels. The restoration of immune function has in turn produced significant decreases in the incidence of virtually all the AIDS-defining complications, with resultant declines in hospitalizations, inpatient costs, and mortality (KAPLAN et al. 2000). An analysis of trends in the incidence of opportunistic infections among HIV-infected patients in the United States is instructive. As can been seen from the curves in Fig. 3.3, declines in most of the defined opportunistic infections were evident before the introduction of protease inhibitors ushered in the era of HAART in late 1995. These declines were probably due to the more widespread use of prophylaxis regimens in persons known to be HIV infected. Clearly though, the rate of decline in opportunistic infections increased sharply as the use

Table 3.1. Drug regimens for primary prophylaxis against opportunistic infections in patients with HIV infection

Pathogen	Treatment regimen
Pneumocystis carinii	Trimethoprim-sulfamethoxazole, 1 double-strength tablet orally per day or 1 single-strength tablet orally per day
Toxoplasma gondii	Trimethoprim-sulfamethoxazole, 1 double-strength tablet orally per day
Mycobacterium tuberculosis	
Isoniazid-sensitive source case (if known)	Isoniazid, 300 mg orally per day, plus pyridoxine, 50 mg orally per day, for 9 months
Isoniazid-resistant source case (if known)	Rifampin, 600 mg orally per day, plus pyrazinamide, 200 mg/kg orally per day, for 2 months
Multidrug-resistant (isoniazid and rifampin)	Choice of drugs requires consultation with experts
M. avium complex	Azithromycin, 1200 mg orally once a week; or clarithromycin, 500 mg orally twice a day

Recommendations for primary prophylaxis of opportunistic infections in HIV-infected persons. This table lists the first-choice regimens for various infections. Alternative treatments are available for selected situations. These recommendations are frequently updated as additional information becomes available

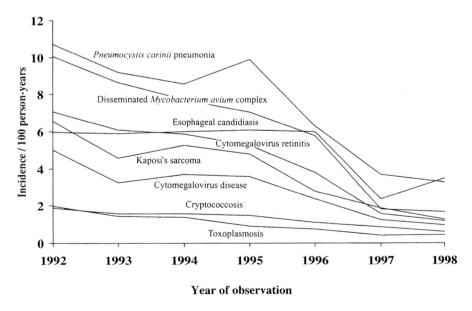

Fig. 3.3. Incidence of various opportunistic infections in HIV-infected patients over time. Declines in the numbers of new infections from the mid-1990s onward reflect the impact of improved prophylactic strategies against opportunistic infections and the effect of highly active antiretroviral regimens. (From KAPLAN 2000)

of HAART became more widespread. These declines are attributable to the improvements in immune function that occurred when improved antiretroviral therapy effectively suppressed HIV replication.

Prior to the availability of HAART, guidelines for the use of prophylaxis against opportunistic infections recommended that once prophylaxis was initiated, it be continued lifelong and that the threshold for initiation of prophylaxis be based on the lowest measured CD4+ lymphocyte count in any individual patient. The rationale for these recommendations was that the degree of immunologic damage incurred was not likely to be correctable and therefore the risk of opportunistic infections remained fixed based on the lowest CD4+ lymphocyte count. The marked decrease in opportunistic infections seen in patients responding to HAART therapy indicated that significant immune reconstitution occurred following effective suppression of HIV. Consequently, the guidelines for prophylaxis against opportunistic infections have recently been revised to acknowledge this fact (CDC 1999). The most recent version of these guidelines suggests that clinicians consider stopping primary prophylaxis for *Pneumocystis carinii* if the CD4+ lymphocyte count increases to >200 cells/µl for at least 3–6 months. Also, clinicians should consider stopping primary prophylaxis for *M. avium* complex disease in patients in whom the CD4+ lymphocyte count has increased to >100 cells/µl for 3–6 months and who also have had sustained HIV suppression while on antiretroviral therapy. Finally, the new recommendations suggest that secondary prophylaxis for cytomegalovirus retinitis can be stopped if patients have CD4+ lymphocyte counts >100–150 cells/µl for 3–6 months, if they can be followed regularly by an ophthalmologist, if the lesions were not directly sight-threatening, and if vision in the other eye is adequate. It is likely that further revisions in these guidelines will occur as additional information is accumulated regarding the impact of HAART on the risk of opportunistic infections.

While all this is undoubtedly good news, it is important to realize that HIV remains an enormously difficult problem. More that 90% of HIV-infected persons worldwide live in areas where health care resources are insufficient for even the most basic HIV care, much less able to pay for antiretroviral drugs. Even among HIV-infected persons fortunate enough to have access to HAART, less than half are able to achieve durable suppression of HIV replication. The reasons for this are complex and include such things as side-effects associated with the drugs,

dosing schedules that are difficult to adhere to, and the evolution of drug resistance in the virus. Thus the challenge of HIV infection remains daunting.

3.5 Conclusion

The HIV pandemic is now estimated to have infected more than 50 million persons worldwide with no evidence of it having peaked. The repeated cycles of viral replication that are the hallmark of this infection induce an inexorable decline in immune function that ultimately leads to acquisition of the opportunistic infections that define AIDS. Improvements in the understanding of risks for such infections have produced better strategies for the use of prophylaxis to prevent new opportunistic infections from occurring. Even more dramatic improvements have been induced with the successful use of highly active antiretroviral therapy which can reconstitute immune function in some patients. These developments have greatly improved the outlook for many HIV-infected persons. Unfortunately, effective treatment is available for only a fraction of those who are HIV infected and is successful for only a portion of them. It is certain that HIV and its complications will remain an important medical problem for the foreseeable future.

References

Alcabes P, Munoz A, Vlahov D, Friedland GH (1993) Incubation period of human immunodeficiency virus. AIDS 15:303–318

Bacchetti P, Moss AR (1989) Incubation period of AIDS in San Francisco. Nature 338:251–253

Centers for Diseases Control (1982) Update on acquired immunodeficiency syndrome (AIDS) – United States. MMWR Morb Mortal Wkly Rep 31:507–514

Centers for Disease Control and Prevention (1999) USPHS/IDSA guidelines for the prevention of opportunistic infections in persons infected with human immunodeficiency virus. MMWR Morb Mortal Wkly Rep 48(RR-10):1–66

Chaisson RE, Sterling TR, Gallant JE (2000) General clinical manifestations of human immunodeficiency virus infection (including oral, cutaneous, renal, ocular, and cardiac diseases). In: Mandell GL, Bennett JE, Dolin R (eds) Principles and practice of infectious diseases. Churchill Livingstone, Philadelphia, pp 1398–1415

Cooper DA, Tindall B, Wilson EJ, et al. (1988) Characterization of T lymphocyte responses during primary HIV infection. J Infect Dis 157:889–896

Crowe SM, Carlin JB, Stewart KI, et al. (1991) Predictive value of CD4 lymphocyte numbers for the development of opportunistic infections and malignancies in HIV-infected persons. J Acquir Immune Defic Syndr 4:770–776

Fauci AS (1993) Multifactorial nature of human immunodeficiency virus disease: implications for therapy. Science 262:1011–1018

Fauci AS, Panteleo G, Stanley S, et al. (1996) Immunopathogenic mechanisms of HIV infection. Ann Intern Med 124:654–663

Gottlieb MS, Schroff R, Schanker, et al. (1981) *Pneumocystis carinii* pneumonia and mucosal candidiasis in previously healthy homosexual men: evidence of a new acquired cellular immunodeficiency. N Engl J Med 305:1425–1431

Kahn JO, Walker BD (1998) Acute human immunodeficiency virus type 1 infection. N Engl J Med 339:33–39

Kaplan JE, Hanson D, Dworkin MS, et al. (2000) Epidemiology of human immunodeficiency virus-associated opportunistic infections in the United States in the era of highly active antiretroviral therapy. Clin Infect Dis 30:S5–S14

Klatzmann D, Champagne E, Chamaret S, et al. (1984) T-lymphocyte T4 molecule behaves as the receptor for human retrovirus LAV. Nature 312:767–768

Kovacs JA, Masur H (2000) Prophylaxis against opportunistic infections in patients with human immunodeficiency virus infection. N Engl J Med 342:1416–1429

Masur H, Michelis MA, Greene GB, et al. (1981) An outbreak of community-acquired *Pneumocystis carinii* pneumonia: initial manifestation of cellular immune dysfunction. N Engl J Med 305:1431–1438

Mellors JW, Rinaldo CR, Phalguni G, et al. (1996) Prognosis in HIV-1 infection predicted by quantity of virus in plasma. Science 272:1167–1170

Metroka CE, Cunningham-Rundles S, Pollack MS, et al. (1983) Generalized lymphadenopathy in homosexual men. Ann Intern Med 99:585–591

Palella FJ, Delaney KM, Moorman AC, et al. (1998) Declining morbidity and mortality among patients with advanced human immunodeficiency virus infection. N Engl J Med 338:853–860

Phair J, Munoz A, Detels R, et al. (1990) The risk of *Pneumocystis carinii* pneumonia among men with human immunodeficiency virus type 1. N Engl J Med 322:161–165

Quinn T (1997) Acute primary HIV infection. JAMA 278:58–62

Rutherford GW, Lifson AR, Hessol NA, et al. (1990) Course of HIV-1 infection in a cohort of homosexual and bisexual men: an 11-year follow-up study. BMJ 301:1183–1188

4 The Pathologic Patterns of AIDS

Marijke R. Canninga-Van Dijk and Jan G. Van den Tweel

4.1 Introduction

Infection with the human immune deficiency virus (HIV) results in a variety of pathologic lesions, leading to multisystem disease (Klatt 1989, 1992; Lucas 1995; Lucas et al. 1993, 1996). Although some of the effects are the direct results of HIV infection, the majority of the lesions are due to secondary infections with opportunistic organisms (Lyon et al. 1996). In addition, a considerable number of proliferative lesions, both benign and malignant, occur as a direct result of the immunodeficiency status of the patient, and the intense therapy also has its drawbacks (John et al. 1998, Paxton and Janssen 2000).

We shall first discuss the most important opportunistic infections and tumors (Table 4.1, Centers for Disease Control and Prevention 1992) that are associated with HIV infections. In the second half of the chapter we will give an overview of the most important pathologic lesions of the relevant organ systems.

4.2 Opportunistic Infections

The main causes of opportunistic infections are bacteria, viruses, protozoa, and fungi. Most of these infections are seen in all kinds of patients with immun-

M.R. Canninga-Van Dijk, MD
J.G. Van den Tweel, MD, PhD
Department of Pathology, H04.312, University Medical Center, PO Box 85500, 3508 GA Utrecht, The Netherlands

Table 4.1. The 1987 and 1992 CDC lists for the case definition of AIDS

Viral infections
    CMV
    Herpes simplex
    JC virus
    Molluscum contagiosum
Bacterial infections
    Recurrent bacterial pneumonia (commonly *Strep. pneumoniae*)
    Mycobacterium tuberculosis
    Nontuberculosis mycobacteriosis (particularly *M. avium-intracellulare* complex)
    Systemic nontyphoid *Salmonella* infections (notably *S. enteritidis* and *S. typhimurium*)
Fungal infections
    Severe *Candida* infection
    Cryptococcus neoformans
    Histoplasma capsulatum
    Coccidioides immitis
Protozoal infections
    Pneumocystis carinii
    Toxoplasma gondii
    Cryptosporidium parvum
    Isospora belli
Tumors
    Kaposi's sarcoma
    Primary cerebral lymphoma
    High-grade non-Hodgkin B cell lymphoma
    Carcinoma (invasive) of the cervix
Other conditions
    HIV-wasting syndrome (fever, weight loss, diarrhea)
    HIV-associated dementia

odeficiency diseases, whatever the reason. However, patients with HIV show these diseases more frequently. The opportunistic infections affect many organ systems, but mainly the respiratory tract, the digestive tract, and the central nervous system (CNS). The pattern of infections in AIDS patients has changed in the last decade (LYON et al. 1996). The general aspects of these infections are discussed in the first part of this chapter, while the organ-specific aspects will be dealt with under the respective organs.

4.2.1
Bacterial Infections

4.2.1.1
Mycobacterium tuberculosis

Although strictly speaking tuberculosis is not an opportunistic infection, its incidence and the number of AIDS patients dying from tuberculosis have increased (BARNES et al. 1991). Especially the extrapulmonary forms of tuberculosis are occurring with increasing frequency as a complication of HIV infection. Morphologically the granulomas display caseous necrosis with identifiable acid-fast microorganisms, as is also seen in non-HIV-infected patients. The extrapulmonary dissemination of this disease is regarded as diagnostic of AIDS. It is suggested that the disease is probably the result of reactivation of a previous infection rather than being a primary infection (RACE et al. 1998). If the disease is disseminated, it involves the respiratory tract (Fig. 4.1), spleen, lymph nodes, liver, and genitourinary tract. The bone marrow, gastrointestinal tract, and kidneys are less commonly involved.

4.2.1.2
Mycobacterium avium-intracellulare

The most frequent atypical mycobacterial infection is caused by *Mycobacterium avium-intracellulare*. The infection is characterized by single cells, small clusters or large groups of histiocytes that are filled with small rods. In massive infections the lymph node has a homogeneous yellow color, similar to the color of microbiologic culture plates. Although the microorganisms can be seen using hematoxylin and eosin (H&E) staining, they are better visible with special stains such as Ziehl-Neelsen, periodic acid-Schiff, Giemsa, and metaminamine silver. The size of the macrophages/histiocytes can be up to 50 μm. As well as the lymph nodes, the spleen (Fig. 4.2) and liver are frequently affected. Other organs that are affected by this infection include the bone marrow, the gastrointestinal tract, and the respiratory tract (Fig. 4.3). It is rarely found in the CNS, skin, and heart. Even widespread *Mycobacterium avium-intracellulare* infection is infrequently a cause of death.

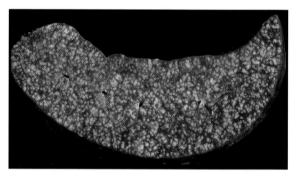

Fig. 4.2. Cut surface of the spleen, massively infiltrated by *Mycobacterium avium*

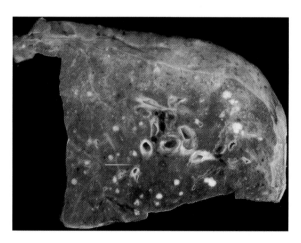

Fig. 4.1. Cut surface of a lung with diffuse small foci of tuberculosis

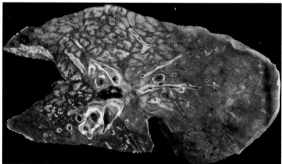

Fig. 4.3. Cut surface of a lung that is distally massively infiltrated by *Mycobacterium avium*

4.2.2
Viral Infections

4.2.2.1
Cytomegalovirus Infection

Cytomegalovirus (CMV) is a virus of the herpes family. It is a worldwide ubiquitous pathogenic agent that only gives rise to serious complications in immunodeficient patients, either by primary infection or after reactivation of a latent infection. Approximately 50% of HIV patients develop CMV infections in the course of their disease. The organs most frequently affected are the adrenals, respiratory tract, and gastrointestinal tract, followed by the CNS and the retina. CMV is most often identified within the endothelial cells or histiocytic clusters. The infected cells are enlarged and show large violaceous to dark red, intranuclear inclusions, surrounded by a thin clear halo (Fig. 4.4). Usually CMV infection is not an aggressive disease. Often it is unclear whether such lesions represent a pathologic condition or a symbiotic relationship.

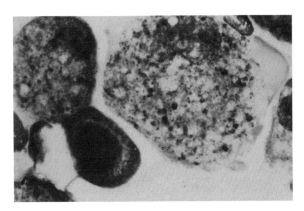

Fig. 4.4. Cytologic preparation of a lung infected by *Pneumocystis carinii* (cloudy areas) and cytomegalovirus (large nuclear inclusion surrounded by a halo (*lower left*)

4.2.2.2
Herpes Simplex Virus and Herpes Zoster Virus

Herpes zoster and herpes simplex usually present as a mucocutaneous disease (Fox et al. 1999). Other localizations are very uncommon. Particularly the perianal region is frequently involved. Oropharyngeal and esophageal infections are less common. Macroscopically the lesions manifest as vesicles or ulcers. Under the microscope the infected cells show eosinophilic intranuclear inclusions. Secondary infections of ulcers are commonly seen.

4.2.2.3
Human Papilloma Virus

Human papilloma virus, a DNA virus, is found in many proliferative epithelial lesions. In AIDS patients it is seen in association with dysplasia and with carcinomas of the anorectal epithelium and also with condylomata acuminata. It is also seen in hairy leukoplakia, a white lesion that is usually present on the lateral border of the tongue. Currently, however, there is more evidence for Epstein-Barr virus (EBV) involvement in the etiology of this lesion.

4.2.3
Protozoal Infections

Protozoal infections are important sources of significant disease in immunocompromised patients. Among them, the three most important ones are *Pneumocystis carinii*, *Cryptosporidium*, and *Toxoplasma gondii*.

4.2.3.1
Pneumocystis carinii

Infection by *Pneumocystis carinii* is often one of the first symptoms of AIDS. The protozoa consist of small cysts that eventually rupture and release up to eight protozoites. After rupturing, they differentiate into trophozoites. These trophozoites form new cysts and repeat the cycle of the microorganism. The microscopic picture is very characteristic. The lungs, the organs that are most often involved, show cloudy alveoli (Fig. 4.4) owing to extensive growth of the protozoa (GAL et al. 1987). Although the H&E sections are rather specific, the microorganisms can be stained by Grocott staining and by methylene blue. These staining methods confirm the expected diagnosis. Extrapulmonary localizations are rare, although this disease can be found in hilar lymph nodes and very occasionally in other organs (RADIN et al. 1990).

4.2.3.2
Cryptosporidium

Cryptosporidium infection usually presents in the gastrointestinal tract. There are no specific gross pathologic lesions. The microorganisms are small, 2–6 μm in diameter, and are usually found along the mucosal brush border of the stomach and the small and large intestine. They can be recognized by Ziehl-Neelsen staining since they are acid-fast. Rarely these organisms are seen in other organs, such as the biliary system and the respiratory tract.

4.2.3.3
Toxoplasma gondii

Toxoplasmosis is an infectious disease that is quite common in a wide variety of animals, especially mammals and birds. It is a very common parasitic infection in the Western world and many children are infected annually at birth. In adults the disease usually manifests as a lymphadenopathy. *Toxoplasma gondii* infection by itself is not an opportunistic infection. In HIV patients the CNS is often involved (TSCHIRHART and KLATT 1988). Extracerebral toxoplasmosis is infrequent in AIDS. While the respiratory tract and gastrointestinal tract are sometimes involved, such involvement is usually found only at autopsy. Microscopically, the disease is diagnosed by finding cysts that measure ca. 50 μm and are filled with bradyzoites. Free protozoa are very difficult to find. Only ruptured cysts can induce an inflammatory response.

4.2.3.4
Other Protozoa

Other protozoal infections that should be mentioned here are *Isospora belli* and *Microsporidium* (SCHWARTZ et al. 1996). Their pathology is usually located in the small intestine. Sometimes regional lymph nodes are also involved.

4.2.4
Fungi

4.2.4.1
Cryptococcus neoformans

Cryptococcus neoformans organisms are small, sometimes budding, yeasts with a diameter of approximately 4–7 μm. The cells have a prominent capsule that can be easily recognized using routine histologic stains. The organisms form pale, mucoid areas in affected tissues. Sometimes the capsule of the organism is missing and epithelioid granulomas with giant cells are present. In this case the organisms appear small and may be confused with *Candida* and histoplasmosis. The CNS is frequently involved, as is the lung. In disseminated disease, other organs can also be affected, e.g., lymph nodes, spleen, bone marrow, and liver.

4.2.4.2
Candida albicans

Candida albicans is a ubiquitous yeast that can be found in the skin and in the oral cavity of healthy individuals. To fulfill the criteria for candidiasis, the fungus must invade the mucosa of the esophagus and the respiratory tract. The gross manifestation of these organisms is by white plaques or patches. The involvement of other organs is very rare.

Histologically, the invading fungi are surrounded by granulocytes. The fungus is characterized by buds and pseudohyphae without branching or true septations. Although *Candida* can be demonstrated in many patients with AIDS, it is a rare cause of death.

4.2.4.3
Other Fungal Infections

Among other fungi, *Aspergillus fumigatus* can cause considerable organ damage (Fig. 4.5). *Histoplasma capsulatum* and *Coccidioides* are also frequently encountered in AIDS patients.

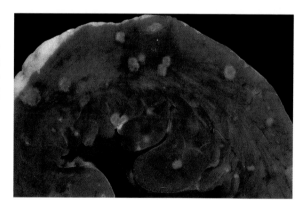

Fig. 4.5. Cut surface of the left ventricular myocardium with many small areas of *Aspergillus* infection

4.3
Neoplasms

Patients with AIDS have a high incidence of malignancies, compared with patients in the same age group without this disorder. Malignant lymphomas, Kaposi's sarcoma, and squamous epithelial tumors deserve special attention here.

4.3.1
Malignant Lymphomas

Approximately 3% of HIV-positive patients present with a non-Hodgkin lymphoma. The risk of developing lymphoma is increased 100-fold 6–8 years after the infection, and the risk approaches 1% per year once the diagnosis of AIDS has been established (BIGGAR and RABKIN 1992; LEVINE 1991; LUCAS et al. 1993; LUXTON et al. 1991). The most common lymphoma in this group of patients is the diffuse large B cell lymphoma in the WHO classification. These tumors tend to be extranodal and involve the lungs, intestines, and CNS (Fig. 4.6). The risk of developing a primary cerebral lymphoma is increased approximately 1,000 times in HIV-positive patients, compared with a normal population. Most of the lymphomas are EBV associated. Since there are various genetic mutations in these lymphomas, the pathogenetic pathways along which the lymphomas develop are probably variable.

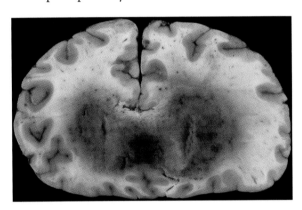

Fig. 4.6. Cross-section of the frontal brain with an extensive localization of a diffuse large B-cell lymphoma

A second B cell lymphoma that is associated with HIV infections is the primary effusion B cell lymphoma (DEPOND et al. 1997). This tumor develops in the pleura, the pericardium, and the peritoneal cavity and is associated with human herpes virus HHV8 infection.

Hodgkin's disease (AMES et al. 1991; GOLD et al. 1991) is also reported to be associated with HIV infection but is not considered a criterion for the diagnosis of AIDS, in contrast to non-Hodgkin lymphomas. Most patients present with advanced disease (82% with stage 3 or 4) and with mixed cellularity histology. In contrast to the normal response to therapy, HIV patients react poorly to conventional therapy and more than two-thirds will die within 1 year of diagnosis. A statistical analysis by GOLD and col-

leagues of a large group of patients revealed that HIV-associated Hodgkin's disease has a strong tendency to occur outside of the normal age range for Hodgkin's disease (GOLD et al. 1991).

4.3.2
Lymphoproliferative Disorders

Due to the immunosuppressed state of the patient, lymphoproliferative lesions are seen in this group, and are similar to lesions in patients with organ transplants. The lymphoproliferative disorders may involve nodal and extranodal structures, especially the mucosa of the gut and the brain (KNOWLES 1999). Some of them transform into a malignant lymphoma. Also Castleman's disease (especially the plasma cell type) is associated with HIV infection and may eventually progress into a non-Hodgkin lymphoma. Now that HIV patients live longer, lymphoproliferative disorders and malignant lymphomas are becoming a bigger problem and present diagnostic and clinical challenges.

4.3.3
Kaposi's Sarcoma

Kaposi's sarcoma is a mesenchymal tumor, probably of vascular origin, that manifests in the skin, the mucous membranes of the bronchial tree, the oropharyngeal and gastrointestinal mucosa (Fig. 4.7), and the lymphatic tissue, with a preference for MALT (ENSOLI et al. 1991; HAVERKOS et al. 1990; PALCA 1992; ROTH et al. 1992; TAPPERO et al. 1993). It is a reactive proliferation of endothelial cells and shows a strong relation

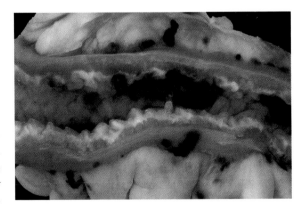

Fig. 4.7. Mucosal aspect of the ileum with extensive localizations of a Kaposi's sarcoma. This tumor is also present in the serosal surface

with human herpes virus HHV8 (CESARMAN and KNOWLES 1999; CHANG et al. 1994). The presence of HHV8 increases the risk that patients will develop Kaposi's sarcoma. The tumor is also described in HIV-seronegative individuals and in patients receiving immunosuppressive therapy. Since the tumor usually develops simultaneously in different organs, this suggests a multifocal genesis. The early lesions of this disease are small red nodules having a diameter of 1–2 mm. Later in the disease, macular and plaque-like lesions occur. Histologically, the cytonuclear pleomorphism is slight to moderate and mitoses can be found. The tumor cells may show erythrophagocytosis. The lesions show expansile growth along existing vessels in the deeper layers and surrounding support tissues of organs, especially the lung, the liver, the heart, and the kidneys.

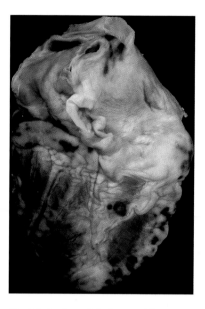

Fig. 4.8. Surface of the heart with many small areas of Kaposi's sarcoma in a patient with generalized Kaposi's sarcoma

4.3.4
Squamous Epithelial Tumors

Squamous cell carcinoma of the cervix was made an AIDS-defining disease in 1992. Strangely enough, although there is a clear increase in cervical intraepithelial neoplasms among HIV-positive women, there is no marked increase in the occurrence of carcinomas. A parallel is seen in HIV-positive gay men. They display more anal interepithelial neoplasms, but this does not lead to more invasive anal carcinomas. In contrast, there is a definite increase in invasive and in situ conjunctival squamous cell carcinomas in HIV patients (WADDELL et al. 1996). Bowen's disease, squamous cell carcinoma, and basal cell carcinoma of the skin are also reported to occur with increased frequency.

4.4
Organ System Pathology

4.4.1
Cardiovascular System

All parts of the heart can be involved in HIV disease, although gross abnormalities are rare. If a tumor, is present it is usually a malignant lymphoma. Approximately 20% of patients with malignant lymphoma show cardiac involvement. Kaposi's sarcoma is rare (Fig. 4.8).

Pericarditis is usually of tuberculous origin in countries where that infection is common. Bacterial

endocarditis and subsequent myocardial abscesses are usually found in patients who use i.v. drugs. Protozoal and viral infections may occur. HIV itself can also cause myocardial damage (GRODY et al. 1990). In the later stages of the disease, dilated cardiomyopathy, predominantly of the left ventricle, is seen and is a cause of congestive heart failure in those patients (BARBARO et al. 1999; COHEN et al. 1986). The etiology of this disorder is drug use and nonspecific damage complicating a septic shock.

Sometimes arterial aneurysms, often multiple, are seen in association with HIV infection (NAIR et al. 1999). This is especially true in South Africa, where HIV infections have a high prevalence.

In addition, vascular complications associated with the use of HIV protease inhibitors have been reported (BEHRENS et al. 1998).

4.4.2
Pulmonary Tract

The respiratory tract is frequently involved in patients with AIDS. Infections of the lung are a major cause of death in AIDS patients. X-rays mostly reveal diffuse bilateral interstitial and alveolar infiltrates (MCKENNA et al. 1986). The clinical features of the different diseases can be indistinguishable, although infections generally cause more diffuse interstitial patterns and malignancies a more nodular appearance. Among the infections, *Pneumocystis carinii*

(PCP) and CMV are the most prominent. Most AIDS patients will have at least one episode of PCP during their disease. PCP was originally a major cause of death in AIDS patients, but the disease is now under good control. The pathologic features of PCP are those of widespread involvement of the alveolar spaces with a gross appearance of pneumonic consolidation with scattered areas of hemorrhage or congestion. Later in the disease, the surface develops a slimy appearance and finally it turns dry, as a result of fibrosis and organization (Fig. 4.9). Bronchoscopy and bronchiolar lavage are the best diagnostic procedure.

CMV is an important cause of diffuse alveolar damage and adult respiratory distress syndrome (ARDS). Clinically and morphologically, it is very difficult to distinguish infections causing ARDS. Microscopically, viral inclusions can be found in endothelial cells and pneumocytes. There are some case reports of a role of HIV in primary pulmonary hypertension (PELLICELLI et al. 1998). Tumors are rare although malignant lymphomas (including the effusion type) and Kaposi's sarcoma occur in the lungs.

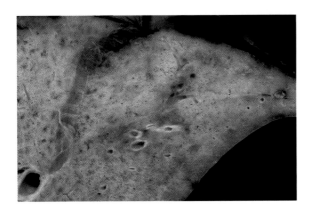

Fig. 4.9. Lung lobe with a consolidated aspect. The dry cut surface is characteristic of *Pneumocystis carinii* infection

4.4.3
Gastrointestinal Tract

A wide range of opportunistic infections can involve the gastrointestinal (GI) tract in HIV-positive patients. In many cases, such infections serve to establish the diagnosis of AIDS according to the official criteria (Table 4.1). The mouth and the esophagus are often involved by invasive candidiasis. The stomach and the upper gastrointestinal tract frequently show the presence of cryptosporidiosis and microsporidiosis. Patients often suffer from diarrhea,

weight loss, and malabsorption. The microorganisms live intracellularly in an extracytoplasmic niche of the surface epithelial cells. Microscopically the only morphologic abnormality is atrophy of the microvilli. For the diagnosis of microsporidiosis, electron microscopic examination is very helpful.

CMV infection is also an important cause of gastrointestinal disease. The virus is present in endothelial cells, causing local vascular damage and consequent necrosis of the mucous membrane.

Mycobacterium avium infection results in small yellow plates with a characteristic macroscopic appearance. An inflammatory infiltrate is usually absent microscopically. Often the regional lymph nodes are also infected.

Kaposi's sarcoma occurs frequently in the GI tract and can be present from the mouth to the anus. Malignant lymphoma of the GI tract is also a frequent complication of HIV infection; as already mentioned, the tumor is usually a diffuse large B-cell lymphoma.

The hepatobiliary system is involved by opportunistic infections or neoplasms in approximately 30% of AIDS patients (CAPPELL 1991; HINNANT et al. 1989). Clinically these are of minor importance since they almost never result in hepatic failure. Among the infections that are found are *Mycobacterium avium*, *Cryptococcus*, and *Histoplasma*. Hepatitis is at present an increasing complication (BRAU et al. 1997; LESENS et al. 1999). Kaposi's sarcoma is rare and, when present, is located in the connective tissue surrounding the large portal venous branches and the large biliary tracts (Fig. 4.10). Malignant lymphomas of the liver are rarely seen as primary tumors (CACCAMO et al. 1986); they usually occur in association with lymphomas elsewhere.

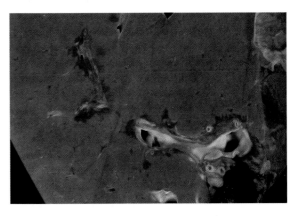

Fig. 4.10. Cut surface of the liver with surrounding vessels and ducts infiltrated by Kaposi's sarcoma

4.4.4
Hematopoietic Organs

Lymphadenopathy is often seen in patients with AIDS. Usually an AIDS-specific reaction to HIV is seen, characterized by extreme follicular hyperplasia with many starry sky macrophages. Later in the disease, an architectural destruction of the lymph node takes place, with fragmentation and disappearance of follicles and finally depletion of lymphoid tissue (ÖST et al. 1989).

The mesenteric lymph nodes are often involved in *Mycobacterium avium* infections.

As has been previously stated, malignant lymphomas are an important cause of lymphadenopathy, although extranodal lymphomas are more frequent than nodal ones.

The bone marrow usually shows dysplastic features of the hematopoiesis (BAIN 1997; SUN et al. 1989), resulting in peripheral cytopenias. In addition, opportunistic infections can be found, although they are infrequent. EBV infection of HIV patients may result in a hemophagocytic syndrome (ALBRECHT et al. 1997).

4.4.5
Central Nervous System

The CNS can be affected by HIV infection (BUDKA 1989; EVERALL et al. 1999) with the clinical manifestation of an HIV encephalopathy/AIDS dementia complex or of secondary lesions, including infections and localizations of malignant tumors, especially lymphoma.

The morphologic spectrum of HIV encephalopathy is the result of multiple perivascular accumulations of multinucleated giant cells with inflammatory reactions and necrosis or of diffuse white matter damage of cerebral and cerebellar hemispheres.

Among the opportunistic infections, toxoplasmosis is the most frequent, being localized in the cerebral hemispheres, the basal ganglia, and the brainstem (Fig. 4.11). The gross appearance is multiple areas of ill-defined necrosis, microscopically accompanied by a mild inflammatory infiltrate with many macrophages and large numbers of *Toxoplasma gondii* tachyzoites in the periphery of the necrotic areas. In addition, fungal infections may be seen, mainly caused by *Cryptococcus neoformans*, *Candida* species, and *Aspergillus*.

An important viral infection in HIV-positive patients is polyomavirus (JC virus or SV 40), which leads to so-called progressive multifocal leukoen-

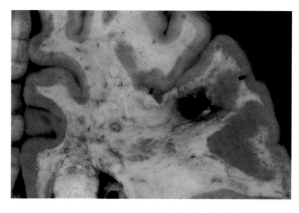

Fig. 4.11. Parietal lobe of the cerebellum with a hemorrhagic area due to infection by toxoplasmosis

cephalopathy. This disease is characterized by multiple confluent areas of demyelination in both hemispheres, the cerebellum, and the brainstem. Viral inclusion bodies are detected both in cells of astrocytic origin and in cells of oligodendroglial origin.

In addition, CMV (Fig. 4.12) causes both encephalitis and microglial nodules. Sometimes herpes simplex virus type I is reported. Destruction of retinal cells due to CMV causes "cotton wool" spots in the retina.

Non-Hodgkin lymphomas are the most frequent tumors to be located in the CNS. They show a predominant perivascular involvement of the brain.

4.4.6
The Skin

The first cutaneous manifestation of HIV infection, occurring in approximately 23% of patients, is acute HIV exanthema (GOLDMAN et al. 1995). This macu-

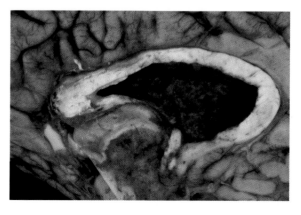

Fig. 4.12. Section of the brain with a hemorrhagic aspect of the third ventricle as the result of a CMV infection

lar, roseoliform dermatosis represents the acute se-roconversion reaction. A skin biopsy shows perivas-cular infiltrates of lymphocytes with usually mild epidermal changes.

Cutaneous diseases occurring at a later stage can be classified into three categories: infections, neo-plasms, and noninfectious dermatoses. In addition to the bacterial, viral, protozoal, and fungal infec-tions discussed in the first part of this chapter, ar-thropod infections (scabies and demodicosis) can be seen in the skin. Scabies is caused by *Sarcoptes sca-biei*, a mite penetrating the skin. In HIV-positive pa-tients, scabies usually presents with an extremely heavy infestation with mites, resulting in keratotic and psoriasiform lesions. This severe manifestation is known as Norwegian scabies. *Demodex follicu-lorum* and *Demodex brevis* are follicle mites, often found in normal human skin. They are found at a higher rate in patients with rosacea, which is usually restricted to the face. In immunocompromised pa-tients, *Demodex* can cause a widespread eruption. Histopathology shows mites in the stratum corneum (scabies) or in the hair follicles (demodicosis).

A bacterial infection that should be mentioned in this chapter is bacillary angiomatosis (LeBoit et al. 1989), a vascular proliferation that most commonly involves the skin but can also affect other organs such as liver, bone and brain. It is caused by *Bartonel-la henselae* and *Bartonella quintana*. The skin le-sions resemble Kaposi's sarcoma. It is very impor-tant to recognize bacillary angiomatosis and distinguish it from Kaposi's sarcoma because of the good response of the former to antibiotic therapy. Under the microscope one sees a proliferation of blood vessels in combination with a mixed infiltrate with many neutrophils. A viral infection limited to the skin is molluscum contagiosum: pearly, umbili-cated papules caused by a poxvirus. Histopathology shows large eosinophilic intracytoplasmic inclu-sions in keratinocytes.

Neoplasms of the skin (Kaposi's sarcoma, lympho-ma, Bowen's disease, and squamous and basal cell car-cinoma) have already been discussed in the first part of this chapter. In a few case reports, HIV positivity has been mentioned as a risk factor for the develop-ment of malignant melanoma (Rivers et al. 1989).

The noninfectious dermatoses are mostly "com-mon" dermatoses that present with increased fre-quency and often increased severity in HIV-posi-tive patients. A frequent skin disease among these patients is seborrheic dermatitis. Scaly, erythema-tous and sometimes papular lesions develop on the face, scalp, chest, and genitalia. Histologically there

is mild parakeratosis with slight spongiosis. HIV-associated eosinophilic folliculitis (Rosenthal et al. 1991) presents with erythematous, follicular papules on the head, neck, and chest (Fig. 4.13). There is a follicular and dermal infiltrate with many lymphocytes and eosinophils. Small eosinophilic pustules may be seen in the hair follicle epithelium. Many photosensitivity reactions like granuloma annulare, (pseudo)porphyria cutanea tarda, and chronic actinic dermatitis can occur in HIV-positive patients. Cutaneous drug eruptions can show a lot of different clinical patterns: exanthematous eruptions, maculopapular lesions, and also the severe blisters of Stevens-Johnson syndrome and toxic epidermal necrolysis (TEN). These drug eruptions most often entail vacuolar changes of the epidermal basal layer with necrotic keratinocytes. The superficial infil-trate consists of lymphocytes, mixed with a vari-able number of eosinophils. In Stevens-Johnson syndrome, TEN, and their less severe variant, erythe-ma multiforme, there is a subepidermal blister with clusters of necrotic keratinocytes in the overlying epidermis. The infiltrate is lymphocytic and superfi-cial. In TEN the infiltrate is very sparse or even ab-sent. AIDS-relared muscocutaneous disorders will be described in detail in chapter 13.

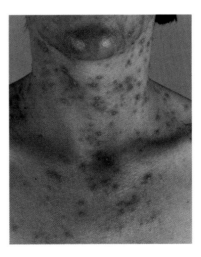

Fig. 4.13. Follicular papules on the face, neck, and chest in a patient with eosinophilic folliculitis

References

Albrecht H, Schafer H, Stellbrink H-J, et al. (1997) Epstein-Barr virus-associated hemophagocytic syndrome. A cause of fever of unknown origin in HIV infection. Arch Pathol Lab Med 121:853–858

Ames ED, Conjalka MS, Goldberg AF, et al. (1991) Hodgkin's disease and AIDS. Hematol Oncol Clin North Am 5:343–356

Bain B (1997) The haematological features of HIV infection. Br J Haematol 99:1–8

Barbaro G, Di Lorenzo G, Grisorio B, Barbarini G (1999) Incidence of dilated cardiomyopathy and detection of HIV in myocardial cells of HIV-infected patients. N Engl J Med 339:1093–1099

Barnes PF, Bloch AB, Davidson PT, et al. (1991) Tuberculosis in patients with human immunodeficiency virus infection. N Engl J Med 324:1644–1650

Behrens G, Schmidt H, Meyer D, et al. (1998) Vascular complications associated with the use of HIV protease inhibitors. Lancet 351:1958–1959

Biggar RJ, Rabkin CS (1992) The epidemiology of acquired immunodeficiency syndrome-related lymphomas. Curr Opin Oncol 4:883–893

Brau N, Leaf HL, Wieczorek RL, et al. (1997) Severe hepatitis in three AIDS patients treated with indinavir. Lancet 349:924–925

Budka H (1989) Human immunodeficiency virus (HIV)-induced disease of the central nervous system: pathology and implications for pathogenesis. Acta Neuropathol (Berl) 77:225–236

Caccamo D, Pervez NK, Marchevsky A (1986) Primary lymphoma of the liver in the acquired immunodeficiency syndrome. Arch Pathol Lab Med 110:553–555

Cappell MS (1991) Hepatobiliary manifestations of the acquired immunodeficiency syndrome. Am J Gastroenterol 86:1–15

Centers for Disease Control and Prevention (1992) 1993 revised classification system for HIV infection and expanded surveillance case definition for AIDS among adolescents and adults. MMWR Morb Mortal Wkly Rep 41 [RR-17]:1–19

Cesarman E, Knowles DM (1999) The role of Kaposi's sarcoma-associated herpesvirus (KSHV/HHV8) in lymphoproliferative diseases. Semin Canc Biol 9:165–174

Chang Y, Cesarman E, Pessin MS, et al. (1994) Identification of herpes virus like sequences in AIDS-associated Kaposi's sarcomas. Science 266:1865–1869

Cohen IS, Anderson DW, Virmani R, et al. (1986) Congestive cardiomyopathy in association with the acquired immunodeficiency syndrome. N Engl J Med 315:628–630

DePond W, Said JW, Tasaka T, et al. (1997) Kaposi's sarcoma-associated herpesvirus and HHV8 (KSV/HHV8)-associated lymphoma of the bowel. Report of two cases in HIV+ve men with secondary effusion lymphoma. Am J Surg Pathol 21:719–724

Ensoli B, Barillari G, Gallo RC (1991) Pathogenesis of AIDS-associated Kaposi's sarcoma. Hematol Oncol Clin North Am 5:281–295

Everall IP, Heaton RK, Marcotte TD, et al. (1999) Cortical synaptic density is reduced in mild to moderate HIV neurocognitive disorder. Brain Pathol 9:209–217

Fox PA, Barton SE, Francis N, et al. (1999) Chronic erosive herpes simplex virus infection of the penis, a possible immune reconstitution disease. HIV Med 1:10–18

Gal AA, Klatt EC, Koss MN, et al. (1987) The effectiveness of bronchoscopy in the diagnosis of *Pneumocystis carinii* and cytomegalovirus pulmonary infections in acquired immunodeficiency syndrome. Arch Pathol Lab Med 111:238–241

Gold JE, Altarac D, Ree HJ (1991) HIV-associated Hodgkin disease: a clinical study of 18 cases and review. Am J Hematol 39:93–99

Goldman GD, Milstone LM, Shapiro PE (1995) Histologic findings in acute HIV exanthem. J Cutan Pathol 22:371–373

Grody WW, Cheng L, Lewis W (1990) Infection of the heart by the human immunodeficiency virus. Am J Cardiol 66:203–206

Haverkos HW, Freidman-Kien AE, Drotman DP, et al. (1990) The changing incidence of Kaposi's sarcoma among patients with AIDS. J Am Acad Dermatol 22:1250–1253

Hinnant K, Schwartz A, Rotterdam H, et al. (1989) Cytomegalovirus and cryptosporidial cholecystitis in two patients with AIDS. Am Surg Pathol 107:133–137

John M, Mallal S, French M (1998) Emerging toxicity with long-term antiretroviral therapy. J HIV Ther 3:58–61

Klatt EC (1989) Diagnostic findings in patients with acquired immune deficiency syndrome. J Acquir Immune Defic Syndr 5:459–465

Klatt EC (1992) Practical AIDS Pathology. ASCP Press, Chicago

Knowles DM (1999) Immunodeficiency-associated lymphoproliferative disorders. Mod Pathol 12:200–217

LeBoit PE, Berger TG, Egbert BM, et al. Bacillary angiomatosis. The histopathology and differential diagnosis of a pseudoneoplastic infection in patients with human immunodeficiency virus disease. Am J Surg Pathol 1989; 13:909–920

Lesens O, Deschenes M, Steben M, et al. (1999) Hepatitis C virus is related to progressive liver disease in HIV+ve haemophiliacs and should be treated as an opportunistic infection. J Infect Dis 179:1254–1258

Levine AM (1991) Epidemiology, clinical characteristics, and management of AIDS-related lymphoma. Hematol Oncol Clin North Am 5:331–342

Levine AM (1992) AIDS-associated malignant lymphoma. Med Clin North Am 76:253–268

Lucas SB (1995) Tropical pathology of the female genital tract and ovaries. In: Fox H (ed) Haines and Taylor obstetrical and gynaecological pathology. Churchill Livingstone, Edinburgh, pp 1209–1231

Lucas SB, Hounnou A, Paecock CS, et al. (1993) The mortality and pathology of HIV disease in a West African city. AIDS 7:1569–1579

Lucas SB, Peacock CS, Hounnou A, et al. (1996) Disease in children infected with HIV in Abidjan, Côte d'Ivoire. Br Med J 312:335–338

Luxton JC, Thomas JA, Crawford DH (1991) Aetiology and pathogenesis of non-Hodgkin lymphoma in AIDS. Cancer Surv 10:103–109

Lyon R, Haque AK, Asmuth DM, et al. (1996) Changing patterns of infection in patients with AIDS: a study of 279 autopsies of prison inmates and nonincarcerated patients at a University Hospital in Eastern Texas, 1984–1993. Clin Infect Dis 23:241–247

McKenna RJ, Campbell A, McMurtrey MJ, et al. (1986) Diagnosis of interstitial lung disease in patients with acquired immunodeficiency syndrome (AIDS): a prospective comparison of bronchial washing, alveolar lavage, transbronchial lung biopsy and open-lung biopsy. Ann Thorac Surg 41:318–321

Nair R, Abdool-Carrim ACR, Robbs J (1999) Arterial aneurysms in patients with HIV: a distinct clinicopathological entity? J Vasc Surg 29:600–607

Öst A, Baroni CD, Biberfeld P, et al. (1989) Lymphadenopathy in HIV-infection: histological classification and staging. Acta Pathol Microbiol Immunol Scand Suppl 8:7–15

Palca J (1992) Kaposi's sarcoma gives on key fronts. Science 225:1352–1355

Paxton LA, Janssen RS (2000) The epidemiology of HIV infection in the era of HAART. J HIV Ther 5:2–4

Pellicelli AM, Palmieri F, D'Ambrosio C, et al. (1998) Role of HIV in primary pulmonary hypertension – case reports. Angiology 49:1005–1011

Race EM, Adelson-Mitty J, Barlam TF, et al. (1998) Focal mycobacterial lymphadenitis following initiation of protease-inhibitor therapy in patients with advanced HIV-1 disease. Lancet 351:252–255

Radin DR, Baker EL, Klatt EC, et al. (1990) Visceral and nodal calcification in patients with AIDS-related *Pneumocystis carinii* infection. AJR 154:27–31

Rivers JK, Kopf AW, Postell AH (1989) Malignant melanoma in a man seropositive for the human immunodeficiency virus. J Am Acad Dermatol 20:1127–1128

Rosenthal D, LeBoit PE, Klumpp L, Berger TG. Human immunodeficiency virus-associated eosinophilic folliculitis. Arch Dermatol 1991; 127:206–209

Roth WK, Brandsetter H, Sturzl M (1992) Cellular and molecular features of HIV-associated Kaposi's sarcoma. AIDS 6:895–913

Schwartz DA, Sobottka I, Leitch GJ, et al. (1996) Pathology of microsporidiosis. Arch Pathol Lab Med 120:173–188

Sun NCJ, Shapshak P, Lachant NA, et al. (1989) Bone marrow examination in patients with AIDS and AIDS-related complex. Am J Clin Pathol 92:589–594

Tappero JW, Conant MA, Wolfe SF, et al. (1993) Kaposi's sarcoma. Epidemiology, pathogenesis, histology, clinical spectrum, staging criteria and therapy. J Am Acad Dermatol 72:245–261

Tschirhart DL, Klatt EC (1988) Disseminated toxoplasmosis in the acquired immunodeficiency syndrome. Arch Pathol Lab Med 112:1237–1241

Waddell KM, Lewallen S, Lucas SB, et al. (1996) Carcinoma of the conjunctiva and HIV infection in Uganda and Malawi. Br J Opthalmol 80:503–508

5 CNS Manifestations of AIDS

Michelle L. Hansman Whiteman and Alan J. Holz

CONTENTS

5.1 Introduction

The World Health Organization estimates that nearly 40 million individuals are currently infected with human immunodeficiency virus (HIV). AIDS has emerged as a leading cause of death in portions of the developed and developing worlds (MERTENS and LOW-BEER 1996). Neurologic dysfunction is a frequent sequela of HIV infection. An estimated 31%–63% of AIDS patients will develop clinical neurologic complications (BERGER et al. 1987b; BRITTON and MILLER 1984; LEVY et al. 1985) and autopsy series have demonstrated CNS involvement in 73%–87% of cases (LEVY et al. 1985; JORDAN et al. 1985). In 10%–20% of AIDS patients, CNS symptomatology is the initial manifestation of HIV-related disease (BERGER et al. 1987b; LEVY et al. 1985).

It is thus clear that imaging of the CNS is of critical importance in the care of these patients. The most frequent signs and symptoms of neurologic disorder in AIDS patients include headache, encephalopathy, seizures, ataxia, and focal motor or sensory deficit. These signs and symptoms are nonspecific, however, in determining a definitive diagnosis. Neuroimaging is therefore essential to the diagnosis and management of CNS disorders in patients with HIV infection.

The imaging modalities most commonly used to document CNS pathology are computed tomography (CT) and magnetic resonance (MR) imaging. Many of these studies employ the use of contrast agents, as a number of infectious and neoplastic diseases will show enhancement. The CT study remains a good screening examination, especially in the detection of mass effect or hydrocephalus. MR imaging, with its greater resolution and multiplanar capability, is better for detection of subtle pathology and meningeal disease and is much more accurate than CT in the depiction of white matter abnormalities. A technique which can increase the conspicuity of lesions on CT is the double-dose delayed study (DDD). A double dose of contrast (78 g iodinated contrast via bolus/drip infusion) is administered with a 1-h interval before scanning (POST et al. 1985). The DDD studies enable visualization of a greater number of lesions as compared to a single-dose contrast CT. In addition, the lesions often show a greater degree of enhancement and larger size on the DDD examinations (POST et al. 1985) compared with routine contrast studies.

In addition to CT and MR imaging, MR angiography (MRA) can be helpful in evaluation of vascular disease and diffusion MR imaging can be used to evaluate acute infarction. Conventional angiography is rarely required. Nuclear medicine studies can also provide useful information in defining mass lesions. Thallium-201 (^{201}Tl) brain single-photon emission computed tomography (SPECT) can be used to differentiate a high-grade tumor from an inflammatory process and is therefore commonly used to differentiate suspected toxoplasmosis from CNS lymphoma. MR spectroscopy, a modality still under investigation, may hold the key to providing a more specific diagnosis, and preliminary results have been promising.

M.L. HANSMAN WHITEMAN, MD; A.J. HOLZ, MD
Department of Radiology, University of Miami School of Medicine, 1115 NW 14th Street, Miami, FL 33136, USA

Both clinical and pathologic series have studied the range of neurologic disorders encountered in this population. One clinical study found that the most common neurologic disorders (in descending order) were *Toxoplasma* encephalitis, cryptococcal meningitis, subacute encephalitis, peripheral neuropathy, and cytomegalovirus (CMV) retinitis. Less commonly encountered were metabolic encephalopathy, progressive multifocal leukoencephalopathy (PML), myopathy, CNS lymphoma, and tuberculous meningitis (BERGER et al. 1987b). In contrast, autopsy series have found the most common pathologic entities to include (in descending order) vacuolar myelopathy, subacute encephalitis, CMV encephalitis, *Toxoplasma* encephalitis, and CNS lymphoma, with cryptococcal meningitis, PML, varicella-zoster encephalitis, and herpes simplex ventriculitis somewhat less frequent (PETITO 1988; PETITO et al. 1986).

The ensuing pages address the most commonly encountered CNS manifestations associated with HIV infection, with a descriptive analysis of the radiographic appearance of these disorders using a variety of neuroimaging techniques. Both cerebral and spinal cord pathology will be discussed.

5.2
Infection

5.2.1
Viral Disease

5.2.1.1
HIV Infection

In the absence of superimposed infection or neoplasm, HIV infection has been implicated as a direct cause of encephalopathy, myelopathy, peripheral neuropathy, and myopathy (BAILEY et al. 1988; LEVY et al. 1985; PETITO 1988). Within the brain, macrophages and multinucleated giant cells appear to be the primary targets of infection by HIV and are closely related to the progressive encephalopathy seen in AIDS patients (GABUZDA et al. 1986; GARTNER et al. 1986). Polymorphic microglia are also frequently infected.

The most common CNS disorder seen in AIDS patients is subacute encephalitis (LEVY et al. 1985; NIELSEN et al. 1984). This is present in 28% of adult AIDS autopsies (PETITO et al. 1986). The clinical presentation includes progressive dementia with motor and/or behavioral dysfunction (NAVIA et al. 1986a).

Difficulty with concentration and memory is often followed by apparent apathy and social withdrawal (Ho et al. 1989). Headache is also a common complaint. The pathologic correlate of HIV encephalopathy appears to be myelin pallor in association with HIV-infected multinucleated giant cells (POST et al. 1988a), microglial nodules, gliosis, and vacuolar degeneration (Ho et al. 1985). These multinucleated giant cells contain retrovirus particles on electron microscopy and their presence strongly correlates with the AIDS dementia complex (ADC) (NAVIA et al. 1986b). The multinucleated giant cells may be scattered within the cortex, basal ganglia, and white matter (EPSTEIN et al. 1985; PETITO 1988). Diffuse atrophy is usually present. Lesions are present initially within the white matter, and with progression of disease there is involvement of the basal ganglia and cortex as well.

HIV infection may also directly cause an acute encephalitis (CARNE et al. 1985) and acute or chronic meningitis (BERGER et al. 1987b; Ho et al. 1985). This viral meningitis usually presents with headache, fever, and meningeal signs. Imaging studies are usually negative (LEVY et al. 1984, 1985).

In general, the clinical diagnosis of HIV encephalitis significantly antedates conventional radiographic evidence of disease (OLSEN et al. 1988; POST et al. 1988b). CT may be negative or will often reveal only atrophy. White matter lesions are less frequently seen on CT (LEVY et al. 1985, 1986).

The effects of cerebral HIV infection are certainly more evident on MR imaging than on CT. Atrophy is the most common finding and can be seen to progress on serial MR studies (POST et al. 1988b; CHRYSIKOPOULOUS et al. 1990). Hyperintense lesions without mass effect are seen in the periventricular white matter and centrum semiovale on T2-weighted and FLAIR (fast-fluid attenuated inversion-recovery) images and correspond to foci of demyelination and vacuolation (BOWEN and POST 1991) (Fig. 5.1). Lesions vary from scattered, isolated, unilateral foci to large, confluent bilateral involvement (BOWEN and POST 1991). These lesions are far less conspicuous on T1-weighted images (usually inapparent) than are the lesions of PML, which are often quite hypointense and well demarcated on T1-weighted images (WHITEMAN et al. 1993a). This is often a helpful differentiating feature. The lesions of HIV demyelination, in general, tend to be somewhat more symmetric than those of PML. These areas of abnormal hyperintensity on T2-weighted images do not enhance on corresponding postcontrast T1-weighted images.

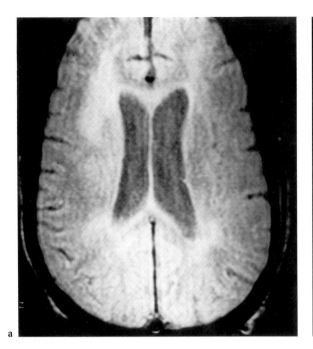
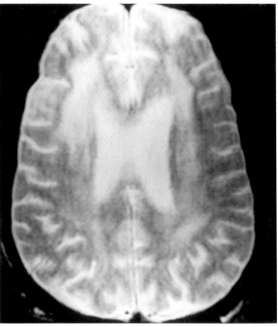

a   b

Fig. 5.1a, b. HIV encephalitis. Proton density (**a**) and T2-weighted (**b**) MR images from a patient with pathologically proven HIV encephalitis demonstrate confluent areas of signal abnormality throughout the periventricular white matter. There is also extension to the subcortical white matter, particularly in the right frontal region. Ex vacuo ventricular enlargement is indicative of associated atrophy in this 43-year-old patient. The white matter lesions were inapparent on T1-weighted images and did not enhance after gadolinium administration

A multicenter AIDS cohort study revealed sulcal prominence and scattered signal abnormalities within the white matter on T2-weighted images in 63% of asymptomatic HIV-seropositive homosexual men compared with 48% of seronegative homosexual men (McArthur et al. 1989). In another study, MR imaging was abnormal in about 50% of patients with AIDS-related complex and 69% of patients with AIDS (Grant et al. 1987). These abnormalities included atrophy as well as white matter disease. Patchy areas of T2 signal hyperintensity became more diffuse, confluent, and homogeneous with clinical progression from subtle cognitive deficits to gross dementia (Grant et al. 1987). Zidovudine therapy has shown partial reduction of HIV-related white matter disease on serial MR studies, with associated improvement in cognitive function (Olsen et al. 1988).

Patients who are HIV seropositive but asymptomatic will most often have negative imaging studies or only minor abnormalities. Initial and repeat MR studies were obtained at 2–4 years on asymptomatic seropositive patients (Post et al. 1993). Eighty percent were normal and remained normal while 20% had minor abnormalities which were static and stable (Post et al. 1993). Another study confirmed that abnormal MR results were only seen in a minority of

asymptomatic HIV-seropositive patients (approximately 13%) whereas 46% of those who were symptomatic had abnormal studies (Post et al. 1992). Increasing cerebral atrophy and white matter disease paralleled the development of clinical neurologic dysfunction (Post et al. 1992).

A number of advanced neuroimaging techniques have also been used to evaluate the effects of HIV infection on the CNS. It is apparent that functional abnormalities can be detected before structural or even behavioral changes are observed. These functional abnormalities are often multifocal, and subcortical structures, such as the basal ganglia, are frequently affected in the early stages of infection (Navia and Gonzalez 1997). Nuclear imaging studies may suggest the presence of cerebral dysfunction prior to the development of any changes on CT or MR imaging. Iodine-123 iodoamphetamine SPECT of patients with ADC has shown multiple focal cortical perfusion abnormalities to be present prior to any evidence of disease on CT or MR imaging (Pohl et al. 1988; Yudd et al. 1987). Technetium-99m hexamethylpropylene amine oxime has also shown regional abnormalities of cerebral blood flow in patients with ADC, and several of these patients also had normal imaging studies (Tatsch et al. 1990).

Fluorodeoxyglucose positron emission tomography (FDG-PET) has shown alterations in cerebral glucose metabolism in patients with HIV infection (NAVIA et al. 1985). A general decrease in cortical metabolism was associated with progressive ADC. Other investigators have found a relative subcortical hypermetabolism during the early stages of cognitive impairment whereas cortical and subcortical hypometabolism were characteristic of patients in the later stages of disease (ROTTENBERG et al. 1987). FDG-PET abnormalities were significantly correlated with cerebral atrophy and ADC stage (ROTTENBERG et al. 1996). The decrease in cerebral metabolism seen in association with ADC has been shown to be reversible in response to zidovudine (BRUNETTI et al. 1989; YARCHOAN et al. 1987).

MR spectroscopy provides an in vivo biochemical assessment of intracranial pathology. To obtain this information, a conventional MR scan is acquired to localize the region of interest, and a voxel is placed in this location. Prior to acquisition of the MR signal from the voxel, the local magnetic field has to be adjusted (shimmed). In addition, the signal from water must be suppressed since it is approximately 10,000 times greater than the signal from any of the metabolites (CHANG and ERNST 1997). The MR signal from the voxel is then converted, via Fourier transformation, into a spectrum based upon the differential resonance frequencies of the nuclei in different metabolites (CHANG and ERNST 1997).

As with conventional MR imaging, MR spectroscopy can be obtained at different echo times (TE). At short TE, the spectroscopy signals are less attenuated by T2 decay and J-coupling, enabling visualization of multiple metabolites. Signals from lipids, glutamate, glutamine, and myo-inositol can typically be seen only at short TE (CHANG and ERNST 1997). With a long TE, the proton spectrum shows fewer overlapping metabolite peaks than are seen with a short TE. For example, signals from lactate and lipids overlap at short TE, whereas with a long TE the lipid signal is greatly attenuated, allowing clear observation of the lactate signal (CHANG and ERNST 1997).

Typical MR spectra can be obtained in 15–20 min (WEBB et al. 1994). The common metabolite peaks observed from a normal brain include *N*-acetyl aspartate (NAA), a neuronal marker that resonates at 2.02 ppm (parts per million), glutamate, glutamine, total creatine (Cr) at 3.0 ppm, choline compounds (Cho) at 3.2 ppm and myo-inositol, a possible marker of glial cell proliferation which resonates at 3.56 ppm (CHANG and ERNST 1997). Excess lactate (at 1.3 ppm) and lipids (1.0–2.5 ppm) are evident only in pathologic states.

There is an emerging body of information regarding proton spectroscopy in AIDS patients. One study compared the cerebral proton spectra from 103 HIV-positive patients with those from a control group (CHONG et al. 1993). Reduced NAA/Cho and NAA/Cr ratios were seen in patients from the study group who had neurologic impairment. NAA is a neuronal marker and thus the reduced ratios suggest that neuronal loss or dysfunction may play a role in ADC. The reduced ratios correlated with the presence of diffuse disease on MR imaging but not with focal lesions (CHONG et al. 1993). Of the 103 HIV-seropositive patients, 11 had normal MR imaging with abnormal spectroscopy and 22 had normal spectra but abnormal MR imaging. Thus, the information provided by these techniques appears to be complementary.

In a subset of 25 HIV-positive patients with normal MR studies who underwent clinical neurologic evaluation, the NAA/Cr was 16% lower in patients with an abnormal neurologic examination. Thus, spectroscopy seemed to indicate subtle biochemical alterations in patients with clinical evidence of neurologic disease (CHONG et al. 1993) that were inapparent on MR imaging.

Other authors have confirmed that changes in NAA can be identified in areas that appear normal on conventional MR imaging studies, suggesting that neuronal loss or damage precedes detectable atrophy (JARVIK et al. 1993; MENON et al. 1990; MEYERHOFF et al. 1993). Other investigators have also encountered reductions in NAA with the NAA/Cr ratio decreased by approximately 20% in AIDS patients as compared with age-matched controls (PALEY et al. 1995). Improvement in NAA has been reported in two patients with progressive ADC in response to treatment with zidovudine (VION-DURY et al. 1995). Thus, some of the spectroscopic abnormalities appear to be reversible.

In addition to the drop in NAA levels seen with advancing dementia, there is also an increase in the Cho/Cr ratio which is seen earlier in the course of cerebral HIV infection (TRACEY et al. 1996). Elevations in myo-inositol have also been seen in the early stages of CNS infection with HIV (NAVIA and GONZALEZ 1997). These changes most often involve the white matter or deep gray structures.

5.2.1.2
Pediatric HIV

It is estimated that 1,500–2,000 HIV-infected infants are born each year in the United States and that there are 15,000–20,000 HIV-infected infants and children presently in the United States (GWINN et al. 1991). More than 90% of pediatric AIDS cases are a result of congenital infection via maternal-infant transmission (vertical acquisition) (Centers for Disease Control and Prevention 1996). Maternal-infant transmission occurs in utero, intrapartum, or postpartum via breast-feeding. A 25% rate of mother to infant infection has been estimated (BOYER et al. 1994; JANSSEN 1996). Maternal factors associated with an increased risk of transmission include low CD4 counts, high viral titers, advanced HIV disease, premature rupture of membranes, increased exposure of infant to maternal blood, premature delivery, and low vitamin A (ABRAMS et al. 1995; BOYER et al. 1994). Perinatal transmission can be reduced significantly by treating HIV-infected pregnant mothers with zidovudine (CONNOR et al. 1994). About 23% of HIV-infected infants develop AIDS by age 1 year and 40% by the age of 4 years (European Collaborative Study 1994).

Pediatric HIV infection may result in a progressive encephalopathy with loss of motor milestones, intellectual ability, and the development of weakness and pyramidal tract signs (BELMAN et al. 1984; EPSTEIN et al. 1985). While neurologic dysfunction in adult AIDS patients is often a result of an opportunistic infection, the primary manifestation of neurologic dysfunction in pediatric AIDS patients is encephalopathy. The encephalopathy may present as an unrelenting progressive encephalopathy, as a progressive encephalopathy with intervening plateau periods, or as a static encephalopathy (CIVITELLO 1993; TAM et al. 1995). Children with progressive encephalopathy usually become symptomatic in the first 2–3 years of life, often associated with severe immunodeficiency. The progressive encephalopathy, also known as HIV-1-associated progressive encephalopathy, is estimated to occur in 23%–50% of HIV-infected children (LOBATO et al. 1995; EPSTEIN et al. 1988). Other manifestations include microcephaly, movement disorders, spasticity, seizures, and ataxia. Mood and behavioral problems are common (BELMAN 1990; BELMAN et al. 1988). This pediatric subacute encephalitis is most likely a direct result of the HIV infection (SHARER et al. 1985). Histopathological examination reveals large multinucleated giant cells infected with HIV, along with inflammatory cell infiltrates, microglial nodules, and extensive calcific vasculopathy, primarily involving small vessels of the basal ganglia, but also seen in the pons and cerebral white matter (BELMAN et al. 1985; SHARER et al. 1985). During the acute phase of HIV infection, there may be damage to the walls of small and medium-sized arteries with calcium deposition in the arterial walls and adjacent brain (BELMAN et al. 1985; SHARER et al. 1985). Diminished brain volume is probably due to myelin loss or reduced myelination as neuronal loss is uncommon (SZE et al. 1987).

CT scans of these children most often show progressive atrophy and ventricular enlargement (BELMAN et al. 1985). White matter hypodensity is infrequent. Calcification is often present in the basal ganglia, bilaterally, and may also be seen in the white matter of the frontal lobes (BELMAN et al. 1985; EPSTEIN et al. 1988) (Fig. 5.2). The calcifications are related to the underlying calcific vasculopathy which is common in pediatric AIDS patients but is not seen in adult AIDS patients (STATES et al. 1997). Enhancement within the basal ganglia has also been reported (EPSTEIN et al. 1988). Patchy white matter disease which becomes more confluent as it progresses may be seen on MR studies in conjunction with progression of dementia. As with CT, serial MR studies reveal progressive atrophy. The basal ganglia calcification may appear as hypointense signal on MR

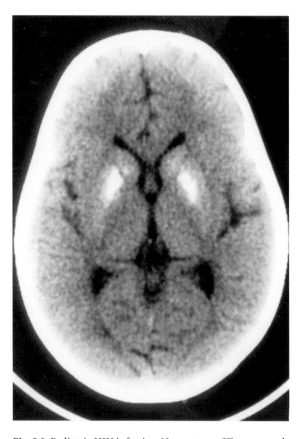

Fig. 5.2. Pediatric HIV infection. Noncontrast CT scan reveals bilateral basal ganglia calcification in this HIV-infected child. Mild, diffuse atrophy is also noted

imaging. T2 signal abnormalities (hyperintensity) may be seen in the basal ganglia on MR imaging while CT is negative (BELMAN 1997). The extent of cerebral atrophy appears to correlate well with the severity of encephalopathy, cognitive dysfunction, and behavioral changes. White matter disease and atrophy are seen more frequently in children with clinical evidence of HIV-associated progressive encephalopathy than in those who are HIV positive but neurologically intact (BELMAN et al. 1985, 1988). Serial studies obtained after treatment with antiretroviral therapy can show a reversal of atrophy in association with clinical improvement (MINTZ and EPSTEIN 1992).

FDG-PET studies of infected children have shown diffuse as well as more focal hypometabolism, with subcortical hypermetabolism also seen in those children with progressive encephalopathy (DEPAS et al. 1995; PIZZO and WILFERT 1994).

MR spectroscopy has shown decreased NAA/Cr ratios in subcortical structures of pediatric AIDS patients, with a greater decrease in those children with AIDS encephalopathy (LU et al. 1996; PAVLAKIS et al. 1995).

Although toxoplasmosis, PML, CMV, and *Candida albicans* have all been reported in the pediatric HIV population (DICKSON et al. 1989; BELMAN et al. 1984), opportunistic infections of the CNS are far less common than in adults (BELMAN et al. 1984). Approximately 15% of the imaging studies performed on pediatric AIDS patients reveal a focal abnormality related to opportunistic infection or CNS lymphoma (EPSTEIN et al. 1988; PETITO 1988). Primary CNS lymphoma is the most common intracerebral mass lesion in children with AIDS (BELMAN et al. 1988), being seen in up to 4% of cases (STATES et al. 1997). As in the adult cases of primary CNS lymphoma, there is solid or more often heterogeneous or peripheral enhancement due to central necrosis. Lesions are often multicentric and there may be subependymal spread or involvement of the corpus callosum.

Cerebrovascular disease is also seen in the pediatric AIDS population. An HIV-related arteriopathy may be seen with fusiform dilatation of the circle of Willis. This arteriomegaly may be seen as an incidental finding, or may be found in association with ischemia or hemorrhage (SHAH and ZIMMERMAN 1996). The ectatic vessels are well demonstrated on contrast CT studies and appear as prominent signal voids on T2-weighted MR images. MR angiography is also useful in evaluation of these patients (Fig. 5.3). Histopathologic examination of the vessels reveals a diffuse vasculitis with infected mononuclear cells throughout the arterial wall, destruction of the elastic lamina, and subintimal fibrosis (SHAH and ZIMMERMAN 1996).

Fibrosing sclerosis is an inflammatory, fibrosing vasculopathy which has also been seen in HIV-infected children (STATES et al. 1997) and is thought to be a direct result of primary HIV CNS infection. Ischemic infarction is seen in the basal ganglia or frontal lobes, and MR angiography may reveal focal areas of vascular stenosis or occlusion (STATES et al. 1997). Histopathologic studies reveal luminal obliteration or stenosis with endothelial proliferation, damage to the elastic lamina, medial thickening, and inflammation of both the media and the adventitia (JOSHI et al. 1987; SHAH and ZIMMERMAN 1996).

5.2.1.3
Cytomegalovirus

Cytomegalovirus is a frequent pathogen in the AIDS population, not only within the CNS, but throughout the body. CMV more commonly presents outside the CNS, involving the respiratory tract, liver, gastrointestinal tract, genitourinary tract, or hematopoietic system (POST et al. 1988a). Nearly 90% of adults have antibodies to CMV and the virus exists in a latent form in the vast majority of the population (LEESTMA 1985). Reactivation usually results in a subclinical or mild infection mimicking mononucleosis (BOYD 1980). In a minority of immunocompromised patients, however, reactivation can result in disseminated infection, necrotizing meningoencephalitis, and/or ependymitis (POST et al. 1986a; BRITTON and MILLER 1984). Neurologic manifestations of CMV also include cranial neuropathy, retinitis, myelitis, polyradiculopathy, and mononeuritis multiplex (McCUTCHEN 1995). CMV retinitis affects 20%–40% of patients with AIDS (DANNER 1995; JABS 1995).

Approximately 15%–30% of adult AIDS autopsies reveal CMV within the CNS (BALE 1984; NAVIA et al. 1986b). CMV may coexist with other lesions, and thus may be clinically silent (POST et al. 1986a). The pathologic hallmark of CMV is the "owl's eye," an enlarged cell with a distended nucleus containing eosinophilic viral inclusions and surrounded by a halo, resulting in the characteristic appearance (POST et al. 1986a). CMV most often involves the ependyma, but rarely can cause extensive destruction of gray and white matter (POST et al. 1988a). CMV intranuclear inclusions are also found in the spinal cord, spinal nerves, and retina (POST et al. 1986a).

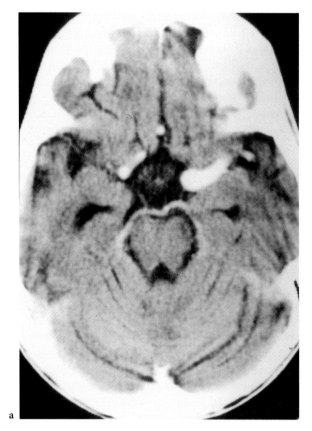

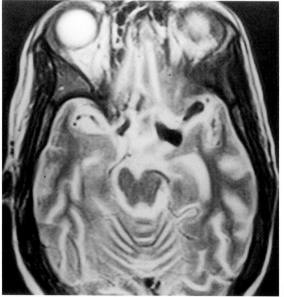

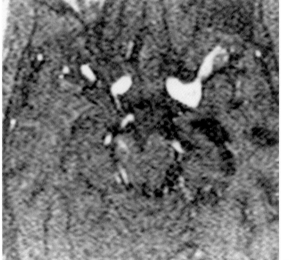

Fig. 5.3a–c. Pediatric HIV-related arteriomegaly. a Contrast-enhanced CT study reveals diffuse enlargement of the left middle cerebral artery. b T2-weighted image from a different child demonstrates enlargement of the M1 and M2 segments of the left middle cerebral artery with a prominent flow void. Note also parenchymal atrophy. c 3D time of flight MRA (same patient as in b) again reveals ectasia and enlargement of the left middle cerebral artery. The right middle cerebral artery is also affected, but to a lesser degree

CMV meningoencephalitis may be seen in patients with HIV infection, as well as in immunocompetent adults, and the disease may be subclinical (NAVIA et al. 1986b; BALE 1984). Less often, symptoms develop over days to months with fever, altered mental status, confusion, memory loss, and progressive dementia (POST et al. 1986a). This is most commonly seen in transplant patients (SCHNECK 1965) and AIDS patients. In some cases there is diffuse brain involvement, not simply limited to the subependymal regions (LEESTMA 1985; LEVY et al. 1984). CSF evaluation and complement fixation blood titers are nonspecific, and thus the clinical diagnosis can be difficult (BRITTON and MILLER 1984).

CT is often insensitive in the imaging of CMV encephalitis (POST et al. 1986). Atrophy is the most frequent finding, and rarely, white matter hypodensity may be present (BRITTON and MILLER 1984; LEVY et al. 1984). Periventricular and subependymal enhancement may also be seen occasionally on CT, especially with the DDD technique (POST et al. 1988a; RAMSEY and GEREMIA 1988).

CMV infection of the CNS is better delineated with MR imaging (POST et al. 1986). In addition to atrophy, increased signal may be present in the periventricular white matter on T2-weighted images (RAMSEY and GEREMIA 1988). Less often, subependymal enhancement may be seen (Fig. 5.4), providing a valuable diagnostic clue (POST et al. 1986a). Fat-suppressed MR im-

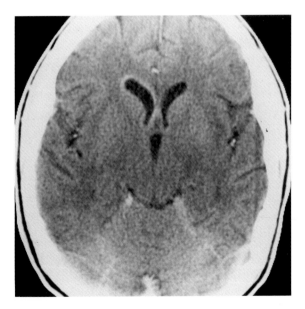

Fig. 5.4. CMV infection, confirmed by polymerase chain reaction (PCR). Contrast-enhanced axial CT demonstrates thin periventricular enhancement surrounding the right frontal horn. CSF was PCR positive for CMV

aging with gadolinium may reveal a thickened and enhancing choroid/retina in patients with CMV retinitis (TIEN et al. 1991b), which is a hemorrhagic retinitis frequently seen in AIDS patients.

5.2.1.4
Herpes Simplex Virus

In patients with AIDS, CNS infection with herpes simplex virus (HSV-1 and HSV-2) has been reported (JORDAN and ENZMANN 1991; POST et al. 1988a) but is infrequent, occurring in only 2% of AIDS autopsy cases (PETITO et al. 1986). In the general population, HSV-1 infection can result in a necrotizing encephalitis, most often affecting the temporal and frontal lobes. In the AIDS population, however, HSV infection more often results in diffuse involvement rather than the temporal/frontal predilection which is seen in immunocompetent hosts (JORDAN and ENZMANN 1991). Both mild and severe forms of encephalitis have been reported and may coexist with other infections (LEVY et al. 1985, 1986). In adults, this usually is a result of viral reactivation. CSF findings are nonspecific, and HSV is rarely cultured. Polymerase chain reaction (PCR), a DNA amplification technique, may be more helpful in establishing a diagnosis (ROWLEY et al. 1990). On MR imaging, areas of involvement demonstrate low signal on T1-weighted images and hyperintensity on T2-weighted images.

Hemorrhage may be seen, appearing as foci of increased signal on the T1-weighted images (LIZERBRAM and HESSELINK 1997). HSV-1 in AIDS patients may involve the brainstem and cerebellum, which are not usually involved in patients who are immunocompetent (HAMILTON et al. 1995). Postcontrast images reveal variable gyriform enhancement (LIZERBRAM and HESSELINK 1997). SPECT imaging can reveal increased perfusion of involved areas of the brain, even when CT and MR studies are negative (MASDEU et al. 1995). Treatment is with intravenous acyclovir or vidarabine.

5.2.1.5
Varicella-Zoster Virus

Varicella-zoster virus (VZV) is the cause of two distinct clinical entities, varicella (chicken pox) and herpes zoster infection (shingles) (TIEN et al. 1993). Both result in similar histopathological changes in the skin (WHITLEY and SCHLITT 1991). CNS infection can be seen in both syndromes and can result in hemorrhagic necrosis with intranuclear inclusions (WHITLEY and SCHLITT 1991). Varicella-zoster encephalitis is seen in about 2% of AIDS autopsies on neuropathological examination (PETITO et al. 1986). Complications of zoster infection include encephalitis, neuritis, myelitis, and/or herpes ophthalmicus (TIEN et al. 1993). Although these complications rarely follow a course of shingles in immunocompetent adult patients, there is an increased risk of CNS involvement in patients who are immunocompromised (TIEN et al. 1993). While cranial and peripheral nerve palsies are the most common neurologic disorders associated with zoster infection in healthy patients, diffuse encephalitis is the most frequent CNS complication seen in the immunosuppressed (REICHMAN 1978) (Fig. 5.5). Latent virus residing in the ganglia of cranial nerves (especially V and VII) can reactivate and, with retrograde extension, traverse the brainstem and incite an encephalitis. Fever, meningism, and altered mental status in a patient with shingles suggests the diagnosis (TIEN et al. 1993). CT may be negative (DAVIDSON and STEINER 1985), while MR imaging may reveal signal abnormalities within the brainstem and/or cortical gray matter (TIEN et al. 1993).

5.2.1.6
Progressive Multifocal Leukoencephalopathy

Progressive multifocal leukoencephalopathy (PML) is a progressive demyelinating disease resulting from CNS infection with a papovavirus. The causative

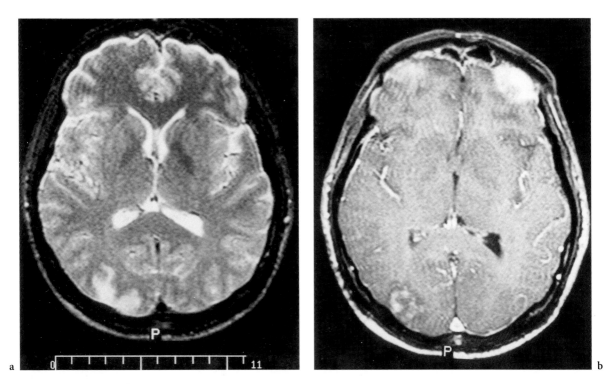

Fig. 5.5a, b. Varicella-zoster encephalitis (autopsy proven). **a** T2-weighted axial image reveals abnormal signal involving the cortex and subcortical region of the right occipital lobe. There is only slight mass effect. **b** Postgadolinium T1-weighted axial MR image reveals patchy enhancement in the right occipital lobe. CSF cultures were nondiagnostic. A biopsy was performed but only revealed necrosis and inflammation. The patient's clinical condition deteriorated rapidly. Postmortem examination revealed herpes zoster encephalitis, with multiple areas of parenchymal necrosis, including the right occipital lobe

agent is the JC virus, which belongs to the papova family of CNS viruses (papilloma, polyoma, vacuolating virus) (RICHARDSON 1988). PML was initially described by Astrom et al. in 1958 (BROOKS and WALKER 1984). Electron microscopy later revealed innumerable virus-like particles within inclusion bodies of oligodendrocytic nuclei (SILVERMAN and RUBINSTEIN 1965). In 1971, the virus was isolated from the postmortem brain of a patient with PML by using this tissue as a source of inoculum in cell cultures (PADGET et al. 1971). The initials of this donor patient were JC, and the virus was thus termed the JC virus. The target of this virus is the oligodendrocyte which forms and maintains the myelin sheath (POST et al. 1986b). Infection of the oligodendrocyte causes cytolytic destruction and results in myelin loss (MAJOR et al. 1992). Intranuclear inclusions consisting of JC virus particles (MAZLO and TARISKA 1980) and enlarged, multinucleated astrocytes are consistent features of PML. Over time, microscopic foci of scattered demyelination enlarge and coalesce (MAJOR et al. 1992). Gross inspection of the brain reveals a gray or brownish discoloration of the white matter as a result of extensive myelin loss.

Antibodies to the JC virus are nearly ubiquitous among the adult population worldwide (WALKER 1985). The virus appears to infect approximately 80% of the human population before adulthood without producing overt illness (GREENFIELD 1984). The virus typically remains latent unless there is reactivation due to immunodeficiency (WALKER 1985). Prior to the era of AIDS, PML was seen in association with other immunodeficiencies, such as renal transplantation, autoimmune disease, sarcoidosis, tuberculosis, Whipple's disease, and lymphoproliferative disorders (BROOKS and WALKER 1984). Patients on chemotherapy are also at increased risk for PML. Currently, 55%–85% of PML cases are seen in AIDS patients (BERGER et al. 1987a; KRUPP et al. 1985), and PML may have a stronger association with AIDS than with any other immunosuppressive disorder (STONER et al. 1986). PML is present in about 5% of patients with AIDS at autopsy (WHITEMAN et al. 1993a).

The clinical presentation of PML includes memory loss, personality change, visual deficits, altered mental status, and cognitive and speech disturbances, as well as motor and sensory abnormalities (BROOKS and WALKER 1984). There is progressive neurologic declinc, with a mean survival of 4 months (BERGER et al. 1987). The most frequent symptoms of PML are hemiparesis, visual impairment, and altered mentation (BERGER et al. 1987a). Patients with posterior fossa involvement may exhibit ataxia, dysarthria, and dysmetria (JONES et al. 1982). PML may, in fact, be the initial manifestation of AIDS in up to 47% of patients who present with PML (WHITEMAN et al. 1993a). CSF studies are usually normal, although an elevated opening pressure or an increased CSF protein may be seen. Although the radiographic appearance is often quite characteristic, definitive diagnosis may require brain biopsy. Alternatively, detection of JC virus in CSF using PCR can provide diagnostic confirmation. There is currently no effective therapy for PML.

CT studies reveal focal white matter hypodensity without mass effect and usually without enhancement. Both periventricular and subcortical white matter may be affected. Patchy enhancement is seen on occasion. Serial studies demonstrate progressive disease.

MR imaging is much more sensitive than CT to the lesions of PML (Fig. 5.6) and is better able to define the extent and number of lesions present (WHITEMAN et al. 1993a). On T2-weighted images, hyperintense signal is seen in the periventricular and/or subcortical white matter. Lesions may be small initially but usually progress to larger areas of involvement (Fig. 5.7). The lesions are often multifocal and bilateral, but are asymmetric, and can be unilateral. There is no mass effect and lesions rarely enhance. If enhancement is

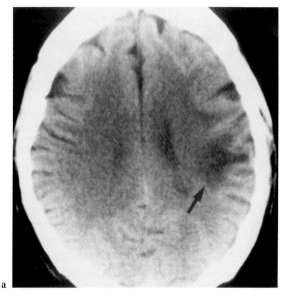

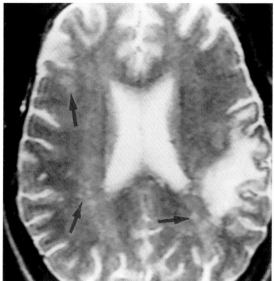

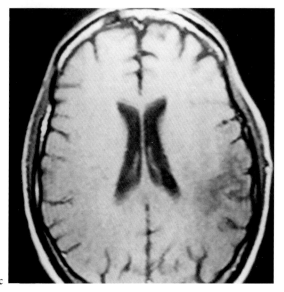

Fig. 5.6a–c. PML in an HIV-seropositive patient. a Noncontrast axial CT image reveals focal hypodensity without mass effect in the subcortical white matter (*arrow*). b T2-weighted axial MR image reveals a larger area of involvement, with hyperintense signal but without mass effect. The overlying cortex is spaced. Smaller foci of abnormal signal (*arrows*) may represent early involvement by PML or HIV encephalitis (same patient as in **a**). c T1-weighted axial MR image without contrast of the same patient reveals a fairly well defined area of hypointensity, compatible with PML. This is in contradistinction to HIV encephalitis, where the lesions are usually isointense and inapparent on T1-weighted images

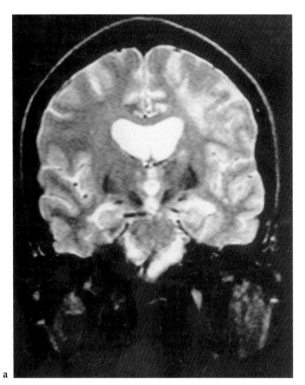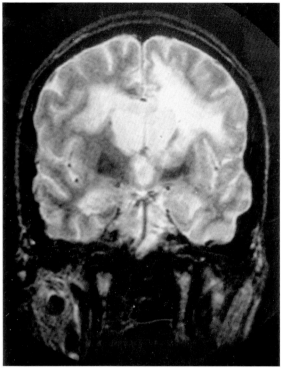

a   b

Fig. 5.7a, b. PML: progression of disease (pathologically proven). **a** Coronal T2-weighted MR image reveals subcortical involvement in the left parietal region without mass effect. There is also ex vacuo dilatation of the ventricles. **b** Same patient, 3 months later. There has been considerable progression of disease. T2 signal hyperintensity now involves the periventricular white matter, the internal capsule, and the corpus callosum, and there is extension into the right cerebral hemisphere as well. The subcortical involvement on the left is also more extensive

present, it is faint and peripheral (WHITEMAN et al. 1993a). The subcortical lesions of PML follow the gray-white interface, resulting in a "scalloped" appearance which is quite characteristic (Fig. 5.8). Any lobe may be affected by PML, but the frontal and parietal/occipital regions are those most commonly involved (WHITEMAN et al. 1993a). On T1-weighted images the lesions of PML are usually hypointense to the parenchyma and sharply circumscribed, which may help to differentiate these lesions from those of HIV encephalitis, which are isointense and less apparent on T1-weighted images.

PML can be seen to affect the deep gray structures; this is due to involvement of very small myelinated fibers that course through the basal ganglia and adjacent structures (WHITEMAN et al. 1993a). Involvement of the posterior fossa is seen in about one-third of PML cases (WHITEMAN et al. 1993a) (Fig. 5.9). Usually, there are concomitant supratentorial lesions but PML may be confined to the posterior fossa in approximately 10% of cases (SZE et al. 1987).

Radiographically, PML may be difficult to distinguish from HIV demyelination. In general, HIV demyelination is more diffuse, symmetric, and periventricular in location, whereas PML is more often asymmetric, multifocal, and subcortical in location. On T1-weighted images, PML is usually hypointense while HIV demyelination is isointense. Early in the course of disease, however, it may be very difficult to differentiate these two disorders. Both are bright on T2-weighted images. Clinical correlation is quite helpful, since the clinical picture usually associated with HIV demyelination is one of dementia and global dysfunction whereas PML will often present with focal neurologic deficits (WHITEMAN et al. 1993b).

MR spectroscopy has been used to evaluate the biochemical alterations present in PML. Using both STEAM (stimulated echo acquisition mode) and PRESS (point resolved spectroscopy) techniques (BOTTOMLEY 1987; FRAHM et al. 1987), studies have found a decreased NAA and Cr, an increased Cho, excess lactate and lipids, and an occasional increase in myo-inositol (CHANG et al. 1997). These findings seem to parallel the pathologic features of PML, with neuronal loss (decreased NAA), cell membrane and myelin breakdown (causing an increase in Cho), and

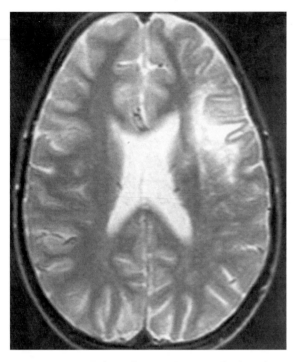

Fig. 5.8. PML (pathologically proven). T2-weighted axial MR image demonstrates the characteristic appearance of PML. There is focal, asymmetric signal hyperintensity present in the subcortical white matter without mass effect. Extension to the gray/white interface results in this "scalloped" appearance. There was no enhancement of the lesion after gadolinium administration

increased glial activity (causing increased myo-inositol). The rise in Cho and myo-inositol appears early in the course of the disease, and with disease progression there is progressive decrease in NAA (progressive neuronal loss) and eventual decrease in all the metabolites (CHANG et al. 1997).

5.2.2
Bacterial Disease

5.2.2.1
Syphilis

Between 1986 and 1989, the incidence of syphilis increased sharply in both men and women, largely as a consequence of AIDS (TIEN et al. 1992). Several studies have documented an increased incidence of positive serology for syphilis in HIV-positive patients compared with non-HIV-positive patients (KATZ et al. 1993). One study found that 44% of patients diagnosed with neurosyphilis over a 42-month period were also HIV seropositive (KATZ and BERGER 1989). The causative agent is *Treponema pallidum*, a spirochete.

Syphilis is a chronic infection with three well-characterized stages. Primary syphilis is indicated by a chancre (ulcer or sore) at the site of inoculation and regional adenopathy. The secondary form,

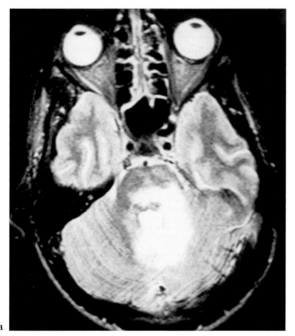

a

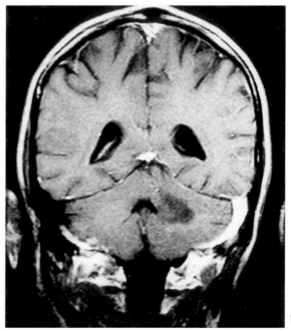

b

Fig. 5.9a, b. PML: infratentorial (biopsy proven). **a** There is extensive involvement of the brainstem and cerebellum, bilaterally, on this axial T2-weighted image. Abnormal hyperintense signal is seen without mass effect, and is greater on the left than on the right. **b** Postcontrast T1-weighted coronal image reveals marked hypointensity of the lesion on the left. There is no enhancement

which represents hematologic dissemination in those patients who go untreated, manifests as a maculopapular rash on the palms of the hands or soles of the feet. It is classically seen 2–8 weeks after appearance of the chancre; however, the progression from primary to secondary syphilis in AIDS patients often occurs much sooner, with a more rapid involvement of the CNS. About one-third of patients with secondary syphilis progress to tertiary syphilis and approximately one-third of these will develop neurosyphilis (KNOX et al. 1976). This disease progression is hastened in HIV-seropositive patients.

In those patients with AIDS, the course of neurosyphilis appears to be accelerated (KATZ et al. 1993) and the disease may be more aggressive (KATZ et al. 1993). One study of patients with neurosyphilis found those who were also HIV positive were younger and more likely to have features of secondary syphilis (rash, fever, adenopathy, headache, meningitis) compared to those who were HIV negative (KATZ et al. 1993). In the same study, the patients who were HIV positive were more likely to have syphilitic meningitis and an abnormal CSF compared to those with neurosyphilis who were HIV negative (KATZ et al. 1993).

Neurosyphilis can occur weeks to decades after initial syphilitic infection and may be seen in the secondary or tertiary stages (HARRIS et al. 1997). Neurosyphilis is most often asymptomatic. AIDS patients with neurosyphilis who become symptomatic most often present with hemiparesis and visual disturbance (KATZ and BERGER 1989) as well as fever, rash, weight loss, and headache (KATZ et al. 1993). A number of CSF studies can be obtained to confirm the diagnosis including Venereal Disease Research Laboratory (VDRL), PCR, and the intrathecal *Treponema pallidum* antibody (ITPA) index (HARRIS et al. 1997).

Symptomatic neurosyphilis may be meningovascular or parenchymatous and the parenchymatous manifestations include both general paresis and tabes dorsalis. In non-AIDS patients, the usual interval from initial infection with syphilis to symptom onset is 5–10 years for meningovascular syphilis, 20 years for general paresis, and 25–30 years for tabes dorsalis. This time course appears accelerated in HIV-positive patients (KATZ et al. 1993). AIDS patients with symptomatic neurosyphilis most commonly present with either acute syphilitic meningitis or meningovascular neurosyphilis (KATZ and BERGER 1989). Acute syphilitic meningitis may present with hydrocephalus, cranial neuropathy, and/or formation of gummas (TIEN et al. 1992), whereas meningovascular neurosyphilis is charac-

terized by headache and vascular disease resulting in focal neurologic deficit.

In meningovascular syphilis there is widespread meningeal thickening and perivascular lymphocytic infiltrates surround small blood vessels (PARKER and DYER 1985). The vascular disease can be characterized as Heubner's endarteritis or Nissl-Alzheimer endarteritis. Heubner's endarteritis, which is the more common type, affects the large and medium-sized vessels whereas Nissl-Alzheimer arteritis primarily affects small vessels (BOWEN and POST 1991). Both types may result in vascular occlusion, ischemia, and infarction (TIEN et al. 1992).

Syphilitic gummas result from an intense localized leptomeningeal inflammatory reaction with spread to the subjacent brain parenchyma (BOWEN and POST 1991). These gummas are a manifestation of tertiary syphilis (HARRIS et al. 1997). Gummas are seen quite rarely, but when present are most often seen over the cerebral convexities, adherent to both dura and cerebral cortex. Lesions vary from 1 mm to 4 cm in size and are usually solitary, though they can be multiple (PARKER and DYER 1985). Spirochetes are rarely present within the lesions (PARKER and DYER 1985).

CT studies of patients with neurosyphilis are often unremarkable. One-third of studies are negative and one-third show only cerebral atrophy (IHMEIDAN et al. 1989). Small infarcts resulting from vasculitis can be seen on CT, but are better demonstrated on MR imaging. Areas of ischemic injury appear bright on T2-weighted images and postgadolinium images can show enhancement in regions of subacute infarction (Fig. 5.10). Acute infarction can be readily identified with diffusion imaging. Meningeal enhancement may also be present and is seen on MR imaging to much better advantage than on CT. MRA may be helpful to document vascular occlusion or narrowing, although conventional angiography remains the gold standard for evaluation of vasculitis (Fig. 5.11).

On imaging studies, gummas appear as a mass lesion at the brain surface with nodular or ring enhancement. There is usually adjacent meningeal enhancement and these lesions may be associated with extensive vasogenic edema. Treatment of syphilis in patients with HIV infection requires the administration of intravenous high-dose aqueous penicillin G for 10–14 days.

5.2.2.2
Mycobacteria

In the United States, tuberculosis (TB) had been on the decline for a number of years; however, in 1986 the incidence of TB increased (RIEDER et al. 1989a,

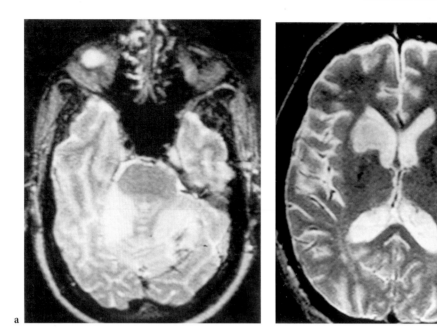

Fig. 5.10a, b. Neurosyphilis: subacute infarction. **a** T2-weighted axial MR image reveals abnormal signal hyperintensity involving the superior cerebellar hemispheres bilaterally. **b** Coronal T1-weighted postgadolinium image demonstrates enhancement in multiple areas of subacute infarction. In this HIV-positive patient, meningovascular neurosyphilis was the cause for the multiple infarctions

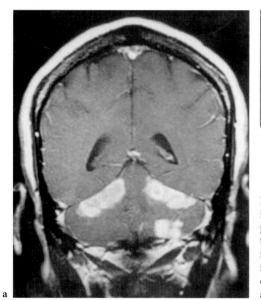

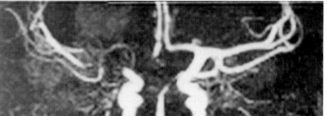

Fig. 5.11a, b. Meningovascular neurosyphilis. **a** T2-weighted axial MR image reveals an acute infarct in the right caudate head in this AIDS patient with neurosyphilis. There is mild mass effect on the right frontal horn. **b** Coronal maximum intensity projection from a 3D time-of-flight MRA reveals diffuse, severe narrowing of the right supraclinoid internal carotid artery and proximal MCA with a loss of flow-related enhancement. There is an occlusion of the A1 segment of the right anterior cerebral artery which contributed to the infarct seen in **a**

b), in large part due to the AIDS epidemic. There has been an increase in extrapulmonary manifestations of TB as well (MEHTA et al. 1991) and up to 70% of AIDS-related TB cases have extrapulmonary evidence of TB (SATHE and REICHMAN 1989). Extrapulmonary TB (including CNS TB) is currently included in the US Centers for Disease Control and Prevention criteria for a diagnosis of AIDS in an HIV-seroposi-

tive patient (SATHE and REICHMAN 1989). The incidence of *Mycobacterium* tuberculosis and *Mycobacterium avium-intracellulare* complex (MAC) in AIDS patients varies considerably with the type of population and geographic location. About 5%–9% of patients with AIDS also have TB (Centers for Disease Control 1987; LOUIE et al. 1986). However, HIV-positive intravenous drug users have a 20% incidence of

TB (SUNDERAM et al. 1986). The relative risk of TB is more than 100 times greater in AIDS patients as compared with the general population. CNS TB occurs in 2%–5% of all patients with TB (BERENGUER et al. 1992; CURLESS and MITCHELL 1991) and in 10% of those with AIDS-related TB (BERENGUER et al. 1992; BISHBURG et al. 1986).

Reactivation of latent tuberculosis is the major mechanism for TB in AIDS patients, although 10%–30% of cases are due to primary infection (KHAN et al. 1977; SELWYN et al. 1989). TB usually presents early in the course of HIV infection and thus usually precedes other AIDS-defining opportunistic infections (PITCHENIK et al. 1984). CD4 cell counts are often relatively higher in HIV patients with TB than in those patients with other infections. Thus, TB often develops in HIV-infected patients before full-blown AIDS is apparent (RIEDER et al. 1989a). Unlike TB, MAC disease is usually diagnosed when there is a much greater degree of immunodeficiency, well after the development of AIDS (SATHE and REICHMAN 1989).

CNS TB may take a variety of forms, including tuberculous meningitis, abscess, cerebritis, and tuberculoma. A subacute encephalitis can be seen with MAC (BISHBURG et al. 1986). Leptomeningitis is the most frequent form of CNS TB encountered in HIV-seropositive patients (VILLORIA et al. 1992), although overall, *Cryptococcus* is a more common cause of meningitis in AIDS patients. Fever, headache, and altered mental status are the most frequent symptoms (VILLORIA et al. 1992). Meningeal signs may be absent in one-third of patients with AIDS-related TB meningitis.

Tuberculous meningitis creates a thick gelatinous exudate which involves the basal cisterns. Arteries which course through this exudate may be affected, producing spasm, thrombosis, and resulting infarction (Fig. 5.12). Arteritis is seen in approximately 28%–41% of cases with basilar meningitis (LEIGUARDA et al. 1988). The middle cerebral artery and small perforating branches to the basal ganglia are most commonly involved (SHELLER and DESPREZ 1986).

In patients with TB meningitis, CSF typically reveals a pleocytosis with a low glucose and slightly elevated protein, although this may be inconsistent in patients with AIDS. Elevated adenosine deaminase levels (>9 u/l CSF) in the CSF suggest tuberculous meningitis, which may be very helpful in establishing an early diagnosis since cultures may take several weeks (RIBERA et al. 1987). If TB is suspected, PCR testing of the CSF may also provide a prompt diagnosis, and can generally be obtained within 48 h. The mortality rate for AIDS patients treated for TB meningitis is about 21% (BERENGUER et al. 1992).

Imaging findings associated with TB meningitis include enhancement of the basal cisterns (which is often quite intense), granulomas, abscess, calcifications, meningeal enhancement above the basal cisterns, and infarction as well as hydrocephalus, usually of the communicating type (Fig. 5.13). A study of 35 patients with AIDS-related CNS TB found hydrocephalus in 51%, meningeal enhancement in 45%, parenchymal disease

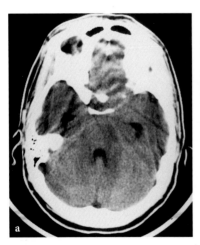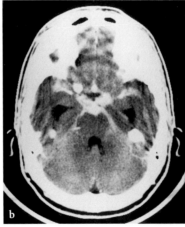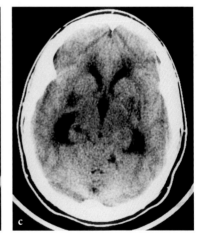

Fig. 5.12a–c. Tuberculous meningitis (culture proven), hydrocephalus, and basal ganglia infarction. **a, b** Pre- and postcontrast axial CT demonstrates intense enhancement of the basilar cisterns in this patient with TB meningitis. There is also dilatation of the temporal horns due to a communicating hydrocephalus. **c** Noncontrast axial CT (same patient as in **a** and **b**) again reveals hydrocephalus, as well as hypodensities in both basal ganglia which are the result of recent infarction. Small vessels which course through the thick tuberculous exudate in the basal cisterns undergo thrombosis with subsequent infarction, as is seen in this example

in 37%, vascular complications in 23%, and a normal study in 23% (VILLORIA et al. 1992).

Parenchymal TB includes abscess, cerebritis, and granulomas. Granulomas (tuberculomas) may result from hematogenous spread of systemic infection or may evolve from extension of a meningitis into adjacent parenchyma (PARKER and DYER 1985). The granuloma is composed of a central zone of solid caseation necrosis, surrounded by a capsule of collagenous tissue, epithelioid cells, multinucleated giant cells, and mononuclear inflammatory cells (BOWEN and POST 1991). Few tubercle bacilli are seen on smears (WHITENER 1978) but may be present in the center or within the capsule (DASTUR 1972). There is surrounding edema and astrocytic proliferation (DASTUR 1972). Tuberculomas may be solitary or multiple, supra- or infratentorial and can be found in the parenchyma, subarachnoid space, or subdural or epidural space (BOWEN and POST 1991). Most commonly, there is involvement of the corticomedullary junction and periventricular region, and the majority of lesions are supratentorial (VILLORIA et al. 1992). Parenchymal disease may occur in conjunction with meningitis or alone (Fig. 5.14).

Contrast CT of a tuberculoma reveals a ring-enhancing lesion corresponding to the central necrosis and peripheral organization which underlies the lesion (GUPTA et al. 1988). A "target sign" may be seen with central calcification or punctate enhancement surrounded by a zone of hypodensity and a surrounding rim of enhancement (VAN DYK 1988). Tuberculomas may be single or multiple. Healed tuberculomas no longer enhance, but may calcify and are therefore more evident on CT than MR imaging (JINKINS 1991). Full resolution of cerebral tuberculomas requires months to years of medical therapy and the length of time to complete resolution is directly related to the size of the original lesion (JINKINS 1991).

On MR imaging without contrast, granulomas are isointense on T1-weighted images and may have a slightly hyperintense rim (possibly secondary to paramagnetic substances within the rim) (GUPTA et al. 1988). They are variable in signal on T2-weighted images. Some are iso- or hypointense, and this relative hypointensity may be due to the presence of paramagnetic free radicals produced by macrophages (SZE and ZIMMERMAN 1988). Alternatively, the low T2 signal

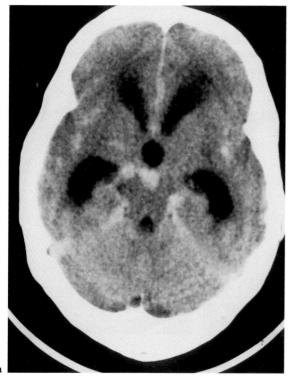 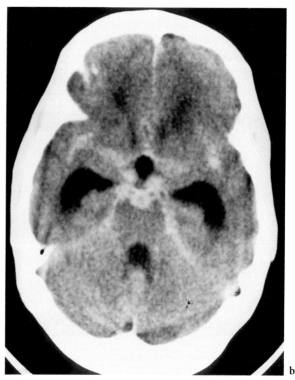

a   b

Fig. 5.13a, b. TB meningitis, hydrocephalus. Postcontrast axial CT images reveal diffuse enhancement throughout all the basal cisterns as well as within the sylvian fissures. As a result of this gelatinous exudate there is a marked communicating hydrocephalus, which is often seen in patients with TB meningitis

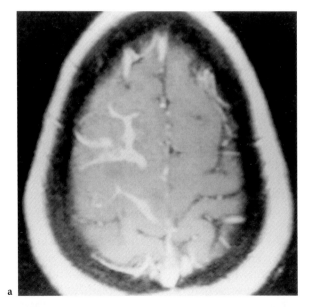

a

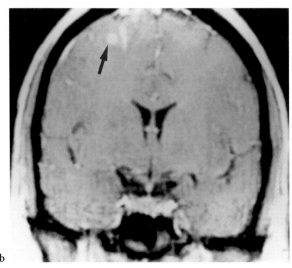

b

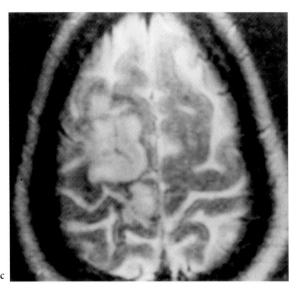

c

may be due to the mature tuberculoma, which is of greater density than adjacent brain (GUPTA et al. 1988). Other granulomas, however, are hyperintense on T2-weighted images, possibly due to central lique-factive necrosis in these lesions (BOWEN and POST 1991). There is usually mass effect and edema sur-rounding the tuberculoma, which is more prominent in the early stages of formation (GUPTA et al. 1988). Postgadolinium images reveal intense nodular and/or ring enhancement (BOWEN and POST 1991).

Tuberculous abscess is rare. In contrast to the solid caseation seen in granulomas (with few tubercle ba-cilli), the abscess contains semiliquid pus which is teeming with tubercle bacilli (WHITENER 1978). The wall of a TB abscess lacks the giant cell epithelioid granulomatous reaction of a tuberculoma (WOUTERS et al. 1985). The abscess may derive from liquefactive breakdown of a more typical caseating tuberculoma (WOUTERS et al. 1985). TB abscesses tend to be larger than granulomas and have a more accelerated clinical course (YANG et al. 1987). The imaging appearance is similar to that of a bacterial abscess (SZE and ZIM-MERMAN 1988), although there may be less edema as compared with a pyogenic abscess. CT studies reveal a hypodense lesion with edema and mass effect.

Postcontrast images reveal ring enhancement that is usually uniform and thin but occasionally may be thick and irregular. On T2-weighted images the cen-tral region of pus and liquefactive necrosis is bright while the rim of inflammation is usually iso- to hy-pointense. Rim enhancement is also seen on contrast MR studies. TB abscesses are often multiloculated (BISHBURG et al. 1986; POST et al. 1985). While tuber-culomas may be solitary or multiple, TB abscesses are usually solitary. Treatment of CNS tuberculosis in HIV-seropositive patients requires a minimum of a three-drug regimen and may require a five-drug regimen. This therapy must be continued for a mini-mum of 9 months. Sensitivity testing should be per-formed in all cases, as *M. tuberculosis* may show mul-tidrug resistance.

Fig. 5.14a–c. TB meningitis, TB granuloma (culture proven). **a** Postcontrast T1-weighted axial MR image through the vertex reveals extensive meningeal enhancement in this patient with TB meningitis. **b** T1-weighted coronal image (same pa-tient as in **a**) reveals linear meningeal enhancement near the vertex as well as a small nodular focus of enhancement (*ar-row*), which likely represents a granuloma. **c** T2-weighted axial MR image through the vertex (same patient) reveals hyperintense signal in the parenchyma. The gyriform nature of this signal abnormality suggests the possibility of an early cerebritis which is likely due to extension of infection from the meninges to the parenchyma

5.2.2.3
Nocardia

The primary immunological defect in AIDS patients is one of cell-mediated immunity rather than humoral immunity. This may account for the relative paucity of bacterial CNS infections seen in this group. *Nocardia* is a true bacteria, not a fungus. This aerobic gram-positive filamentous rod is variably acid fast and exhibits branching and beading of the filaments, which can break up to form bacillary or coccobacillary forms (BARNICOAT et al. 1989). *Nocardia* accounts for less than 2% of all infections seen in patients with AIDS (UTTAMCHANDANI et al. 1994). It is also seen in other patients with a variety of immunosuppressive disorders, including autoimmune diseases, cancer, transplant patients, and others (ADAIR et al. 1987; BARNICOAT et al. 1989). Most of the AIDS-related cases of *Nocardia* infection have been due to *N. asteroides* (UTTAMCHANDANI et al. 1994). Infection most often results from inhalation into the lungs, as *Nocardia* is a common soil organism. Direct inoculation as a result of trauma is a less common route of infection. *Nocardia* is usually seen in HIV-positive patients with advanced disease and low CD4 cell counts (JAVALY et al. 1992; UTTAMCHANDANI et al. 1994). In HIV-positive patients, there seems to be a greater incidence of *Nocardia* infection among intravenous drug users (JAVALY et al. 1992; UTTAMCHANDANI et al. 1994). The most common site of infection is the lungs, which are involved in 81% of patients (PALMER et al. 1974). The CNS is the second most common site, accounting for 15%–30% of cases (BEAMAN et al. 1976). CNS infection is often a result of hematogenous spread from pulmonary infection (BROSS and GORDON 1991) or other primary site. In one study of HIV-related *Nocardia* infection, more than 40% presented with *Nocardia* as their initial opportunistic infection (JAVALY et al. 1992). Symptoms of CNS *Nocardia* infection are nonspecific and include fever, headache, confusion, and/or seizures.

The most common manifestation of CNS *Nocardia* infection is brain abscess, which is often multiple (BEAMAN et al. 1976). Meningitis is seen less commonly. Cerebral *Nocardia* abscess is associated with an 80% mortality rate (PRESANT et al. 1973), and survival depends on proper antimicrobial therapy, the degree of immunodeficiency, and prompt surgical intervention when necessary (FRAZIER et al. 1975).

Contrast CT reveals a ring-enhancing lesion which may be multiple or multiloculated (LEBLANG et al. 1995). There is surrounding edema and mass effect. The appearance on MR imaging is typical of an abscess with central low signal on T1-weighted images and high signal on T2-weighted images, with a surrounding capsule, extensive edema, and mass effect (Fig. 5.15).

Culture of *Nocardia* requires 2–4 weeks of incubation, often resulting in a delayed diagnosis if clinical suspicion is not high. A timely diagnosis is only feasible if the treating clinicians maintain a high level of suspicion. The diagnosis of *Nocardia* infection should be suspected in a patient with an intracranial lesion and a cavitary lung infiltrate (LEBLANG et al. 1995). Trimethoprim-sulfamethoxazole (TMP-SMX) is the current treatment of choice (LEBLANG et al. 1995). Prolonged therapy is needed, as rapid relapse may occur if treatment is prematurely discontinued, and the disease may then become resistant to medical therapy (UTTAMCHANDANI et al. 1994). TMP-SMX is used as prophylaxis against *P. carinii* pneumonia and this is probably protective against *Nocardia* infection. This may account, in part, for the low incidence of *Nocardia* infection in AIDS patients.

5.2.2.4
Bacillary Angiomatosis

Bacillary angiomatosis is a multisystem infectious disease occurring primarily in HIV-infected patients. The causative agent is a gram-negative bacillus, *Bartonella* (previously *Rochalimaea*) *henselae*, a rickettsia-like organism (SLATER et al. 1992). This disorder presents with cutaneous lesions of angiomatous tender papules that may, on occasion, resemble Kaposi's sarcoma (LE BOIT et al. 1989). Systemic signs and symptoms include fever, chills, night sweats, and weight loss (BARON et al. 1990). Lytic bone lesions can be seen in multiple locations which may become clinically symptomatic before the cutaneous manifestations are evident (BARON et al. 1990). In addition to bone involvement, the liver, spleen, conjunctiva, lymph nodes, and respiratory tract may be involved (BARON et al. 1990). The bone lesions are often painful and bone scan is positive at both symptomatic and asymptomatic foci (BARON et al. 1990). CT demonstrates the lytic lesions well, which are multifocal. Since AIDS-related Kaposi's sarcoma does not involve the osseous structures, the presence of a cutaneous lesion in association with a painful bone lesion should suggest the diagnosis of bacillary angiomatosis (BARON et al. 1990). Effective treatment is with erythromycin.

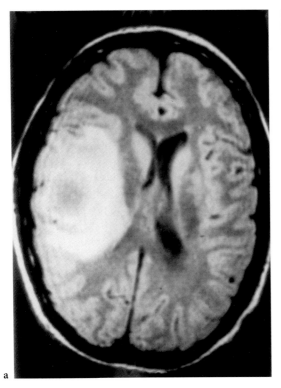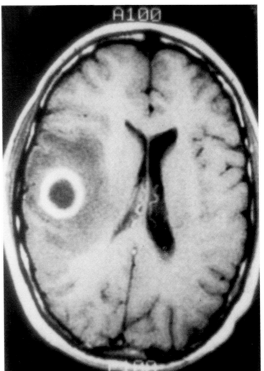

a b

Fig. 5.15a, b. *Nocardia* abscess (pathologically proven). **a** Proton density axial MR image reveals a lesion with extensive edema in the right cerebral hemisphere. There is mass effect and mild shift of the midline. The central portion of the abscess is of lower signal intensity than the surrounding edema on this proton density image. **b** Postcontrast T1-weighted axial image reveals the typical, smooth ring enhancement associated with an abscess, although the ring in this case is somewhat thick. The central purulent portion of the abscess is hyperintense to CSF

5.2.3
Fungal Disease

Fungal disease may affect the immunocompetent host as well as the immunosuppressed. Fungi which generally involve an immunocompromised host include *Aspergillus, Candida*, and *Mucor*. Fungi which may occur in the normal host as well as the immunocompromised host include *Cryptococcus, Coccidioides immitis* (causing coccidiomycosis), *Histoplasma capsulatum* (causing histoplasmosis), and *Blastomyces dermatitidis* (causing blastomycosis) (Lyons and Andriole 1986). *Aspergillus, Cryptococcus, Candida*, and *Mucor* are ubiquitous, whereas the other fungi are endemic to specific geographic locations (Kobayshi 1980).

The configuration of the fungal form determines to a large degree the type of mycotic involvement seen within the CNS (Parker and Dyer 1985). Fungi growing as yeast cells (*Cryptococcus, Histoplasma*) are small enough to spread hematogenously to the microvasculature of the meninges, penetrate the vessel walls, and incite an acute or chronic leptomenin-

gitis (Parker and Dyer 1985). Less often, parenchymal disease, such as granuloma or abscess, is seen.

Fungi growing as hyphae (*Aspergillus, Mucor*) or pseudohyphae (*Candida*) have less access to the meningeal circulation by virtue of their larger size. These hyphae form mycelial colonies capable of vascular invasion and obstruction of large, medium, and small arteries, resulting in infarction and cerebritis (Parker and Dyer 1985). Pseudohyphae are adherent yeast cells and their progeny are somewhat smaller than true hyphae.

5.2.3.1
Cryptococcus

Cryptococcus neoformans is the most frequent fungus associated with CNS infection in AIDS patients (De La Paz and Enzmann 1988). Clinically, it is seen in about 10% of AIDS patients in the United States (Ennis and Saag 1993). In 45% of those with both AIDS and cryptococcal infection, it is the initial manifestation of their immunodeficiency (Davenport et al. 1992). Inhalation is the route of infection. A subacute basilar granulomatous meningitis results (DE LA PAZ and ENZMANN 1988), with headache being the most common and often the only symptom (LEVY et al. 1985). Other clinical signs and symptoms include altered mentation, fever, neck stiffness, and seizures (BRITTON and MILLER 1984). Diagnosis can be made via India ink preparation of the CSF, via detection of cryptococcal antigen in the CSF, or by fungal CSF culture.

CT examination of AIDS patients with cryptococcal meningitis is often unremarkable, but may reveal atrophy or communicating hydrocephalus (LEVY et al. 1984). Meningeal enhancement is rare, but can occur (POST et al. 1985) (Fig. 5.16). MR imaging may be negative as well, but may reveal meningeal enhancement on postgadolinium images. Cryptococcal meningitis carries a mortality rate of 17% (ENNIS and SAAG 1993). Treatment is with amphotericin B and flucytosine.

Parenchymal infection with *Cryptoccocus* may occur via hematogenous dissemination or from spread of meningeal disease to adjacent parenchyma (BOWEN and POST 1991). The parenchymal disease is variable in appearance, and the literature is often confusing on this issue. Four patterns of parenchymal disease may be encountered: (a) parenchymal mass lesions (cryptococcomas), (b) dilated Virchow-Robin spaces, (c) parenchymal/leptomeningeal nodules, and (d) a mixed pattern. Symptoms are often muted, probably due to an inability to mount a significant cell-mediated immune response (SZE et al. 1987).

Cryptococcomas represent a collection of inflammatory cells, fungal organisms, and gelatinous mucoid material (MATHEWS et al. 1992). The relative proportion of each constituent may vary, and thus lesions in immunocompetent patients may appear solid, whereas the cryptococcomas seen in AIDS patients have an appearance termed "gelatinous pseudocyst" (MATHEWS et al. 1992).

Virchow-Robin spaces are perivascular spaces that can become filled with fungus and associated mucoid material. Fungal invasion results in enlargement of these perivascular spaces, best seen in the basal ganglia region. Parenchymal/leptomeningeal nodules are small granulomas (SZE et al. 1987). These are uncommon in AIDS patients.

Infrequently, CT may reveal hypodense lesions with solid or ring enhancement (ZUGER et al. 1986). Peripheral, small enhancing nodules can occasionally be seen, consistent with granulomas, which may contain punctate calcifications. More commonly, small hypodensities without enhancement are seen in the basal ganglia, corresponding to dilated perivascular spaces which are engorged with fungal organisms and mucoid material. Larger, cystic masses are also seen in the region of the basal ganglia, the so-called gelatinous pseudocysts (Fig. 5.17). These may have septations, and are often bilateral and asymmetric. There is mild mass effect but no significant enhancement.

On MR imaging, the dilated Virchow-Robin spaces are isointense to CSF, and may be seen in the mid-

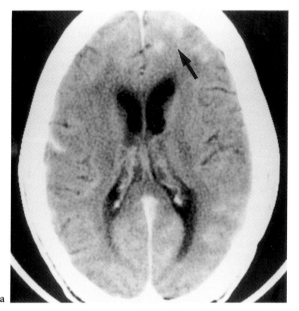
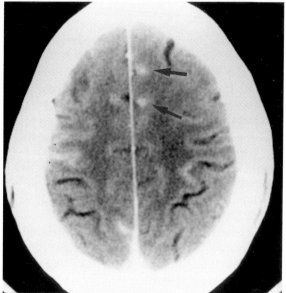

a   b

Fig. 5.16a, b. Cryptococcal meningitis. Axial postcontrast CT images reveal curvilinear enhancement in this patient with cryptococcal meningitis. Nodular enhancement (*arrows*) is also noted, which may represent small granulomas

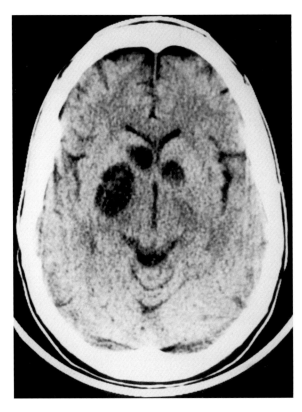

Fig. 5.17. "Gelatinous pseudocysts" in a patient with crypto-coccal infection. Axial CT scan without contrast demon-strates the typical appearance of these lesions in AIDS pa-tients. These cystic masses contain fungal elements, inflam-matory cells, and gelatinous mucoid material. The inflamma-tory response to cryptococcal infection is often muted in AIDS patients and thus the gelatinous pseudocysts have minimal mass effect and usually do not enhance. Internal septations are often seen, as in the largest lesion on the right

brain (TIEN et al. 1991a) as well as the basal ganglia, without enhancement (Fig. 5.18). Miliary enhancing parenchymal/leptomeningeal nodules can be seen (TIEN et al. 1991a), consistent with granulomas.

Hydrocephalus and enhancement are more com-monly seen in immunocompetent patients with CNS cryptococcosis than in AIDS patients with crypto-coccosis (TIEN et al. 1991a). The paucity of hydro-cephalus in AIDS patients is again attributed to a rel-ative lack of inflammatory leptomeningeal reaction.

5.2.3.2
Mucor

Mucormycosis is a phycomycosis of the genus *Mucor*. CNS involvement is most often seen in diabetics as well as other immunocompromised patients, and has

been reported in association with AIDS (CUADRADO et al. 1988). Mucormycosis is usually of the rhinoce-rebral type (craniofacial), with spread along perivas-cular and perineural channels (Fig. 5.19). Extension across the cribriform plate may result in frontal lobe infection, and disease at the orbital apex can extend into the cavernous sinus (BOWEN and POST 1991). Paranasal sinus disease is often present, but need not be severe for CNS spread to occur. Intracranial exten-sion can result in abscess and/or infarction, and may occur at a site remote from the primary focus due to vascular dissemination. Vascular invasion results in occlusion and infarction.

5.2.3.3
Aspergillosis

CNS aspergillosis is seen only rarely in patients with AIDS. CNS infection may result from direct extension from the paranasal region or from hematogenous spread. *Aspergillus* hyphae are angioinvasive, result-ing in vascular invasion, occlusion, and hemorrhagic infarction (BOWEN and POST 1991). Septic infarcts may be seen and usually involve the anterior circula-tion (BOWEN and POST 1991). Focal cerebritis and abscess formation may also occur (BOWEN and POST 1991). Within the paranasal sinus region, both *Mucor* and *Aspergillus* may appear markedly hypointense on T1- and T2-weighted images, possibly due to the pres-ence of metallic ions such as iron, manganese, and magnesium. When present, this hypointense signal in the paranasal sinuses can provide a helpful diagnostic clue, suggesting the presence of fungal disease.

5.2.3.4
Candidiasis

Outside the CNS, *Candida* is a common pathogen in AIDS patients, but it is rarely seen in the CNS. When present, *Candida* infection has a variable appear-ance, ranging from meningitis and meningoenceph-alitis to abscess, microabscess, and granulomas (DE LA PAZ and ENZMANN 1988; LEVY et al. 1985).

The microabscess appears on CT as an iso- or hy-podense lesion with multiple punctate enhancing nodules seen on contrast studies (DE LA PAZ and EN-ZMANN 1988). A "target" appearance can be seen on MR imaging, with a central hypointensity and sur-rounding hyperintensity on T2-weighted images (SZE and ZIMMERMAN 1988).

Granulomas may be seen as hyperdense nodules on CT (DE LA PAZ and ENZMANN 1988), with sur-rounding edema and nodular or ring enhancement.

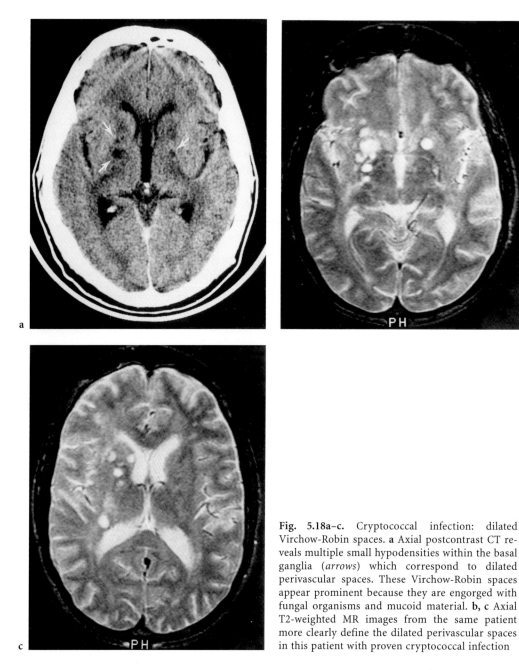

Fig. 5.18a–c. Cryptococcal infection: dilated Virchow-Robin spaces. **a** Axial postcontrast CT reveals multiple small hypodensities within the basal ganglia (*arrows*) which correspond to dilated perivascular spaces. These Virchow-Robin spaces appear prominent because they are engorged with fungal organisms and mucoid material. **b, c** Axial T2-weighted MR images from the same patient more clearly define the dilated perivascular spaces in this patient with proven cryptococcal infection

5.2.4
Parasitic Disease

5.2.4.1
Toxoplasma Encephalitis

Opportunistic infections of the CNS are a common manifestation of HIV infection. Cerebral toxoplasmosis is seen in 10%–34% of AIDS autopsies (MARTINEZ et al. 1995; PETITO et al. 1986). *Toxoplasma* encephalitis results from infection by *Toxoplasma*

gondii, an obligate intracellular protozoan with a worldwide distribution (BOWEN and POST 1991). In the United States, seropositivity for adults ranges from 20% to 70% (LEVY et al. 1985; PARKER and DYER 1985). Initial infection is usually subclinical, or may produce a benign illness with self-limiting lymphadenopathy, with or without fever (KRICK and REMINGTON 1978). Following the acute infection, the parasite assumes a latent form, the encysted bradyzoite. Any tissue previously infected may harbor these cysts. With a decline in cell-mediated im-

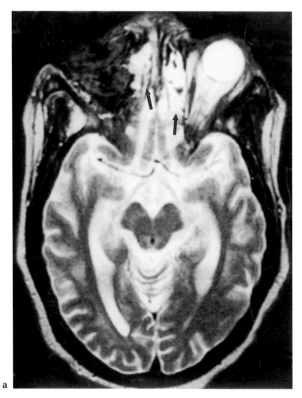

a

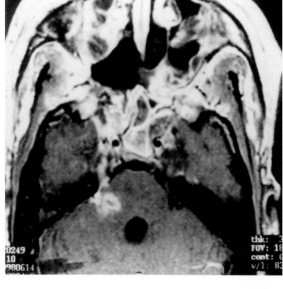

b

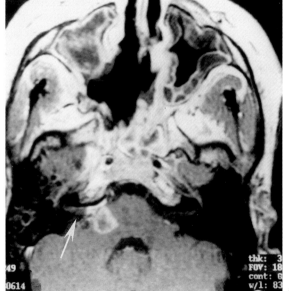

c

Fig. 5.19a–c. Mucormycosis in an HIV-infected patient. **a** T2-weighted axial MR images demonstrates hypointense signal in the right orbit status post orbital exenteration for mucormycosis. Hyperintense signal is seen in the ethmoid air cells, indicating inflammatory disease (*arrows*). **b** Postcontrast axial T1-weighted image reveals irregular enhancement throughout the maxillary and sphenoid sinuses with extensive opacification. Postsurgical changes are seen involving the medial walls of both maxillary sinuses. There is abnormal widening of the right cavernous sinus due to fungal invasion with perineural extension to Meckel's cave as well as along the cisternal segment of cranial nerve V. There is additional perineural extension along the 5th nerve into the brainstem. **c** Postcontrast T1-weighted axial image also reveals perineural extension of mucormycosis from the brainstem into the internal auditory canal, along the 7th–8th nerve complex (*white arrow*)

munity, the cysts rupture, releasing the invasive, free tachyzoites. Thus, in most cases, *Toxoplasma* encephalitis represents a recrudescence of infection rather than a newly acquired infection (LUFT and REMINGTON 1992)

The major mode of transmission for *Toxoplasma* is via raw meat (LEVY et al. 1986). Transmission is also possible via transfusions, bodily secretions, raw milk, organ transplantation, contaminated needles, cat feces, and in utero exposure (LEVY et al. 1986). Prior to the era of AIDS, fulminant necrotizing encephalitis

resulting from toxoplasmosis was seen only in patients with disorders that resulted in significant immunodeficiency, such as malignancy, organ transplantation, collagen vascular disease, or treatment with steroids, chemotherapy, or radiation therapy (KRICK and REMINGTON 1978; VIETZKE et al. 1968).

In AIDS patients, *Toxoplasma* results in a progressive and often fatal encephalitis if untreated (LEVY et al. 1985; POST et al. 1983). It is usually seen when CD4 cell counts fall below 100 cells/mm^3 (GIRRARD et al. 1993) Clinical symptoms include altered mental status, confusion, lethargy, fever, headache, seizure, and focal neurological deficit (LEVY et al. 1985; POST et al. 1983). Toxoplasmosis is the most commonly reported CNS infection in AIDS patients who present with altered mentation, fever, seizure, and/or focal neurological deficit (DE LA PAZ and ENZMANN 1988; POST et al. 1983). It is also the most common cause of an intracerebral mass lesion in patients with HIV infection (MCARTHUR 1987).

CSF findings in toxoplasmosis are nonspecific. Because seropositivity for *Toxoplasma* is so widespread, a positive titer is nondiagnostic, indicating only past or recent exposure. A negative titer in a patient with an intracranial mass lesion suggests that other diagnostic possibilities should be considered but does not completely exclude toxoplasmosis. Up to 22% of AIDS patients with *Toxoplasma* encephalitis may not have detectable anti-*Toxoplasma* IgG antibodies (PORTER and SANDE 1993).

Pathologically, *Toxoplasma* encephalitis contains three distinct zones without a capsule (POST et al. 1983). The center is avascular and necrotic, with few organisms. The intermediate zone contains an intense inflammatory reaction with patchy areas of necrosis. There are numerous free intracellular and ex-

tracellular tachyzoites and encysted forms are rare. This zone is engorged with blood vessels. There is endothelial cell swelling and proliferation with cuffing of venules by lymphocytes, plasma cells, and macrophages (POST et al. 1983). The peripheral zone contains more encysted forms (bradyzoites) and fewer free tachyzoites. Leptomeningitis is present only directly adjacent to a region of encephalitis. Vascular involvement can lead to small vessel thrombosis and necrosis without arteritis of the larger vessels (POST et al. 1983). Pathological diagnosis is based upon hematoxylin and eosin (H&E) stains or Giemsa stains. In difficult cases, electron microscopy of formalin-fixed material or standard immunoperoxidase procedures may be used (POST et al. 1983).

The imaging appearance of *Toxoplasma* encephalitis is often characteristic, although nonspecific. On noncontrast CT, lesions are iso- to hypodense with surrounding edema and mass effect. There is a predilection for the basal ganglia (in 75%–88%) and the corticomedullary junction (POST et al. 1983). Lesions may vary in size from <1 cm to over 3 cm (POST et al. 1983). Hemorrhage is uncommon. Postcontrast CT studies reveal ring, solid, and/or nodular enhancement (Fig. 5.20). Ring enhancement is the most com-

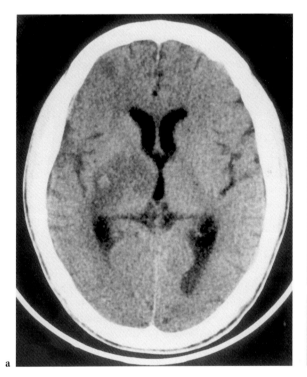
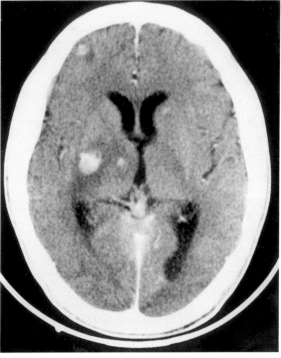

a   b

Fig. 5.20a, b. Toxoplasmosis. **a** Noncontrast axial CT scan reveals hypodensity in the right basal ganglia, with mass effect and minimal midline shift. Within the hypodensity is a lesion which is isodense. **b** Postcontrast scan reveals enhancement of the isodense lesion as well as several other enhancing lesions

mon pattern. The ring is usually thin and smooth, but may be thick and irregular, especially in larger lesions (POST et al. 1983). The double dose delayed (DDD) technique for administration of contrast has been found to significantly increase the number and size of lesions detected on CT imaging (POST et al. 1985). The DDD technique, using 200 cc of intravenous contrast and a 1-h delay, permits maximal enhancement of CNS toxoplasmosis (POST et al. 1985).

The radiographic appearance of toxoplasmosis correlates well with the pathological findings. The central hypodensity often seen on CT images corresponds to the central area of avascular necrosis. The ring-enhancing portion of the lesion appears to correlate with the region of intense inflammation, and the peripheral zone corresponds to the surrounding edema (POST et al. 1983). Pathologic-radiologic correlation has shown that the extent of these lesions is often greater than the area seen as enhancement on CT (POST et al. 1983).

MR imaging without and with gadolinium is more sensitive than contrast CT in the detection of *Toxoplasma* encephalitis (LEVY et al. 1985, 1986). MR imaging may be positive when the CT is negative (LEVY et al. 1985, 1986), or MR images may reveal a greater number of lesions when the CT is positive. On T2-weighted images, active lesions are of variable signal intensity. Some lesions are iso- to hypointense centrally, with surrounding high signal edema (SZE et al. 1987). Other lesions may show central hyperintensity, indistinguishable from the surrounding edema (Fig. 5.21). On T1-weighted images, the lesions are iso- to hypointense centrally, with surrounding edema which appears hypointense. Postgadolinium imaging (0.1 mm/kg) reveals ring or nodular enhancement of active lesions, clearly distinguishable from the surrounding low signal edema. Hemorrhage is uncommon. Toxoplasmosis is usually multifocal. Only 14% of patients with toxoplasmosis have a solitary lesion on contrast MR studies (PORTER and SANDE 1993). Thus, if only a single lesion is detected on a good-quality MR study, other diagnoses should be considered although toxoplasmosis remains a possibility.

Toxoplasma encephalitis is effectively treated with pyrimethamine and sulfadiazine or pyrimethamine and clindamycin, with dramatic clinical improvement (LUFT et al. 1993). Serial CT or MR studies demonstrate a decrease in the number and size of lesions, with a reduction in edema and mass

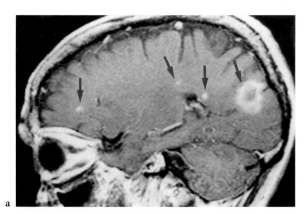
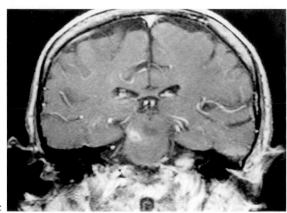
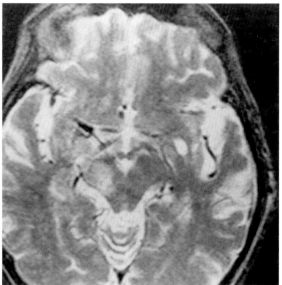

Fig. 5.21a–c. Toxoplasmosis. **a** Parasagittal T1-weighted postgadolinium MR reveals multiple foci of enhancement, with both ring and nodular patterns of enhancement (*arrows*). **b** T1-weighted postcontrast coronal image reveals an enhancing lesion in the midbrain with only slight mass effect. **c** T2-weighted axial image of same patient as in **b**. A hyperintense lesion with mild mass effect is present in the right cerebral peduncle

effect. These changes are evident within 2–4 weeks after initiation of therapy (Post et al. 1985), but full resolution may require 6 months (Levy et al. 1985, 1986). Larger lesions tend to resolve more slowly. Treated *Toxoplasma* lesions have a variable appearance on CT. Areas of previous involvement may revert to normal, may reveal focal encephalomalacia, or may calcify (Post et al. 1985) (Fig. 5.22). Healed, calcified lesions may be more obvious on CT, but may show foci of hypointensity on T1- and T2-weighted images, corresponding to the foci of calcification. These may be more evident on gradient echo T2-weighted MR images. Mineralization of some lesions can result in bright signal foci on T1- and T2-weighted images, presumably due to paramagnetic species (e.g., manganese, iron, copper) (Atlas et al. 1988). Despite complete radiographic resolution, *Toxoplasma* encephalitis is likely to recur in the presence of persistent cellular immunodeficiency if treatment is discontinued. This is because medical therapy is effective against the free tachyzoites but not the encysted forms of toxoplasmosis. Thus, the parasite is never entirely eradicated and lifelong maintenance therapy is required (Post et al. 1985).

In the past, early biopsy of enhancing CNS lesions was advocated in order to establish a diagnosis and promptly institute appropriate treatment (Levy et al. 1984, 1985). More recently, these cases have been handled conservatively. Because toxoplasmosis is fairly common in AIDS patients, those who present with typical clinical and radiographic findings are placed on anti-*Toxoplasma* medication and repeat imaging is obtained in 10–14 days. Consistent clinical and radiographic improvement is presumptive evidence of *Toxoplasma* infection. However, lesions should be followed to complete resolution as multiple pathologies may be present in a given patient. Lack of improvement on medical therapy may indicate the need for biopsy, since the etiology may actually be due to CNS lymphoma or other infection. It is difficult to accurately assess lesion activity if the patient is on steroids. Steroid therapy can reduce enhancement, edema, and mass effect, simulating a response to treatment.

Primary CNS lymphoma can be radiographically indistinguishable from toxoplasmosis. Both can present as single or multifocal lesions. Treatment of these disorders, however, is radically different, and thus it is imperative that a correct diagnosis be established as quickly as possible. Thallium-201 (^{201}Tl) brain SPECT imaging has become invaluable in making this distinction. Thallium, a potassium analogue, is taken up by metabolically active tissue, such as tumor (i.e., lymphoma) but not by infection (i.e., toxoplasmosis) (Ruiz et al. 1994). There is active uptake of ^{201}Tl by tumors via the cell membrane ATPase system, with sodium extruded from the cell in exchange for ^{201}Tl (Ruiz et al. 1997). A positive ^{201}Tl brain SPECT study suggests the presence of a CNS tumor, and in HIV-positive patients most likely indi-

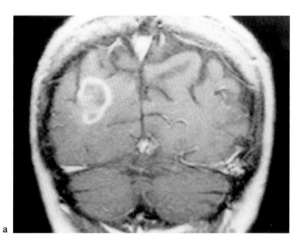

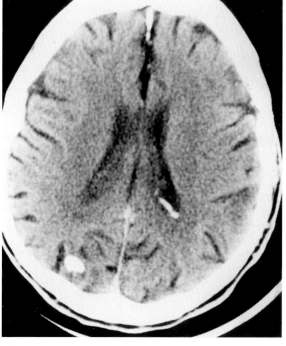

Fig. 5.22a, b. Treated toxoplasmosis. **a** Postcontrast coronal MR image reveals a large ring-enhancing lesion in the right occipital lobe, with mild mass effect. **b** This postcontrast CT scan was obtained several months later, after treatment for toxoplasmosis. A calcification is seen at the site of the previous ring-enhancing lesion, and there is no residual enhancement

cates a primary CNS lymphoma (RUIZ et al. 1994). This study can be obtained quickly and can preclude the need for 10–14 days of trial therapy and reevaluation. Positive scans often result in biopsy for definitive diagnosis. Negative thallium scans are presumed to be due to either toxoplasmosis or other infectious cause (Fig. 5.23). These patients are followed on anti-*Toxoplasma* treatment with repeat imaging usually obtained in 10–14 days. Again, continued clinical and radiographic improvement is presumptive evidence for *Toxoplasma* infection. The sensitivity of thallium studies is limited by resolution, and lesions

under 6–8 mm in size may not be detected (RUIZ et al. 1994).

FDG-PET imaging has also been used to distinguish CNS neoplasm from infection. Several studies have found the standardized uptake values on FDG-PET scanning to be significantly greater for CNS lymphoma than for toxoplasmosis, allowing distinction between these two causes of cerebral mass lesions (O'DOHERTY et al. 1997; VILLRINGER et al. 1995).

Advances in MR spectroscopy have resulted in the development of a diagnostic tool which can be used

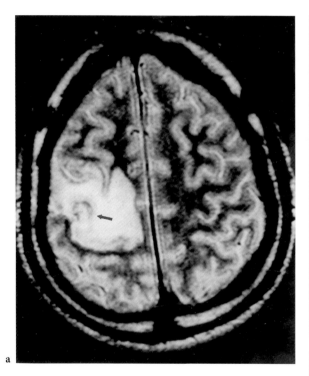

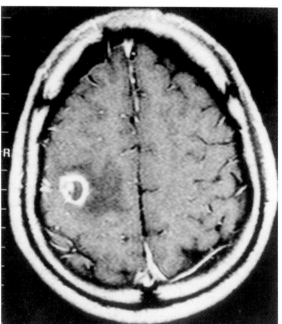

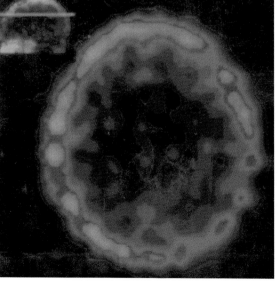

Fig. 5.23a–c. Toxoplasmosis: negative ^{201}Tl study. **a** T2-weighted axial MR scan reveals extensive edema at the right frontoparietal junction. Within the edema is a hypointense focus (*arrow*) which corresponds to the ring-enhancing lesion seen in **b**. **b** Postgadolinium MR demonstrates a ring-enhancing lesion at the same site, with mass effect and surrounding hypointense edema. **c** [201]Tl brain SPECT was obtained to differentiate between neoplasm and infection. This corresponding image from the study does not reveal any significant uptake at the site of the lesion, and is therefore compatible with an inflammatory process. The patient was treated with anti-*Toxoplasma* therapy and showed both clinical and radiographic response to treatment. (In contrast, see Fig. 5.31 for a positive ^{201}Tl brain SPECT study in a patient with lymphoma.)

not only to distinguish inflammatory from neoplastic CNS disorders, but also to provide specific information regarding biochemical alterations. MR spectroscopy does not require injection of a radiopharmaceutical (as does ^{201}Tl and FDG-PET) and can be performed on clinical MR scanners as part of the overall MR examination.

MR spectroscopy can be useful in distinguishing between toxoplasmosis and CNS lymphoma in HIV-seropositive patients. In toxoplasmosis, the lactate and lipid peaks are markedly elevated while all other normal brain metabolites are virtually absent (CHANG et al. 1995). This pattern is consistent with the anaerobic acellular environment within an abscess and the inflammatory response which surrounds the abscess. Unfortunately, this pattern is not completely specific and has also been observed within the necrotic portion of brain neoplasms (CHANG and ERNST 1997).

In contrast, the spectroscopic pattern in lymphoma shows a mild to moderate increase in lactate and lipids, a markedly elevated choline peak, and preservation of some normal metabolites. It is essential, however, that the voxel for spectroscopic analysis of a lymphoma be placed over the cellular portion of the lesion (CHANG and ERNST 1997) as the necrotic center can simulate the findings seen in toxoplasmosis. Since there is overlap in spectroscopic patterns, the results must be correlated with other clinical and radiographic information.

Perfusion MR imaging has also been used to distinguish between toxoplasmosis and lymphoma in AIDS patients. One prospective study of 13 patients (ERNST et al. 1998) found decreased perfusion in lesions of toxoplasmosis and increased perfusion in CNS lymphoma. Regional cerebral blood volume (rCBV) was determined by using dynamic echo-planar MR imaging during bolus injection of a gadolinium chelate. The rCBV was decreased in lesions of toxoplasmosis and increased within lymphoma. Thus, a number of different techniques are currently available which enable distinction between tumor and infection when conventional imaging reveals a nonspecific mass lesion.

5.2.4.2
Cysticercosis

Cysticercosis is the most common parasitic infection of the human CNS worldwide, and is seen in both immunocompetent and immunodeficient patients from endemic regions (DAVIS and KORNFELD 1991). It is not an opportunistic infection per se, but cysticercosis is seen in AIDS patients from endemic areas and therefore must be recognized and correctly diagnosed. Endemic locations include Mexico, Central and South America, India, and China (DAVIS and KORNFELD 1991). Cases have also been reported from Eastern Europe, Portugal, Africa, and Asia. Immigration has resulted in an increased prevalence of this disorder in the United States.

The causative agent is *Taenia solium*, a pork tapeworm. Humans can be the definitive hosts (infected with a tapeworm) or the intermediate host (infected with cysticercus, the larval form). When humans ingest inadequately cooked pork containing the larvae of *T. solium* (cysticerci), they become definitive hosts for the tapeworm (DAVIS and KORNFELD 1991). The cysticercus develops in the small intestine into a tapeworm, 1–8 m in length. Eggs are then passed into the stool (DAVIS and KORNFELD 1991). If these ova contaminate food or water that is then eaten by a pig, the life cycle continues with the pig as the intermediate host (DAVIS and KORNFELD 1991).

Similarly, if the contaminated food or water is ingested by humans, they can become intermediate hosts. Within the stomach, the outer shell of the ova is dissolved to release the oncosphere. The oncosphere (primary larva) penetrates the gastrointestinal mucosa, enters the bloodstream, and may lodge in any tissue but shows a predilection for the brain (DAVIS and KORNFELD 1991). The oncosphere may burrow into the brain parenchyma, meninges, ependyma, and/or choroid plexus. There are four types of neurocysticercosis – parenchymal, subarachnoid, intraventricular, and mixed (CARBAJAL et al. 1977). The parenchymal type is probably the most common.

The initial infection of the brain by the larva is usually asymptomatic and results in a small edematous lesion (LOPES-HERNANDEZ 1983). The secondary larvae (cysticerci) then develop into cysts, which are usually apparent about 2–3 months after the original host ingestion of ova (DAVIS and KORNFELD 1991). Each cyst contains a protoscolex and the cysts measure 3–18 mm in diameter (ESCOBAR 1983). While alive, the cyst provokes a minimal surrounding inflammatory reaction and remains viable for 2–6 years after infestation (DAVIS and KORNFELD 1991). During this period, the patient is often asymptomatic, although seizures can occur.

However, as the cyst dies, it incites an inflammatory reaction in the adjacent tissues. Antigens and metabolic products leak out as the cyst is dying, and the clear fluid of the cyst becomes turbid and gelatinous (DAVIS and KORNFELD 1991). An edematous reaction is produced, and the patient is often symptomatic with either seizures or focal neurological signs. The cyst eventually collapses, degenerates, and may calcify (DAVIS and KORNFELD 1991).

If the oncospheres lodge in the meninges or choroid plexus, infection may arise within the ventricular system and/or subarachnoid space. In the subarachnoid space, the cysts may appear multiloculated and can vary in size from 5 mm to 9 cm (DAVIS and KORNFELD 1991). This is known as the racemose form. The protoscolex is absent in the racemose type of infection (MCCORMICK 1985). Chronic meningitis and/or ventriculitis can result, possibly from leakage of cysticercosis antigens into the CSF, with an accompanying inflammatory response (DAVIS and KORNFELD 1991). This can result in hydrocephalus (LOBATO et al. 1981). The racemose cyst does not usually calcify after degeneration.

In an untreated patient, a single cysticercosis lesion takes about 2–10 years to resolve. In endemic regions, there may be recurrent ingestion of ova; thus intracranial cysts may be seen in different stages of evolution. CSF is abnormal in about 50% of cases. A lymphocytic pleocytosis may be present (DAVIS and KORNFELD 1991).

The imaging findings in cysticercosis are quite characteristic. The initial infection results in a focal edematous lesion which appears hypodense on CT and hyperintense on T2-weighted MR images and does not usually enhance significantly (KRAMER et al. 1989). The formation of mature cysts is known as the vesicular stage. These are clearly evident on CT or MR imaging. The cyst wall is thin and smooth with little, if any, edema. The scolex is seen as a focal nodule within the cyst and is often better appreciated on MR imaging than on CT (Fig. 5.24). The cysts at this stage are isointense to CSF on all MR sequences and of fluid density on CT. A greater number of lesions may be seen on MR studies as compared with CT.

As the larva dies, the surrounding inflammatory response can result in formation of a fibrous capsule that may appear as ring enhancement on imaging studies. Degenerating cysts may appear hyperintense on both T1- and T2-weighted images, owing to the debris and proteinaceous material accumulating within the cyst (SPICKLER et al. 1989). This is the colloidal vesicular stage. Surrounding edema appears bright on T2-weighted images and hypodense on CT (Fig. 5.25). In the granular nodular stage, the cyst retracts, forming a granulomatous lesion which can demonstrate ring or nodular enhancement (CHANG et al. 1991).

As the lesion becomes mineralized, it enters the final nodular calcified stage, where the granulomatous nodules are replaced by gliosis and may calcify (CHANG et al. 1991). These calcified lesions may be

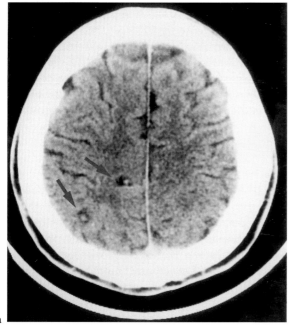
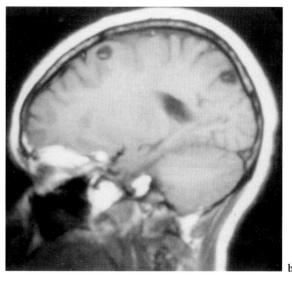

Fig. 5.24a, b. Cysticercosis: vesicular stage. **a** Noncontrast axial CT reveals small cystic lesions in the right cerebral hemisphere without mass effect (*arrows*). Note central hyperdense scolex. **b** T1-weighted parasagittal MR in another patient demonstrates two separate cystic lesions without edema or mass effect. Punctate signal within the cysts corresponds to the scolex, which is usually well visualized on MR

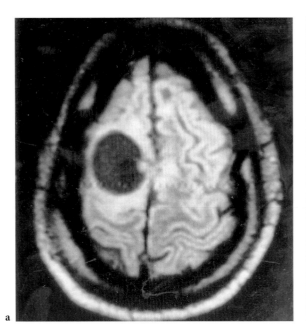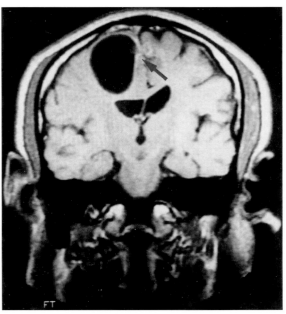

a   b

Fig. 5.25a, b. Cysticercosis: early colloidal vesicular stage. **a** Proton density image reveals a large cystic lesion near the right vertex. A mural nodule is seen along the medial border, corresponding to the scolex. Surrounding hyperintense edema is seen, indicating that the lesion is beginning to degenerate. Leakage of metabolic products into the surrounding tissues incites this edematous reaction. The cyst remains isointense to CSF, as it has only just begun to degenerate. Later, the proteinaceous fluid within the degenerating cyst will become hyperintense to CSF. **b** Same patient as in **a**. This large cyst demonstrates faint peripheral enhancement (*arrow*) as it begins to degenerate

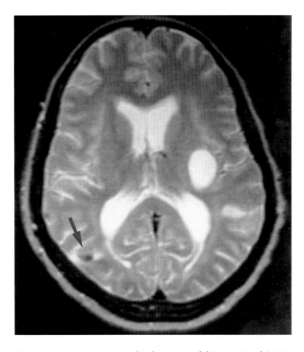

Fig. 5.26. Cysticercosis: multiple stages of disease. On this T2-weighted axial MR image, there is a cystic lesion without mass effect or edema in the left basal ganglia, typical of the vesicular stage. Focal hypointensity (*arrow*) on the right indicates a lesion in the nodular calcified stage, which is often seen better on CT

easier to identify on CT, although T2-weighted gradient-echo MR sequences are also helpful in detecting the calcifications, which appear as punctate foci of very hypointense signal (Fig. 5.26).

Intraventricular and subarachnoid cysts are often best visualized on MR imaging. On CT, the lesions are isodense to CSF. On MR imaging, the cysts are usually close to CSF in signal but are readily identified by the distortion of the subarachnoid spaces and cisterns. The racemose cysts can be quite extensive, and often difficult to treat. The cerebellopontine angle and suprasellar cisterns are the most common locations. A chronic meningitis may result, with cisternal enhancement and hydrocephalus (BOWEN and POST 1991).

The diagnosis of neurocysticercosis is based on a combination of clinical, radiographic, and serological indicators. Treatment is with praziquantel or albendazole. The subarachnoid cysts do not respond as well as the parenchymal cysts to therapy. Because treatment results in crenation of the cyst, the inflammatory response often transiently worsens, with increased edema and enhancement. Symptoms may therefore worsen for a period of time before the patient shows clinical or radiographic improvement.

5.3
Neoplasm

5.3.1
Primary CNS Lymphoma

Primary CNS lymphoma is the most common neo-plasm of the CNS in HIV-positive patients. It is iden-tified in 6% of all AIDS autopsies and is seen in 6.4% of AIDS patients presenting with neurologic dysfunc-tion (PETITO et al. 1986). CNS lymphoma in an HIV-seropositive individual is considered an AIDS-defin-ing condition (SAFAI et al. 1992). Patients are usually profoundly immunocompromised, with CD4 cell counts <50 cells/mm³. There is a strong association between primary CNS lymphoma and the Epstein-Barr virus (EBV) (MACMAHON et al. 1991). Reactiva-tion of a latent lymphocyte infection with EBV in patients with impaired cellular immunity is thought to play a significant role in the pathogenesis of prima-ry CNS lymphoma (SMIRNIOTOPOULOS et al. 1997).

Primary CNS lymphoma is usually of B cell origin. The most common types of AIDS-related lymphomas are large cell immunoblastic lymphoma (30%) and the small, noncleaved cell type (60%) (ROSENBLUM et al. 1988). Lesions are usually central in location, most often involving the basal ganglia, corpus callosum, periventricular regions, and cerebellar vermis. How-ever, AIDS-related CNS lymphoma can also occur more peripherally, and are more likely than non-AIDS-related lymphomas to be seen in peripheral lo-cations. Subependymal spread may also be seen.

Primary CNS lymphoma may appear as solitary or multiple masses, or with meningeal disease. Clini-cal studies suggest that 50%–75% of patients with CNS lymphoma have multiple lesions, whereas au-topsy data reveal multicentric disease to be present in almost 100% (FORSYTH and DEANGELIS 1996).

Clinical symptoms include focal neurological defi-cit, confusion, lethargy, and memory loss, and seizures may be seen in up to one-third of cases (ROSENBLUM et al. 1988). Other symptoms include nonspecific headache, nausea, and vomiting. B symptoms (fever, night sweats, weight loss) are seen more frequently in AIDS-related CNS lymphoma than in non-AIDS lym-phomas (REMICK et al. 1990). AIDS-related CNS lym-phomas have a greater male predominance and a younger age at presentation (34 years vs 59 years) than CNS lymphoma in patients who are HIV negative (REMICK et al. 1990). CSF protein is usually increased and a pleocytosis may be present (REMICK et al. 1990). CSF cytology is positive in 20%–25% of AIDS-related CNS lymphoma (REMICK et al. 1990). EB virus DNA

may be detected in the CSF of some AIDS patients with CNS lymphoma and may thus confirm a suspect-ed diagnosis of lymphoma (DINA 1991).

Imaging is suggestive, although nonspecific. AIDS-related CNS lymphomas may appear hy-podense or hyperdense on noncontrast CT. Non-AIDS lymphomas are usually hyperdense, probably due to the cellularity of these lesions (JIDDANE et al. 1986). The hypodensity seen in AIDS-related lym-phomas may be due, in part, to the greater degree of necrosis present in such lesions. Edema and mass effect are present, but to a variable degree. The pat-tern of edema cannot be used to reliably distin-guish between toxoplasmosis and lymphoma. Hemorrhage and calcification are rare (ZIMMER-MAN 1990).

Postcontrast CT usually reveals somewhat hetero-geneous enhancement and may demonstrate a ring-enhancing lesion owing to central necrosis within the mass (Fig. 5.27). This is in contrast to non-AIDS lymphomas, which usually enhance in a more homo-geneous fashion. The ring-enhancing lesions are of-ten indistinguishable from those of toxoplasmosis. Periventricular enhancement suggests subependy-mal tumor spread, which can be a valuable clue to the radiographic diagnosis of CNS lymphoma (Fig. 5.28). Lesions may be single or multiple.

On MR imaging, lymphomatous lesions which are not necrotic will often appear isointense or slightly hyperintense to parenchyma on T2-weighted imag-es, (Fig. 5.29), likely as a result of the cellularity of these tumors. Necrotic lesions will have a central portion that is bright on T2-weighted images, and a rim which is less bright on the T2-weighted images. This rim often shows dense and irregular enhance-ment after gadolinium administration. The nonne-crotic lesions will enhance more homogeneously (Fig. 5.30). As with CT, there is variable mass effect and edema, and again, lesions may be solitary or, more often, multiple. If there is meningeal involve-ment; this will be much better visualized on postgad-olinium MR imaging than on contrast CT.

HIV-positive patients who present with symp-toms suggestive of an intracranial mass lesion un-dergo CT imaging, usually with the DDD technique or MR imaging. If an enhancing mass lesion is iden-tified, ²⁰¹Tl brain SPECT is often obtained to differ-entiate between an inflammatory process and a neo-plasm (see preceding section on toxoplasmosis). A positive ²⁰¹Tl brain SPECT study indicates the pres-ence of tumor, which in this clinical setting is most compatible with primary CNS lymphoma. A biopsy is then obtained for confirmation (Fig. 5.31). If the

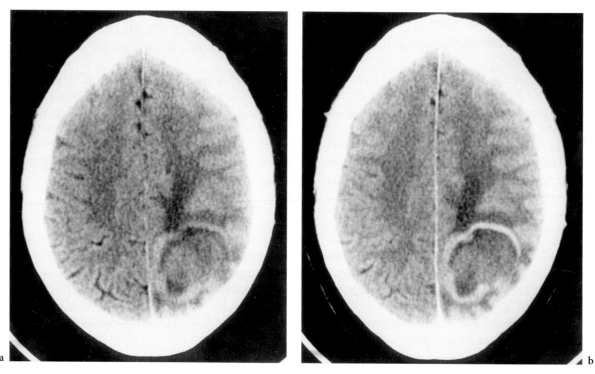

Fig. 5.27a, b. Forty-year-old female with AIDS-related primary CNS lymphoma. **a** Noncontrast axial CT image reveals a left parietal mass with a slightly hyperdense rim. Within this rim are areas of hypodensity and more centrally, an area of isodense soft tissue. Surrounding edema and mass effect are present. **b** Postcontrast image of the same patient demonstrates irregular rim enhancement. The central portion, containing debris and necrosis, does not enhance. This patient had a ^{201}Tl SPECT brain scan which showed focal uptake consistent with a high-grade neoplasm, such as lymphoma

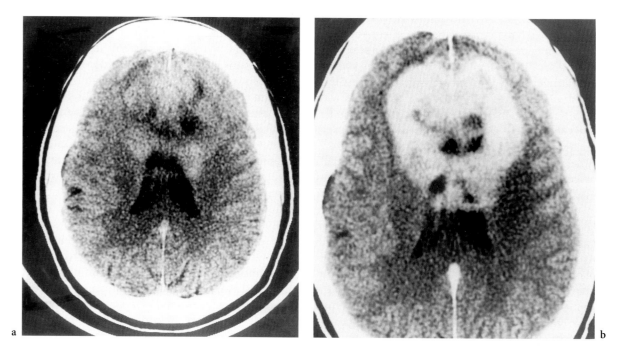

Fig. 5.28a, b. Periventricular enhancement in a patient with primary CNS lymphoma. **a** Noncontrast axial CT reveals mass effect in the frontal region, bilaterally, and patchy areas of hyperdensity as well as iso- and hypodensity. **b** Postcontrast image reveals intense, thick, periventricular enhancement involving the subependymal regions as well as the corpus callosum

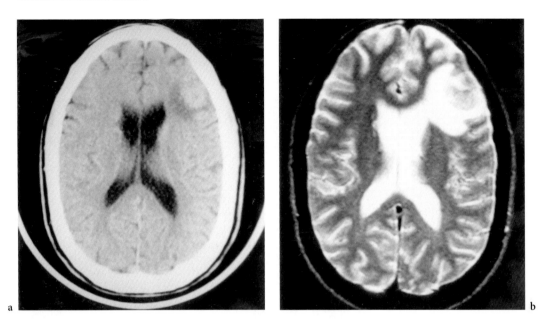

Fig. 5.29a, b. Primary CNS lymphoma in an HIV-seropositive patient. a Noncontrast axial CT reveals a slightly hyperdense lesion in the left frontal lobe with surrounding edema. b T2-weighted axial MR image of the same patient reveals the lesion to be only slightly hyperintense to gray matter with surrounding hyperintense edema

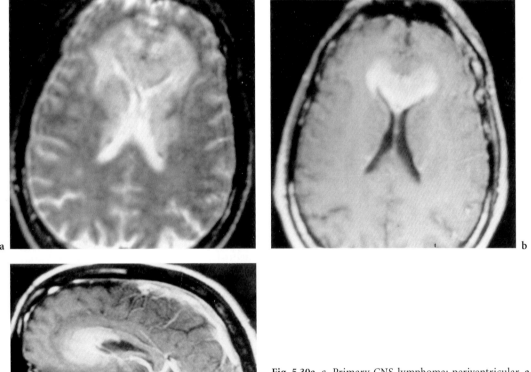

Fig. 5.30a–c. Primary CNS lymphoma: periventricular. a T2-weighted axial MR image reveals mild hyperintensity in the periventricular regions bilaterally with involvement of the corpus callosum and some deformation of the left frontal horn. b, c Sagittal (b) and axial (c) postgadolinium MR images demonstrate extensive periventricular enhancement with infiltration and expansion of the genu of the corpus callosum and involvement of the subependymal region as well

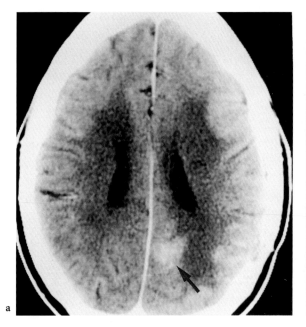
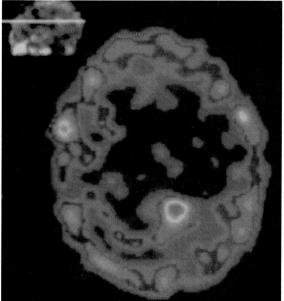

a   b

Fig. 5.31a, b. Primary CNS lymphoma: positive ^{201}Tl brain SPECT (biopsy proven). **a** Postcontrast axial CT reveals a focal area of enhancement in the left parasagittal region (*arrow*). There is adjacent edema and mild mass effect. **b** ^{201}Tl brain SPECT at corresponding level demonstrates focal uptake consistent with a high-grade neoplasm. Biopsy was then performed, confirming the presence of lymphoma. (compare with Fig. 5.23, a negative SPECT study in a patient with toxoplasmosis)

SPECT study is equivocal, other modalities such as spectroscopy may be used to enable this important distinction.

Until the results of ^{201}Tl brain SPECT imaging are available, the patient is placed on antitoxoplasmosis medication. If the SPECT study is more suggestive of an inflammatory process, the therapy is continued and the patient is reimaged in 10–14 days. Significant clinical and radiographic improvement is presumptive evidence for *Toxoplasma* encephalitis. A lack of consistent improvement suggests other etiologies, such as viral, fungal, or mycobacterial disease.

When the initial CT or MR study is obtained, there may be quite extensive edema and mass effect. In addition to the antitoxoplasmosis medications, the patient may be given steroids to reduce the mass effect and edema. The addition of steroids can confuse the radiologic picture and this caveat must be kept in mind. An inflammatory lesion which is not toxoplasmosis may respond to the steroid therapy with a reduction in enhancement, mass effect, and edema. There will appear to be radiographic improvement; however, this is a response to the steroids and not the antitoxoplasmosis therapy. Thus, consistent and persistent improvement needs to be documented as the steroids are tapered down. Additionally, lymphoma can have a transient response to steroid therapy as well, with a reduction in enhance-

ment, mass effect, and edema. This improvement due to steroids can be misinterpreted as a response to the antitoxoplasmosis treatment, when, in fact, the underlying lesion is a lymphoma. This is why additional imaging modalities such as ^{201}Tl SPECT or spectroscopy are necessary, i.e., so that a neoplastic process can be identified quickly and accurately and the appropriate therapy initiated.

As mentioned earlier, MR spectroscopy reveals a fairly characteristic spectral pattern for primary CNS lymphoma with a mild increase in lactate and lipids, a marked elevation in choline, and preservation of some normal metabolites (Fig. 5.32). In contrast, lactate and lipid peaks are markedly elevated in toxoplasmosis, while all other normal metabolites are virtually absent (CHANG et al. 1995). The spectral pattern obtained should allow for discrimination between toxoplasmosis and lymphoma, despite a similar appearance on conventional MR imaging. However, it is essential that the spectroscopy voxel be placed on the cellular portion of a suspected lymphoma, rather than the necrotic portion, as placement over an area of necrosis can produce spectral results which overlap with those of toxoplasmosis.

FDG-PET has also been used to differentiate CNS lymphoma from non-neoplastic lesions. As indicated in Sect. 5.2.4.1, standardized uptake values are significantly greater for lymphoma as compared to toxoplas-

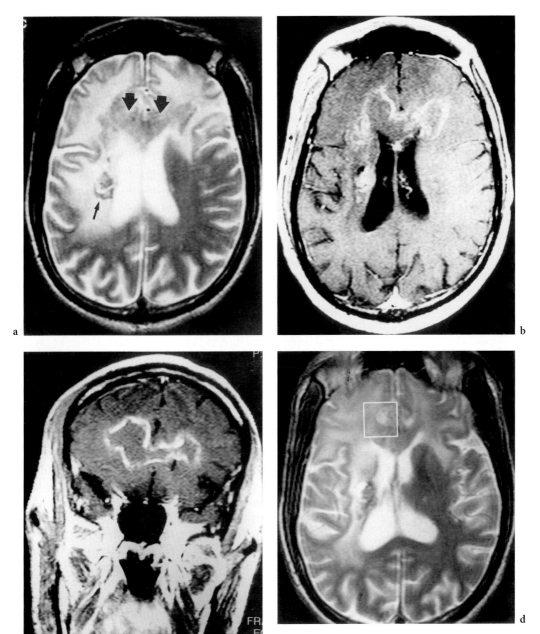

Fig. 5.32a–e. Primary CNS lymphoma – spectroscopic evaluation. **a** T2-weighted axial MR demonstrates abnormal hyperintensity diffusely throughout the white matter of the frontal lobes and in the right corona radiata. There is an isointense mass lesion present in the corpus callosum which narrows the frontal horns of both lateral ventricles (*large arrows*). There is a focal area of hypointense signal along the lateral margin of the right lateral ventricle which is due to a previously treated lesion of toxoplasmosis (*small arrow*). **b** Postcontrast axial MR reveals irregular rim enhancement of the lesion in the corpus callosum. The lesion appears somewhat more extensive on the right. Hyperintense signal is also seen at the site of the prior *Toxoplasma* lesion, adjacent to the right lateral ventricle. **c** Coronal postcontrast image again reveals irregular rim enhancement of the corpus callosum mass with a greater extent of disease on the right. **d, e** MR spectra obtained from the right frontal region using PRESS technique and an 8.0-cc voxel (**d**) reveals a pattern consistent with lymphoma (**e**). There is an elevated choline peak and a depression of the NAA peak. The metabolite peak marked as "lac" on the spectrum is actually due to a combination of lipids and lactate, and in this patient, is primarily due to elevated lipids

mosis, enabling distinction between these two disorders (O'DOHERTY et al. 1997; VILLRINGER et al. 1995).

Overall, the median survival for treated patients with AIDS-related primary CNS lymphoma is 3–4 months (LEVY and ROTHHOLTZ 1997). Supportive care alone results in survival of 1–2 months (LEVY and ROTHHOLTZ 1997). Radiation is the primary treatment modality for these patients. Treatment with high-dose intravenous zidovudine (in combination with other medications) has had promising results (RAEZ et al. 1999). Treatment with chemotherapy is limited by the underlying immunodeficiency in AIDS patients (REMICK et al. 1990). Neurosurgical involvement is primarily directed toward biopsy. The multicentric nature of CNS lymphoma renders surgical therapy an impractical option.

In addition to primary CNS lymphoma, there may be secondary spread of a systemic lymphoma to the central nervous system. This is seen in approximately 20% of AIDS-related systemic lymphoma (SZE et al. 1987). This is usually via meningeal spread and is therefore much better demonstrated with contrast MR imaging than with CT. Symptoms of cranial nerve neuropathy and radiculopathy may result from meningeal spread of disease, in addition to headache and mental status change (SZE et al. 1987).

5.4
AIDS-Related Diseases of the Spine and Spinal Cord

The incidence of spinal infection and spinal neoplasm has been on the rise in recent years. This is due in large part to the increasing population of immunocompromised patients, particularly those with AIDS. In less than two decades, HIV and the AIDS epidemic has spread to more than 190 countries, and all continents (MERTENS and LOW-BEER 1996). Sequelae of HIV-related spinal infection include destruction of vertebral bodies and disc spaces with resultant deformity and neural compromise. Disease may also involve the paraspinal tissues, spinal cord, and nerves, producing potentially permanent neurologic damage. In patients with HIV infection, spinal cord disease is rare in the absence of brain involvement (PETITO 1997). Approximately 7% of AIDS patients appear to have clinical evidence of myelopathy, whereas about 50% of autopsy cases have spinal cord abnormalities (HENIN et al. 1992; MCARTHUR 1987).

HIV-related spinal cord pathology includes vacuolar myelopathy tract pallor, myelitis, opportunistic infection, and neoplasm. Infectious agents include bacterial, fungal, viral, and parasitic pathogens. Lymphoma is the primary neoplastic process involving the spinal cord in AIDS patients. In general, infection presents acutely while spinal cord tumors tend to present more insidiously.

5.4.1
Myelitis

Myelitis indicates a nonspecific inflammation of the spinal cord. Clinical signs include progressive weakness, hypoflexia, and urinary bladder and anal sphincter disturbances. Bacterial infection of the spinal cord is usually a result of systemic bacteremia. A respiratory infection, usually staphylococcal or streptococcal in origin, is the most common source. Sequential imaging studies of the spinal cord suggest that the progression from infectious myelitis to frank cord abscess parallels the evolution from cerebritis to abscess which is seen in the brain (MURPHY et al. 1998). Early MR imaging findings in infectious myelitis include an increase in cord diameter and diffuse, ill-defined hyperintensity on T2-weighted images with poorly defined enhancement on postcontrast T1-weighted images. In later stages, imaging may reveal decreased signal abnormalities on T2-weighted images with well-defined ring enhancement seen following contrast administration, corresponding to intramedullary abscess formation. Following antibiotic therapy, serial scans may show a progressive decrease in the size of the enhancing lesion and associated edema (MURPHY et al. 1998).

Between 1985 and 1991 an estimated 40,000 new cases of TB occurred as a direct result of the AIDS epidemic (SHARIF et al. 1995). TB is estimated to be approximately 500 times more common in AIDS patients than in HIV-negative individuals. Of those patients with AIDS-related TB, approximately 10% have CNS involvement (THURNHER et al. 1997). As with TB elsewhere in the spine, infection is usually the result of hematogenous spread from a primary pulmonary site. Pathologically, mature tuberculomas have a central area of solid caseous necrosis and a capsule of collagenous tissue, epithelioid cells, multinucleated giant cells, and mononuclear inflammatory cells. MR imaging features of intramedullary tuberculomas vary depending on whether the granuloma is noncaseating, caseating with a solid center, or caseating with a liquid center. Noncaseating granulomas are usually hypointense on T1-weighted images and hyperintense on T2-weighted images, and

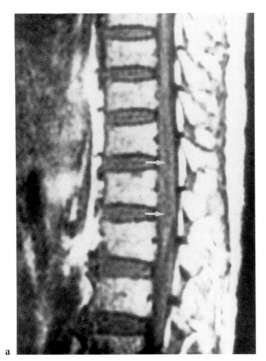
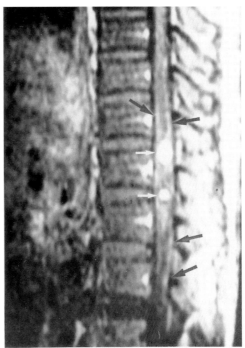

a   b

Fig. 5.33a, b. Noncaseating TB granulomas, TB myelitis. **a** Sagittal T1-weighted MR of the thoracolumbar junction reveals patchy areas of hypointense signal in the conus and lower thoracic spinal cord (*arrows*). **b** After gadolinium administration (and partial fat suppression), there is intense enhancement of two focal nodules within the distal cord and conus (*white arrows*). These are compatible with noncaseating tuberculomas. In addition, there is mild expansion of the conus and less intense enhancement of the distal cord and conus, compatible with myelitis. Note also leptomeningeal enhancement along the surface of the spinal cord as well as some of the nerve roots (*black arrows*)

enhance homogeneously (Fig. 5.33). Caseating granulomas with a solid center are hypointense to isointense on T1-weighted images and isointense to hypointense on T2-weighted images, and demonstrate peripheral enhancement following contrast administration. Caseating granulomas with a liquid center are generally hypointense on T1-weighted images and hyperintense on T2-weighted images, and enhance peripherally (JINKINS et al. 1995; WHITEMAN 1997). The varied appearance of intramedullary tuberculomas implies that these lesions are often indistinguishable from pyogenic infections as well as granulomatous diseases such as spinal sarcoidosis or even intramedullary tumors (GERO et al. 1991).

Other granulomatous infections that affect immunocompromised hosts include those due to fungal agents, such as *Aspergillus, Cryptococcus, Coccidioides immitis, Blastomyces dermatitidis*, and *Histoplasma capsulatum. Cryptococcus* is reported to involve the CNS in approximately 5%–10% of AIDS patients. As with TB, CNS involvement is almost always due to hematogenous spread from a primary pulmonary infection (THURNHER et al, 1997). Coccidiomycosis is endemic in the southwest, blastomy-

cosis in the southeast, and histoplasmosis in the midwestern United States. These infections may be seen in AIDS subpopulations in these regions.

Viral infection of the spinal cord is seen almost exclusively or with increased incidence and severity in AIDS patients. Most have associated brain lesions. About 29% of adult AIDS autopsies demonstrate vacuolar myelopathy (POST et al. 1988a). A recent review by PETITO (1997) found vacuolar myelopathy to be the most common cord pathology in AIDS patients. The neuropathologic findings are similar to those seen with subacute combined degeneration; however, there is no definitive evidence of vitamin B_{12} deficiency in these patients (ROBERTSON et al. 1993). Vacuolar myelopathy is identified microscopically as patchy vacuolation in the white matter of the spinal cord, in association with lipid-laden macrophages. The vacuoles develop from splitting of the myelin lamellae by intramyelinic edema (LIZERBRAM and HESSELINK 1997). This may occur with or without tract pallor, in which a loss of myelin staining occurs without vacuolation or the presence of numerous macrophages (QUENCER and POST 1997; SANTOSH et al. 1995). Both conditions typically involve the dorsal columns and lateral corticospinal tracts of the cervical and thoracic cord. The mid and lower thoracic spine is most often affected (PETITO et al. 1985). T2-weighted MR imaging reveals abnormal intramedullary hyperintensity in approximately two-thirds of patients (SANTOSH et al. 1995), without associated cord enlargement or contrast enhancement (Fig. 5.34). Patients with vacuolar myelopathy generally have a steadily progressive spastic ataxic paraparesis and urinary incontinence, while those with isolated tract pallor have a sensory neuropathy (QUENCER and POST 1997). The clinical correlate to vacuolar myelopathy is HIV-1 associated myelopathy (JANSSEN et al. 1991).

HIV myelitis is far less common that vacuolar myelopathy and is seen in 5%–8% of AIDS patients (PETITO 1997). In HIV myelitis, discrete microglial nodules with multinucleated giant cells involve either the gray or the white matter. This is most often

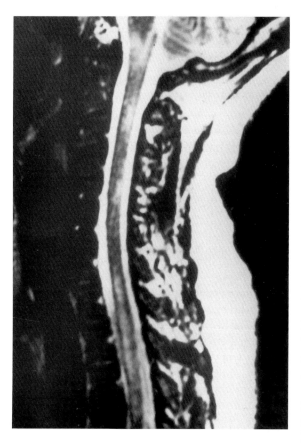

Fig. 5.34. HIV-related signal abnormality of the spinal cord. Sagittal T2-weighted MR image (with partial fat suppression) demonstrates multiple patchy areas of signal abnormality throughout the cervical and upper thoracic spinal cord. There is no cord expansion and there was no enhancement on contrast images. CSF cultures were positive for HTLV III

seen in patients with severe HIV encephalitis (QUENCER and POST 1997) which then extends to the cord, resulting in HIV encephalomyelitis.

Opportunistic viral infections are primarily those of the herpes family including cytomegalovirus (CMV) and herpes simplex virus (HSV) 1 and 2. CMV has been shown pathologically to infect endothelial cells in the periphery of the lumbar and thoracic cord, including the posterior columns and dorsal roots (QUENCER and POST 1997; THURNHER et al. 1997). It may produce tract pallor, myeloradiculitis, or polyradiculopathy. Clinically, a rapidly ascending polyradiculoneuropathy can be seen with a polymorphonuclear CSF pleocytosis (VINTERS et al. 1989). Symptoms at presentation consist of radicular pain, rapidly progressive paraparesis, and urinary retention (WHITEMAN et al. 1994). Deep tendon reflexes are reduced or absent. There is rapid development of a distal flaccid paraparesis, which ascends.

In addition to urinary retention, there is sensory alteration in the lumbar and sacral dermatomes ("saddle anesthesia") (WHITEMAN et al. 1994). Leg and/or back pain is a frequent complaint. The upper extremities are minimally affected.

Diagnosis of CMV polyradiculomyelitis is chiefly based upon the clinical examination and imaging findings (Fig. 5.35). CSF cultures are often negative. PCR (polymerase chain reaction), a DNA amplification technique, can provide a rapid diagnosis in many cases (CINQUE et al. 1992; GOZLAN et al. 1992). Treatment is with ganciclovir, although foscarnet is used if symptoms appear resistant to ganciclovir. Recovery is variable, depending on the degree of involvement and the duration of symptoms.

In patients with CMV infection, unenhanced MR images are often unremarkable, but may occasionally display thickening of the conus and cauda equina. Postcontrast images frequently demonstrate enhancement of the conus, nerve roots, and leptomeninges of the cord (Fig. 5.36). HSV may pathologically affect similar regions of the spinal cord and present with similar symptoms; however, unlike CMV, it has not been described as having clearly identifiable imaging characteristics (THURNHER et al. 1997).

Toxoplasmosis is the primary parasitic infection in AIDS patients. *Toxoplasma gondii* is an obligate intracellular organism, which may produce a self-limited subclinical infection in immunocompetent individuals (REDDY et al. 1995). With immunosuppression, there is reactivation of latent infection. In AIDS patients, toxoplasmosis is rarely found in the spinal cord, but when present, often coexists with brain lesions. In one autopsy study of 138 AIDS pa-

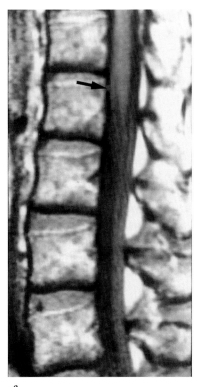

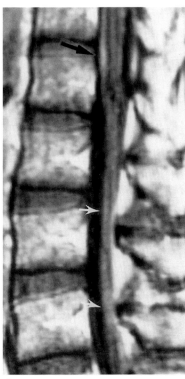

a   b

Fig. 5.35a, b. CMV polyradiculomyelitis. **a** Noncontrast sagittal T1-weighted MR image reveals slight thickening of the ventral nerve roots (*arrow*) but is otherwise unremarkable. **b** Postgadolinium MR image reveals enhancement of the nerve roots (*arrows*)

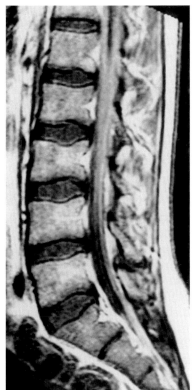

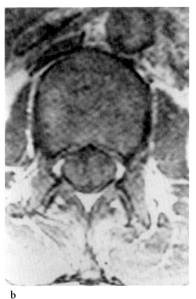

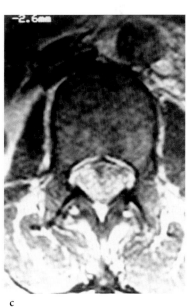

a   b   c

Fig. 5.36a–c. CMV polyradiculomyelitis. **a** Postcontrast T1-weighted sagittal MR image reveals diffuse enhancement of the cauda equina. **b, c** Precontrast (**b**) and postcontrast (**c**) axial images of the same patient as in **a** reveal intense diffuse enhancement of the cauda equina, which also appears thickened and somewhat clumped

tients, cerebral toxoplasmosis was detected in 32 patients, while spinal cord infection with *Toxoplasma* was found in only one patient (HENIN et al. 1992). MR imaging of *Toxoplasma* infection of the spinal cord reveals hypointensity to isointensity on T1-weighted images, hyperintensity on T2-weighted images, and fairly homogeneous enhancement following contrast administration (Fig. 5.37). In the cord, as in the brain, it is difficult to distinguish toxoplasmosis from lymphoma, which may have similar imaging findings. Occasionally, CSF cytology may provide a diagnosis. To date, nuclear scanning with ^{201}Tl SPECT has not been successful in imaging the spinal cord. However, one may favor the diagnosis of spinal lymphoma in a patient with coexisting brain and cord lesions who has a positive ^{201}Tl brain SPECT examination (QUENCER and POST 1997).

5.4.2
Arachnoiditis

Arachnoiditis or leptomeningitis is a broad term denoting inflammation of the meninges and subarach-

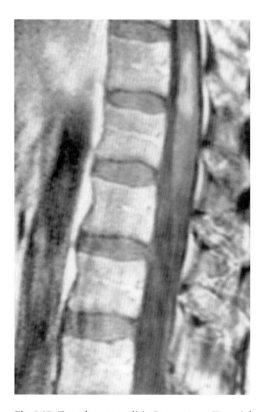

Fig. 5.37. *Toxoplasma* myelitis. Postcontrast T1-weighted sagittal MR reveals focal enhancement within the distal spinal cord in this patient with *Toxoplasma* infection

noid space. In immunocompromised patients etiologies include both neoplastic and infectious causes. Carcinomatous meningitis can result from hematogenous spread of malignancy as well as CSF seeding from primary CNS tumors. CNS lymphomas in AIDS patients are almost always of the B cell type. They may be primary, arising within the neuraxis, or secondary (metastatic) from systemic lymphoma. Although the incidence of primary CNS lymphoma is much greater in AIDS patients than in the general population, the spine is much more likely to be affected by secondary spread of lymphoma arising outside the CNS (THURNHER et al. 1997). With regard to infection, etiologies include bacterial, viral, fungal, and parasitic agents.

Spinal tuberculous meningitis usually arises by dissemination of intracranial tuberculous meningitis through the subarachnoid space. However, infection may also spread to the meninges hematogenously from a source outside the CNS or via intraspinal extension of a discitis/osteomyelitis (GUPTA et al. 1994; WHITEMAN 1997). Pathologically, subarachnoid infection produces meningeal inflammation leading to congestion and inflammatory exudate. Adhesions form between fibrin-coated nerve roots and meninges, resulting in root tethering, blockage of CSF flow, and the formation of CSF loculations. The spinal cord may also be involved as a complication of arachnoiditis. Vascular involvement due to inflammation or compression by fibrous tissue may produce cord ischemia, infarction, myelomalacia, and/or cavitation (SHARMA et al. 1997).

T1-weighted MR images reveal an indistinct or absent cord outline due to an increase in signal intensity of the surrounding CSF, which approaches the signal of the cord. This may be due to an elevation in CSF protein content, the presence of inflammatory exudate, or the formation of microadhesions along the surface of the cord. T2-weighted images, particularly those with MR myelographic technique (heavily T2-weighted FSE with fat suppression), often demonstrate CSF loculations and adhesions in the cervical and thoracic regions with obliteration of the subarachnoid space. In the lumbar region, nerve root fusion may produce irregularly thickened, clumped nerve roots which may occasionally be misinterpreted as a tethered cord (pseudocord) or thickened filum terminale. Peripheral adherence of nerve roots to the thecal sac leads to the "featureless" or "empty" sac (JOHNSON and SZE 1990).

Contrast enhancement in lumbar arachnoiditis has a variable appearance. The presence of enhancement may be due to development of a vascular network within the fibrous stroma proliferating in the subarachnoid space. Three patterns of enhancement have been described. The most common is a smooth, linear layer of enhancement outlining the surface of the cord and nerve roots. Next is a nodular pattern with discrete foci of enhancement seen along the surface of the cord and nerve roots. The least common pattern consists of diffuse, thick intradural enhancement which completely fills the subarachnoid space (Fig. 5.38). Unfortunately, no enhancement pattern is characteristic of any specific infectious agent or neoplasm (GERO et al. 1991; GUPTA et al. 1994).

5.4.3
Discitis/Osteomyelitis

Disease of the spinal column in AIDS patients includes both infectious and neoplastic processes. Bacterial infections, for example those caused by *Staphylococcus aureus* and *M. tuberculosis*, are the most common cause of discitis, osteomyelitis, epidural phlegmon/abscess, and paraspinal abscess in AIDS

patients. A prospective cohort study of infants born to HIV-infected mothers concluded that the rate of invasive bacterial infection is higher in HIV-infected children than in their peers (GLAZER and HU 1996). Infection is usually spread hematogenously and therefore begins in the most richly vascularized structure in the spine. In children, this is the disc space, while in adults the cancellous bone adjacent to the cartilaginous end plates receives the greatest blood supply.

Imaging studies performed in patients with pyogenic infection of the spine show disc space narrowing with osteolytic destruction of the adjacent vertebral end plates. In contrast to degenerated, desiccated discs, which are hypointense on T2-weighted MR images, infected, edematous discs are hyperintense on T2-weighted acquisitions. The adjacent vertebral marrow is replaced by inflammatory tissue, seen as abnormal hypointensity on T1-weighted images and hyperintensity on T2-weighted sequences (Fig. 5.39). Postcontrast images demonstrate peripheral or diffuse enhancement of the disc space and enhancement of the adjacent vertebral end plates (THURNHER et al.

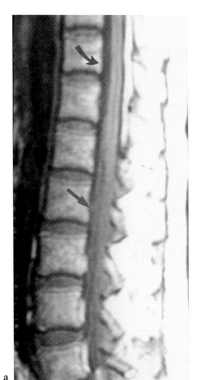
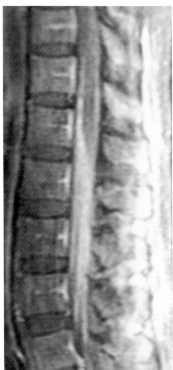
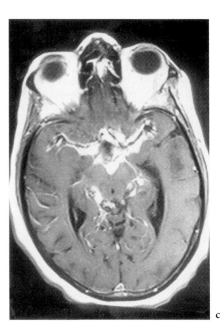

a   b   c

Fig. 5.38a–c. Tuberculous arachnoiditis/intracranial meningitis. **a** Noncontrast T1-weighted sagittal MR demonstrates slight hyperintensity of the CSF in the lumbar region (*straight arrow*) as compared with the normal appearance of the CSF in the thoracic region (*curved arrow*). **b** Postcontrast image with fat suppression demonstrates diffuse enhancement of the lumbar subarachnoid space and cauda equina, with leptomeningeal enhancement seen along the surface of the conus. **c** Axial T1-weighted postcontrast intracranial image from the same patient reveals an extensive basilar meningitis with enhancement seen diffusely throughout the basal cisterns

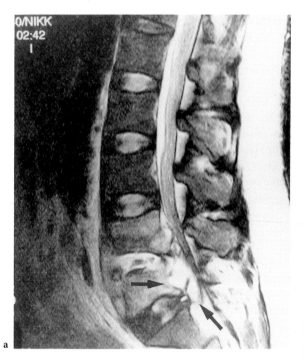

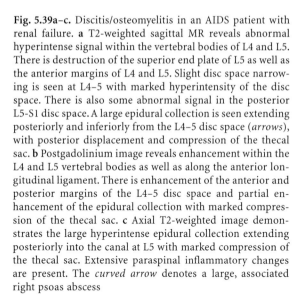

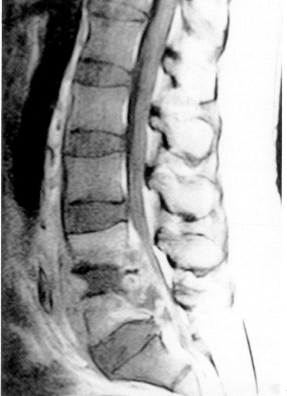

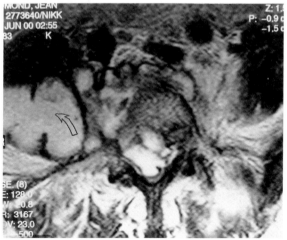

Fig. 5.39a–c. Discitis/osteomyelitis in an AIDS patient with renal failure. **a** T2-weighted sagittal MR reveals abnormal hyperintense signal within the vertebral bodies of L4 and L5. There is destruction of the superior end plate of L5 as well as the anterior margins of L4 and L5. Slight disc space narrowing is seen at L4–5 with marked hyperintensity of the disc space. There is also some abnormal signal in the posterior L5-S1 disc space. A large epidural collection is seen extending posteriorly and inferiorly from the L4–5 disc space (*arrows*), with posterior displacement and compression of the thecal sac. **b** Postgadolinium image reveals enhancement within the L4 and L5 vertebral bodies as well as along the anterior longitudinal ligament. There is enhancement of the anterior and posterior margins of the L4–5 disc space and partial enhancement of the epidural collection with marked compression of the thecal sac. **c** Axial T2-weighted image demonstrates the large hyperintense epidural collection extending posteriorly into the canal at L5 with marked compression of the thecal sac. Extensive paraspinal inflammatory changes are present. The *curved arrow* denotes a large, associated right psoas abscess

1997). Tuberculous infections are more insidious and may have a better prognosis than pyogenic infections (Fig. 5.40). The intervertebral disc spaces are often preserved until late in the disease process. A lack of proteolytic enzymes in the mycobacterium has been proposed as one of the causes of relative preservation of the disc compared with pyogenic infection. Hematogenous spread of tuberculous bacilli is thought to begin in the anterior and inferior portions of the vertebral body. L1 is the most common site of infec-

tion. Untreated infection may spread beneath the longitudinal ligaments, destroying multiple vertebrae and resulting in a gibbus deformity.

Spread of infection into the epidural or paraspinal region may accompany infectious spondylitis. Again, *Staphylococcus aureus* is the most common organism in both immunocompetent and immunocompromised patients. Collections are typically isointense or hypointense to the spinal cord on T1-weighted images and hyperintense on T2-weighted images. Homoge-

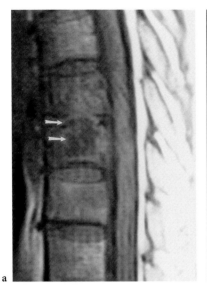
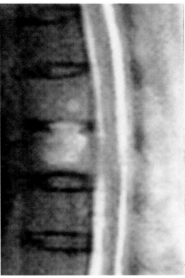
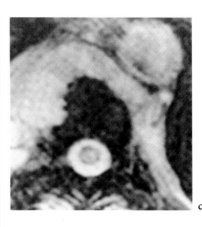

a

b

c

Fig. 5.40a–c. Tuberculous discitis/osteomyelitis. **a** Noncontrast T1-weighted MR image reveals abnormal hypointensity within a thoracic vertebral body, extending superiorly into the adjacent disc space (*arrows*). The disc space is narrowed. **b** T2-weighted sagittal MR with fat suppression again reveals abnormal signal in the vertebral body and disc space. **c** Axial T2-weighted image from another patient with TB discitis/osteomyelitis demonstrates erosive changes of the vertebral body on the right, associated with a large pre- and paravertebral collection in this patient with Pott's disease

neous enhancement is typical of phlegmon, whereas peripheral enhancement surrounding a nonenhancing center is more indicative of a liquefactive abscess. In contrast to acute/subacute abscesses which contain frank pus, chronic abscesses may be filled with granulation tissue and thus enhance more homogeneously. Paraspinal abscess formation is strongly suggestive of tuberculosis, especially when calcification and/or bilaterality is present (THURNHER et al. 1997).

Spinal lymphoma affecting AIDS patients may be osseous, epidural, leptomeningeal, or intramedullary in location (Fig. 5.41). Lymphomatous bone marrow involvement has been reported in approximately 22% of patients with AIDS (SAFAI et al. 1992). The normal bright signal of marrow on T1-weighted images is replaced by hypointense soft tissue, which also enhances after gadolinium administration. These areas are usually slightly hyperintense on T2-weighted images. MR imaging of spinal cord lymphoma may reveal an enlarged cord with intramedullary iso- to hyperintensity on T2-weighted images, hypointensity on T1-weighted images, and patchy enhancement following contrast administration. In contrast to the brain, where primary CNS lymphoma is seen fairly often in AIDS patients, spinal cord involvement is rare, and has been identified in only 2%4% of a postmortem series (PETITO 1997).

Epidural lymphoma is almost always due to direct extension of lymphoma from affected vertebral bodies

rather than from hematogenous spread (LI et al. 1992). The epidural soft tissue mass can produce compression of the thecal sac or frank cord compression, and may also extend into the neural foramina (Fig. 5.42).

Leptomeningeal spread of lymphoma may occur as a result of hematogenous spread or from CSF

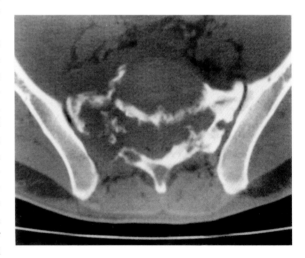

Fig. 5.41. Lymphoma of the sacrum. Axial CT image through the sacrum demonstrates an extensive lytic and destructive process with epidural extension into the spinal canal. Biopsy revealed lymphoma. This was the patient's initial manifestation of AIDS. He was not previously known to be HIV positive, although subsequent testing determined that he was HIV seropositive

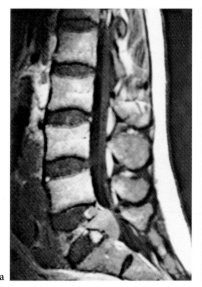

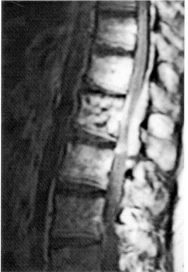

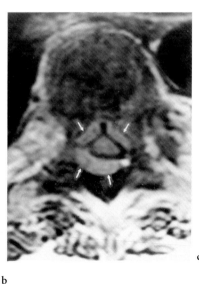

a

b

c

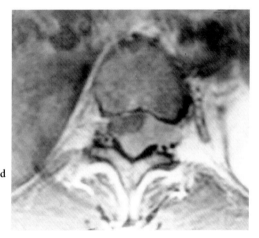

d

Fig. 5.42a–d. Epidural lymphoma. **a** T1-weighted postcontrast sagittal MR image reveals marked compression of the L5 vertebral body due to lymphoma. There is a large associated posterior epidural soft tissue component which extends into the canal and causes significant sac compression. **b** Postcontrast T1-weighted sagittal MR of another patient with osseous and epidural lymphoma reveals loss of stature and abnormal signal in several vertebral bodies. There is nearly circumferential epidural soft tissue encasing and compressing the thoracic spinal cord. **c** T1-weighted axial MR image without contrast of another patient with epidural lymphoma. Slightly hyperintense epidural soft tissue is seen surrounding the thecal sac (*arrows*), with sac compression and mild deformity of the cord. **d** T1-weighted postgadolinium axial image of another patient with epidural lymphoma shows a mildly enhancing mass in the canal with displacement of the sac to the right and moderate sac compression. There is also extension into the left neural foramen

seeding within the subarachnoid space. Pial enhancement may be seen along the surface of the cord, and multiple enhancing nerve roots may be visualized within the thecal sac (Fig. 5.43). The nerve roots may also appear thickened and clumped.

References

Abrams EJ, Matheson PB, Thomas PA, et al. (1995) Neonatal predictors of infection status and early death among 332 infants at risk of HIV-1 infection monitored prospectively from birth, New York City perinatal HIV transmission collaborative study group. Pediatrics 96:451–458

Adair JC, Beck AC, Apfelbaum RI, et al. (1987) Nocardial cerebral abscess in the acquired immunodeficiency syndrome. Arch Neurol 44:548–550

Atlas SW, Grossman RI, Hackney DB, et al. (1988) Calcified intracranial lesions: detection with gradient echo acquisition rapid MR imaging. AJNR 9:253–259

Bailey R, Baltch A, Venkatish R, et al. (1988) Sensory motor neuropathy associated with AIDS. Neurology 38:886–891

Bale JF Jr (1984) Human cytomegalovirus infection and disorders of the nervous system of patients with the acquired immune deficiency syndrome. Arch Neurol 41:310–320

Barnicoat MJ, Wierzbicki AS, Norman PM (1989) Cerebral nocardiosis in immunosuppressed patients: five cases. Q J Med 268:689–698

Baron AL, Steinbach LS, LeBoit PE, et al. (1990) Osteolytic lesions and bacillary angiomatosis in HIV infection: radiological differentiation from AIDS-related Kaposi sarcoma. Radiology 177:77–81

Beaman B, Burnside J, Edwards B, et al. (1976) Nocardial infection in the United States, 1972–1974. J Infect Dis 134:286–289

Belman AL (1990) AIDS and pediatric neurology. Neurol Clin North Am 8:571–603

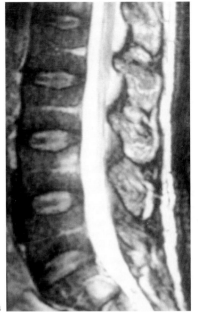
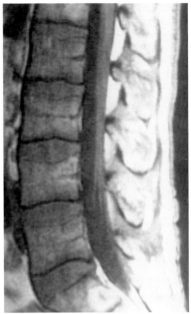
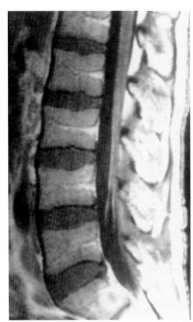

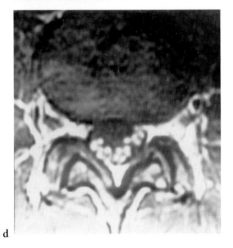

Fig. 5.43a–d. Lymphomatous meningitis in an HIV-seropositive patient. **a** On this T2-weighted sagittal MR image, the nerve roots appear unremarkable. The lesion in the posterior aspect of S1 is likely a fat island or hemangioma. **b, c** Precontrast (**b**) and postcontrast (**c**) T1-weighted sagittal images reveal smooth, linear enhancement along the nerve roots of the cauda equina. **d** Postcontrast axial T1-weighted image reveals prominent, diffuse enhancement of the nerve roots of the cauda equina, which also appear slightly thickened

Belman AL (1997) Pediatric neuro-AIDS, update. Neuroimaging Clin North Am 7:593–613

Belman AL, Novick B, Ultmann MH, et al. (1984) Neurological complications in children with acquired immune deficiency syndrome. Ann Neurol 16:414

Belman AL, Ultmann MH, Horoupian D, et al. (1985) Neurological complications of infants and children with acquired immune deficiency syndrome. Ann Neurol 18:560–566

Belman AL, Diamond G, Dickson D, et al. (1988) Pediatric AIDS: neurologic syndromes. Am J Dis Child 142:29–35

Berenguer J, Moreno S, Laguna F, et al. (1992) Tuberculous meningitis in patients infected with the human immunodeficiency virus. N Engl J Med 326:668–672

Berger JR, Kaszowitz B, Post MJD, et al. (1987a) Progressive multifocal leukoencephalopathy associated with human immunodeficiency virus infection. A review of the literature with a report of sixteen cases. Ann Intern Med 107:78–87

Berger JR, Moskowitz L, Fischl M, et al. (1987b) Neurological disease as the presenting manifestation of acquired immunodeficiency syndrome. South Med J 80:683–686

Bishburg E, Sunderama G, Reichman LB, et al. (1986) Central nervous system tuberculosis with the acquired immunodeficiency syndrome and its related complex. Ann Intern Med 105:210–213

Bottomley PA (1987) Spatial localization in NMR spectroscopy in vivo. Ann NY Acad Sci 508:333

Bowen BC, Post MJD (1991) Intracranial infection. In: Atlas SW (ed) Magnetic resonance imaging of the brain and spine. Raven, New York, pp 501–538

Boyd JF (1980) Adult cytomegalic inclusion disease. Scott Med J 25:266–269

Boyer PJ, Dillon M, Navaie M, et al. (1994) Factors predictive of maternal-fetal transmission of HIV-1: preliminary analysis of zidovudine given during pregnancy and/or delivery. JAMA 271:1925–1930

Britton CB, Miller JR (1984) Neurological complications of acquired immunodeficiency syndrome (AIDS). Neurol Clin 2:315–339

Brooks BR, Walker DL (1984) Progressive multifocal leukoencephalopathy. Neurol Clin 2:299–313

Bross JE, Gordon G (1991) Nocardial meningitis: case reports and review. Rcv Infect Dis 13:160–165

Brunetti A, Berg C, DiChiro G, et al. (1989) Reversal of brain metabolic abnormalities following treatment of AIDS dementia complex with 3'-azido-2,3' dideoxythymidine (AZT, zidovudine): PET-FDG study. J Nucl Med 30:567–597

Carbajal JR, Palacios E, Azar-kia B, et al. (1977) Radiology of cysticercosis of the central nervous system including computed tomography. Radiology 125:127–131

Carne CA, Tedder RS, Smith A, et al. (1985) Acute encephalopathy coincident with seroconversion for anti-HTLV-III. Lancet 2:1206–1208

Centers for Disease Control (1983) Primary resistance to anti-tuberculous drugs – United States. MMWR Morb Mortal Wkly Rep 32:521–523

Centers for Disease Control (1987) Tuberculosis and acquired immunodeficiency syndome – New York City. MMWR Morb Mortal Wkly Rep 36:785–795

Centers for Disease Control and Prevention (1996) HIV/AIDS surveillance report. 8:1–33

Chang K-H, Lee JH, Han MH, et al. (1991) The role of contrast-enhanced MR imaging in the diagnosis of neurocysticercosis. AJNR 128:509–512

Chang L, Ernst T. (1997) MR spectroscopy and diffusion weighted MR imaging in focal brain lesions in AIDS. Neuroimag Clin North Am 7:409–429

Chang L, Miller B, McBride D, et al. (1995) Brain lesions in patients with AIDS: H-1 MR spectroscopy. Radiology 197:527

Chang L, Ernst T, Tornatore C, et al. (1997) Metabolite abnormalities in progressive multifocal leukoencephalopathy: a proton magnetic resonance spectroscopy study. Neurology 48:836–845

Chong WK, Sweeney B. Wilkinson I, et al. (1993) Proton spectroscopy of the brain in HIV infection: correlation with clinical, immunological, and MR imaging findings. Radiology 188:119–124

Chrysikopoulous HS, Press GA, Grafe MR, et al. (1990) Encephalitis caused by human immunodeficiency virus: CT and MR imaging manifestations with clinical and pathological correlation. Radiology 175:185–191

Cinque P, Vago L, Brytting M, et al. (1992) Cytomegalovirus infection of the central nervous system in patients with AIDS: diagnosis by DNA amplification from cerebrospinal fluid. J Infect Dis 166:1408–1411

Civitello LA (1993) Neurologic manifestations of HIV infection in infants and children. Pediatr AIDS HIV Infection 4:227–234

Connor EM, Sperling RS, Gelber R, et al. (1994) Reduction of maternal-infant transmission of human immunodeficiency virus type I with zidovudine treatment. N Engl J Med 331:1173–1180

Cuadrado LM, Guerrero A, et al. (1988) Cerebral mucormycosis in two cases of acquired immunodeficiency syndrome. Arch Neurol 45:109–111

Curless RG, Mitchell CD (1991) Central nervous system tuberculosis in children. Pediatr Neurol 7:270–274

Danner SA (1995) Management of cytomegalovirus disease. AIDS 9 (Suppl 2):S3–S8

Dastur DK (1972) Neurotuberculosis. In: Minckler J (ed) Pathology of the nervous system, vol 3. McGraw-Hill, New York, pp 2412–2422

Davenport C, Dillon WP, Sze G (1992) Neuroradiology of the immunosuppressed state. Radiol Clin North Am 30:611–637

Davidson HD, Steiner RE (1985) Magnetic resonance imaging of infections of the central nervous system. AJNR 6:499–504

Davis LE, Kornfeld M (1991) Neurocysticercosis: neurological, pathogenic, diagnostic and therapeutic aspects. Eur Neurol 31:229–240

De La Paz RL, Enzmann D (1988) Neuroradiology of acquired immunodeficiency syndrome. In: Rosenblum ML, et al. (eds) AIDS and the nervous system. Raven, New York, pp 121–153

Depas G, Chiron C, Tardieu M, et al. (1995) Functional brain imaging in HIV-1-infected children born to seropositive mothers. J Nucl Med 36:2169–2174

Dickson DW, Belman Al, Park YD, et al. (1989) Central nervous system pathology in pediatric AIDS: an autopsy study. APMIS 8 (Suppl): 40–57

Dina TS (1991) Primary central nervous system lymphoma versus toxoplasmosis in AIDS. Radiology 179:823–828

Ennis DM, Saag MS (1993) Cryptococcal meningitis in AIDS. Hosp Pract (Off Ed) 28:99–102

Epstein LG, Sharer LR, Joshi VV (1985) Progressive encephalopathy in children with acquired immune deficiency syndrome. Ann Neurol 17: 488–496

Epstein LG, Sharer LR, Goudsmit J (1988) Neurological and neuropathological features of human immunodeficiency virus infection in children. Ann Neurol 23 (Suppl 6): 19–23

Ernst TM, Chang L, Witt MD, et al. (1998) Cerebral toxoplasmosis and lymphoma in AIDS: perfusion MR imaging experience in 13 patients. Radiology 208:663–669

Escobar A (1983) The pathology of neurocysticercosis. In: Palacios E, Rodriguez-Carbajal J, Taveras JM (eds) Cysticercosis of the central nervous system. Charles C. Thomas, Springfield, pp 27–59

European Collaborative Study (1994) Natural history of vertically acquired human immunodeficiency virus-1 infection. Pediatrics 94:815–819

Forsyth PA, DeAngelis LM (1996) Biology and management of AIDS-associated primary CNS lymphomas. Hematol Oncol Aspects HIV Infect 10:1125–1135

Frahm J, Merboldt KD, Hanicke W (1987) Localized proton spectroscopy using stimulated echoes. J Magn Reson B72:502

Frazier AR, Rosenow EC, Roberts GD (1975) Nocardiosis. A review of 25 cases occurring during 24 months. Mayo Clin Proc 50:657–663

Gabuzda DH, Ho DD, dela Monte SM, et al. (1986) Immunohistochemical identification of HTLV-III antigen in brains of patients with AIDS. Ann Neurol 20:289–295

Gartner S, Markovits P, Markovits DM, et al. (1986) Virus isolation from and identification of HTLV-III/LAV-producing cells in brain tissue from a patient with AIDS. JAMA 256:2365–2371

Gero B, Sze G, Sharif H (1991) MR imaging of intradural inflammatory diseases of the spine. AJNR 12:1009–1019

Girrard PM, Landman R, Gandebout C, et al. (1993) Dapsone-pyrimethamine compared with aerosolized pentamidine as primary prophylaxis against Pneumocystis carinii pneumonia and toxoplasmosis in HIV infection. N Engl J Med 328:1514–1520

Glazer PA, Hu SS (1996) Pediatric spinal infections. Orthop Clin North Am 27:111–122

Gozlan J, Salord J-M, Roullet E, et al (1992) Rapid detection of cytomegalovirus DNA in cerebrospinal fluid of AIDS patients with neurologic disorders. J Infect Dis 166:1416–1421

Grant I, Atkinson JH, Hesselink JR, et al. (1987) Evidence for early central nervous system involvement in the acquired immunodeficiency syndrome (AIDS) and the human immunodeficiency virus (HIV) infections. Ann Intern Med 107:828–836

Greenfield JG (1984) Greenfield's Neuropathology, 4th edn. Wiley, New York, pp 261–288

Gupta RK, Jena A, Sharma DK, et al. (1988) MR imaging of intracranial tuberculomas. J Comput Assist Tomogr 12:280–285

Gupta RK, Gupta S, Kumar S, et al. (1994) MRI in intraspinal tuberculosis. Neuroradiology 36:39–43

Gwinn M, Pappaioanou M, George JR, et al. (1991) Prevalence of HIV infection in childbearing women in the United States. JAMA 265:1704–1708

Hamilton RL, Achim C, Grafe MR (1995) Herpes simplex virus brainstem encephalitis in an AIDS patient. Clin Neuropathol 14:45–50

Harris DE, Enterline DS, Tien RD (1997) Neurosyphilis in patients with AIDS. Neuroimaging Clin North Am 7:215–221

Henin D, Smith TW, DeGirolami U, et al. (1992) Neuropathology of the spinal cord in the acquired immunodeficiency syndrome. Hum Pathol 23:1106–1114

Ho DD, Rota TR, Schooler RT (1985) Isolation of HTLV-III from cerebrospinal fluid and neuronal tissue of patients with neurological syndromes related to the acquired immunodefiency syndrome. N Engl J Med 313:1493–1497

Ho DD, Bredesen DE, Vinters HV, et al. (1989) The acquired immunodeficiency syndrome (AIDS) dementia complex. Ann Intern Med 111:400

Ihmeidan IH, Post MJD, Katz D, et al. (1989) Radiographic findings in HIV+ patients with neurosyphilis. AJNR 10:896

Jabs DA (1995) Ocular manifestations of HIV infection. Trans Opththalmol Soc 93:623–683

Janssen RS (1996) Epidemiology and neuroepidemiology of human immunodeficiency virus infection. In: Berger JR, Levy RM (eds) AIDS and the nervous system, 2nd edn. Lipponcott-Raven, Philadelphia, pp 13–37

Janssen RS, Cornblath DR, Epstein LG, et al. (1991) Nomenclature and research case definitions for neurological manifestations of human immunodeficiency virus-type I (HIV-1) infection: report of a working group of the American Academy of Neurology Task Force. Neurology 41:778–785

Jarvik JG, Lenkinski R, Grossman R, et al. (1993) Proton MR spectroscopy of HIV-infected patients: characterization of abnormalities with imaging and clinical correlation. Radiology 186:739–744

Javaly K, Horowitz HW, Wormser GP (1992) Nocardiosis in patients with human immunodeficiency virus infection. Report of 2 cases and review of the literature. Medicine 71:128–138

Jiddane M, Nicole F, Diaz P, et al. (1986) Intracranial malignant lymphoma. Report of 30 cases and review of the literature. J Neurosurg 65:592–599

Jinkins JR (1991) Computed tomography of intracranial tuberculosis. Neuroradiology 33:126–135

Jinkins RJ, Gupta R, Chang KH, et al. (1995) MR imaging of central nervous system tuberculosis. Radiol Clin North Am 33:771–785

Johnson CE, Sze G (1990) Benign lumbar arachnoiditis: MR imaging with gadopentetate dimeglumine. AJNR 11:763–770

Jones HR, Hedley-Whyte T, Friedberg SR, et al. (1982) Primary cerebellopontine progressive multifocal leukoencephalopathy diagnosed premortem by cerebellar biopsy. Am Neurol 11:199–202

Jordan BD, Navia BA, Petito C, et al. (1985) Neurological syndromes complicating AIDS. Front Radiat Ther Oncol 19:82–87

Jordan J, Enzmann DR (1991) Encephalitis. Neuroimag Clin North Am 1:17–38

Joshi VV, Power B, Conner E, et al. (1987) Arteriopathy in children with acquired immune deficiency syndrome. Pediatr Pathol 7:261–275

Katz DA, Berger JR (1989) Neurosyphilis in acquired immunodeficiency syndrome. Arch Neurol 46:895–898

Katz DA, Berger JR, Duncan RC (1993) Neurosyphilis, a comparative study of the effects of infection with human immunodeficiency virus. Arch Neurol 50:243–249

Khan MA, Kovnat DM, Bachus B, et al. (1977) Clinical and roentgenographic spectrum of pulmonary tuberculosis in the adult. Am J Med 62:31–38

Knox JM, Musher D, Guzick ND (1976) The pathogenesis of syphilis and related treponematoses. In: Johnson RC (ed) The biology of parasitic spirochetes. Academic Press, San Diego, pp 249–259

Kobayshi GS (1980) Fungi. In: Davis BD, Dulbecco R, Eisen HN, Ginsbert HS (eds) Microbiology. Harper & Row, New York, pp 817–850

Kramer LD, Locke GE, Byrd SE, et al. (1989) Cerebral cysticercosis: documentation of the natural history with CT. Radiology 171:459–462

Krick JA, Remington JS (1978) Current concepts in parasitology. Toxoplasmosis in the adult – an overview. N Engl J Med 298:550–553

Krupp LB, Lipton RB, Swerdlow ML, et al. (1985) Progressive multifocal leukoencephalopathy: clinical and radiographic features. Ann Neurol 17:344–349

LeBlang SD, Whiteman MLH, Post MJD, et al. (1995) CNS nocardia in AIDS patients: CT and MRI with pathologic correlation. J Comput Assist Tomogr 19:15–22

LeBoit PE, Berger T, Egbert BM, et al. (1989) Bacillary angiomatosis: the histopathology and differential diagnosis of a pseudoneoplastic infection in patients with HIV infection. Am J Surg Pathol 13:909–920

Leestma JE (1985) Viral infections of the nervous system. In: Davis RL, Robertson DM (eds) Textbook of neuropathology. Williams & Wilkins, Baltimore, pp 704–787

Leiguarda R, Berthier M, Starkstein S, et al. (1988) Ischemic infarction in 25 children with tuberculous meningitis. Stroke 19:200–204

Levy RM, Rothholtz V (1997) HIV-1 related neurologic disorders, neurosurgical implications. Neuroimag Clin North Am 7:527–559

Levy RM, Pons VG, Rosenblum ML (1984) Central nervous system mass lesions in the acquired immunodeficiency syndrome (AIDS). J Neurosurg 61:9–16

Levy RM, Bredesen DE, Rosenblum ML (1985) Neurological manifestations of the acquired immunodeficiency syndrome (AIDS): experience at UCSF and review of the literature. J Neurosurg 62:475–495

Levy RM, Rosenbloom S, Perrett LV (1986) Neuroradiological findings in the acquired immunodeficiency syndrome (AIDS): a review of 200 cases. AJNR 7:833–839

Li MH, Holtas S, Larsson EM (1992) MR imaging of spinal lymphoma. Acta Radiol 33:338–342

Lizerbram EK, Hesselink JR (1997) Viral infections. Neuroimaging Clin North Am 7:261–280

Lobato MN, Caldwell MB, Ng P, et al. (1995) Encephalopathy in children with perinatally acquired immunodeficiency syndrome virus infection: pediatric spectrum of disease clinical consortium. J Pediatr 126:170–175

Lobato RD, Lamas E, Portillo JM, et al. (1981) Hydrocephalus in cerebral cysticercosis. J Neurosurg 55:786–793

Lopes-Hernandez A (1983) Clinical manifestations and sequential computed tomographic scans of cerebral cysticercosis in childhood. Brain Dev 5:269–277

Louie E, Rice LB, Holzman RS (1986) Tuberculosis in non-Haitian patients with acquired immunodeficiency syndrome. Chest 90:542–545

Lu D, Pavlakis SG, Frank Y (1996) Magnetic spectroscopy of the basal ganglia in normal children and children with AIDS. Radiology 199:423–428

Luft BJ, Remington JS (1992) Toxoplasmic encephalitis in acquired immune deficiency syndrome. Clin Infect Dis 15:211–222

Luft BJ, Hafner R, Korzun AH, et al. (1993) Toxoplasmic encephalitis in patients with the acquired immunodeficiency syndrome. N Engl J Med 329:995–1000

Lyons RW, Andriole VT (1986) Fungal infections of the CNS. Neurol Clin 159–170

MacMahon EME, Glass JD, Hayward SD, et al. (1991) Epstein Barr virus (EBV) in acquired immune deficiency syndrome-related primary central nervous system lymphoma. Lancet 338:969–973

Major EO, Amemiya K, Tornatore CS, et al. (1992) Pathogenesis and molecular biology of progressive multifocal leukoencephalopathy. the JC virus-induced demyelinating disease of the human brain. Clin Microbiol Rev 5:49–73

Martinez AJ, Sell M, Mitrovis T, et al. (1995) The neuropathology and epidemiology of AIDS: a Berlin experience: a review of 220 cases. Pathol Res Pract 191:427–443

Masdeu JC, Van Heertum FL, Abdel-Dayem H (1995) Viral infections of the brain. J Neuroimaging (Suppl 1): 40–44

Mathews VP, Alo PL, Glass JD, et al. (1992) AIDS-related CNS cryptococcosis: radiological-pathological correlation. AJNR 13:1477–1486

Mazlo M, Tariska I (1980) Morphological demonstration of the first phase of polyomavirus replication in oligodendroglia cells of human brain in progressive multifocal leuko-encephalopathy (PML). Neuropathology 49:133–143

McArthur JC (1987) Neurologic manifestations of acquired immune deficiency syndrome. Medicine 66:407–437

McArthur JC, Cohen BA, Selnes OA, et al. (1989) Low prevalence of neurological and neuropsychological abnormalities in otherwise healthy HIV-1 infected individuals : results from the Multicenter AIDS Cohort Study. Ann Neurol 26:601–611

McCormick GF (1985) Cysticercosis: review of 230 patients. Bull Clin Neurosci 50:76–101

McCutchen JA (1995) Cytomegalovirus infections of the nervous system in patients with AIDS. Clin Infect Dis 20:747–754

Mehta JB, Dutt A, Harrill L, et al. (1991) Epidemiology of extrapulmonary tuberculosis. A comparative analysis with pre-AIDS era. Chest 99:1134–1138

Menon DK, Baudouin CJ, Tomlinson D, et al. (1990) Proton MR spectroscopy and imaging of the brain in AIDS: evidence of neuronal loss in regions that appear normal with imaging. J Comput Assist Tomogr 14:882–885

Mertens TE, Low-Beer D (1996) HIV and AIDS: where is the epidemic going? Bull World Health Org 74:121–129

Meyerhoff DJ, MacKay S, Poole N, et al. (1993) Reduced brain N-acetylaspartate suggest neuronal loss in cognitively impaired human immunodeficiency virus-seropositive individuals: in vivo H magnetic resonance spectroscopic imaging. Neurology 43:509–515

Mintz M, Epstein LG (1992) Neurologic manifestations of pediatric acquired immunodeficiency syndrome: clinical features and therapeutic appoaches. Semin Neurol 12:51–56

Murphy KJ, Brunberg JA, Quint DJ, et al. (1998) Spinal cord infection: myelitis and abscess formation. AJNR 19:341–348

Navia BA, Gonzalez RG (1997) Functional imaging of the AIDS dementia complex and the metabolic pathology of the HIV-1 infected brain. Neuroimag Clin North Am 7:431–445

Navia BA, Rottenberg DA, Sidtis J, et al. (1985) Regional cerebral glucose metabolism in AIDS dementia complex. Neurology 35:226

Navia BA, Jordan BD, Price RW (1986a) The AIDS dementia complex 1. Clinical features. Ann Neurol 19:517–524

Navia BA, Cho E-S, Petito CK, et al. (1986b) The AIDS dementia complex: II Neuropathology. Ann Neurol 19:525–535

Nielsen SL, Petito CK, Urmacher CD, et al. (1984) Subacute encephalitis in acquired immune deficiency syndrome : a postmortem study. Am J Clin Pathol 82:678–682

O'Doherty MJ, Barrington SF, Campbell M, et al. (1997) PET scanning and the human immunodeficiency virus-positive patient. J Nucl Med 38:1575–1583

Olsen WL, Longo FM, Mills CM, et al. (1988) White matter disease in AIDS: findings at MR imaging. Radiology 169:445–448

Padget BL, Walker DL, ZuRheim GM, et al. (1971) Cultivation of papova-like virus from human brain with progressive multifocal leukoencephalopathy. Lancet 1:1257–1260

Paley M, Wilkinson ID, Hall-Craggs MA (1995) Short echo time proton spectroscopy of the brain in HIV infection/AIDS. Magn Reson Imaging 13:871–875

Palmer DL, Harvey RL, Wheeler JK (1974) Diagnostic and therapeutic considerations in Nocardia asteroides infection. Medicine 53:391–401

Parker JC Jr, Dyer MC (1985) Neurological infection due to bacteria, fungi and parasites. In: Davis RL, Robertson DM (eds) Textbook of neuropathology, Williams & Wilkins, Baltimore, pp 632–703

Pavlakis SG, Lu D, Frank Y, et al. (1995) Magnetic resonance spectroscopy in childhood AIDS encephalopathy. Pediatr Neurol 12:277–282

Petito CK (1988) Review of central nervous system pathology in human immunodeficiency virus infection. Ann Neurol 23 (Suppl):54–57

Petito CK (1997) The neuropathology of human immunodeficiency virus infection of the spinal cord. In: Berger JR, Levy RM (eds) AIDS and the nervous system, 2nd edn. Lippincott-Raven, Philadelphia, pp 451–459

Petito CK, Navia BA, Cho E-S, et al. (1985) Vacuolar myelopathy pathologically resembling subacute combined degeneration in patients with the acquired immunodeficiency syndrome. N Engl J Med 312:874–879

Petito CK, Cho E-S, Lemann W, et al. (1986) Neuropathology of acquired immunodeficiency syndrome (AIDS): an autopsy review. J Neuropathol Exp Neurol 45:635–646

Pitchenik AE, Cole C, Russell BW, et al. (1984) Tuberculosis, atypical mycobacteriosis, and the acquired immunodeficiency syndrome among Haitian and non-Haitian patients in South Florida. Ann Intern Med 101:641–645

Pizzo PA, Wilfert CM (1994) Antiretroviral treatment for children with HIV infection. In: Pizzo PA, Wilfert CM, Preston T (eds) Pediatric AIDS: the challenge of HIV infection in infants, children and adolescents, 2nd edn. Williams & Wilkins, Baltimore, pp 651–687

Pohl P, Vogl G, Fill H, et al. (1988) Single photon emission computed tomography in AIDS dementia complex. J Nucl Med 29:1382–1386

Porter SB, Sande MA (1993) Toxoplasmosis of the central nervous system in the acquired immunodeficiency syndrome. N Engl J Med 2:1643–1648

Post MJD, Chan JC, Hensley GT, et al. (1983) *Toxoplasma* encephalitis in Haitian adults with acquired immunodeficiency syndrome: a clinical-pathological-CT correlation. AJR 140:861–868

Post MJD, Kursunoglu SJ, Hensley GT, et al. (1985) Cranial CT in acquired immunodeficiency syndrome: spectrum of diseases and optimal contrast enhancement technique. AJNR 6:743–754

Post MJD, Hensley GT, Moskowitz LB, et al. (1986a) Cytomegalic inclusion virus encephalitis in patients with AIDS: CT, clinical and pathological correlation. AJR 146:1229–1234

Post MJD, Sheldon JJ, Hensley GT, et al. (1986b) Central nervous system disease in acquired immunodeficiency syndrome: prospective correlation using CT, MR imaging and pathological studies. Radiology 158:141–148

Post MJD, Berger JR, Hensley GT (1988a) The radiology of central nervous system disease in the acquired immunodeficiency syndrome. In: Taveras JM, Ferrucci JT (eds) Radiology: diagnosis – imaging – intervention, vol 3. Lippincott, Philadelphia, pp 1–26

Post MJD, Tate LG, Quencer RM, et al. (1988b) CT, MR and pathology in HIV encephalitis and meningitis. AJNR 9:469–476

Post MJD, Levin BE, Berger JR, et al. (1992) Sequential cranial MR findings of asymptomatic and neurologically symptomatic HIV positive subjects. AJNR 13:359–370

Post MJD, Berger JR, Duncan R, et al. (1993) Asymptomatic and neurologically symptomatic HIV-seropositive subjects: results of long-term MR imaging and clinical follow up. Radiology 188:727–733

Presant CA, Wiernik PH, Serpick AA (1973) Factors affecting survival in nocardiosis. Am Rev Respir Dis 108:1444–1448

Quencer RM, Post MJD (1997) Spinal cord lesions in patients with AIDS. Neuroimag Clin North Am 7:359–373

Raez L, Cabral L, Cai JP, et al. (1999) Treatment of AIDS-related primary central nervous system lymphoma with zidovudine, ganciclovir, and interleukin 2. AIDS Res Hum Retroviruses 15:713–719

Ramsey RG, Geremia GK (1988) CNS complications of AIDS: CT and MR findings. AJR 151:449–454

Reddy S, Leite CC, Jinkins JR (1995) Imaging of infectious disease of the spine. Spine: State of the Art Reviews 9:119–139

Reichman RC (1978) Neurological complications of varicella-zoster infection. Am Intern Med 89:375–388

Remick SC, Diamond C, Migliozzi JA, et al. (1990) Primary central nervous system lymphoma in patients with and without the acquired immune deficiency syndrome. A retrospective analysis and review of the literature. Medicine 69:345–360

Ribera E, Martinez-Vasquez JM, Ocana I, et al. (1987) Activity of adenosine deaminase in cerebrospinal fluid for the diagnosis and follow-up of tuberculosis meningitis in adults. J Infect Dis 155:603–607

Richardson EP Jr (1988) Progressive multifocal leukoencephalopathy 30 years later. N Engl J Med 318:315–317

Rieder HL, Cauthen GM, Bloch AB, et al. (1989a) Tuberculosis and acquired immunodeficiency syndrome – Florida. Arch Intern Med 149:1268–1273

Rieder HL, Cauthen GM, Kelly GD, et al. (1989b) Tuberculosis in the United States. JAMA 262:385–389

Robertson CR, Stern RA, Hall CD, et al. (1993) Vitamin B-12 deficiency and nervous system disease in HIV infection. Arch Neurol 50:807–811

Rosenblum ML, Levy RM, Bredensen DE et al. (1988) Primary central nervous system lymphomas in patients with AIDS. Ann Neurol 23:S13–S16

Rottenberg DA, Moeller JR, Strother SC, et al. (1987) The metabolic pathology of the AIDS dementia complex. Ann Neurol 22:700–706

Rottenberg DA, Sidtis JJ, Strother SC, et al. (1996) Abnormal cerebral glucose metabolism in HIV-1 seropositive subjects with and without dementia. J Nucl Med 37:1133–1141

Rowley AH, Whitley RJ, Lakemar FD, et al. (1990) Rapid detection of herpes simplex virus DNA in cerebrospinal fluid of patients with herpes simplex encephalitis. Lancet 335:440–441

Ruiz A, Ganz WI, Post MJD, et al. (1994) Use of thallium-201 brain SPECT to differentiate cerebral lymphoma from *Toxoplasma* encephalitis in AIDS patients. AJNR 15:1885–1894

Ruiz A, Post MJD, Ganz WI, et al. (1997) Nuclear medicine applications to the neuroimaging of AIDS. Neuroimag Clin North Am 7:499–511

Safai B, Diaz B, Schwartz J, et al. (1992) Malignant neoplasms associated with human immunodeficiency virus infection. CA Cancer J Clin 42:74–96

Santosh CG, Bell JE, Best JJK (1995) Spinal tract pathology in AIDS: postmortem MRI correlation with neuropathology. Neuroradiology 37:134–138

Sathe SS, Reichman LB (1989) Mycobacterial disease in patients infected with the human immunodeficiency virus. Clin Chest Med 10:445–463

Schneck SA (1965) Neuropathological features of human organ transplantation. I. Possible cytomegalovirus infection. J Neuropathol Exp Neurol 24:415–429

Selwyn PA, Hartel D, Lewis VA, et al. (1989) A prospective study of the risk of tuberculosis among intravenous drug users with human immunodeficiency virus infection. N Engl J Med 320:545–550

Shah S, Zimmerman RA (1996) Cerebrovascular complications of pediatric CNS HIV disease. AJNR 17:1913–1917

Sharer LR, Epstein LG, Joshi VV, et al. (1985) Neuropathological observations in children with AIDS and with HTLV-III infection of brain. J Neuropathol Exp Neurol 44:350

Sharif HS, Morgan JL, Al Shahed MS, et al. (1995) Role of CT and MR imaging in the management of tuberculous spondylitis. Radiol Clin North Am 33:787–803

Sharma A, Goyal M, Mishra NK (1997) MR imaging of tubercular spinal arachnoiditis. AJR 168:807–812

Sheller JR, DesPrez RM (1986) CNS tuberculosis. Neurol Clin 4:143–158

Silverman L, Rubinstein LJ (1965) Electron microscopic observations on a case of progressive multifocal leukoencephalopathy. Acta Neuropathol (Berl) 5:215–224

Slater LN, Welch DF, Min W-F (1992) *Rochalimacea henselae* causes bacillary angiomatosis and peliosis hepatis. Arch Intern Med 152:602

Smirniotopoulos JG, Koeller KK, Nelson AM, et al. (1997) Neuroimaging – autopsy correlations in AIDS. Neuroimag Clin North Am 7:615–637

Spickler EM, Lufkin RB, Teresi L, et al. (1989) High signal intraventricular cysticercosis on T1 weighted MR imaging. AJNR 10 (Suppl):64

States LJ, Zimmerman RA, Rutstein RM (1997) Imaging of pediatric central nervous system HIV infection. Neuroimag Clin North Am 7:321–339

Stoner G, Ryschkewitsch CF, Walker DL, et al. (1986) JC papovavirus large tumor (T)-antigen expression in brain tissue of acquired immune deficiency syndrome (AIDS) and non-AIDS patients with progressive multifocal leukoencephalopathy. Proc Natl Acad Sci USA 23:2271–2275

Sunderam G, McDonald RJ, Maniatis T, et al. (1986) Tuberculosis as a manifestation of the acquired immunodeficiency syndrome (AIDS). JAMA 256:362–366

Sze G, Zimmerman RD (1988) The magnetic resonance imaging of infection and inflammatory diseases. Radiol Clin North Am 26:839–859

Sze G, Brant-Zawadzki MN, Norman D, et al. (1987) The neuroradiology of AIDS. Semin Roentgenol 22:42–53

Tam D, Shapiro SM, Snead RW (1995) Neurologic and psychiatric manifestations of pediatric AIDS. Immunol Allergy Clin North Am 15:288–305

Tatsch K, Schielke E, Einhaupl KM, et al. (1990) Tc-99m HMPAO SPECT in early stages of HIV infection. J Nucl Med 31:827

Thurnher MM, Jinkins RJ, Post MJD (1997) Diagnostic imaging of infections and neoplasms affecting the spine in patients with AIDS. Neuroimag Clin North Am 7:341–357

Tien RD, Chu PK, Hesselink JR, et al. (1991a) Intracranial cryptococcosis in immunocompromised patients: CT and MR findings in 29 cases. AJNR 12:283–289

Tien RD, Chu PK, Hesselink JR, et al. (1991b) Intra- and paraorbital lesions: value of fat suppression MR imaging with paramagnetic contrast enhancement. AJNR 12:245–247

Tien RD, Gean-Marton AD, Mark AS (1992) Neurosyphilis in HIV carriers: MR findings in six patients. AJR 158:1325–1328

Tien RD, Feldberg GJ, Osumi AK (1993) Herpesvirus infections of the CNS: MR findings. AJR 161:167–176

Tracey I, Carr CA, Guimaraes AR, et al. (1996) Brain choline-containing compounds are elevated in HIV-positive patients before the onset of AIDS dementia complex: a proton magnetic resonance spectroscopic study. Neurology 46:783–788

Uttamchandani RB, Daikos GL, Reyes RR, et al. (1994) Nocardiosis in 30 patients with advanced human immunodeficiency virus infection. Clinical features and outcome. Clin Infec Dis 18:348–353

Van Dyk A (1988) CT of intracranial tuberculosis with specific reference to the "target sign". Neuroradiology 30:329–336

Vietzke WM, Gelderman AH, Grimley PM, et al. (1968) Toxo-

plasmosis complicating malignancy. Experience at the National Cancer Institute. Cancer 21:816–827

Villoria MF, delaTorre J, Munoz L, et al. (1992) Intracranial tuberculosis in AIDS: CT and MRI findings. Neuroradiology 34:11–14

Villringer K, Jager H, Dichgans M, et al. (1995) Differential diagnosis of CNS lesions in AIDS patients by FDG-PET. J Comput Assist Tomogr 19:532–6

Vinters HV, Kwok MK, Ho HW, et al. (1989) Cytomegalovirus in the nervous system of patients with the acquired immune deficiency syndrome. Brain 112:245–268

Vion-Dury J, Nicoli F, Salvan A-M, et al. (1995) Reversal of brain metabolic alterations with zidovudine detected by proton localized magnetic resonance spectroscopy. Lancet 345:60–61

Walker DL (1985) Progressive multifocal leukoencephalopathy. In: Vinken PJ, Bruyn GW, Klawans HL (eds) Handbook of clinical neurology, vol 47. Demyelinating diseases. Elsevier Science, Amsterdam, pp 503–524

Webb P, Sailasuta N, Kohler SJ, et al. (1994) Automated single-voxel proton MR spectroscopy: technical development and multisite verification. Magn Reson Med 31:365

Whiteman MLH (1997) Neuroimaging of central nervous system tuberculosis in HIV-infected patients. Neuroimag Clin North Am 7:199–214

Whiteman MLH, Post MJD, Berger JR, et al. (1993a) Progressive multifocal leukoecnephalopathy in 47 HIV-seropositive patients: neuroimaging with clinical and pathological correlation. Radiology 187:233–240

Whiteman MLH, Post MJD, Bowen BC, et al. (1993b) AIDS-related white matter diseases. Neuroimag Clin North Am 3:331–359

Whiteman MLH, Dandapani BK, Shebert RP, et al. (1994) MRI of AIDS-related polyradiculomyelitis. J Comput Assist Tomogr 18:7–11

Whitener DR (1978) Tuberculous brain abscess: report of a case and review of the literature. Arch Neurol 35:148–155

Whitley RJ, Schlitt M (1991) Encephalitis caused by herpesviruses, including B virus. In: Scheld WM, Whitley RJ, Durack DT (eds) Infection of the central nervous system. Raven, New York, pp 41–86

Wouters EFM, Hupperts RMM, Vreeling FW, et al. (1985) Successful treatment of tuberculous brain abscess. J Neurol 23:118–119

Yang PJ, Reger KM, Seeger JF, et al. (1987) Brain abscess: an atypical CT appearance of CNS tuberculosis. AJNR 8:919–920

Yarchoan R, Berg G, Brouwers P, et al. (1987) Response of human immunodeficiency virus-associated neurological disease to 3'-azido-2,3'dideoxythymidine. Lancet 1:132–135

Yudd AP, Van Heertum RL, O'Connell RA, et al. (1987) SPECT brain scanning in patients with HIV positive encephalopathy. J Nucl Med 30:811

Zimmerman RA (1990) Central nervous system lymphoma. Radiol Clin North Am 28:697–721

Zuger A, Louis E, Holzman RS, et al. (1986) Cryptococcal disease in patients with the acquired immunodeficiency syndrome. Diagnostic features and outcome of treatment. Ann Intern Med 104:234–240

6 Imaging of Spinal Cord Lesions and the Peripheral Nervous System in AIDS

R. A. MEULI and P. P. MAEDER

CONTENTS

6.1 Introduction

In the past the occurrence of a myelopathy in patients with AIDS was reported with some frequency, although certainly much less often than neurologic diseases related to the brain or peripheral nerves. In a series of 186 AIDS patients with neurologic disease, McARTHUR (1987) diagnosed only 13 spinal cord lesions (7%). In other series, the prevalence of clinical myelopathy varied from 2% to 22% (LEVY et al. 1985). Int the experience of our AIDS clinic in charge of about 500 HIV-positive patients, including 150 with AIDS, 42 definite clinical diagnoses of AIDS-associated myelopathy were recorded within a 6-year period (1991–1996), with an incidence of 5% per year. Since 1997, the spectacular improvement in the treatment of HIV has significantly decreased the number of AIDS patients and thus AIDS-associated spinal cord abnormalities.

Various pathologic processes need to be considered in the differential diagnosis of myelopathy in AIDS patients (Table 6.1). In our unpublished clinical series of 42 patients mentioned above, the final diagnosis was vacuolar myelopathy in 24%, viral infection in 38%, toxoplasmosis in 5%, and postinfectious inflammatory myelitis in 2%. In 31% of patients, it was not possible to demonstrate the infectious agent or to proceed to a neuropathologic examination. Surprisingly, spinal cord lesions are commonly found at autopsy. PETITO and co-workers (1985, 1993, 1997) found histologic lesions in 50% of 178 spinal cords in AIDS patients at autopsy. In this series, vacuolar myelopathy was present in 29%, HIV myelitis in 5%, viral infection in 8%, other infections in 7%, and lymphoma in 2%. In a recent review of neuropathologic AIDS autopsies including 475 spinal cord examinations, BUDKA (1997) recorded 22.5% with vacuolar myelopathy, 6% with HIV myelitis, 5.8% with viral infections, 4.1% with fungal bacterial and protozoal infections, and 2.3% with lymphoma.

The clinical picture of these patients is variable: presentation can be abrupt or slowly progressive. Accurate data about the incidence of clinical signs and symptoms of myelopathy in AIDS patients are not available. The discrepancy in incidence between clinical presentation and neuropathologic data may have several explanations. Spinal cord symptoms often remain undetected when they co-exist with other signs of encephalopathy. This is especially true when

Table 6.1. Classification of HIV-associated myelopathy

Vacuolar myelopathy[a]
HIV myelitis
Viral infections[a]
Cytomegalovirus[a]
Varicella-zoster virus
Herpes simplex virus
Other opportunistic infections
Toxoplasmosis
Cryptococcosis
Candida
Tuberculosis
Treponemal infection
Other
Neoplasm
Primary lymphoma

[a]The most common myelopathies

R.A. MEULI, MD; P.P. MAEDER, MD
Department of Radiology, University Hospital, CHUV, 1011 Lausanne, Switzerland

the level of the sensory deficit is not clear, as in most cases of vacuolar myelopathy. Clinical signs may also be missed or misinterpreted in terminally ill patients with major systemic complications of HIV disease.

Peripheral nerve disease is frequently associated with AIDS. Various peripheral neuropathies are described, a painful peripheral neuropathy being the most frequent (FULLER et al. 1993). The incidence of peripheral nerve syndromes in AIDS patients is much higher than the incidence of myelopathy. However, radiologic imaging plays little role in the diagnosis and management of these syndromes. Yet, peripheral nerve syndromes frequently coexist with central nervous system dysfunction, leading to complex clinical signs. In such cases imaging of the brain and spinal cord may help in understanding the dominant pathology (myelopathy or peripheral neuropathy).

Magnetic resonance imaging (MRI) is by far the best imaging modality for AIDS patients with a clinical diagnosis of myelopathy. When available, MRI should be the first imaging study. Myelography, computed tomography (CT), and CT-myelography may efficiently detect extradural lesions, but most intramedullary processes will be overlooked. Advanced techniques of high-field MRI with appropriate surface coils are required to efficiently detect and characterize intramedullary lesions. The use of contrast agent (gadolinium) is also mandatory for both detection and characterization of the lesions.

This chapter will review the neuropathology, clinical appearance, and imaging features of the most common lesions of the spinal cord encountered in AIDS patients.

6.2
Vacuolar Myelopathy

Vacuolar myelopathy (VM) was recognized and described in AIDS patients in 1985 (PETITO et al. 1985) and is the major cause of spinal cord disease related to HIV infection. It usually appears in cases of advanced immune deficiency but rarely is the initial illness in AIDS patients. Accompanying peripheral neuropathy and dementia can frequently be observed. Key features of VM are summarized in Table 6.2.

The clinical picture (EPSTEIN and GENDELMAN 1993) is one of progressive development of spastic paraparesis within a few weeks or months. Sensory ataxia due to loss of joint position sense is observed in 20% of cases. Sphincter impairment may be present, often without a clear sensory level.

Table 6.2. Key features of vacuolar myelopathy

Epidemiologic features
   Occurs in the advanced stage of AIDS
Involves 5%–10% of AIDS patients clinically
   Present in up to 50% of autopsies in adult cases
   Often not recognized clinically
   Rarely an initial presentation of AIDS
   Very unusual in children
Clinical features
   Slowly progressive spastic paraparesis over
   the course of weeks or months (100%)
   Knee hyperreflexia (93%)
   Gait ataxia related to joint position sense loss (60%)
   Sphincter impairment (>50%)
   No clear sensory level
   Associated with distal sensory neuropathy and dementia
   Antiretroviral therapy has little efficacy
MRI features
   The best MRI technique is needed
   T2 hyperintensity in the posterior and lateral columns
surrounding gray matter
   No enhancement after gadolinium injection

VM is much more frequently diagnosed at autopsy than clinically. In an autopsy-based case-control study of 215 AIDS autopsies, DAL PAN et al. (1994) observed VM in 46.5% of cases. Fifty-six of these VM cases had undergone detailed neurologic examination but only 15 of them (26.8%) had signs and symptoms of myelopathy. The presence of symptomatic myelopathy was related to pathologic severity according to the criteria of PETITO et al. (1985). VM was also strongly associated with systemic infection.

Histologic investigation reveals a spongy degeneration of the lateral and posterior columns of the spinal cord, predominantly affecting the middle and lower thoracic region. The vacuolations arise from swelling between layers of the myelin sheets. Macrophage infiltration and reactive astrocytosis are accompanying findings. Multinucleated giant cells similar to those seen in HIV encephalopathy may occasionally be present (Fig. 6.1).

The cause of VM is unknown, but several hypotheses have been proposed. Although the myelopathy observed in vitamin B_{12} deficiency is strikingly similar, in AIDS patients with VM the vitamin B_{12} serum level and metabolites are usually normal (GRAY et al. 1988). This suggests a possible metabolic role of vitamin B_{12} metabolites, perhaps related to high consumption by macrophages. Another suggestion is that VM is due to a direct infection by HIV, but HIV is rarely detected in the cord, except within the macrophages. A mechanism in which infected macrophages initiate neurotoxicity amplified by a cell-to-cell interaction with astrocytes has

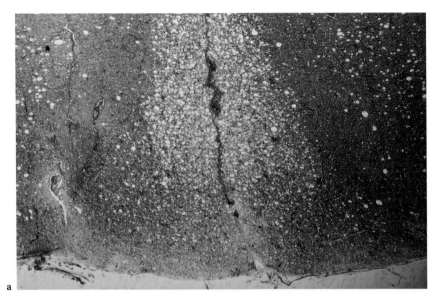

a

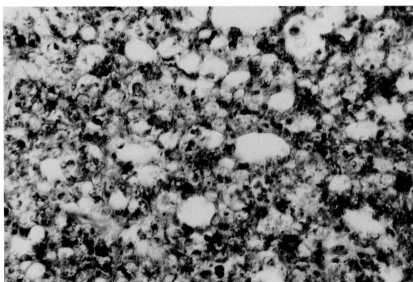

b

Fig. 6.1a, b. Vacuolar myelopathy. a Photomicrograph (hematoxylin-eosin technique) reveals vacuolar degeneration of the posterior columns of the spinal cord at the thoracic level. b Higher magnification of a with the Loyer technique for myelin demonstrates that the vacuolations arise from swelling between the layers of the myelin sheets

also been suggested (EPSTEIN and GENDELMAN 1993; TYOR et al. 1993; TAN et al. 1995). Tumor necrosis factor (TNF)-a produced in excess by the macrophages due to diminishing production of cytokines such as interleukin-4 and -10 by CD4-infected T cells has been proposed as the mechanism of neurotoxicity. This has been suggested as a unifying hypothesis for the pathogenesis of HIV-associated dementia complex, vacuolar myelopathy, and sensory neuropathy (TYOR et al. 1995). A further hypothesis is that other opportunistic infections not readily identified may be involved. In support of this theory is the fact that VM is rare in HIV-infected children (DICKSON et al. 1989), who have fewer opportunistic infections than adults.

Imaging of VM is difficult. MRI is the only way to observe the vacuolar changes limited to the posterior and lateral columns of the spinal cord. Standard spine MRI is usually not sufficient; rather, high-resolution spin-echo T2-weighted images (512 matrix for transverse and 1024 matrix for sagittal sections) using flow compensation is required. With this technique, hyperintensity can be observed in the posterior and lateral portions of the cord surrounding gray matter. Abnormalities are seen on multiple contiguous slices (Fig. 6.2). There is no enhancement after gadolinium injection. When observed, this pattern is sufficiently specific to differentiate VM from other spinal cord lesions (SANTOSH et al. 1995).

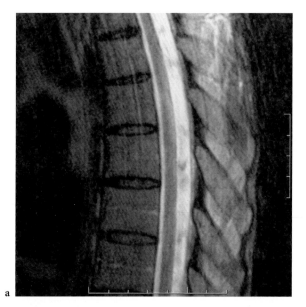

a

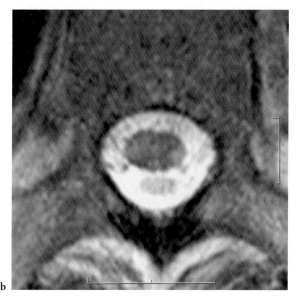

b

Fig. 6.2a, b. Vacuolar myelopathy. High-resolution fast spin-echo T2-weighted images [1024 matrix for sagittal (**a**) and 512 matrix for transverse sections (**b**) using flow compensation]. Hyperintensity can be observed in the white matter confined to the posterior and lateral portions of the cord. There is no enhancement after gadolinium injection. When observed, this pattern is sufficiently specific to differentiate VM from other spinal cord lesions

6.3
HIV Myelitis

HIV myelitis is seen in association with HIV leu-koencephalopathy in 5%–8% of AIDS patients as determined by neuropathologic examination (PETITO 1997). Usually, encephalitis is more extensive and

severe than myelitis. Unusual cases of HIV myelitis without brain involvement are reported (PETITO 1997). HIV myelitis by itself is generally considered to be asymptomatic and has been observed as early as at the time of HIV seroconversion (DENNING et al. 1987). A self-limiting paraparesis may occur and carries a good prognosis. To our knowledge, no articles detailing the imaging findings of this type of myelitis have been published.

6.4
Herpes Group Viruses

Herpes group viruses include varicella-zoster virus (VZV), cytomegalovirus (CMV), and herpes simplex virus (HSV). All of them may cause a spinal cord syndrome. Key features of myelitis related to the herpes group viruses are summarized in Table 6.3. The neurologic deficit begins with ipsilateral motor signs followed by spinothalamic and inconsistent posterior column damage. The course of the myelitis is faster than with VM, and most patients end up with complete paraplegia. Generally VZV myelitis is seen

Table 6.3. Key features of myelitis related to herpes group viruses

Clinical features
Begins with ipsilateral motor signs followed by damage to the spinothalamic tract
Isolated posterior column damage is unusual (opposite to VM)
The course of the myelitis is more rapid than for VM
Patients rapidly develop paraplegia with sensory loss
VZV typically induces a vesicular rash restricted to a dermatome, followed 1–3 weeks later by the myelitis
Cases with isolated VZV myelitis have been described
CMV can begin with lower extremity and sacral paresthesia
CMV occurs only with a CD4 count of <50 cells/mm³
CMV myelitis is generally associated with CMV retinitis
Frequently CMV radiculitis and myelitis occur simultaneously
MRI features of VZV and HSV myelopathy
Hyperintense intramedullary lesions on T2-weighted images
Lesions can be diffuse or focal
Size of the spinal cord is normal
Contrast enhancement is variable
MRI features of CMV myelopathy
T1-weighted images after contrast injection show a strong enhancement of the pia lining the cord and the conus medullaris, cauda equina, and lumbar nerve roots
Intramedullary lesion similar to VZV

within 1–3 weeks of reactivation of the virus with a typical dermatomal vesicular rash (GILDEN et al. 1994). However, cases with isolated myelitis have also been described. CMV myelitis occurs only in patients with severe immunodeficiency resulting in CD4 T lymphocyte counts of less than 50 cells/mm^3. It must be suspected when a rapid onset of ascending myelitis is observed. Myelitis and radiculitis frequently occur simultaneously and myelitis is also associated with retinitis. HSV also causes a spinal cord syndrome. It is frequently detected as a co-infection with CMV (PETITO 1993). At pathologic examination, inflammation, infarction, hemorrhage, demyelination, and necrosis may be present at different stages and in various locations (Fig. 6.3). With CMV, microglial nodules are present; some of them contain giant cells with typical CMV inclusions

(Fig. 6.4). CSF shows a pleocytosis usually absent in VM.

MRI easily detects hyperintense intramedullary lesions on T2-weighted images in advanced cases of necrotizing myelitis (Fig. 6.5). Lesions can be diffuse or focal, and contrast enhancement is generally observed. Plain T1-weighted images, myelography, and CT-myelography are usually normal, showing no cord swelling. When the myeloradiculitis is predominant, T1-weighted images after contrast injection reveal strong enhancement of the pia lining the cord, the conus medullaris, cauda equina, and lumbar nerve roots (Fig. 6.4) (TALPOS et al. 1991; MAHIEUX et al. 1989; CHRÉTIEN et al. 1993; GRAFE and WILEY 1989). This MRI pattern is similar for all viruses of the herpes group but is also indistinguishable from some other causes of myelitis.

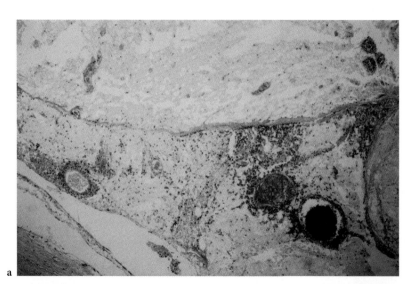

a

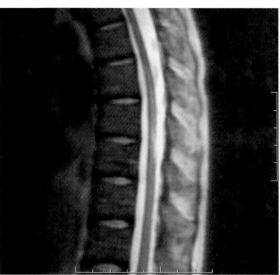

b

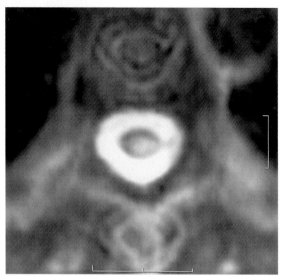

c

Fig. 6.3a–c. Varicella-zoster virus (VZV). a A transverse section of the spinal cord at the thoracic level. The hematoxylin-eosin stained section shows complete necrosis of the spinal cord parenchyma. In addition, meningitis and a leptomeningeal vessel with vasculitis and secondary thrombosis are present. b Sagittal and c transverse T2-weighted MR images easily detect hyperintense intramedullary lesions involving gray and white matter. Contrast enhancement was not demonstrated in this case but may be present in advanced forms with severe necrosis. This MRI pattern is similar for all viruses of the herpes group

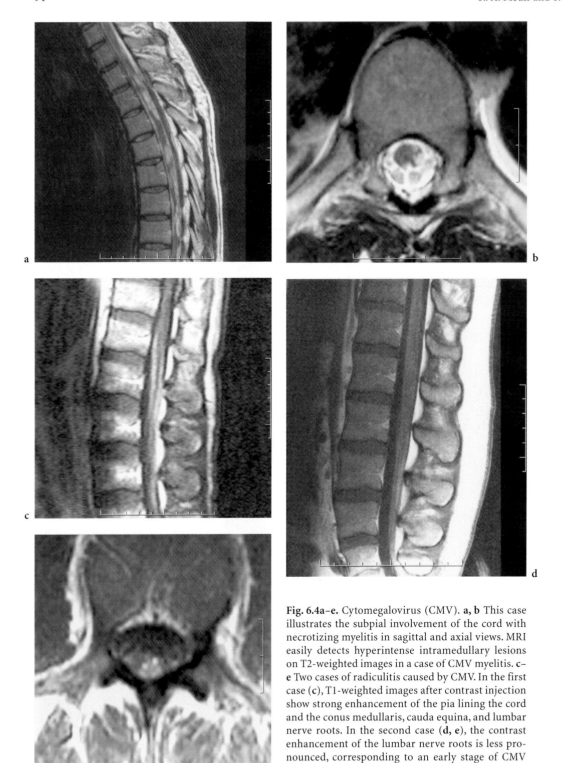

Fig. 6.4a–e. Cytomegalovirus (CMV). **a, b** This case illustrates the subpial involvement of the cord with necrotizing myelitis in sagittal and axial views. MRI easily detects hyperintense intramedullary lesions on T2-weighted images in a case of CMV myelitis. **c–e** Two cases of radiculitis caused by CMV. In the first case (**c**), T1-weighted images after contrast injection show strong enhancement of the pia lining the cord and the conus medullaris, cauda equina, and lumbar nerve roots. In the second case (**d, e**), the contrast enhancement of the lumbar nerve roots is less pronounced, corresponding to an early stage of CMV radiculomyelitis

Final diagnosis is based on identification of the virus. For this purpose, polymerase chain reaction (PCR) of CSF is, for the time being, the most sensitive technique. A prompt and precise diagnosis of myelitis related to herpes group viruses is important because clinical improvement or at least stabilization of the disease can be achieved by treatment with acyclovir or ganciclovir.

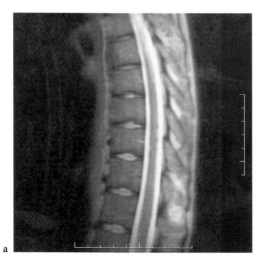
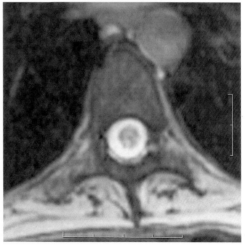

Fig. 6.5a, b. Herpes simplex virus (HSV) myelitis. MRI detects hyperintense intramedullary lesions on T2-weighted images. Lesions can be diffuse or focal and contrast enhancement may be present. This MRI pattern is similar for all viruses of the herpes group. HSV is frequently detected as a co-infection of CMV. Final diagnosis is based on identification of the virus

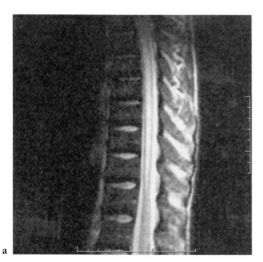
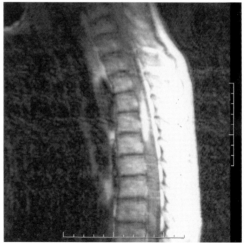

Fig. 6.6a, b. Toxoplasmosis. MRI shows focal enlargement of the spinal cord with increased T2 signal (**a**) and homogeneous contrast enhancement (**b**). Toxoplasmosis is the most frequent cause of intracerebral mass lesion in patients with AIDS. Rarely an isolated spinal cord form has been reported

6.5
Other Infections

Other infections or inflammatory processes can cause intramedullary lesions and spinal cord syndrome. Human T cell lymphotropic virus types I and II (HTLV-I and HTLV-II) can be responsible for a slowly evolving spastic paraplegia with essentially normal spinal MRI (BERGER et al. 1991; MCARTHUR et al. 1990). Toxoplasmosis is the most frequent cause of intracerebral mass lesions in patients with AIDS. An isolated spinal cord form has occasionally been

reported (RESNICK et al. 1995; POON et al 1992). MRI shows focal enlargement of the spinal cord with increased T2 signal and homogeneous contrast enhancement (Fig. 6.6). These features are nonspecific as diseases such as non-Hodgkin's lymphoma enters into the differential diagnosis. *Mycobacterium tuberculosis* can result in meningoradiculitis or intramedullary tuberculoma (MELHEM and WANG 1992; WOOLSEY et al. 1988). On MRI, spinal cord tuberculoma appears slightly expansive, with heterogeneous signal intensity on T2- and T1-weighted postcontrast images. Syphilis has also been clinically described as a rare cause of treatable myelitis without an imaging description (BERGER 1992). Multiple sclerosis can be a preexisting disease and spinal cord demyelinated lesions may appear during the course of AIDS. Among seven HIV-positive patients with multiple sclerosis, BERGER et al. (1989) described the first onset of the disease as concomitant with the demonstration of HIV seropositivity in three cases.

6.6
Spinal and Epidural Lesions

In AIDS patients, infections and tumors of the spine must be considered when spinal cord neurologic deficits are discovered. Epidural abscesses are unusual; they are more frequently encountered in intravenous drug addicts, owing to the frequent occurrence of bacteremia. They can originate from the epidural space or can spread from a spondylodiscitis. *Staphylococcus aureus* is the most common organism detected in such abscesses, but *Mycobacterium tuberculosis*, *Nocardia*, and *Aspergillus* have also been described (WOODS and GOLDSMITH 1990). The classical clinical picture is that of a febrile patient with back pain who develops a paraparesis within 24–72 h. A more subacute onset over weeks or months is also possible, depending on the infecting agent and the immune response of the patient. Tumors are rare; lymphoma and plasmocytoma are usually mentioned in the differential diagnosis. Kaposi's sarcoma occurring as a lytic vertebral lesion has also been described (ISSENBARGER and ARONSON 1994).

MRI with injection of gadolinium is the first choice for imaging in such cases. Features of abscesses or tumors are similar to those observed in non-AIDS patients (MARK 1996; SZE 1996). Myelography or CT-myelography usually discloses an extradural compression. Plain radiographs of the spine may also help to localize the involved portion of the spine.

6.7
Management Plan

Radiologic and neurologic textbooks (HARRISON and MCARTHUR 1995) propose the rapid use of MRI as the first imaging technique in the presence of a spastic paraplegia in order to exclude an epidural compressive process. It should precede CSF examination, which may be hazardous if a large epidural abscess is present. In cases without signs of extradural compression, a careful examination of the cord itself should be conducted with high-resolution fast spin-echo T2-weighted images in the transverse and sagittal planes. Contrast enhancement with gadolinium should be used systematically. In a recent clinical study, CHONG et al. (1999) studied 21 patients with a clinical diagnosis of AIDS-associated myelopathy. Spinal cord atrophy was recorded in 15 cases. Six patients presented with abnormal T2 hyperintensity of the spinal cord. In our own experience with 42 patients with AIDS-associated myelopathy, 16 (38%) presented with intrinsic spinal cord signal abnormality. T2 hyperintensity of the spinal cord was observed in 20% (2/10) of the cases of VM, in 50% (8/16) of the cases of myelitis related to herpes group viruses, and in 13% (3/) of the cases of myelopathy of unknown etiology. In this group of patients, high-resolution MRI was not used in many cases, which may explain the low sensitivity for detection of VM.

In practice, MRI should be able to discriminate between extradural compression, VM, or more extensive necrotic-hemorrhagic cord lesions. CSF culture is necessary to detect common infectious organisms. PCR of the CSF will assess the possibility of myelitis related to herpes group viruses. Correlation of clinical findings, MRI findings, and laboratory results is important to ensure a precise final diagnosis. In many cases, a specific antibiotic or antiviral treatment may improve or stabilize the neurologic deficit (HARRISON and MCARTHUR 1995).

References

Berger JR (1992) Spinal cord syphilis associated with human immunodeficiency virus infection: a treatable myelopathy. Am J Med 92:101–103

Berger JR, Sheremata WA, Resnick L, et al. (1989) Multiple sclerosis-like illness occurring with human immunodeficiency virus infection. Neurology 39:324–329

Berger JR, Svenningsson A, Raffanti S, et al. (1991) Tropical spastic paraparesis-like illness occurring in a patient dually infected with HIV-1 and HTLV-II. Neurology 41:85–87

Budka H (1997) Neuropathology of myelitis, myelopathy, and spinal infections in AIDS. In: Donovan Post MJ (ed) Neuroimaging of AIDS II. Neuroimaging Clin North Am 7:639–650

Chong J, Di Rocco A, Tagliati M, et al. (1999) MR findings in AIDS-associated myelopathy. AJNR 20:1412–1416

Chrétien F, Gray F, Lescs MC, et al. (1993) Acute varicella-zoster virus ventriculitis and meningo-myelo-radiculitis in acquired immunodeficiency syndrome Acta Neuropathol (Berl) 86:659–665

Dal Pan GJ, Glass JD, McArthur JC (1994) Clinicopathologic correlations of HIV-1-associated vacuolar myelopathy: an autopsy-based case-control study. Neurology 44:2159–2164

Denning DW, Anderson J, Rudge P, et al. (1987) Acute myelopathy associated with primary infection with human immunodeficiency virus. Br Med J 294:143–144

Dickson DW, Belman AL, Kim TS, et al. (1989) Spinal cord pathology in pediatric acquired immunodeficiency syndrome Neurology 39:227–235

Epstein LG, Gendelman HE (1993) Human immunodeficiency virus type 1 infection of the nervous system: pathogenetic mechanisms. Ann Neurol 33:429–436

Fuller GN, Jacobs JM, Gulloff RJ (1993) Nature and incidence of peripheral nerve syndromes in HIV infection. J Neurol Neurosurg Psychiatry 56:372–381

Gilden DH, Beinlich BR, Rubinstien et al (1994) Varicella-zoster virus myelitis: An expanding spectrum. Neurology 44:1818–1823

Grafe MR, Wiley CA (1989) Spinal cord and peripheral nerve pathology in AIDS: the roles of cytomegalovirus and human immunodeficiency virus. Ann Neurol 25:561–566

Gray F, Gherardi R, Scaravilli F (1988) The neuropathology of the acquired immune deficiency syndrome (AIDS). Brain 111:245–266

Harrison MJG, McArthur JC (1995) AIDS and Neurology. Clinical Neurology and Neurosurgery Monographs. Churchill Livingstone, Edinburgh London New York

Issenbarger DW, Aronson NE (1994) Lytic vertebral lesions: an unusual manifestation of AIDS-associated Kaposi's sarcoma. Clin Infect Dis 19:751–755

Levy RM, Dale PD, Bredesen E, et al. (1985) Neurological manifestations of the acquired immuno-deficiency syndrome (AIDS): experience at UCSF and review of the literature. J Neurosurg 62:475–495

Mahieux F, Gray F, Fenelon G, et al. (1989) Acute myeloradiculitis due to cytomegalovirus as the initial manifestation of AIDS. J Neurol Neurosurg Psychiatry 52:270–274

Mark AS (1996) Infectious and inflammatory diseases of the spine. In: Atlas SW (ed) Magnetic resonance imaging of the brain and spine, 2nd edn. Lippincott-Raven, Philadelphia New York, pp 1207–1264

McArthur JC (1987) Neurological manifestations of AIDS. Medicine 66: 407–437

McArthur JC, Griffin JW, Cornblath DR, et al. (1990) Steroid-responsive myeloneuropathy in a man dually infected with HIV-1 and HTLV-I. Neurology 40:938–944

Melhem ER, Wang H (1992) Intramedullary spinal cord tuberculoma in a patient with AIDS. AJNR 13:986–988

Petito CK (1993) Myelopathies. In: Scaravilli F (ed) The neuropathology of HIV infection. Springer, London, pp 187–199

Petito CK (1997) The neuropathology of human immunodeficiency virus infection of the spinal cord. In: Berger JR, Levy RM (eds) AIDS and the nervous system, 2nd edn. Lippincott-Raven, Philadelphia New York, pp 451–460

Petito CD, Navia BA, Cho ES, et al. (1985) Vacuolar myelopathy pathologically resembling subacute combined degeneration in patients with acquired immune deficiency syndrome. N Engl J Med 312:874–879

Poon TP, Tcherkoff V, Pares GF, et al. (1992) Spinal cord *Toxoplasma* lesion in AIDS: MR findings. J Comput Assist Tomogr 16:817–819

Resnick DK, Comey CH, Welch WC, et al. (1995) Isolated toxoplasmosis of the thoracic spinal cord in a patient with acquired immunodeficiency syndrome. J Neurosurg 82:493–496

Santosh CG, Bell JE, Best JJK (1995) Spinal tract pathology in AIDS: postmortem MRI correlation with neuropathology. Neuroradiology 37:134–138

Sze G (1996) Neoplastic disease of the spine and spinal cord. In: Atlas SW (ed) Magnetic resonance imaging of the brain and spine. Lippincott-Raven, Philadelphia New York, pp 1339–1386

Talpos D, Tien RD, Hesselink JR (1991) Magnetic resonance imaging of AIDS-related polyradiculopathy. Neurology 41:1995–1997

Tan SV, Guiloff RJ, Scaravilli F (1995) AIDS-associated vacuolar myelopathy. A morphometric study. Brain 118:1247–1261

Tyor WR, Glass JD, Baumrind N, et al. (1993) Cytokine expression of macrophages in HIV-1-associated vacuolar myelopathy. Neurology 43:1002–1009

Tyor WR, Wesselingh SL, Griffin JW, et al. (1995) Unifying hypothesis for the pathogenesis of HIV-associated dementia complex, vacuolar myelopathy, and sensory neuropathy. J Acquir Immune Defic Syndr Hum Retrovirol 9:379–388

Woods GL, Goldsmith C (1990) *Aspergillus* infection of the central nervous system in patients with acquired immunodeficiency syndrome. Arch Neurol 47:181–184

Woolsey RM, Chambers TJ, Chung HD, et al. (1988) Mycobacterial meningomyelitis associated with human immunodeficiency virus infection. Arch Neurol 45:691–693

7 Chest Radiology in AIDS

Linda B. Haramati and Elizabeth R. Jenny-Avital

L.B. Haramati, MD
Department of Radiology, Albert Einstein College of Medicine and Montefiore Medical Center, 111 East 210th Street, Bronx, New York 10467, USA
E.R. Jenny-Avital, MD
Department of Medicine, Division of Infectious Diseases, Albert Einstein College of Medicine, Jacobi Medical Center, 1400 Pelham Parkway South, Bronx, New York 10461, USA

7.1 Introduction

Human immune deficiency virus (HIV) infection is a heterogeneous condition whose most advanced expression, AIDS, is associated with a number of well-characterized opportunistic infections and neoplasms. However, clinically asymptomatic HIV infection accounts for a longer duration of HIV infection than does symptomatic AIDS, except for a minority of patients who progress rapidly to AIDS. Although asymptomatic HIV-infected patients do not have AIDS-related opportunistic infections or CD4 cell counts of less than 200 cells/mm^3, they do have demonstrable immunologic abnormalities. Another interesting group of HIV-infected patients have experienced substantial immune reconstitution as a result of highly active antiretroviral therapy (HAART). These patients generally have very low CD4 cell counts, which rise during treatment with HAART (Palella et al. 1998). The newly reconstituted CD4 cell count seems to protect against the opportunistic infections that occur with lower CD4 cell counts (Schneider et al. 1999). Paradoxically, some patients develop localized inflammatory reactions soon after HAART is begun, as the viral load is abruptly decreasing. These "immune reconstitution phenomena" are often targeted against a preexisting infection such as tuberculosis (Narita et al. 1998) or Mycobacterium avium complex infection (Race et al. 1998).

HIV-infected patients without AIDS have subtle immunologic derangements which coexist alongside the usual risk factors for lung disease. The interplay between the patient's perturbed immune system and various infectious agents and environmental factors likely accounts for the variety of cardiopulmonary manifestations increasingly linked to HIV infection. Bacterial pneumonia, tuberculosis, cardiomyopathy (Barbaro et al. 1998), pulmonary hypertension (Opravil et al. 1997), lymphocytic interstitial pneumonitis (Travis et al. 1992), and emphysema (Diaz et al. 2000) are all linked to HIV but do not occur at a predictable level of immune dysfunction.

Table 7.1. Intrathoracic infections and neoplasms occurring with increased prevalence in HIV infection

Clinical setting	Condition	Radiographic findings	Epidemiology and associations
	Common		
First AIDS-defining opportunistic infection (CD4 <200 cells/mm^3)	*Pneumocystis carinii* pneumonia	Bilateral symmetric, perihilar granular, reticular or airspace opacities Air cysts, pneumothorax Pleural effusions and lymphadenopathy uncommon	Very common in USA Prevented by antibiotic prophylaxis
	Cryptococcosis	Single/multiple nodules, consolidation, +/- cavitation	Common in USA and developing countries Meningitis far more common
	Histoplasmosis[a]	Normal or diffuse, small, ≤3 mm lung nodules	Endemic: Ohio, Mississippi River valleys, Caribbean, Central America
	Coccidioidomycosis[a]	Diffuse nodular or reticulonodular parenchymal opacities Focal consolidation, hilar adenopathy, pleural effusions	Desert of southwest USA, parts of South America
	Penicilliosis[a]	Localized diffuse reticular opacities, consolidation	Southeast Africa, associated with characteristic skin lesions
	Less common		
	Nocardiosis	Large consolidation, diffuse interstitial pattern, mass, +/- cavitation	Southern USA, rural areas
	Uncommon		
	Toxoplasmosis	Bilateral coarse nodular and reticulonodular opacities	Europe, cat exposure
	Rhodococcosis	Dense consolidation, cavitation, pleural effusion, empyema	Present in soil, causes disease in farm animals
	Bacillary angiomatosis	Endobronchial lesions, parenchymal nodules, lymphadenoma	Reservoir in cats
	Blastomycosis	Focal airspace opacities or masses Diffuse nodular opacities	Midwest, South Central USA
Subsequent opportunistic infection seen in long standing advanced HIV	Aspergillosis	Chronic necrotizing: thick-walled cavity Disseminated disease: bilateral nodules/masses	Preexisting lung disease Steroids, neutropenia, antibiotics
	Cytomegalovirus	Reticular, reticulonodular opacities	
	Pseudomonas, other gram-negative pneumonia	Consolidation, cavitation	
	Kaposi's sarcoma	Coarsening bronchovascular bundles Ill-defined nodules with perihilar predominance	Seropositive for HHV-8 Male homosexual, Africa
	Strongyloidiasis	Hyperinfection syndrome: bilateral miliary nodules, reticular interstitial opacities	Tropical, subtropical regions
	Mycobacterium avium complex	Lymphadenopathy, parenchymal consolidation, small or large pulmonary nodules, +/- cavitation	
	Nontuberculous mycobacteria	Similar to tuberculosis	
Any CD4	Tuberculosis	Consolidation, nodules, lymphadenopathy, cavitation infrequent at low CD4, +/- pleural effusions	Prior exposure Developing countries
	Bacterial pneumonia	Lobar consolidation	Smoking, intravenous drug use
	Cardiomyopathy[a]	- cardiac silhouette Pulmonary venous congestion	Infection with cardiotropic viruses
	Pulmonary hypertension	Enlarged central pulmonary arteries	
	Emphysema (precocious)	Severe emphysema	Smoking
	Lymphoma	Lung nodules and masses Pleural effusions	Epstein-Barr virus infection

[a]Occurs in persons who have resided in endemic areas

Among patients with AIDS, opportunistic infections occur largely as a result of reactivation of infections acquired remotely. Thus they vary with the patients' geographic and exposure history (Table 7.1). The most overt example of this is the frequent occurrence of *Pneumocystis carinii* pneumonia in North America and Europe in contrast to its rarity in Africa, presumably due to differences in environmental distribution of *Pneumocystis carinii*. The endemic mycoses with geographically limited distributions cause fungal disease in patients who live or have lived in the region of endemicity. This is true for coccidioidomycosis, histoplasmosis, and penicilliosis. A history of past exposure to tuberculosis and to certain animals (e.g., cats – bacillary angiomatosis) is relevant to the occurrence of disease due to those agents. Infections due to agents that reside in soil such as *Nocardia* and *Rhodococcus* are seen more often in patients who live or have lived in rural locales. Sometimes laboratory tests can also be used to determine past exposure to relevant infectious agents: PPD for tuberculosis or *Toxoplasma* serology for *T. gondii*. The HIV risk factor may be relevant in predicting the types of opportunistic conditions that complicate AIDS. For example, human herpes virus 8 (HHV-8), the virus associated with Kaposi's sarcoma, is sexually transmitted, more common in gay men, and endemic in Africa.

7.2
Bacterial Infections

HIV-infected patients are prone to developing bacterial infections in the chest, including both tracheobronchitis (McGuinness et al. 1997) and pneumonia (Hirschtick et al. 1995). At CD4 cell counts above 200 cells/mm^3, the infections are usually caused by common pathogens (Shah et al. 1997). Two or more episodes of bacterial pneumonia in a single year are AIDS-defining in an HIV-infected person regardless of CD4 cell count.

7.2.1
Tracheobronchitis

Tracheobronchitis is common in HIV infection, especially in cigarette smokers. A specific microbial etiology is often not identified with either acute or chronic tracheobronchitis. However, usual respiratory viruses, *Chlamydia*, and *Mycoplasma* are often implicated.

Tracheobronchitis is usually not evident on chest radiographs. Subtle findings such as peribronchial thickening and "increased markings" may, however, be present. On computed tomography (CT), bronchial wall thickening, mucoid impaction, and small centrilobular nodules are typical features (McGuinness et al. 1997) (Fig. 7.1). Bronchiectasis occurs with increasing frequency in AIDS patients and may be re-

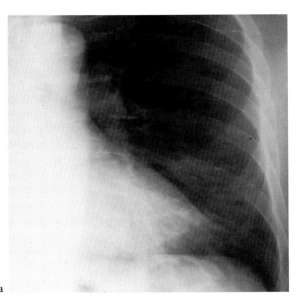

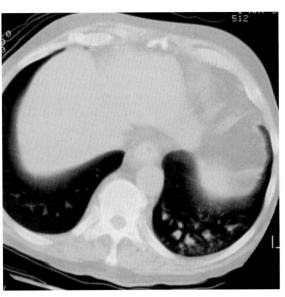

a   b

Fig. 7.1a, b. A 55-year-old man with AIDS and persistent cough and bronchitis. **a** Cone-down view from a PA chest radiograph demonstrates tubular opacity in the left lower lobe. **b** Chest CT at the lung basis demonstrates tubular "v" and "y" shaped opacities in the left lower lobe consistent with mucoid impaction

lated to repeated episodes of bronchitis and pneumonia, although it has been described in AIDS without previously documented infections and may, at times, be a more direct effect of HIV on the bronchi.

7.2.2
Pneumonia

Bacterial pneumonia caused by the usual pathogens is common at all stages of HIV infection but more so as immunodeficiency progresses. Additional risk factors for the occurrence of bacterial pneumonia such as cigarette smoking, intranasal drug use, periodic unconsciousness due to drugs, alcohol, or seizures, depressed sensorium due to neurologic disease, and poor dentition are commonly operative in addition to HIV infection.

Pneumococcal pneumonia is still the most important cause of acute bacterial pneumonia and presents as a "typical pneumonia." Bacteremic pneumococcal pneumonia is more common with HIV infection than in those without immunosuppression, although bacteremic pneumococcal pneumonia is not uncommon in normal hosts. In general, when AIDS patients develop bacterial pneumonia, it is more frequently multilobar and is more frequently associated with bacteremia than in the non-AIDS population.

Certain bacterial pathogens are associated with pneumonias occurring at low CD4 counts. This includes *Pseudomonas aeruginosa*, enteric gram-negative rods, *Rhodococcus equi*, and *Nocardia* species (FURMAN et al. 1996). Pneumonias due to these pathogens are often associated with cavitation (Fig. 7.2).

Septic emboli, caused by bacterial endocarditis and usually due to *Staphylococcus aureus*, occur in bacteremic intravenous drug abusers. Such patients are acutely ill, complain of marked pleuritic chest pain, and have fever and leukocytosis. Chest radiographic and CT findings include bilateral focal pulmonary parenchymal opacities with a peripheral predominance (Fig. 7.3). The opacities are often wedge shaped and develop cavitation. Pleural effusions and cardiomegaly may be present.

Routine antimicrobial prophylaxis against *Pneumocystis carinii* with trimethoprim/sulfamethoxazole in patients with a CD4 cell count of less than 200 cells/mm³ and against *Mycobacterium avium* complex with a macrolide antibiotic in patients with a CD4 cell count of less than 50 cells/mm³ reduce the occurrence of bacterial pneumonia. Such antibiotics also change the spectrum and antimicrobial susceptibility of the patient's flora.

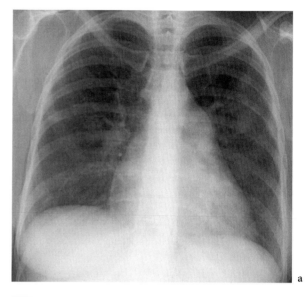

a

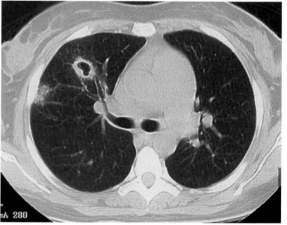

b

Fig. 7.2a, b. A 37-year-old woman with AIDS, CD4=5/mm³, presenting with cough and fever. She was diagnosed with *Pseudomonas* pneumonia. **a** PA chest radiograph demonstrates vague bilateral upper lobe opacities. Additionally, there is cardiomegaly. The central pulmonary arteries are prominent, consistent with pulmonary arterial hypertension. **b** Chest CT at the level of the right upper lobe bronchus 1 week later demonstrates a 2-cm-thick walled cavity in the anterior segment of the right upper lobe. There is a focal area of consolidation posterolateral to the cavity

7.2.3
Nocardiosis

Nocardiosis is caused by a soil-borne aerobic actinomycete, a higher bacterium, usually acquired by inhalation. *Nocardia* causes disseminated infection in a variety of immunocompromised hosts such as those with lymphoreticular malignancies, those with organ transplants, and those receiving immunosuppressive treatments. *Nocardia*, especially *N. brasiliensis*, can

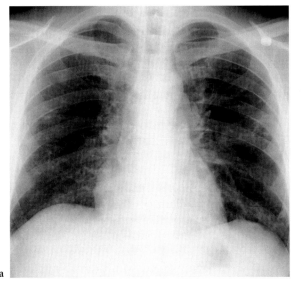

a

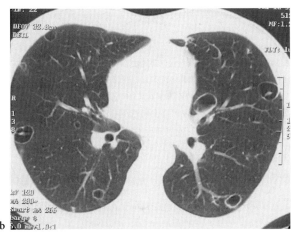

b

Fig. 7.3a, b. A 39-year-old HIV-infected man, an intravenous drug user, with a CD4 count of 59/mm³. Blood cultures were positive for *Staphylococcus aureus*. **a** PA chest radiograph demonstrates multiple bilateral lung nodules, many cavitaries, consistent with septic emboli. Splenomegaly is present. **b** Chest CT demonstrates multiple bilateral cavities with a dramatic peripheral predominance, typical for septic emboli

cause skin and soft tissue infections in immunocompromised hosts. *Nocardia* is not common in AIDS. When it does occur, it is more commonly reported from southern and rural regions of the United States, possibly reflecting differential exposure to soil-borne pathogens compared to urban areas. In AIDS patients, *Nocardia* infection, usually *N. asteroides*, commonly involves the lungs; it may concomitantly involve the CNS or soft tissues. Less frequently, only extrapulmonary sites are involved. Most of the *Nocardia* species which cause disseminated disease respond clinically to trimethoprim/sulfamethoxazole, so that routine prophylaxis against *Pneumocystis carinii* pneumonia

prevents nocardiosis. Nocardiosis in AIDS typically presents in patients with a low CD4 cell count and it may be a first opportunistic infection heralding HIV infection (UTTAMCHANDANI et al. 1994).

Radiographically, *Nocardia* presents with large areas of consolidation involving several lobes, a diffuse interstitial pattern, or a solitary well-defined mass. Cavitation within a consolidated area is also common. Pleural or pericardial effusion and mediastinal lymphadenopathy may occur (KRAMER and UTTAMCHANDANI 1990) (Fig. 7.4). An upper lobe predominance is described and the radiographic findings may be mistaken for tuberculosis (BANI-SADR et al. 1995).

7.2.4
Rhodococcosis

Rhodococcosis is caused by infection with *Rhodococcus equi*, a gram-positive rod which resides in soil and is known to cause pneumonia in horses, pigs, and other farm animals. Human infection is uncommon and occurs exclusively in immunocompromised hosts, including AIDS patients with CD4 cell counts of less than 200 cells/mm³ (HARVEY and SUNSTRUM 1991). Patients typically have a history of animal or soil exposure. The clinical presentation is usually subacute with symptoms developing over weeks. The radiographic manifestations of rhodococcal pneumonia

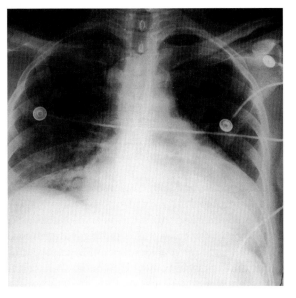

Fig. 7.4. A 39-year-old woman with late-stage AIDS diagnosed with pericarditis due to *Nocardia asteroides*. AP chest radiograph demonstrates a globularly enlarged cardiac silhouette consistent with pericardial effusion

include parenchymal consolidation, usually accompanied by cavitation (SHAPIRO et al. 1992). Pleural effusions and empyema frequently complicate rhodococcal pneumonia. Lymphadenopathy may be present (MUNTANER et al. 1997).

Diagnosis is by identification of the organism in culture from respiratory specimens and, in many cases, blood. This pathogen resembles nonpathogenic diphtheroids and so it may be spuriously dismissed as normal flora. In some cases, calcified phagolysosomes, the pathognomonic finding of malakoplakia, are evident (KWON and COLBY 1994; SUPPARATPINYO et al. 1994). Prolonged treatment with appropriate antibiotics can be successful.

7.3
Zoonoses

7.3.1
Bacillary Angiomatosis

Bartonella henselae and *Bartonella quintana* are both causes of the clinical syndromes of bacillary angiomatosis and peliosis in HIV-infected patients. Bacillary peliosis also occurs in other immunocompromised patients. *B. henselae* is the organism almost exclusively associated with cat scratch disease and it is capable of causing high-grade bacteremia in cats without causing illness in the animal. *B. quintana* is the agent of trench fever and is transmitted by the human body louse (KOEHLER et al. 1997).

Bacillary angiomatosis is a neovascular proliferative disorder that was initially described to involve skin and lymph nodes in HIV-infected patients but has since been described to involve visceral organs including the liver, spleen, and lungs. The most common manifestation of bacillary angiomatosis is skin disease – subcutaneous or dermal purplish nodules that superficially resemble Kaposi's sarcoma. *B. quintana* can cause lytic bone lesions.

In the chest, bacillary angiomatosis can have a varied presentation. Violaceous endobronchial lesions can mimic Kaposi's sarcoma on bronchoscopic inspection of the airways. In the lung, parenchymal nodules are the most common manifestation. Additional findings include pleural effusions, lymphadenopathy and chest wall masses. Because of the vascular nature of these lesions, the lymphadenopathy and chest wall masses frequently densely enhance with intravenous contrast administration when imaged by CT (MOORE et al. 1995).

Because bacillary angiomatosis is a bacterial infection that responds well to antibiotic therapy, familiarity with its varied manifestations is important in leading to an early diagnosis. Diagnosis by blood culture using special techniques can be accomplished when clinical biopsy specimens cannot be obtained.

7.3.2
Pasteurella

Pasteurella multocida is a gram-negative bacterium that is a frequent colonizer of the upper respiratory tract of dogs and cats. Skin and soft tissue infection is the most common manifestation of *Pasteurella* infection and is usually associated with an animal bite or scratch. In patients with normal immunity and underlying lung disease, *Pasteurella* may cause upper and lower respiratory infections often related to a dog or cat bite. In immunocompromised patients, *Pasteurella* can cause pneumonia even in the absence of underlying lung disease (DRABICK et al. 1993). The radiographic findings include focal areas of consolidation which may be complicated by cavitation and pleural effusion (Fig. 7.5).

7.3.3
Bordetella

Another zoonosis that can occur in AIDS patients is infection with *Bordetella bronchiseptica*, a gram-

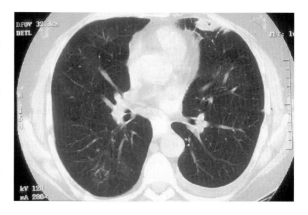

Fig. 7.5. A 50-year-old HIV-infected man, CD4=22/mm³, with leg edema and ulcers. He had a dog at home who licked his legs. He presented with cough and fever and was diagnosed with *Pasteurella multocida* pneumonia. Chest CT of the mid lungs demonstrates a cavitary ovoid nodule in the inferior lingula and patchy bilateral areas of ground glass opacity. There is a small left pleural effusion

negative coccobacillus. *Bordetella* causes respiratory diseases in dogs, cats, and pigs, but rarely in humans with normal immunity. A broad spectrum of illness has been described in AIDS, including upper and lower respiratory infection and disseminated disease. Generally, the patients have advanced stage AIDS and CD4 cell counts of less than 50 cells/mm^3. A history of contact with sick dogs or cats can sometimes be elicited (DWORKIN et al. 1999). Chest radiographic findings include interstitial infiltrates which may be bilateral and focal areas of consolidation (Fig. 7.6). Cavitation has occasionally been described. Diagnosis is accomplished by culture of respiratory specimens.

7.4
Mycobacterial Infections

7.4.1
Tuberculosis

HIV infection is a potent risk factor for the development of tuberculosis (BARNES et al. 1991) throughout its course (JONES et al. 1993). In fact, development of tuberculosis is considered AIDS defining in an HIV-infected person regardless of the CD4 cell count. Histologically, the inflammatory response to tuberculosis varies with the CD4 cell count, with well-formed granulomata and few bacilli seen in patients with preserved CD4 cell counts in contrast to poorly formed granulomata with abundant organisms in patients with low CD4 cell counts (DI PERRI et al. 1996). Similarly, the radiographic appearance of tuberculosis varies with the CD4 cell count (KEIPER et al. 1995). In HIV-infected patients with tuberculosis and CD4 cell counts of more than 200 cells/mm^3, the chest radiograph demonstrates the typical pattern of reactivation tuberculosis (GREENBERG et al. 1994). Airspace disease and consolidation usually involve the apical and posterior segments of the upper lobes and/or the superior segments of the lower lobes. Cavitation is frequent and lymphadenopathy infrequent. As the CD4 count decreases, the radiographic appearance changes. Lung parenchymal disease is more randomly distributed. Lung nodules may be the dominant parenchymal finding in some cases. Cavitation occurs infrequently. Lymphadenopathy is often present and may be unilateral or bilateral (HARAMATI et al. 1997). On contrast-enhanced chest CT, tuberculous lymphadenopathy is usually low attenuation and may be peripherally en-

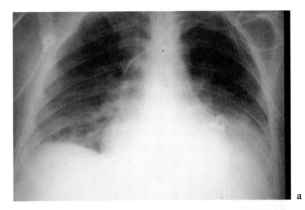

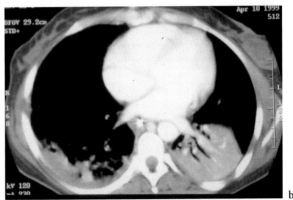

Fig. 7.6a, b. A 36-year-old woman with AIDS and pneumonia due to *Bordetella bronchiseptica*. **a** AP chest radiograph demonstrates dense consolidation of the left lower lobe and patchy opacity in the right lower lobe. **b** Chest CT demonstrates the left greater than right lower lobe lung parenchymal disease. In addition, a small right pleural effusion is evident

hancing (PASTORES et al. 1993). Disseminated tuberculosis is more common in severely immunocompromised patients (Fig. 7.7). Pleural effusions are slightly more prevalent in AIDS-associated tuberculosis as the CD4 count decreases. More significantly, AIDS patients with low CD4 cell counts typically have a higher mycobacterial organism burden, and therefore their tuberculous effusions are more likely to stain positive for acid-fast organisms and culture positive for *Mycobacterium tuberculosis* (RELKIN et al. 1994). Despite the differences in radiographic appearance and increased frequency of disseminated disease as the CD4 cell count decreases, AIDS patients with tuberculosis respond well to antituberculous therapy at all levels of CD4.

Multidrug-resistant tuberculosis can be prevalent in certain populations with AIDS, including noncompliant patients and those from countries where drug-resistant strains are endemic. The radiographic findings are indistinguishable from those of sensitive

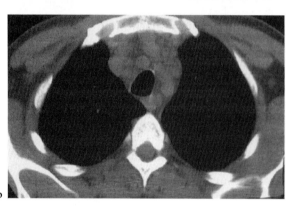

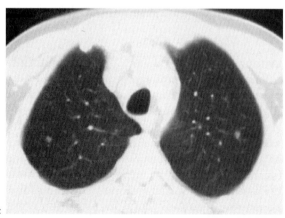

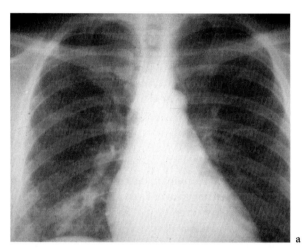

strains of tuberculosis, but there is continued radiographic progression beyond 2 weeks after initiation of conventional antituberculous therapy (Fig. 7.8).

Some AIDS patients with tuberculosis experience a transient worsening of their radiographic findings and symptomatology related to the initiation of HAART. Such paradoxical reactions had been described in the pre-HIV era in association with the initiation of tuberculosis therapy. In both instances, it is believed that the paradoxical reaction is due to an augmented immune response against mycobacte-

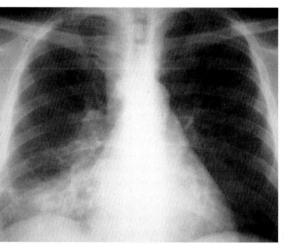

Fig. 7.7a–c. A 43-year-old man with AIDS, CD4=127/mm^3, presenting with fever, cough, and a left neck mass. He was diagnosed with disseminated tuberculosis. The portable chest radiograph was nearly normal. a Contrast-enhanced neck CT demonstrates multiple enlarged lymph nodes in the left neck. The lymph nodes are low attenuation with peripheral enhancement. b Chest CT without intravenous contrast demonstrates numerous mediastinal lymph nodes bilaterally. c Lung windows from the chest CT demonstrate numerous bilateral lung nodules ranging in size from 2 to 5 mm

Fig. 7.8a, b. A 30-year-old man with AIDS, fever, and sweats. Acid-fast bacilli were identified in his sputum and standard antituberculous therapy was initiated. The patient's disease continued to progress and he was ultimately diagnosed with multidrug-resistant tuberculosis. a PA chest radiograph at the time of clinical presentation demonstrates a patchy infiltrate at the right lung base. b Follow-up PA chest radiograph 4 weeks later demonstrates worsening consolidation in the right middle and lower lobes. There is new lymphadenopathy in the right hilum and right paratracheal regions

rial antigens. In the chest, such reactions are manifested as increasing lymphadenopathy, worsening infiltrates, pleural effusion, and the appearance of miliary infiltrates (FISHMAN et al. 2000). This may be confused with drug-resistant tuberculosis. The reaction is self-limited, although steroids may be required to control symptoms.

7.4.2
Mycobacterium avium Complex

Mycobacterium avium complex (MAC) infection in AIDS patients is often a disseminated disease affecting patients with CD4 counts of less than 50 cells/mm^3. The portal of entry is usually the respiratory or gastrointestinal tract. In disseminated disease the organism can be cultured from blood and bone marrow. Patients usually have subacute constitutional symptoms (HORSBURGH 1991). Patients with disseminated MAC will have intrathoracic disease in about 10% of cases. Radiographic findings include lymphadenopathy, parenchymal consolidation, and small or large pulmonary nodules with or without cavitation (KALAYJIAN et al. 1995) (Fig. 7.9).

MAC can also cause pulmonary disease in AIDS patients who do not have disseminated disease. On average, those patients have less advanced AIDS with CD4 cell counts usually >50 cells/mm^3. The usual radiographic findings include areas of consolidation which may be cavitary (HOCQUELOUX et al. 1998). However, the majority of patients with MAC in their sputum do not have disseminated MAC and do not have radiographic abnormalities attributable to MAC.

An immune reconstitution reaction akin to the paradoxical reaction described for tuberculosis can occur with MAC, usually resulting in lymphadenitis. Patients with very low CD4 cell counts develop fever and lymphadenitis in the neck, chest (Fig. 7.10), or abdomen soon after the initiation of HAART as their CD4 cell count rises. This is believed to be an augmented inflammatory response to a MAC infection (RACE et al. 1998).

7.4.3
Other Mycobacterial Infections

HIV-infected patients are generally at risk for developing a variety of mycobacterial infections. In addition to tuberculosis and MAC, uncommon mycobacterial infections occur with some frequency in AIDS patients. The disease may be localized to the lungs, gastrointestinal tract, or other sites, or may be disseminated (ARONCHICK and MILLER 1993).

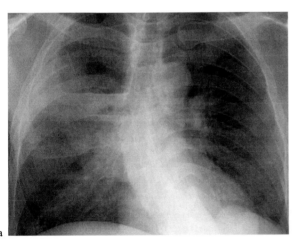
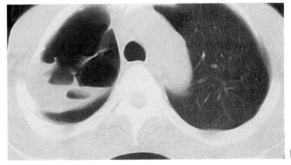
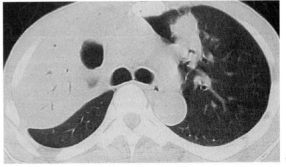

Fig. 7.9a–c. A 52-year-old man with late-stage AIDS, fever, and productive cough. Sputum and needle aspirate yielded the diagnosis of MAC pneumonia. **a** PA chest radiograph demonstrates a large septated cavity with multiple air fluid levels in the right upper lobe. There is adjacent consolidation. **b** Chest CT at the level of the aortic arch demonstrates a septated cavity in the right upper lobe containing multiple air fluid levels. **c** Chest CT at the level of the carina demonstrates consolidation with air bronchograms in the right upper lobe. There is also a cavity medially in the right upper lobe and a focal area of consolidation in the anterior left upper lobe

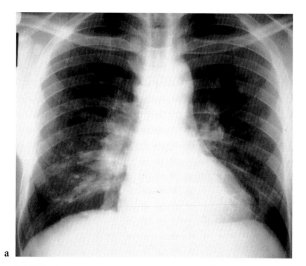

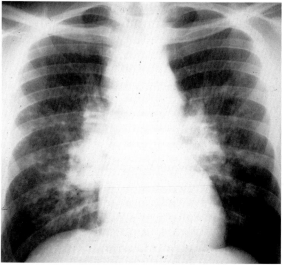

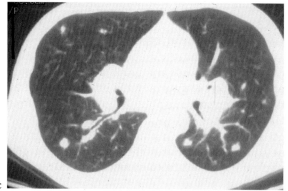

Fig. 7.10a–c. A 34-year-old man with AIDS diagnosed with pulmonary and disseminated MAC disease. **a** PA chest radiograph at the time of diagnosis when the CD4 was 28/mm^3 demonstrates bilateral hilar and mediastinal lymphadenopathy associated with perihilar nodules. **b** Chest CT at the same time as **a** demonstrates bilateral hilar lymphadenopathy and scattered bilateral lung nodules. **c** The patient was started on HAART, leading to a rise in his CD4 from 28/mm^3 to 221/mm^3 in 5 weeks. His symptoms worsened. Follow-up PA chest radiograph demonstrates marked worsening of the lymphadenopathy and lung parenchymal disease. Further evaluation only demonstrated MAC, with the worsening symptoms and radiographic findings consistent with reconstitution lymphadenitis

Organisms that are described in association with HIV infection include *M. kansasii* (FISHMAN et al. 1997), *M. gordonae, M. fortuitum*, and *M. xenopi*, among others. These infections predominate in patients with very low CD4 cell counts. The radiographic picture overlaps with that of tuberculosis (LAISSY et al. 1997) (Fig. 7.11). The growth rate and drug sensitivities vary with the specific mycobacterial organism and must be determined at culture for appropriate therapy.

7.5
Pneumocystis carinii Pneumonia

Widespread effective prophylaxis and HAART have markedly reduced the rate of *Pneumocystis carinii* (PCP) infection in AIDS patients. Despite this decline, PCP remains the most common opportunistic pulmonary infection in patients with AIDS (GATELL et al. 1996). The organism is ubiquitous, but cannot be grown in culture, and its taxonomy is controversial. It was originally considered to be a protozoan, but based on genetic analysis is now thought to more closely resemble a fungus (KUHLMAN 1996). Presenting symptoms are dyspnea and dry cough. Patients with PCP are usually hypoxic and have an elevated serum lactate dehydrogenase (LDH). The typical radiographic features of PCP are bilateral, often symmetric, perihilar, granular, reticular, or airspace opacities (Fig. 7.12) (AMOROSA et al. 1990). Lymphadenopathy and pleural effusions are uncommon radiographic findings in PCP. Lung parenchymal disease may occasionally be focal or nodular, or have an upper lobe predominance. Kerley B lines are uncommon. Air cysts develop in 10%–34% of patients, usually due to pneumatocele formation, and less frequently necrotizing pneumonitis (SANDHU and GOODMAN 1989). The air cysts tend to develop during the course of active infection and decrease in size or even resolve completely after successful treatment. However, pneumothorax complicates the course of infection in about one-third of patients with PCP and air cysts (CHOW et al. 1993).

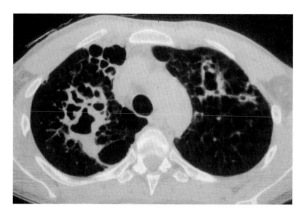

Fig. 7.11. A 45-year-old man with AIDS and *Mycobacterium fortuitum* pneumonia. Chest CT at the level of the aortic arch demonstrates bilateral upper lobe thick-walled cavities. One in the right upper lobe contains a shallow air-fluid level

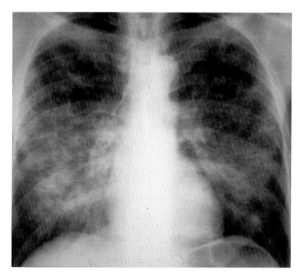

Fig. 7.12. A 41-year-old man with AIDS and *Pneumocystis carinii* pneumonia. AP chest radiograph demonstrates bilateral perihilar hazy granular and reticular opacities. There are bilateral upper lung cysts

The pneumothoraces may be unilateral or less frequently bilateral. On CT, PCP typically appears as ground glass opacity, often with a patchy distribution, although it may be homogeneous (GRUDEN et al. 1997). Air cysts are more readily detected on CT (KUHLMAN et al. 1990).

PCP can, in rare cases, be a disseminated disease. This usually occurs in patients receiving aerosolized pentamidine prophylaxis. The drug has very little systemic absorption and any organ can become infected. Radiographic and CT findings include enlarged lymph nodes, liver, and spleen containing punctate calcifications or areas of low attenuation.

7.6
Fungal Infections

Cellular immunity plays an important role in host defense mechanisms against many fungal infections. Therefore, both endemic (CONCES 1999) and opportunistic fungal infections increase in prevalence in AIDS patients with CD4 counts below 100 cells/mm^3 (CONNOLLY et al. 1999). In patients with fungal infections on HAART, a paradoxical worsening of their clinical and radiographic findings may occur as part of the "immune reconstitution syndrome" as the viral load decreases and CD4 cell count increases (see Fig. 7.14).

7.6.1
Endemic Fungal Infections

7.6.1.1
Histoplasmosis

Histoplasmosis is the most common endemic fungal infection in the United States. It is caused by *Histoplasma capsulatum*, a soil-borne fungus which thrives in regions with moderate temperature and humidity. Infection is caused by inhalation of the organism. In the United States, exposure to *Histoplasma* is greatest in the Ohio and Mississippi River valleys. In immunocompetent adults, histoplasmosis is either asymptomatic or causes a mild flu-like illness, a self-limited febrile pulmonary illness. Disseminated histoplasmosis typically occurs in immunocompromised hosts or children less than 1 year old. In patients who live or have lived in endemic areas, disseminated histoplasmosis is a common initial AIDS-defining opportunistic infection occurring at a CD4 count of less than 200 cells/mm^3 (CONCES 1999). In New York City, histoplasmosis is seen in AIDS patients from Puerto Rico, the Dominican Republic, and Central America. Clinically, patients present with fever, weight loss, and hematologic abnormalities, and about half develop pulmonary involvement. Elevated LDH often causes diagnostic confusion with PCP. Diagnosis is accomplished by culture or histology. A rapid polysaccharide antigen test is also extremely useful.

The chest radiographic findings in AIDS patients with disseminated histoplasmosis may be normal in about half of the cases. When the chest radiograph is abnormal, the most common finding is diffuse small lung parenchymal nodules (Fig. 7.13). Other parenchymal findings include linear, irregular, and airspace opacities. Pleural effusions and lymphadenopathy are uncommon (CONCES et al. 1993).

7.6.1.2
Coccidioidomycosis

Coccidioidomycosis is caused by the dimorphic fungus *Coccidioides immitis. C. immitis* is endemic in the soil in locales with arid climate, hot summers, and low rainfall. This includes the desert areas of the southwest United States, northern Mexico, and discrete areas in South and Central America. AIDS patients are at an increased risk for developing disseminated coccid-

ioidomycosis either on the basis of progressive primary infection or on the basis of reactivation of a previously acquired latent infection (FISH et al. 1990).

In immunocompetent hosts, the majority of infections are inapparent or mild, while a minority develop a febrile respiratory illness. Fungemia, diffuse pulmonary involvement, and extrathoracic infections occur in patients with deficient cell-mediated immunity, including AIDS patients who live or have lived in areas endemic for coccidioidomycosis. In endemic areas, coccidioidomycosis is a common initial AIDS-defining opportunistic infection (SINGH et al. 1996). The usual symptoms are fever, weight loss, and cough, occurring at a mean CD4 count of 100 cells/mm^3. The lung is commonly involved, in 80% of cases in one large study (BRONNIMANN et al. 1987). Meninges, skin, and other extrapulmonary sites may be involved, with or without lung involvement. Diagnosis is accomplished by culture, histology, or, in an appropriate clinical setting, serology.

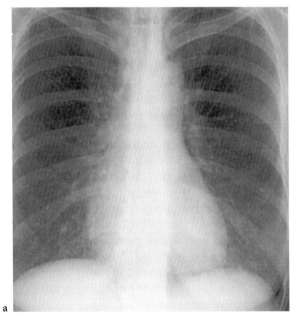

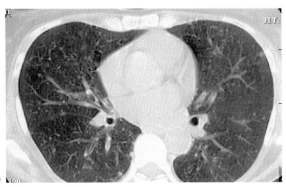

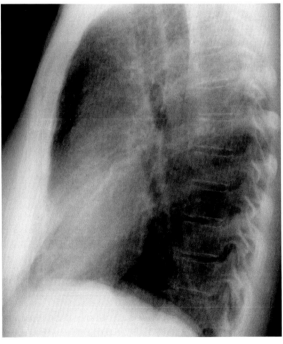

Fig. 7.13a–c. A 54-year-old woman with AIDS and disseminated histoplasmosis. **a, b** PA and lateral chest radiographs demonstrate innumerable small bilateral lung nodules. **c** Chest CT through the mid lungs demonstrates innumerable bilateral lung nodules ranging in size from 2 to 5 mm

The most frequent chest radiographic finding in AIDS patients with coccidioidomycosis is diffuse nodular or reticulonodular lung parenchymal opacities. Focal alveolar infiltrate, discrete nodules, hilar lymphadenopathy, pulmonary cavity, and pleural effusion occur. Those patients with diffuse pulmonary disease usually have lower CD4 cell counts and a high mortality.

7.6.1.3
Blastomycosis

Blastomycosis is the least prevalent of the endemic fungal infections in the United States. Its endemic areas are the southeastern United States and the Ohio and Mississippi River Valley regions. Infection with blastomycosis is not common in AIDS patients (CONCES 1999). When it occurs, it may be localized to the lung or disseminated. The chest radiographic findings of localized disease include focal airspace opacities or masses. The most common chest radiographic finding in disseminated disease is diffuse nodular opacities. Cavitation, lymphadenopathy, and pleural effusions occur less commonly. Disseminated disease often has a fulminant clinical course.

7.6.1.4
Penicilliosis

Penicillium marneffei is a dimorphic fungus endemic to Southeast Asia and the southern part of China. In some parts of Thailand, penicilliosis is the third most common AIDS-related opportunistic infection after extrapulmonary tuberculosis and cryptococcal meningitis. It occurs commonly as an initial AIDS-defining infection. Usual presenting symptoms are fever, weight loss, anemia, and skin lesions – most commonly generalized papules with central umbilication. In one large series (SUPPARATPINYO et al. 1994), chest radiographs were abnormal in 30/80 cases. Predominant abnormalities were diffuse reticular infiltrates and localized alveolar infiltrates. Diffuse alveolar infiltrates, localized interstitial infiltrates, and pleural effusion also occurred.

Diagnosis is accomplished by isolation of the organism in culture or visualization on tissue biopsy or touch preps, almost invariably from extrapulmonary sites. Blood, lymph node, bone marrow, and skin lesions have the highest diagnostic yield.

Importantly, HIV-infected patients who have traveled to or resided in an endemic area for *P. marneffei* (RABAUD et al. 1996) present with penicilliosis in a non-endemic area due to reactivation of remotely acquired disease (JONES and SEE 1992).

7.6.2
Opportunistic Fungal Infections

7.6.2.1
Cryptococcosis

Cryptococcosis is caused by the fungus *Cryptococcus neoformans*. The organism is usually found in soil contaminated by pigeon excreta. In immunocompetent patients, *Cryptococcus neoformans* is minimally pathogenic and occasionally will cause localized pulmonary disease. In AIDS patients, although the initial portal of entry of infection is the lungs, the presenting clinical illness is usually cryptococcal meningitis. The reported rate of cryptococcal pulmonary disease in AIDS patients with cryptococcal meningitis varies, but may be as high as 50% and is often a manifestation of disseminated disease (WASSER and TALAVERA 1987). The pulmonary disease is often clinically inapparent. Chest radiographic findings in AIDS patients with pulmonary cryptococcal disease include single or multiple lung nodules, areas of consolidation with or without cavitation and diffuse reticular opacities (Fig. 7.14). Pleural effusions and lymphadenopathy may be present (MILLER et al. 1990). Definitive diagnosis is by biopsy and culture of a pulmonary lesion. A presumptive diagnosis can be made when a compatible lesion is associated with a positive serum cryptococcal antigen or a positive blood culture.

7.6.2.2
Aspergillosis

Aspergillosis, due to soil-borne ubiquitous *Aspergillus* – usually *A. fumigatus*, causes pulmonary disease in patients with long-standing advanced AIDS. Risk factors associated with aspergillosis in AIDS include: corticosteroid use, antecedent broad-spectrum antibiotics, neutropenia, and longstanding depressed CD4 count. Localized pulmonary disease is more frequent than widespread hematogenous dissemination. Aspergillosis in AIDS patients takes three major forms: invasive disease, chronic necrotizing aspergillosis, and tracheobronchial aspergillosis. Infection typically occurs in patients with preexisting cavitary lung disease or neutropenia and occurs less frequently in AIDS patients than in organ transplant patients (DENNING et al. 1991).

Invasive pulmonary aspergillosis affects patients with advanced AIDS and is fatal in more than half. Although it is diagnosed in only 1%–2% of AIDS patients, autopsy series show a 5% prevalence of disease. Infection occurs by inhalation and the symptoms are

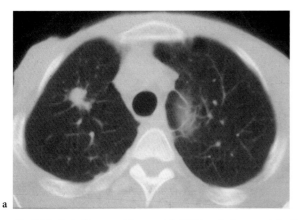
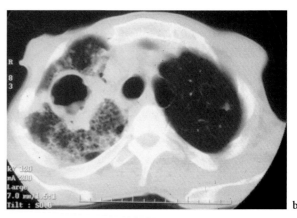

Fig. 7.14a, b. A 65-year-old man with AIDS and a lung nodule diagnosed as cryptococcal disease. **a** Chest CT through the upper lungs demonstrates an irregularly marginated nodule in the right upper lobe associated with subpleural nodularity. There is a left apical bulla. **b** Chest CT 2 months later after initiation of HAART and marked decrease in viral load demonstrates enlargement and cavitation of the right upper lobe nodule associated with surrounding reticular and small nodular opacities and a new left upper lobe nodule. Biopsy revealed granulomatous inflammation and cryptococcosis

usually nonspecific. Diagnosis of invasive aspergillosis requires tissue for diagnosis because the significance of *Aspergillus* in the sputum is uncertain. Some believe that upper airway colonization is frequent while others have demonstrated that identification of *Aspergillus* in respiratory secretions is highly predictive of active disease. The availability of itraconazole, an oral drug, may improve the outcome since early empiric therapy is practical in cases of suspected aspergillosis.

Radiographic findings in invasive pulmonary aspergillosis in AIDS usually include ill-defined nodules or masses, or areas of consolidation. Cavitation or the "air crescent sign" which is often seen in non-AIDS patients with invasive pulmonary aspergillosis, is less common in AIDS. Pleural effusions and lymphadenopathy are not common (STAPLES et al. 1995); systemic dissemination occurs in about one-third of cases.

Chronic necrotizing aspergillosis is the most common form of aspergillosis in AIDS patients. It resembles chronic necrotizing aspergillosis in the non-AIDS population. Patients usually have preexisting upper lobe cavitary disease from *Pneumocystis carinii* pneumonia or from mycobacterial infection. They often develop intracavitary masses ("air crescent sign") which may be mobile (Fig. 7.15). Although cavitary aspergillosis may mimic tuberculosis, cavitary tuberculosis is unusual in markedly immunocompromised patients. Compared to non-AIDS patients, rapid local progression of the cavity is more common. The main complication of chronic necrotizing aspergillosis is hemoptysis, which occurs in almost half the patients and is fatal in 50% of those (MILLER et al. 1994). Systemic dissemination complicates chronic necrotizing aspergillosis in 10%–20% of cases.

Tracheobronchial aspergillosis is uncommon but was initially described in patients with AIDS and takes two forms: obstructing bronchial aspergillosis, which has a more indolent course and presents with cough, fever, and wheezing, and pseudomembranous necrotizing aspergillosis, which is similar but which is associated with tissue invasion. The chest radiograph in patients with tracheobronchial aspergillosis may be normal or only subtly abnormal. Mucoid impaction in lower lobe airways and patchy parenchymal opacities are the main findings.

7.6.3
Miscellaneous Fungal Infections

Candida species are mucosal pathogens which cause thrush and esophagitis but rarely cause invasive disease. Unusual opportunistic fungal infections on occasion cause pulmonary disease in severely immunocompromised AIDS patients. *Torulopsis glabrata* is one such species. Chest radiographic findings include areas of consolidation or lung masses which may be cavitary and may be accompanied by lymphadenopathy.

7.7
Cytomegalovirus Infection

Cytomegalovirus (CMV) is the most common viral pathogen in AIDS patients. It is present in 80% of AIDS patients on autopsy series. CMV disease is usu-

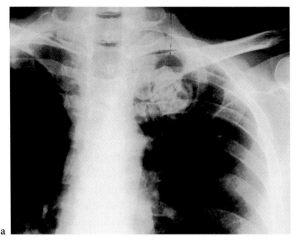

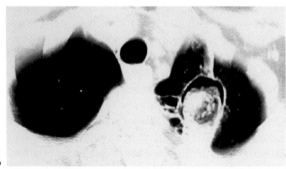

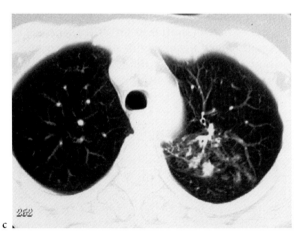

ally recognized as retinitis or enteritis, with pulmonary disease diagnosed less commonly. CMV pneumonia is usually a manifestation of disseminated disease occurring in AIDS patients with CD4 cell counts of less than 50 cells/mm^3. Symptoms are nonspecific and include cough, fever, and dyspnea. The diagnosis relies on identification of cytomegalic cells with intranuclear and intracytoplasmic inclusions in biopsy specimens. CMV pneumonia is preceded by the diagnosis of extrapulmonary CMV disease in two-thirds of AIDS patients (WAXMAN et al. 1997). Radiographic findings of CMV pneumonia are often subtle and include reticular or reticulonodular opacities and peribronchial thickening. Widespread granular opacities, areas of consolidation, and lung nodules or masses are more conspicuous radiographic findings of CMV pneumonia (Fig. 7.16). CT findings include bronchiectasis and a "tree in bud" pattern of branching small centrilobular nodules as well as areas of ground glass attenuation, reticular opacities, lung nodules, and masses (McGUINNESS et al. 1994).

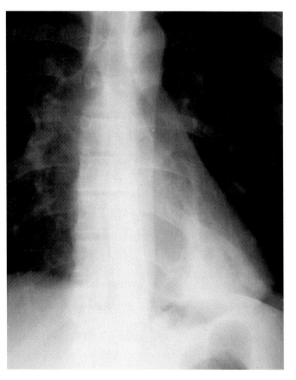

Fig. 7.15a–c. A 38-year-old woman with late-stage AIDS and dementia presenting with hemoptysis. She was diagnosed with chronic necrotizing aspergillosis. **a** Cone-down view from an AP chest radiograph demonstrates a sponge-like mass within a left apical cavity. **b** Chest CT at the apices demonstrates a large dependent sponge-like mass within a left apical cavity associated with an "air crescent" sign. There are band-like linear opacities extending from the cavity to the pleural surface anteriorly, medially, and posteriorly. **c** Chest CT 3 cm lower than in **b** demonstrates irregularly marginated nodules below the inferior aspect of the cavity

Fig. 7.16. A 31-year-old man with AIDS and persistent left lower lobe consolidation. Biopsy of the left lower lobe was diagnostic of CMV pneumonia

7.8
Parasitic Diseases

7.8.1
Toxoplasmosis

Toxoplasmosis is caused by the intracellular protozoan *Toxoplasma gondii*. Cats are the definitive hosts. People become infected with toxoplasmosis by ingesting either inadequately cooked meat containing tissue cysts or sporulated oocytes shed in cat feces. Prior exposure to toxoplasmosis is evident in up to 90% of Europeans, but is less common in the United States. This variation in prevalence is probably related to differences in diet and the presence of cat waste in the environment. AIDS patients who develop toxoplasmosis usually have reactivation of a previously acquired infection as evidenced by prior seropositivity for *Toxoplasma* IgG. The central nervous system is by far the most frequently affected organ system, but the lung is second in frequency. *Toxoplasma* pneumonia may occur in isolation or concomitant with disease in the central nervous system. The clinical signs are nonspecific, although the patients are usually acutely ill with fever, cough with rales, and a CD4 cell count of less than 200 cells/mm^3. Elevated LDH is common, causing diagnostic confusion with PCP. Diagnosis is made by identifying the organism in fluid obtained by bronchoalveolar lavage or in tissue (RABAUD et al. 1996).

Chest radiographic findings in *Toxoplasma* pneumonia consist predominantly of bilateral lung parenchymal disease. Coarse nodular opacities and reticulonodular opacities are most common. Confluent consolidation may also be seen. Pleural effusion is occasionally present. Lymphadenopathy is not typical (GOODMAN and SCHNAPP 1992).

7.8.2
Strongyloidiasis

Strongyloides stercoralis is a roundworm which is endemic in tropical and subtropical regions. In the United States, *Strongyloides* is prevalent in the Appalachian region. Humans are the principal hosts. Infection occurs percutaneously by infectious filariform larvae due to contact with fecally contaminated soil or due to unhygienic conditions resulting in other exposure to feces. Dissemination of the filariform larvae from the skin to the lungs occurs first and may be accompanied by a Löffler syndrome of patchy pneumonitis, respiratory symptoms, and

eosinophilia. Expectorated larvae are ultimately swallowed so that the adult worms may develop in the upper small intestine, where they persist for many years. The adult worms usually produce noninfectious rhabditiform larvae which pass out of the stool. *Strongyloides* infection may be asymptomatic or may produce symptoms related to the skin, the lungs, or, most commonly, the gastrointestinal tract (GENTA 1989).

In the hyperinfection syndrome, the rhabditiform larvae transform into infectious filariform larvae which penetrate the intestinal wall and widely disseminate in the body, often tracking enteric bacteria into the bloodstream, with resultant bacteremia and meningitis (IGRA-SIEGMAN et al. 1981). The hyperinfection syndrome is seen in immunocompromised patients who live or have lived in areas endemic for *Strongyloides* (GUERIN et al. 1995).

Chest radiographic findings in pulmonary strongyloidiasis vary with the severity of infection. Chest radiographs may be normal. More commonly, bilateral miliary nodules or reticular interstitial opacities are seen (Fig. 7.17). Patchy alveolar opacities and lobar consolidation may also be present. In patients with hyperinfection syndrome, bilateral alveolar opacities and even adult respiratory distress syndrome (ARDS) may develop. Diffuse involvement may be mistaken for PCP. Diagnosis is accomplished by wet mount or Papanicolaou stain, sputum examination, or bronchoalveolar lavage (NOMURA and REKRUT 1996).

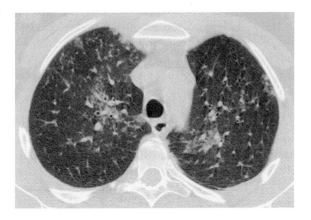

Fig. 7.17. A 42-year-old woman with AIDS presenting with "asthma" and diarrhea. *Strongyloides stercoralis* was present in sputum and stool. Chest CT at the level of the aortic arch demonstrates small nodules and patchy areas of ground glass opacity bilaterally

7.9
Sarcoidosis

Sarcoidosis rarely develops in HIV-infected patients. Case reports from the last decade have described only a few cases of new-onset sarcoidosis in HIV-infected patients, usually in patients with relatively preserved immune systems. Recently, we have observed a number of cases of newly diagnosed sarcoidosis in HIV-infected patients, with the sarcoidosis developing after initiation of HAART and coincident with partial immune reconstitution. Several additional cases have been described in the recent literature (Naccache et al. 1999; Mirmirani et al. 1999). Most of these patients had radiographic findings typical for sarcoidosis, including hilar and mediastinal lymphadenopathy and pulmonary nodules (Fig. 7.18). These cases suggest that sarcoidosis may fall into the spectrum of immune reconstitution phenomena in AIDS patients on HAART.

7.10
Malignancies and Associated Conditions

Proliferation of oncogenic viruses and diminished immune surveillance potentially explain the observations that HIV-infected patients have a higher than expected incidence of several malignancies (Broder and Karp 1992). Kaposi's sarcoma was the disease that initially prompted recognition of the AIDS epidemic in 1981. Shortly thereafter, AIDS-related lymphoma was recognized. Cervical carcinoma, anorectal carcinoma (usually in gay men), and bronchogenic carcinoma have also been linked to HIV infection. Each of these malignancies can have intrathoracic manifestations (White 1996). Cohort studies have revealed declining rates of AIDS-associated malignancies coincident with the widespread use of HAART (Jones et al. 1999).

7.10.1
Kaposi's Sarcoma

Human herpesvirus 8 (HHV-8) has been recently recognized as the sexually transmitted etiology of Kaposi's sarcoma in both classical, endemic and AIDS-related Kaposi's sarcoma. In the United States, HHV-8 and consequently Kaposi's sarcoma occur predominantly in the male homosexual population

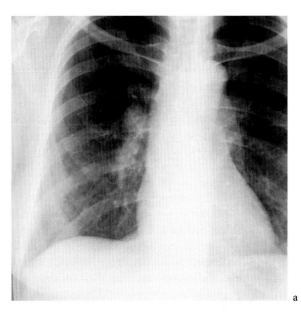

a

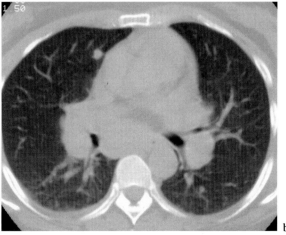

b

Fig. 7.18a, b. A 43-year-old woman with AIDS and a CD4 count of less than 50/mm^3 was begun on HAART. This led to a rise in the CD4 count and a decreased viral load. However, she developed new lymphadenopathy and lung nodules. On biopsy there were noncaseating granulomas. All cultures and special stains were unrevealing and she was diagnosed with sarcoidosis. **a** PA chest radiograph demonstrates mild bilateral hilar and mediastinal lymphadenopathy which had not been present on a chest radiograph 3 months earlier. There is also a poorly defined right lower lobe nodule. **b** Chest CT 1 month later demonstrates a 6-mm nodule in the anterior right upper lobe. There is also extensive bilateral hilar and subcarinal lymphadenopathy that had progressed from the chest radiograph obtained 1 month earlier

and only occasionally in women (Kedes et al. 1997; Haramati and Wong 2000). In Africa, HHV-8 is endemic and Kaposi's sarcoma occurs in both men and women (Martin et al. 1998).

Kaposi's sarcoma presents either as indolent cutaneous disease characterized by typical violaceous skin lesions or as aggressive visceral disease involving the skin, mucous membranes, gastrointestinal tract, and upper and lower respiratory tract. Indolent cutaneous disease has a minimal effect on survival while visceral disease is much more aggressive and is often fatal. Both may respond favorably to HAART. Patients with intrathoracic Kaposi's sarcoma typically have concomitant cutaneous disease (CADRANEL and MAYAUD 1995). Generally, intrathoracic disease progresses in a sequential fashion, with radiographic extent correlating with bronchoscopic extent of disease.

Early chest radiographic findings include coarsening of bronchovascular bundles and peribronchial cuffing. Ill-defined nodules occur later, often with a perihilar predominance. The nodules may be small, large, or coalescent (DAVIS et al. 1987). Kerley B lines and pleural effusions are manifestations of more advanced disease (GRUDEN et al. 1995). Intrathoracic lymphadenopathy is not a prominent feature of Kaposi's sarcoma. On chest CT, nodules and masses are the most common feature of intrathoracic Kaposi's sarcoma. They are usually distributed along the bronchovascular bundles and are often ill-defined (TRAILL et al. 1996; KHALIL et al. 1995) (Fig. 7.19). Pleural effusions and thickened interlobular septa are a manifestation of more advanced disease.

7.10.2
Lymphoma

Lymphoma is a neoplasm that occurs with increased prevalence in HIV-infected patients and is a cause of significant morbidity and morality. AIDS-related lymphoma is frequently a high-grade B cell non-Hodgkin's lymphoma. However, HIV-infected patients are also at increased risk for developing T cell lymphomas, Hodgkin's disease, and polyclonal lymphoma (BRODER and KARP 1992). While the Epstein-Barr virus genome has been identified in most AIDS-related primary brain lymphomas, it is less consistently identified in other AIDS-related lymphomas. A rare type of lymphoma called body cavity lymphoma is associated with infection with HHV-8 (CESARMAN et al. 1995). The incidence of non-central nervous system AIDS-related lymphoma has shown a smaller decline with HAART compared with opportunistic infections, Kaposi's sarcoma, and primary brain lymphoma (GRULICH 1999).

Intrathoracic disease occurs in 10%–50% of patients with AIDS-related lymphoma, depending on the population studied. Extranodal disease predomi-

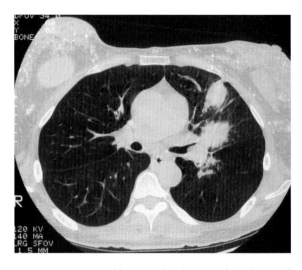

Fig. 7.19. A 52-year-old man with a history of smoking and increasing dyspnea. His HIV risk factor was homosexual contact. Transbronchial biopsy diagnosed Kaposi's sarcoma. Chest CT through the mid lungs demonstrates irregular marginated masses and nodules in the left upper and lower lobes. Note the presence of breast implants and free silicone in both breasts

nates in the chest (BAZOT et al. 1999). The most frequent intrathoracic manifestations of AIDS-related lymphoma are lung parenchymal consolidation, masses, and nodules, which may progress rapidly and may be cavitary (SIDER et al. 1989). Pleural effusions or masses can be seen in two-thirds of cases (EISNER et al. 1996) (Fig. 7.20). Although the disease is predominantly extranodal, lymphadenopathy is present in slightly more than half of cases. Body cavity lymphoma in the chest is manifested as pleural and/or pericardial effusion without associated lymphadenopathy or parenchymal abnormality and with slight thickening of the parietal surface (MORASSUT et al. 1997).

7.10.3
Lymphocytic Interstitial Pneumonia

Lymphocytic interstitial pneumonia (LIP) was described early in the AIDS epidemic in children. It occurs occasionally in adults with AIDS. It is characterized by a polyclonal proliferation of lymphocytes mixed with plasma cells and histiocytes. It is felt to be an immune response to infection with HIV or perhaps the Epstein-Barr virus, in some cases. AIDS-related LIP is not premalignant. The radiographic findings in LIP include reticular and nodular interstitial opacities (Fig. 7.21). Rarely, alveolar opacities may be seen (OLDHAM et al. 1989). On CT, small nodules are the dominant finding, often with a pre-

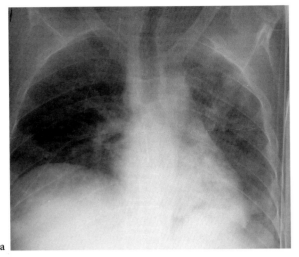

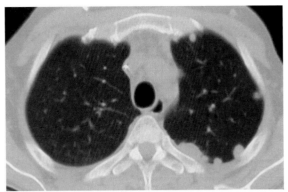

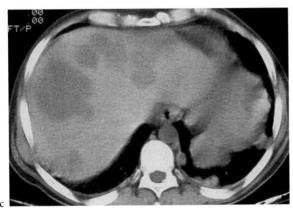

Fig. 7.20a-c. A 41-year-old man with AIDS-related lymphoma. a AP chest radiograph demonstrates multiple bilateral nodules, more numerous on the left. b Chest CT just above the level of the aortic arch demonstrates multiple left-sided pleural nodules. c CT at the level of the diaphragm demonstrates left-sided pleural nodules and masses as well as multiple liver masses

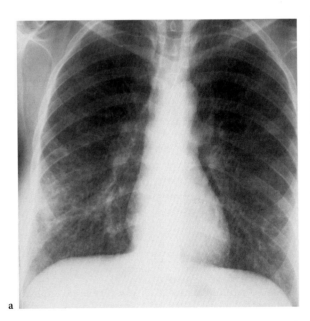

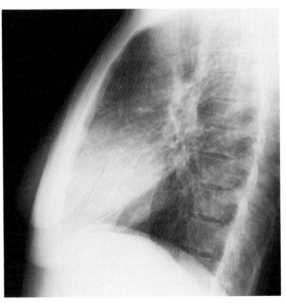

Fig. 7.21a, b. A 25-year-old woman with AIDS, CD4=85/mm³, who complained of dyspnea on exertion. Transbronchial biopsy was diagnostic of lymphocytic interstitial pneumonitis. PA and lateral chest radiographs demonstrate bilateral reticulonodular interstitial opacities

dominance in the peribronchovascular distribution. Areas of ground glass opacity may also be present.

7.10.4
Emphysema

In the late 1980s, precocious emphysema and bullous lung damage associated with advanced immunosuppression and the prior occurrence of pulmonary infections, especially PCP, was described (KUHLMAN et al. 1989). More recent studies, however, have identified a substantial occurrence of precocious emphysema with high-resolution CT among HIV-infected patients without prior pulmonary infections and without advanced HIV infection (DIAZ et al. 2000). The occurrence of precocious emphysema is greatest in those who have smoked the most. Impaired pulmonary diffusion has been correlated with HIV immunosuppression in a variety of studies. Structurally, the impaired diffusion was found to be related to the presence of emphysema rather than to interstitial disease on high-resolution CT (DIAZ et al. 1999). HIV-infected smokers were disproportionately affected compared to HIV-negative smokers and HIV-infected nonsmokers. While it is often emphasized that PCP may present with a normal chest radiograph, it is especially important to consider chronic lung disease as a potential etiology of dyspnea and hypoxia in an afebrile HIV-infected smoker with a relatively preserved CD4 count.

7.10.5
Lung Cancer

There has been some debate about whether or not lung cancer occurs with increased frequency in patients with AIDS (CHAN et al. 1993). The preponderance of evidence does point to such an increase (PARKER et al. 1998). Because lung cancer is most often caused by exposure to cigarette smoking and not by an oncogenic virus, the reason for its increased prevalence in HIV infection is unclear. Some authors speculate that the diminished immune surveillance associated with HIV infection increases the risk of all malignancies. Others suggest that because intravenous drug use is associated with smoking, AIDS patients with that risk factor have high rates of lung cancer.

HIV-infected patients with lung cancer generally present with late-stage, unresectable disease. The dominant cancer cell type is adenocarcinoma. The ra-

diographic appearance of lung cancer in AIDS patients is usually a peripheral or central nodule or mass, similar to the radiographic appearance of lung cancer in the general population (Fig. 7.22). The second most common radiographic appearance is a pleural effusion; in these cases chest CT will often reveal an underlying lung mass that has extended to the pleura at the time of presentation (WHITE et al. 1995).

7.10.6
Cervical Carcinoma and Anal Carcinoma

Cervical carcinoma and anal carcinoma are caused by infection with specific subtypes of the human papilloma virus (HPV) in virtually all cases (BRODER and KARP 1992). Women and homosexual men with AIDS often acquire HIV infection by sexual contact, which is a common route of infection with HPV. Infection with HIV also seems to increase the risk that a woman infected with HPV will develop cervical dysplasia or carcinoma. In some series, cervical dysplasia will be present in up to 50% of HIV-infected women. When cervical carcinoma develops it will often metastasize widely to many sites, including the chest.

Radiologic findings in metastatic cervical and anal carcinoma to the chest include small or large lung nodules, lymphangitic disease, and lymphadenopathy (Fig. 7.23). On contrast-enhanced CT, the lymphadenopathy may be low attenuation and peripherally enhancing. This appearance can also be seen in tuberculosis.

7.11
Cardiovascular Diseases

HIV infection can have a direct effect on the cardiovascular system. It is specifically implicated in AIDS-related cardiomyopathy and pulmonary hypertension. Pericardial effusions in AIDS patients can be due to a variety of etiologies.

7.11.1
Cardiomyopathy

Dilated cardiomyopathy usually occurs as a complication of HIV infection at a moderate stage of disease. In a large prospective clinical and echocardiographic study of asymptomatic patients (CD4 $>400/\text{mm}^3$), cardiomyopathy developed in 8% over 5 years, all

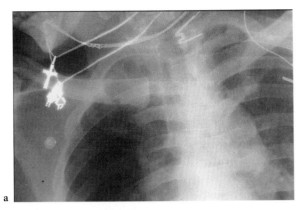

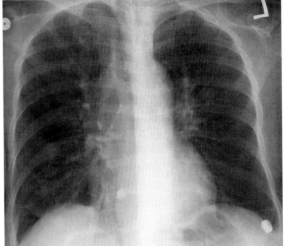

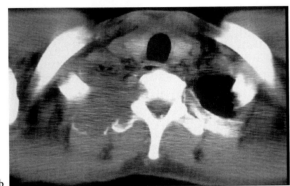

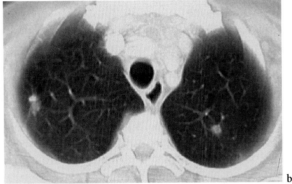

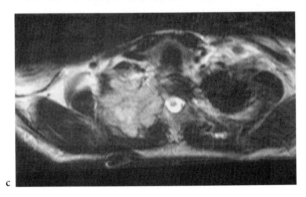

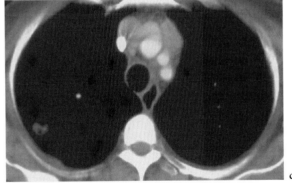

Fig. 7.22a–c. A 47-year-old HIV-infected man presented with right-sided back pain. He was diagnosed with poorly differentiated non-small cell lung cancer. **a** Cone-down view from an AP chest radiograph demonstrates a right apical opacity associated with destruction of the right second posterior rib. **b** Chest CT at the level of the thoracic inlet demonstrates the right apical mass extending through the posterior chest wall with destruction of the second posterior rib and right T2 transverse process. **c** T2-weighted magnetic resonance image of the chest shows the right apical mass to invade the adjacent posterior chest wall musculature

Fig. 7.23a–c. A 56-year-old HIV-infected woman with metastatic cervical carcinoma. **a** PA chest radiograph demonstrates bilateral lung nodules. **b** CT through the upper lungs demonstrates bilateral nodules. **c** Contrast-enhanced CT just above the level of the aortic arch demonstrates anterior mediastinal lymphadenopathy

with CD4 >200/mm³ (Barbaro et al. 1998). It occurs with increasing frequency as the CD4 cell count diminishes. On histologic analysis, myocarditis is usually present (Anderson et al. 1988). HIV nucleic acid can be found in the myocardium of up to 76% of

patients with HIV-associated cardiomyopathy. Other cardiotropic viruses, including Coxsackie virus group B, cytomegalovirus, and Epstein-Barr virus, are occasionally present as well. The patients clinically usually have symptomatic congestive heart failure. On echocardiography, these patients have four-chamber enlargement associated with left and right ventricular hypokinesia. The chest radiographic findings are those of dilated cardiomyopathy with an enlarged cardiac silhouette, with or without pulmonary venous congestion and edema (CORBOY et al. 1987). Abrupt cardiac decompensation with cardiomegaly may be seen in patients with a rapid drop in hematocrit, usually due to zidovudine.

7.11.2
Pulmonary Hypertension

Pulmonary hypertension occasionally complicates the course of HIV infection. In some patients, the pulmonary hypertension is secondary to interstitial fibrosis which may complicate PCP. In patients who use intravenous drugs, pulmonary hypertension may occur as a consequence of foreign body granulomatous vasculitis. However, in some HIV-infected patients, pulmonary hypertension develops in the absence of other predisposing conditions. In this group, infection with HIV itself is the presumed cause of pulmonary hypertension. HIV-associated pulmonary hypertension can occur at any CD4 cell count (OPRAVIL et al. 1997). On chest radiography, the central pulmonary arteries are enlarged and markedly decreased in caliber peripherally (Fig. 7.24). Right ventricular enlargement may be present.

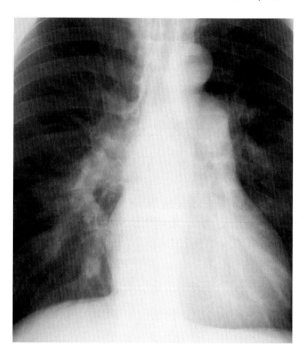

Fig. 7.24. A 48-year-old HIV-infected man with pulmonary hypertension. His pulmonary arterial pressure was 90 mmHg. PA chest radiograph demonstrates markedly enlarged central pulmonary arteries consistent with pulmonary arterial hypertension

7.11.3
Pericardial Effusion

Pericardial effusions occur in 10%–15% of HIV-infected patients (SILVA-CARDOSO et al. 1999). Most are clinically unimportant and are identified incidentally on echocardiography or CT. In 5%–10% of cases, they are hemodynamically significant with diastolic compression of the right atrium seen on echocardiography. Some present with pericardial tamponade (REYNOLDS et al. 1992). The effusions are often idiopathic or related to viral infection or congestive heart failure. However, 30% of patients with tuberculosis (Fig. 7.25) and 40% of those with Kaposi's sarcoma had moderate to severe pericardial effusions in one series. Purulent bacterial pericarditis, fungal pericarditis, and involvement with lymphoma and metastatic carcinoma occasionally will cause AIDS-associated pericardial effusion.

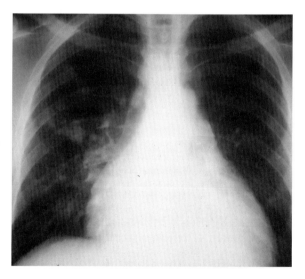

Fig. 7.25. A 25-year-old man with AIDS diagnosed with tuberculosis involving the right lung and pericardium. PA chest radiograph demonstrates a globularly enlarged cardiac silhouette consistent with pericardial effusion. There is also a right perihilar nodular lung parenchymal opacity

References

Amorosa JK, Nahass RG, Nosher JL, Gocke DJ (1990) Radiologic distinction of pyogenic pulmonary infection from *Pneumocystis carinii* pneumonia in AIDS patients. Radiology 175:721–724

Anderson DW, Virmani R, Reilly JM, et al. (1988) Prevalent myocarditis at necropsy in the acquired immunodeficiency syndrome. J Am Coll Cardiol 11:792–799

Aronchick JM, Miller WT Jr (1993) Disseminated nontuberculous mycobacterial infections in immunosuppressed patients. Semin Roentgenol 28:150–157

Bani-Sadr F, Hamidou M, Raffi F, Chamoux C, Caillon J, Freland C (1995) Clinical and bacteriological aspects of nocardiasis. Presse Med 24:1062–1066

Barbaro G, Di Lorenzo G, Grisorio B, Barbarini G (1998) Incidence of dilated cardiomyopathy and detection of HIV in myocardial cells of HIV-positive patients. N Engl J Med 339:1093–1099

Barnes PF, Bloch AB, Davidson PT, Snider DE Jr (1991) Tuberculosis in patients with human immunodeficiency virus infection. N Engl J Med 324:1644–1650

Bazot M, Cadranel J, Benayoun S, Tassart M, Bigot JM, Carette MF (1999) Primary pulmonary AIDS-related lymphoma: radiographic and CT findings. Chest 116:1282–1286

Broder S, Karp JE (1992) The expanding challenge of HIV-associated malignancies. CA Cancer J Clin 42:69–73

Bronnimann DA, Adam RD, Galgiani JN, Habib MP, Petersen EA, Porter B, Bloom JW (1987) Coccidioidomycosis in the acquired immunodeficiency syndrome. Ann Intern Med 106:372–379

Cadranel J, Mayaud C (1995) Intrathoracic Kaposi's sarcoma in patients with AIDS. Thorax 50:407–414

Cesarman E, Chang Y, Moore PS, Said JW, Knowles DM (1995) Kaposi's sarcoma-associated herpesvirus-like DNA sequences in AIDS-related body-cavity-based lymphomas. N Engl J Med 332:1186–1191

Chan TK, Aranda CP, Rom WN (1993) Bronchogenic carcinoma in young patients at risk for acquired immunodeficiency syndrome. Chest 103:862–864

Chow C, Templeton PA, White CS (1993) Lung cysts associated with *Pneumocystis carinii* pneumonia: radiographic characteristics, natural history, and complications. Am J Roentgenol 161:527–531

Conces DJ Jr (1999) Endemic fungal pneumonia in immunocompromised patients. J Thorac Imaging 14:1–8

Conces DJ Jr, Stockberger SM, Tarver RD, Wheat LJ (1993) Disseminated histoplasmosis in AIDS: findings on chest radiographs. Am J Roentgenol 160:15–19

Connolly JE Jr, McAdams HP, Erasmus JJ, Rosado-de-Christenson ML (1999) Opportunistic fungal pneumonia. J Thorac Imaging 14:51–62

Corboy JR, Fink L, Miller WT (1987) Congestive cardiomyopathy in association with AIDS. Radiology 165:139–141

Davis SD, Henschke CI, Chamides BK, Westcott JL (1987) Intrathoracic Kaposi sarcoma in AIDS patients: radiographic-pathologic correlation. Radiology 163:495–500

Denning DW, Follansbee SE, Scolaro M, Norris S, Edelstein H, Stevens DA (1991) Pulmonary aspergillosis in the acquired immunodeficiency syndrome. N Engl J Med 324:654–662

Diaz PT, King MA, Pacht ER, et al. (1999) The pathophysiology of pulmonary diffusion impairment in human immunodeficiency virus infection. Am J Respir Crit Care Med 160:272–277

Diaz PT, King MA, Pacht ER, et al. (2000) Increased susceptibility to pulmonary emphysema among HIV-seropositive smokers. Ann Intern Med 132:369–372

Di Perri G, Cazzadori A, Vento S, et al. (1996) Comparative histopathological study of pulmonary tuberculosis in human immunodeficiency virus-infected and non-infected patients. Tuber Lung Dis 77:244–249

Drabick JJ, Gasser RA Jr, Saunders NB, Hadfield TL, Rogers LC, Berg BW, Drabick CJ (1993) *Pasteurella multocida* pneumonia in a man with AIDS and nontraumatic feline exposure. Chest 103:7–11

Dworkin MS, Sullivan PS, Buskin SE, Harrington RD, Olliffe J, MacArthur RD, Lopez CE (1999) *Bordetella bronchiseptica* infection in human immunodeficiency virus-infected patients. Clin Infect Dis 28:1095–1099

Eisner MD, Kaplan LD, Herndier B, Stulbarg MS (1996) The pulmonary manifestations of AIDS-related non-Hodgkin's lymphoma. Chest 110:729–736

Fish DG, Ampel NM, Galgiani JN, et al. (1990) Coccidioidomycosis during human immunodeficiency virus infection. A review of 77 patients. Medicine 69:384–391

Fishman JE, Schwartz DS, Sais GJ (1997) *Mycobacterium kansasii* pulmonary infection in patients with AIDS: spectrum of chest radiographic findings. Radiology 204:171–175

Fishman JE, Saraf-Lavi E, Narita M, Hollender ES, Ramsinghani R, Ashkin D (2000) Pulmonary tuberculosis in AIDS patients: transient chest radiographic worsening after initiation of antiretroviral therapy. Am J Roentgenol 174:43–49

Furman AC, Jacobs J, Sepkowitz KA (1996) Lung abscess in patients with AIDS. Clin Infect Dis 22:81–85

Gatell JM, Marrades R, el Ebiary M, Torres A (1996) Severe pulmonary infections in AIDS patients. Semin Respir Infect 11:119–128

Genta RM (1989) Global prevalence of strongyloidiasis: critical review with epidemiologic insights into the prevention of disseminated disease. Rev Infect Dis 11:755–767

Goodman PC, Schnapp LM (1992) Pulmonary toxoplasmosis in AIDS. Radiology 184:791–793

Greenberg SD, Frager D, Suster B, Walker S, Stavropoulos C, Rothpearl A (1994) Active pulmonary tuberculosis in patients with AIDS: spectrum of radiographic findings (including a normal appearance). Radiology 193:115–119

Gruden JF, Huang L, Webb WR, Gamsu G, Hopewell PC, Sides DM (1995) AIDS-related Kaposi sarcoma of the lung: radiographic findings and staging system with bronchoscopic correlation. Radiology 195:545–552

Gruden JF, Huang L, Turner J, et al. (1997) High-resolution CT in the evaluation of clinically suspected *Pneumocystis carinii* pneumonia in AIDS patients with normal, equivocal, or nonspecific radiographic findings. Am J Roentgenol 169:967–975

Grulich AE (1999) AIDS-associated non-Hodgkin's lymphoma in the era of highly active antiretroviral therapy. J Acquir Immune Defic Syndr 21 (Suppl 1):S27–S30

Guerin JM, Masmoudi R, Leibinger F (1995) Anguillulase et SIDA. Med Mal Infect 25:1196

Haramati LB, Wong J (2000) Intrathoracic Kaposi's sarcoma in women with AIDS. Chest 117:410–414

Haramati LB, Jenny-Avital ER, Alterman DD (1997) Effect of HIV status on chest radiographic and CT findings in patients with tuberculosis. Clin Radiol 52:31–35

Harvey RL, Sunstrum JC (1991) *Rhodococcus equi* infection in patients with and without human immunodeficiency virus infection. Rev Infect Dis 13:139–145

Hirschtick RE, Glassroth J, Jordan MC, et al. (1995) Bacterial pneumonia in persons infected with the human immunodeficiency virus. Pulmonary Complications of HIV Infection Study Group. N Engl J Med 333:845–851

Hocqueloux L, Lesprit P, Herrmann JL, de La BA, Zagdanski AM, Decazes JM, Modai J (1998) Pulmonary *Mycobacterium avium* complex disease without dissemination in HIV-infected patients. Chest 113:542–548

Horsburgh CR Jr (1991) *Mycobacterium avium* complex infection in the acquired immunodeficiency syndrome. N Engl J Med 324:1332–1338

Igra-Siegman Y, Kapila R, Sen P, Kaminski ZC, Louria DB (1981) Syndrome of hyperinfection with *Strongyloides stercoralis*. Rev Infect Dis 3:397–407

Jones BE, Young SM, Antoniskis D, Davidson PT, Kramer F, Barnes PF (1993) Relationship of the manifestations of tuberculosis to CD4 cell counts in patients with human immunodeficiency virus infection. Am Rev Respir Dis 148:1292–1297

Jones JL, Hanson DL, Dworkin MS, Ward JW, Jaffe HW (1999) Effect of antiretroviral therapy on recent trends in selected cancers among HIV-infected persons. Adult/Adolescent Spectrum of HIV Disease Project Group. J Acquir Immune Defic Syndr 21 (Suppl 1):S11–S17

Jones PD, See J (1992) *Penicillium marneffei* infection in patients infected with human immunodeficiency virus: late presentation in an area of nonendemicity. Clin Infect Dis 15:744

Kalayjian RC, Toossi Z, Tomashefski JF Jr, Carey JT, Ross JA, Tomford JW, Blinkhorn RJ Jr (1995) Pulmonary disease due to infection by *Mycobacterium avium* complex in patients with AIDS. Clin Infect Dis 20:1186–1194

Kedes DH, Ganem D, Ameli N, Bacchetti P, Greenblatt R (1997) The prevalence of serum antibody to human herpesvirus 8 (Kaposi sarcoma-associated herpesvirus) among HIV-seropositive and high-risk HIV-seronegative women. JAMA 277:478–481

Keiper MD, Beumont M, Elshami A, Langlotz CP, Miller WT Jr (1995) CD4 T lymphocyte count and the radiographic presentation of pulmonary tuberculosis. A study of the relationship between these factors in patients with human immunodeficiency virus infection. Chest 107:74–80

Khalil AM, Carette MF, Cadranel JL, Mayaud CM, Bigot JM (1995) Intrathoracic Kaposi's sarcoma. CT findings. Chest 108:1622–1626

Koehler JE, Sanchez MA, Garrido CS, et al. (1997) Molecular epidemiology of *Bartonella* infections in patients with bacillary angiomatosis-peliosis. N Engl J Med 337:1876–1883

Kramer MR, Uttamchandani RB (1990) The radiographic appearance of pulmonary nocardiosis associated with AIDS. Chest 98:382–385

Kuhlman JE (1996) Pneumocystic infections: the radiologist's perspective. Radiology 198:623–635

Kuhlman JE, Knowles MC, Fishman EK, Siegelman SS (1989) Premature bullous pulmonary damage in AIDS: CT diagnosis. Radiology 173:23–26

Kuhlman JE, Kavuru M, Fishman EK, Siegelman SS (1990) *Pneumocystis carinii* pneumonia: spectrum of parenchymal CT findings. Radiology 175:711–714

Kwon KY, Colby TV (1994) *Rhodococcus equi* pneumonia and pulmonary malacoplakia in acquired immunodeficiency syndrome. Pathologic features. Arch Pathol Lab Med 118:744–748

Laissy JP, Cadi M, Cinqualbre A, et al. (1997) *Mycobacterium tuberculosis* versus nontuberculous mycobacterial infection of the lung in AIDS patients: CT and HRCT patterns. J Comput Assist Tomogr 21:312–317

Martin JN, Ganem DE, Osmond DH, Page-Shafer KA, Macrae D, Kedes DH (1998) Sexual transmission and the natural history of human herpesvirus 8 infection. N Engl J Med 338:948–954

McGuinness G, Scholes JV, Garay SM, Leitman BS, McCauley DI, Naidich DP (1994) Cytomegalovirus pneumonitis: spectrum of parenchymal CT findings with pathologic correlation in 21 AIDS patients. Radiology 192:451–459

McGuinness G, Gruden JF, Bhalla M, Harkin TJ, Jagirdar JS, Naidich DP (1997) AIDS-related airway disease. Am J Roentgenol 168:67–77

Miller WT Jr, Edelman JM, Miller WT (1990) Cryptococcal pulmonary infection in patients with AIDS: radiographic appearance. Radiology 175:725–728

Miller WT Jr, Sais GJ, Frank I, Gefter WB, Aronchick JM, Miller WT (1994) Pulmonary aspergillosis in patients with AIDS. Clinical and radiographic correlations. Chest 105:37–44

Mirmirani P, Maurer TA, Herndier B, McGrath M, Weinstein MD, Berger TG (1999) Sarcoidosis in a patient with AIDS: a manifestation of immune restoration syndrome. J Am Acad Dermatol 41:285–286

Moore EH, Russell LA, Klein JS, et al. (1995) Bacillary angiomatosis in patients with AIDS: multiorgan imaging findings. Radiology 197:67–72

Morassut S, Vaccher E, Balestreri L, et al. (1997) HIV-associated human herpesvirus 8-positive primary lymphomatous effusions: radiologic findings in six patients. Radiology 205:459–463

Muntaner L, Leyes M, Payeras A, Herrera M, Gutierrez A (1997) Radiologic features of *Rhodococcus equi* pneumonia in AIDS. Eur J Radiol 24:66–70

Naccache JM, Antoine M, Wislez M, Fleury-Feith J, Oksenhendler E, Mayaud C, Cadranel J (1999) Sarcoid-like pulmonary disorder in human immunodeficiency virus-infected patients receiving antiretroviral therapy. Am J Respir Crit Care Med 159:2009–2013

Narita M, Ashkin D, Hollender ES, Pitchenik AE (1998) Paradoxical worsening of tuberculosis following antiretroviral therapy in patients with AIDS. Am J Respir Crit Care Med 158:157–161

Nomura J, Rekrut K (1996) *Strongyloides stercoralis* hyperinfection syndrome in a patient with AIDS: diagnosis by fluorescent microscopy. Clin Infect Dis 22:736

Oldham SA, Castillo M, Jacobson FL, Mones JM, Saldana MJ (1989) HIV-associated lymphocytic interstitial pneumonia: radiologic manifestations and pathologic correlation. Radiology 170:83–87

Opravil M, Pechere M, Speich R, et al. (1997) HIV-associated primary pulmonary hypertension. A case control study. Swiss HIV Cohort Study. Am J Respir Crit Care Med 155:990–995

Palella FJ Jr, Delaney KM, Moorman AC, et al. (1998) Declining morbidity and mortality among patients with advanced human immunodeficiency virus infection. HIV Outpatient Study Investigators. N Engl J Med 338:853–860

Parker MS, Leveno DM, Campbell TJ, Worrell JA, Carozza SE (1998) AIDS-related bronchogenic carcinoma: fact or fiction? Chest 113:154–161

Pastores SM, Naidich DP, Aranda CP, McGuinnes G, Rom WN (1993) Intrathoracic adenopathy associated with pulmonary tuberculosis in patients with human immunodeficiency virus infection. Chest 103:1433–1437

Rabaud C, May T, Lucet JC, Leport C, Ambroise-Thomas P, Canton P (1996) Pulmonary toxoplasmosis in patients infected with human immunodeficiency virus: a French National Survey. Clin Infect Dis 23:1249–1254

Race EM, Adelson-Mitty J, Kriegel GR, Barlam TF, Reimann KA, Letvin NL, Japour AJ (1998) Focal mycobacterial lymphadenitis following initiation of protease-inhibitor therapy in patients with advanced HIV-1 disease. Lancet 351:252–255

Relkin F, Aranda CP, Garay SM, Smith R, Berkowitz KA, Rom WN (1994) Pleural tuberculosis and HIV infection. Chest 105:1338–1341

Reynolds MM, Hecht SR, Berger M, Kolokathis A, Horowitz SF (1992) Large pericardial effusions in the acquired immunodeficiency syndrome. Chest 102:1746–1747

Sandhu JS, Goodman PC (1989) Pulmonary cysts associated with Pneumocystis carinii pneumonia in patients with AIDS. Radiology 173:33–35

Schneider MM, Borleffs JC, Stolk RP, Jaspers CA, Hoepelman AI (1999) Discontinuation of prophylaxis for Pneumocystis carinii pneumonia in HIV-1-infected patients treated with highly active antiretroviral therapy. Lancet 353:201–203

Shah RM, Kaji AV, Ostrum BJ, Friedman AC (1997) Interpretation of chest radiographs in AIDS patients: usefulness of CD4 lymphocyte counts. Radiographics 17:47–58

Shapiro JM, Romney BM, Weiden MD, White CS, O'Toole KM (1992) Rhodococcus equi endobronchial mass with lung abscess in a patient with AIDS. Thorax 47:62–63

Sider L, Weiss AJ, Smith MD, VonRoenn JH, Glassroth J (1989) Varied appearance of AIDS-related lymphoma in the chest. Radiology 171:629–632

Silva-Cardoso J, Moura B, Martins L, Mota-Miranda A, Rocha-Goncalves F, Lecour H (1999) Pericardial involvement in human immunodeficiency virus infection. Chest 115:418–422

Singh VR, Smith DK, Lawerence J, Kelly PC, Thomas AR, Spitz B, Sarosi GA (1996) Coccidioidomycosis in patients infected with human immunodeficiency virus: review of 91 cases at a single institution. Clin Infect Dis 23:563–568

Staples CA, Kang EY, Wright JL, Phillips P, Muller NL (1995) Invasive pulmonary aspergillosis in AIDS: radiographic, CT, and pathologic findings. Radiology 196:409–414

Supparatpinyo K, Khamwan C, Baosoung V, Nelson KE, Sirisanthana T (1994) Disseminated Penicillium marneffei infection in southeast Asia. Lancet 344:110–113

Traill ZC, Miller RF, Shaw PJ (1996) CT appearances of intrathoracic Kaposi's sarcoma in patients with AIDS. Br J Radiol 69:1104–1107

Travis WD, Fox CH, Devaney KO, et al. (1992) Lymphoid pneumonitis in 50 adult patients infected with the human immunodeficiency virus: lymphocytic interstitial pneumonitis versus nonspecific interstitial pneumonitis. Hum Pathol 23:529–541

Uttamchandani RB, Daikos GL, Reyes RR, Fischl MA, Dickinson GM, Yamaguchi E, Kramer MR (1994) Nocardiosis in 30 patients with advanced human immunodeficiency virus infection: clinical features and outcome. Clin Infect Dis 18:348–353

Wasser L, Talavera W (1987) Pulmonary cryptococcosis in AIDS. Chest 92:692–695

Waxman AB, Goldie SJ, Brett-Smith H, Matthay RA (1997) Cytomegalovirus as a primary pulmonary pathogen in AIDS. Chest 111:128–134

White CS, Haramati LB, Elder KH, Karp J, Belani CP (1995) Carcinoma of the lung in HIV-positive patients: findings on chest radiographs and CT scans. Am J Roentgenol 164:593–597

White DA (1996) Pulmonary complications of HIV-associated malignancies. Clin Chest Med 17:755–761

8 Abdominal AIDS Imaging: Luminal Tract Manifestations

Judy Yee

CONTENTS

8.1
Introduction

It has been close to two decades since the first cases of AIDS were reported in 1981 and the epidemic continues despite the use of multiple new antiviral drug regimens. Most patients with AIDS will have symptoms of gastrointestinal tract disease at some point during the course of their illness. The diagnosis of clinical AIDS is often made by identifying a malignant neoplasm or an opportunistic infection of the gastrointestinal tract. It is essential that physicians are aware of the specific gastrointestinal manifestations of this disease.

8.2
Primary HIV Infection

Patients may develop odynophagia or dysphagia at the time of initial infection by human immune deficiency virus (HIV). Endoscopy and esophagogram

J. YEE, MD
Chief of CT and GI Radiology, VA Medical Center/UCSF, 4150 Clement Street, San Francisco, CA 94121, USA

performed at this time may demonstrate a large, flat ulceration of the lower esophagus surrounded by a thin rim of edema (Fig. 8.1). These lesions have been termed *idiopathic esophageal ulcerations associated with HIV infection* (SOR et al. 1995). Electron microscopy of biopsy specimens of ulcer margins has demonstrated retrovirus-like particles, implicating infection by HIV itself as the etiology (RABENECK et al. 1990). Esophagoscopy and biopsy are necessary to exclude other infectious agents, particularly cytomegalovirus infection, which can cause identical giant esophageal ulcerations in AIDS patients. HIV-related esophageal ulcers have also been found to occur long after the initial seroconversion period (LEVINE et al. 1991). Treatment of these idiopathic esophageal ulcerations with prednisone can result in rapid clinical, endoscopic, and radiographic improvement (WILCOX and SCHWARTZ 1992). HIV also directly infects the lower intestinal tract and has been isolated within intestinal tissues in up to 50% of patients with AIDS (NELSON et al. 1988). *Idiopathic AIDS enteropathy* represents a condition of chronic diarrhea in an HIV-positive patient without other identifiable opportunistic infectious etiology. Barium study or CT scan will show nonspecific mild small bowel wall thickening.

8.3
Malignant Neoplasms of AIDS

8.3.1
Kaposi's Sarcoma

Kaposi's sarcoma (KS) is an endothelial malignant neoplasm that did not occur commonly prior to the AIDS epidemic. Currently, KS is the most common malignancy occurring in AIDS patients. KS typically occurs in homosexual or bisexual AIDS patients rather than other risk categories. KS-associated herpesvirus (KSHV), also known as human herpesvirus 8 (HHV-8), has been identified in KS lesions and

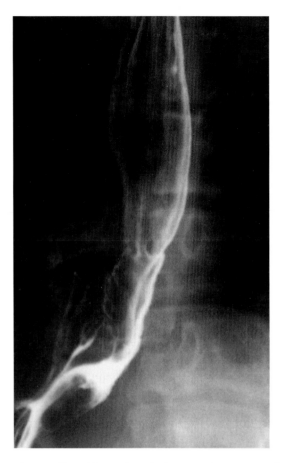

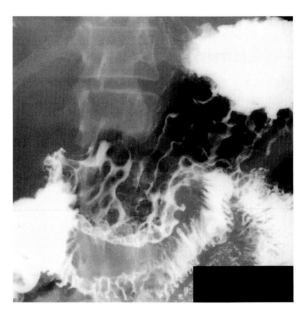

Fig. 8.2. Gastric and duodenal KS. Upper gastrointestinal barium study shows multiple gastric and duodenal nodular lesions secondary to KS in an AIDS patient

Fig. 8.1. Idiopathic esophageal ulceration due to HIV infection. Esophagogram demonstrates a giant flat ulceration of the distal esophagus in an HIV-positive patient. Biopsy specimen revealed no evidence of opportunistic pathogen

there is compelling evidence that this agent is the likely etiology of KS in AIDS patients. About 30%–40% of homosexual men infected with HIV are seropositive for KSHV (GNANN et al. 2000). Almost all patients with KS of any epidemiological type have serological evidence of KSHV infection.

In AIDS patients, KS is particularly aggressive, with multiorgan involvement and widespread cutaneous and nodal spread. The gastrointestinal tract is the third most common site of involvement and the duodenum is the most frequently involved segment of the gastrointestinal tract. KS skin lesions typically antedate the development of gastrointestinal disease. Other sites of KS involvement include the lung, liver, and spleen.

Kaposi's sarcoma lesions of the gastrointestinal tract typically appear as submucosal nodules (Fig. 8.2). These nodules may demonstrate a "bulls-eye" or "target" appearance due to central umbilication. With advanced disease, large polypoid masses and

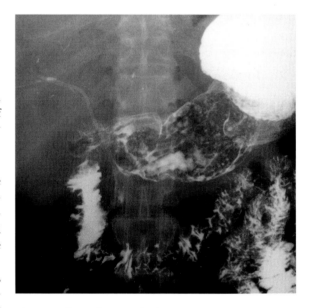

Fig. 8.3. Advanced KS. Multiple gastric masses are present, with one lesion in the proximal antrum demonstrating the target or bull's-eye appearance due to central umbilication. Diffuse involvement of the duodenum has caused biliary obstruction and subsequent placement of a biliary duct stent. A small amount of contrast has refluxed into the intrahepatic biliary tree

irregular fold thickening may be seen (Fig. 8.3). Enteric KS will appear on CT scan as intraluminal nodules or nodular wall thickening which is typically segmental. Diffuse wall thickening is more suggestive of lymphoma or an infectious enteritis. High-attenuation adenopathy on contrast-enhanced CT scan in AIDS patients is suggestive of disseminated KS, which is believed to reflect the vascular nature of this tumor.

8.3.2
AIDS-Related Lymphoma

Malignant lymphoma is a complication of late-stage AIDS. HIV-infected individuals have a greater than 50-fold increased risk of developing non-Hodgkin's lymphoma than the HIV-negative population (BECK et al. 1996). Non-Hodgkin's lymphoma is considered to be an AIDS-defining lesion in HIV-positive patients. HIV-related non-Hodgkin's lymphoma tends to be highly aggressive, and diffuse disease is usually present at the time of diagnosis. Poorly differentiated high-grade, large cell and B cell types are common. AIDS-related lymphoma predominantly presents at extranodal sites, with the gastrointestinal tract and the central nervous system being the most commonly involved sites. The colon, ileum, and stomach are the most frequently involved portions of the gastrointestinal tract, although lesions at unusual sites, such as oral, esophageal, and perianal lesions, as well as multifocal lesions have been reported. HIV-positive patients with lymphoma often have a short survival time and show a poor response to chemotherapy (CAPPELL and BOTROS 1994). Life-threatening complications of gastrointestinal tract lymphoma include bleeding, perforation, and obstruction.

Lymphoma of the gastrointestinal tract often appears as irregular fold thickening on barium studies (Fig. 8.4). CT scan is necessary to demonstrate the extraluminal extent of gastrointestinal tract lymphomatous masses (Figs. 8.5, 8.6). Nonspecific hepatosplenomegaly may also be present. Lymphomatous involvement of the liver and spleen in AIDS patients is suggested by focal homogeneous low-density masses on CT scan or focal hypoechoic lesions on ultrasonography. Abundant retroperitoneal or mesenteric adenopathy is a common manifestation of AIDS-related lymphoma, but may also be due to KS or mycobacterial infection. Numerous small retroperitoneal lymph nodes are often present in AIDS patients but are due to reactive hyperplasia rather than malignancy or an opportunistic infection.

8.4
Opportunistic Infections

8.4.1
Candidiasis

Candida albicans is one of the most common opportunistic infections in AIDS patients and typically involves the oropharynx and esophagus. *Candida*

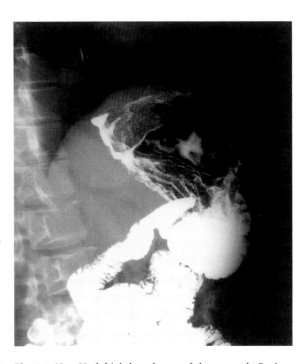

Fig. 8.4. Non-Hodgkin's lymphoma of the stomach. Barium study shows that markedly thickened and irregular folds are present in the fundus of the stomach due to lymphomatous involvement

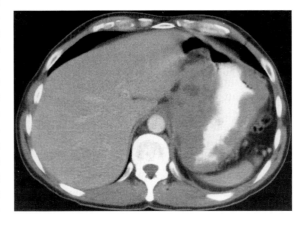

Fig. 8.5. CT scan of gastric lymphoma demonstrates extensive irregular wall thickening of the proximal stomach. Retrocrural adenopathy is also present

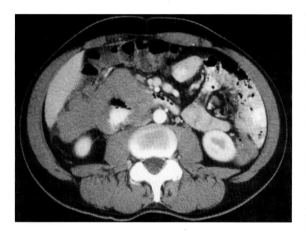

Fig. 8.6. CT scan of enteric lymphoma. There is a large lobu-
lated mass involving the second portion of the duodenum
and extending between the tip of the liver and the right kidney

esophagitis occurring in a seropositive patient de-
fines clinical AIDS in that patient. Patients often
present with dysphagia or odynophagia, but can develop acute retrosternal chest pain. The presence of
oral thrush can help to suggest the presence of candidal esophagitis, although the absence of oral
thrush does not help to exclude the diagnosis of
candidal infection of the esophagus. Although not as
common, oral thrush may occur in the setting of
viral esophagitis or with a combination of candidal
and viral esophagitis.

The appearance on endoscopy is characteristic
(focal or confluent yellowish-white plaques overlying an erythematous mucosa), although medical
therapy is often initiated based on clinical symptoms, especially if typical findings are present on
barium swallow. Radiographic findings of candidal
esophagitis include mucosal plaques and fold thickening (Figs. 8.7, 8.8). Occasionally a cobblestone appearance may be seen secondary to submucosal edema. AIDS patients tend to present in the more
advanced stages of infection. Severe candidal esophagitis appears on esophagogram as a markedly irregular shaggy-appearing esophagus due to barium
trapping within plaques and pseudomembranes in
conjunction with deep ulcerations and mucosal
sloughing (LEVINE et al. 1985).

Systemic infection by *Candida* is rare, and hematogenous dissemination can result in the development of microabscesses in the liver, spleen, and kidneys. Intestinal candidiasis can also occur, although
it is typically difficult to diagnose. Barium findings
are nonspecific and include bowel dilatation or irregular narrowing, thickened folds, and ulcerations.

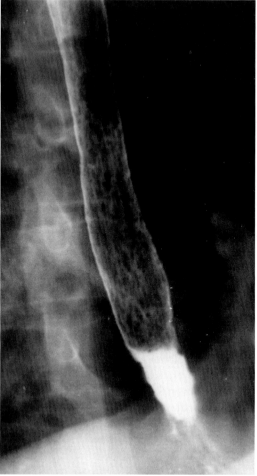

Fig. 8.7. Candidal esophagitis. Barium study shows multiple
mucosal plaques involving the esophagus diffusely

Necrotizing enterocolitis has also been reported as a
complication of *Candida* in an AIDS patient with the
development of bowel ischemia and extensive pneumatosis intestinalis (BALTHAZAR and STERN 1994).

8.4.2
Herpes

The causative agent for herpes esophagitis in AIDS
patients is HSV type 1 or type 2. Odynophagia is the
most common presenting symptom, although patients can also present with dysphagia and rarely
hematemesis. The features of herpes esophagitis best
demonstrated on double-contrast esophagogram
consist of small, discrete, scattered shallow ulcers
which are separated by normal-appearing mucosa
(Fig. 8.9). When viewed en face, these ulcers may
have a diamond or stellate shape and are surrounded

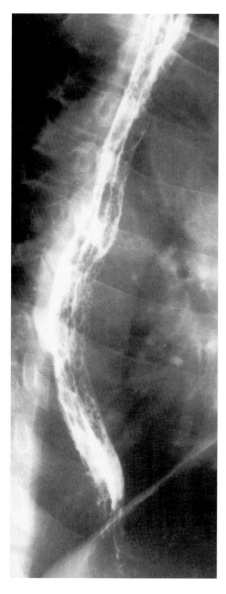

Fig. 8.8. Candidal esophagitis. Extensive involvement of the esophagus with plaque formation and fold thickening

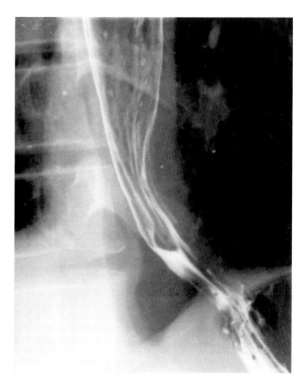

Fig. 8.9. Herpes esophagitis. Multiple small ulcerations, each surrounded by a ring of lucency due to edema, are present in the distal esophagus

by a lucent rim of edema. Plaque-like lesions that are indistinguishable from candidal esophagitis may also be present. Esophagogram abnormalities can almost always be detected in patients with herpes esophagitis, and in greater than half of the cases the specific diagnosis can be made (LEVINE et al. 1988). Endoscopic findings include discrete ulcers with exudate. Biopsy and histologic analysis reveals typical Cowdry-type A intranuclear inclusion bodies (MCBANE and GROSS 1991).

8.4.3
Cytomegalovirus

Cytomegalovirus (CMV) is the most common infection of the gastrointestinal tract of HIV-positive patients. Approximately 30% of AIDS patients develop gastrointestinal CMV disease (GOODGAME 1993), typically later in the course of their disease. Involvement of all portions of the gastrointestinal tract has been described, although infection of the lower intestinal tract occurs most commonly.

Severe odynophagia is the most common presenting symptom of CMV esophagitis. Substernal and midepigastric pain may also occur. CMV infection causes small, well-circumscribed ulcerations of the esophagus with normal appearance of the intervening mucosa. This appearance is similar to herpes esophagitis, but can usually be distinguished from esophageal candidiasis. However, the characteristic finding of CMV esophagitis on endoscopy and esophagogram is a giant (larger than 2 cm), superficial mucosal ulceration with a halo of edema usually located in the middle or distal esophagus (BALTHAZAR et al. 1987). This appearance is identical to the large flat idiopathic esophageal ulcerations associated with HIV infection, and definitive diagnosis can only be made by endoscopic biopsy and histopathologic examination. Less commonly, deep ulcers are found in 8% of cases of CMV esophagitis (WILCOX et al. 1994).

Frequently, CMV gastritis involves the antrum and appears as nodular wall thickening and luminal narrowing (BALTHAZAR et al. 1985). Features of CMV enteritis and colitis are ulcerations that are initially shallow and then become deeper with increasing edema and wall thickening which can mimic inflammatory bowel disease (Fig. 8.10). CT scan will demonstrate extensive bowel wall thickening in involved areas (Fig. 8.11). CMV involvement of the lower gastrointestinal tract may be segmental or the bowel may be involved diffusely. Lymphadenopathy is usually not a prominent feature of CMV enterocolitis. Giant ulcerations of the ileum and colon (9–10 cm) due to CMV infection have also been described (BALTHAZAR and MARTINO 1996).

Gastrointestinal tract ulcerations are believed to be secondary to a CMV-induced vasculitis with ischemic injury of the endothelium. Complications of CMV enterocolitis may be severe and include peritonitis, perforation, and extensive bleeding. Emergency surgery is often necessary when these complications occur in AIDS patients. Ileocecal resection or right-sided hemicolectomy has also been performed for persistent symptomatic cytomegalovirus enterocolitis that is unresponsive to medical therapy in AIDS patients (SODERLUND et al. 1994).

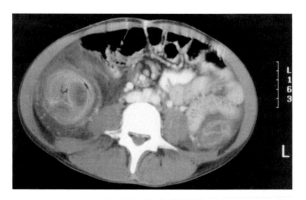

Fig. 8.11. CT scan of CMV colitis shows extensive thickening of the wall of the cecum and descending colon with pericolonic fluid. A small amount of air is present in the wall of the ascending colon, representing pneumatosis

8.4.4
Mycobacterial Infections

8.4.4.1
Mycobacterium tuberculosis

Esophageal tuberculosis is rare and is associated with direct extension from adjacent mediastinal lymph nodes or a lung focus. The middle third of the esophagus is the typical site of tuberculous involvement. The findings on esophagogram and CT scan include traction diverticula, focal extrinsic mass impression, deep ulcerations, and sinus tract and fistula formation. Sinus tracts are to the mediastinum, and bronchoesophageal as well as esophagoesophageal fistulas may occur (GOODMAN et al. 1989). Gastric tuberculosis is also uncommon, although less rare than esophageal involvement. Radiographic and endoscopic findings include ulceration, masses, and outlet obstruction. Histologic findings of acid-fast bacilli and noncaseating granulomas are necessary to confirm the diagnosis of gastrointestinal tract tuberculosis.

The ileocecal area and jejunoileum are the most common sites of tuberculous involvement of the gastrointestinal tract (MARSHALL 1993). Segmental ulcers, wall thickening, strictures, and mass-like lesions of the cecum and terminal ileum may be identified on barium studies and CT scan (BALTHAZAR et al. 1990) (Fig. 8.12). Associated regional low-attenuation necrotic lyphmadenopathy is a helpful diagnostic finding on CT scan. Possible complications of ileocecal tuberculosis include fistula formation, obstruction, perforation, and bleeding.

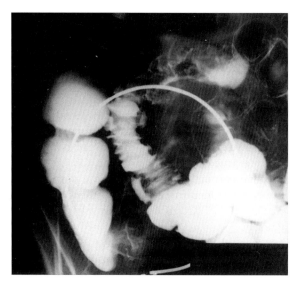

Fig. 8.10. CMV enteritis. Spot film from a barium study shows marked fold thickening with several large ulcerations of the distal ileum

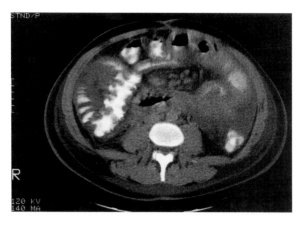

Fig. 8.12. Tuberculous enterocolitis. CT scan demonstrates terminal ileal and cecal wall thickening. Colonoscopic biopsy revealed acid-fast bacilli and noncaseating granulomas

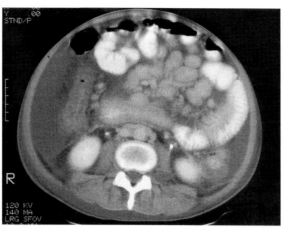

Fig. 8.14. CT scan of a patient with MAC enteritis and CMV colitis. Duodenal wall thickening and bulky mesenteric adenopathy were secondary to MAC infection. Thickening of the wall of the ascending colon was found to be due to CMV

8.4.4.2
Mycobacterium avium Complex

Mycobacterium avium complex (MAC) is the most common opportunistic infection occurring in patients with advanced AIDS.

The most common site of MAC infection of the gastrointestinal tract is the small bowel. Clinically patients will present with diarrhea, fever, and weight loss. Because the pathophysiology and radiographic findings of MAC enteritis mimic Whipple's disease, it is often described as pseudo-Whipple disease. Barium study and CT scan will show mild small bowel dilatation and diffuse, irregular fold thickening (Fig. 8.13). Small bowel loops may appear separated or displaced due to adenopathy. Large mesenteric and retroperitoneal adenopathy is often present (Fig. 8.14) and may appear low density due to necrosis. However, this

pattern of low-density lymphadenopathy has been reported to be more common with *M. tuberculosis* infection (GOODMAN et al. 1989). Marked hepatosplenomegaly is often present. However, low-density MAC microabscesses within the liver and spleen due to hematogenous dissemination are an uncommon finding. Focal hypodense hepatosplenic lesions are more commonly associated with systemic tuberculous infection (RADIN 1991).

8.4.5
Cryptosporidiosis

Cryptosporidiosis is an enteric parasitic infection caused by a small protozoan that produces a profuse diarrhea in AIDS patients. *Cryptosporidium* can cause life-threatening dehydration and electrolyte abnormalities in these patients. The proximal small bowel is the most common site of gastrointestinal tract infection, although extensive involvement of both the large and the small bowel is associated with the most severe diarrheal illness. The diagnosis of intestinal *Cryptosporidium* infection is made by stool examination, although the organism may also be identified by bowel biopsy. There is histologic evidence that *Cryptosporidium* infection causes gastrointestinal tract epithelial cell injury which may be influenced by co-pathogens such as cytomegalovirus (LUMADUE et al. 1998). Fecal-oral contamination and sexual contact are the most common routes of spread in AIDS patients.

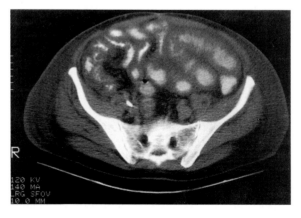

Fig. 8.13. CT scan of MAC enteritis. Small bowel wall thickening is present diffusely. Several small bowel loops in the left abdomen also demonstrate mild dilatation

Fold thickening is most prominent in the duodenum and jejunum although the entire small bowel may be involved (Fig. 8.15). Mild small bowel dilatation as well as barium dilution, fragmentation, and flocculation due to hypersecretion can occur. This may occasionally produce a sprue-like appearance. CT scan findings of small bowel cryptosporidiosis are often nonspecific and show fluid-filled, mildly dilated enteric segments. There is usually no associated lymphadenopathy, in contrast to other infections such as MAC or tuberculosis.

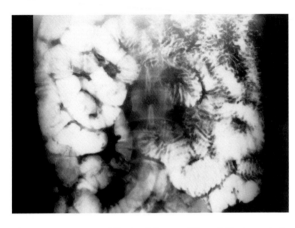

Fig. 8.15. Cryptosporidiosis of the small bowel. Barium study demonstrates fold thickening involving jejunal loops with normal-appearing ileal loops. This pattern is commonly seen with enteric *Cryptosporidium* infection

8.5
Conclusion

AIDS patients often have multiple infections of the gastrointestinal tract that are slow to respond or do not respond to conventional treatments. HIV-related malignancies of the gastrointestinal tract are particularly aggressive, and widespread disease is often present at the time of diagnosis. It is important to recognize the radiographic spectrum of gastrointestinal diseases that occur in AIDS patients since therapy and management decisions often rely on imaging findings.

References

Balthazar EJ, Martino JM (1996) Giant ulcers in the ileum and colon caused by cytomegalovirus in patients with AIDS. AJR 166:1275–1276

Balthazar EJ, Stern J (1994) Necrotizing candida enterocolitis in AIDS: CT features. J Comput Assist Tomogr 18:298–300

Balthazar EJ, Megibow AJ, Hulnick DH (1985) Cytomegalovirus esophagitis and gastritis in AIDS. AJR 144:1201–1204

Balthazar EJ, Megibow AJ, Hulnick D, et al. (1987) Cytomegalovirus esophagitis in AIDS: radiographic features in 16 patients. AJR 149:919–923

Balthazar EJ, Gordon R, Hulnick D (1990) Ileocecal tuberculosis: CT and radiologic evaluation. AJR 154:499–503

Beck PL, Gill MJ, Sutherland LR (1996) HIV-associated non-Hodgkin's lymphoma of the gastrointestinal tract. Am J Gastroenterol 91:2377–2381

Cappell MS, Botros N (1994) Predominantly gastrointestinal symptoms and signs in 11 consecutive patients with gastrointestinal lymphoma: a multicenter, multiyear study including 763 HIV-seropositive patients. Am J Gastroenterol 89:545–549

Gnann JW Jr, Pellett PE, Jaffe HW (2000) Human herpesvirus 8 and Kaposi's sarcoma in persons infected with human immunodeficiency virus. Clin Infect Dis 30:72–76

Goodgame RW (1993) Gastrointestinal cytomegalovirus disease. Ann Intern Med 119:924–935.

Goodman P, Pinero SS, Rance RM, et al. (1989) Mycobacterial esophagitis in AIDS. Gastrointest Radiol 14:103–105

Levine MS, Macones PJ, Laufer I (1985) *Candida* esophagitis: accuracy of radiographic diagnosis. Radiology 154:581–587

Levine MS, Loevner LA, Saul SH, et al. (1988) Herpes esophagitis: sensitivity of double-contrast esophagography. Am J Roentgenol 151:57–62

Levine MS, Loercher G, Katzka DA, et al. (1991) Giant human immunodeficiency virus-related ulcers of the esophagus. Radiology 180:323–326

Lumadue JA, Manabe YC, Moore RD, et al. (1998) A clinicopathologic analysis of AIDS-related cryptosporidiosis. AIDS 12:2459–2466

Marshall JB (1993) Tuberculosis of the gastrointestinal tract and peritoneum. Am J Gastroenterol 88:989–999

McBane RD, Gross JB Jr (1991) Herpes esophagitis: clinical syndrome, endoscopic appearance, and diagnosis in 23 patients. Gastrointest Endosc 37:600–603

Nelson JA, Reynolds-Kohler C, Margaretten W, et al. (1988) HIV detected in bowel epithelium from patients with gastrointestinal symptoms. Lancet 1:259–262

Rabeneck, L, Popovic M, Gartner S, et al. (1990) Acute HIV infection presenting with painful swallowing and esophageal ulcers. JAMA 263:2318–2322

Radin DR (1991) Intraabdominal *Mycobacterium tuberculosis* vs *Mycobacterium avium-intracellulare* infections in patients with AIDS: distinction based on CT findings. AJR 156:487–491

Soderlund C, Bratt GA, Engstrom L, et al. (1994) Surgical treatment of cytomegalovirus enterocolitis in severe human immunodeficiency virus infection. Report of eight cases. Dis Colon Rectum 37:63–72

Sor S, Levine MS, Kowalski TE, Laufer I, Rubesin SE, Herlinger H (1995) Giant ulcers of the esophagus in patients with human immunodeficiency virus: clinical, radiographic, and pathologic findings. Radiology 194:447–451

Wilcox CM, Schwartz DA (1992) A pilot study of oral corticosteroid therapy for idiopathic esophageal ulcerations associated with human immunodeficiency virus infection. Am J Med 93:131–134

Wilcox CM, Straub RF, Schwartz DA (1994) Prospective endoscopic characterization of cytomegalovirus esophagitis in AIDS. Gastrointest Endosc 40:481–484

9 Abdominal AIDS Imaging: Hepatic, Splenic, Biliary, and Pancreatic Manifestations

RICHARD M. GORE, FRANK H. MILLER, VAHID YAGHMAI, JONATHAN W. BERLIN, GERALDINE M. NEWMARK

CONTENTS

9.1 Introduction

The liver, spleen, pancreas, and biliary tract are commonly affected by opportunistic infections, malignancy, and inflammatory disorders during the course of human immune deficiency virus (HIV) infection (Table 9.1). Clinical manifestations of involvement of these organs are protean and usually nonspecific, but it is important to establish a specific diagnosis promptly in these often critically ill patients (TSHIBWABWA et al. 2000). Because of the limitations of physical and laboratory examinations, cross-sectional imaging studies are often obtained to

R. M. GORE, MD; V. YAGHMAI, MD; J. W. BERLIN, MD;
G. M. NEWMARK, MD
Department of Diagnostic Radiology, Evanston Northwestern Healthcare, 2650 Ridge Ave., Evanston, IL 60201, USA
F. H. MILLER, MD
Department of Radiology, Northwestern Memorial Hospital, Northwestern University Medical School, 676 St. Clair, Chicago, IL 60611, USA

Table 9.1. Hepatic splenic, biliary, and pancreatic disease associated with HIV infection

Infection

Bacterial
Salmonella
Rochalimaea
Mycobacterial
M. tuberculosis
M. avium intracellulan complex
M. xenopi

Viral
Cytomegalovirus
Hepatitis B, C, and D
Herpesvirus
Adenovirus
HIV

Fungal
Candida
Cryptococcus
Histoplasma
Aspergillus
Coccidia
Sporothrix

Protozoal
Pneumocystis
Cryptosporidia
Microsporidia
Leishmania
Toxoplasma

Neoplasms
Non-Hodgkin's lymphoma
Kaposi's sarcoma
Metastatic cancer of anal canal

Drug-related
Trimethoprim-sulfamethoxazole
Ketoconazole
Isoniazid
Rifampin
Zidovudine
Pentamidine
Diphenylhydantoin
Prochlorperazine
Didanosine
Fluconazole
Oxacillin
Dideoxyinosine

clarify the clinical situation (DeToma et al. 1999; Wu et al. 1998). This chapter reviews the imaging spectrum of HIV-associated hepatosplenic and pancreaticobiliary disease.

9.2
Neoplasms

The opportunistic neoplasms Kaposi's sarcoma and non-Hodgkin's lymphoma can involve the liver, spleen, bile ducts, gallbladder, and pancreas but are seldom seen alone. Usually there is multisystemic involvement. Kaposi's sarcoma is an AIDS-defining illness and usually occurs early in the disease course (Krown 1997). AIDS-related lymphoma (ARL) typically develops when there is profound immunosuppression (CD4 lymphocyte count <50 mm^3).

Kaposi's sarcoma is the most common neoplasm in patients with AIDS and is seen almost exclusively in homosexual men (Gourevitch 1996). Visceral involvement is often asymptomatic even in the presence of extensive disease, though there may be mild elevation of serum alkaline phosphatase. The Kaposi's sarcoma lesion is a purple nodule macroscopically that microscopically consists of irregularly dilated vascular spaces coated with swollen endothelial cells. Detection of Kaposi's sarcoma on imaging studies is difficult because the tumor spreads via microscopic perivascular infiltration. Distinctive CT features that indicate the diagnosis include the presence of normal or mildly enlarged lymph nodes that have high density approaching the attenuation of enhancing blood vessels due to the hypervascularity of the tumor (Herts et al. 1992). They are usually observed in the groin but can be retroperitoneal, axillary, or pelvic in location. Skin nodules and nodular metastases to the hollow viscera and lung may also be seen (Ferrozzi et al. 1995).

Non-Hodgkin's lymphoma is the second most common AIDS-related malignancy and it is believed to be related to Epstein-Barr virus infection (Wang et al. 1996). The frequency of non-Hodgkin's lymphoma is much higher in patients with AIDS than in the general population, and the disease course also differs. ARLs generally are B cell type centroblastic, lymphoblastic, or immunoblastic and are relatively aggressive, undifferentiated forms of lymphoma (Straus 1997). ARL tends to have a more advanced grade, greater extranodal disease, and a worse prognosis compared with lymphomas occurring in patients without AIDS. The poor prognosis (mean sur-

vival 5–6 months) is also worsened by associated infections (Levine 1992).

9.3
Infections

Infection with HIV causes progressive depletion of T-helper lymphocytes that play a pivotal role in the regulation of the immune system. As a result, AIDS patients are extraordinarily susceptible to opportunistic fungal, viral, protozoan, and mycobacterial infections. Unfortunately, these patients may reveal few systemic signs of infection and laboratory values may be misleading because there may be little fever or associated leukocytosis. Cross-sectional imaging occasionally will reveal large abscesses that are clinically occult. When imaging studies disclose a focal parenchymal mass, imaging-directed percutaneous biopsy (Koegan et al. 1999) may be helpful. When these biopsies are taken, special stains and cultures for mycobacterial, mycotic, and viral organisms should be performed in addition to cytologic evaluation (Jeffrey 1992).

Hepatic, splenic, biliary tract, and pancreatic infections may develop during any stage of HIV disease, from the otherwise asymptomatic state to end-stage immunodeficiency (Schacker et al. 1997). The likely organism infecting a given patient is determined by the degree of immunosuppression (French et al. 1997). Most bacterial diseases, including *Mycobacterium tuberculosis* (MTB), are seen at early or intermediate stages of immunocompromise, when the CD4 lymphocyte count is 200–750 mm^3. Protozoan and fungal infections, such as cryptosporidiosis and *Pneumocystis carinii*, occur when the CD4 lymphocyte count is less than 200 mm^3. *Mycobacterium avium-intracellulare* complex (MAC) and cytomegalovirus (CMV) infections almost always develop in the setting of profound immunosuppression (CD4 lymphocyte count <60 mm^3) (Friedman 1995).

After decades of decreasing incidence, a resurgence of MTB infection has accompanied the AIDS epidemic (Markowitz et al. 1997). MTB infection may develop before other evidence of AIDS and involve the liver, spleen, pancreas, and kidneys without pulmonary involvement (Telzak 1997). Less typical presentations are becoming more prevalent, and extrapulmonary involvement is identified in up to 70% of AIDS patients with MTB, including involvement of the liver, spleen, lymph nodes, central nervous system, bone, gastrointestinal tract, kidney, and soft tissues (HAVLIR and BARNES 1999). The liver is less commonly involved with MTB than MAC. Disseminated MAC infection is insidious, with a relatively late presentation, producing fever, anorexia, lymphadenopathy, hepatosplenomegaly, and elevation of liver function tests (HORSBURGH 1999).

HIV infection is often associated with disseminated hepatitis B and C viruses, CMV, herpes simplex virus, and Epstein-Barr virus due to similar modes of transmission (CAVERT 1997; SORIANO et al. 1999).

All AIDS patients, but particularly those who are intravenous drug abusers, are prone to develop septic emboli and abscesses from a variety of bacteria, most often *Staphylococcus aureus*. The lungs, liver, spleen, and kidneys may also be involved due to hematogenous dissemination. Multiple organisms are often cultured from these abscesses (ALVAREZ et al. 2000).

Candida albicans, Cryptococcus neoformans, Histoplasma capsulatum, and *Coccidioides immitis* infections can cause hepatic, splenic, and pancreatic microabscesses, especially in intravenous drug abusers (MINAMOTO and ROSENBERG 1997). The diagnosis of candidiasis can be difficult because the clinical and radiologic presentation is nonspecific, and this organism may be difficult to culture following biopsy. Additionally, blood cultures are positive in only 50% of patients.

Extrapulmonary *P. carinii* infection is occurring more frequently in AIDS patients owing to their longer life span and the introduction of prophylactic aerosolized pentamidine. Although this therapy produces drug levels sufficient to prevent pulmonary infection, systemic distribution is inadequate, encouraging extrapulmonary disease spread to the liver, spleen, kidneys, lymph nodes, and bone marrow, and, less often, to the adrenal glands, retina, thyroid and parathyroid glands, gallbladder, and pancreas. *P. carinii* pneumonia spreads both hematogenously and lymphogenously. Fortunately, extrapulmonary spread occurs in fewer than 1% of patients. Disseminated disease is usually a premorbid event unless systemic treatment is provided, only a solitary extrapulmonary site is involved, or there is no concurrent active pulmonary infection.

9.4
Hepatosplenic Disease

Nearly 80% of patients with AIDS have abnormal liver function tests at some point of their disease and nearly two-thirds have hepatomegaly and 20% splenomegaly (POLES et al. 1997). The differential diagnosis of these abnormalities is problematic. Although marked elevation of serum alkaline phosphatase levels suggests either biliary tract disease or diffuse hepatic infiltration by mycobacterial infection or lymphoma, elevations of serum transaminases do not correlate with a specific etiology (CHALASANI and WILCOX 1996). Cross-sectional imaging is useful in differentiating the causes of hepatic dysfunction in these patients. It should be remembered that most hepatic disorders that are diagnosed in patients with AIDS signify advanced immunosuppression and occur late in the natural history of the disease when little can be done to improve overall survival (KIM and CELLO 1999).

9.4.1
Mycobacterial Infections

Mycobacterium avium-intracellulare complex is the most common opportunistic pathogen found on liver biopsy in patients with HIV (PANTONGRAG-BROWN et al. 1995). Hepatic involvement usually occurs in the setting of disseminated disease involving lymph nodes, spleen, bone marrow, and/or the gastrointestinal tract so that systemic symptoms may dominate the clinical picture. Liver function tests are often abnormal. Most commonly, there is a marked elevation of the serum alkaline phosphatase, which is thought to arise from microscopic obstruction of smaller biliary ductules by granulomas. Jaundice can occasionally develop from extrahepatic obstruction secondary to porta hepatis and peripancreatic lymphadenopathy. MAC-related granulomas are seen in up to 76% of specimens. These granulomas are poorly formed due to suppressed T cell activity and contain numerous acid-fast organisms. Multidrug antibiotic regimens generally produce an initial response; however, the long-term outcome remains poor owing to the advanced nature of the immunosuppression.

MTB infection occurs in less advanced stages of immunocompromise than does MAC. This accounts for the differences seen histopathologically, which include the presence of caseation and well-formed granulomas. Patients with AIDS are at increased risk for MTB, with the highest incidence in intravenous drug users. Treatment response is good, with median survival of 16 months unless a multidrug-resistant strain is present.

Radiologic evidence of parenchymal involvement is often absent in spite of significant pathologic involvement in MAC. Focal lesions more commonly occur in MTB and this probably relates to the greater attenuation of the host immune status in MAC. MAC may present as multiple hypodense lesions on CT owing to granuloma formation (Rubin 1997). Sonographically multiple tiny echogenic foci in the liver and kidneys similar to extrapulmonary *P. carinii* infection have been reported in patients with MAC infection. Most commonly, however, only hepatosplenomegaly (Fig. 9.1) is seen on imaging studies (Knollmann et al. 1997). A high index of suspicion is required when processing biopsy specimens.

On computed tomography (CT), MTB presents with multifocal lesions in the liver, spleen (Fig. 9.2), kidneys, and pancreas, often associated with enlarged retroperitoneal and mesenteric lymph nodes that usually have central necrosis (Marincili et al. 1986). Concomitant segmental ileocecal wall thick-

ening can also be seen on CT (Suri et al. 1999). Hepatosplenomegaly is more impressive in MAC than in MTB. Low-density lymph nodes are seen in 93% of patients with MTB but only 14% of patients with MAC (Gulati et al. 1999; Radin 1991).

The most common abdominal sonographic and CT (Fig. 9.3) finding in AIDS patients with mycobacterial infection is lymphadenopathy (Chung et al. 1994). Radiologic evidence of parenchymal disease is often absent in spite of significant pathologic involvement; focal lesions occur much more often in MTB than in MAC (Radin 1991). Perhaps the greater attenuation of the host immune status accounts for the absence of focal masses in MAC. Histologically, MAC causes multiple noncaseating granulomas within the lobular parenchyma and portal tracts of the liver (Lefkowitch 1994). MAC may present as multiple hypodense lesions on CT owing to granuloma formation. Sonographically, multiple tiny echogenic foci in the liver and spleen similar to extrapulmonary *P. carinii* infection have been reported (Wetton et al. 1993). Most commonly, however, only hepatosplenomegaly is observed on imaging studies.

A high index of suspicion is required when processing liver biopsy specimens in patients with HIV infection. They should be routinely stained for acid-fast bacilli and cultured for MAC, because caseating granulomatous reaction may be absent in patients with AIDS. In the clinical setting of profound immunosuppression, the presumptive diagnosis of MAC can be made without biopsy if CT demonstrates focal hepatic, splenic, or renal lesions associated with enlarged soft tissue density retroperitoneal or mesenteric lymph nodes and focal jejunal thickening (Radin 1995).

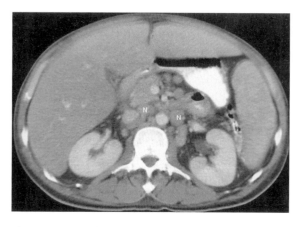

Fig. 9.1. Hepatosplenomegaly associated with MAC. CT scan shows mild hepatosplenomegaly with mesenteric and retroperitoneal lymphadenopathy (*N*)

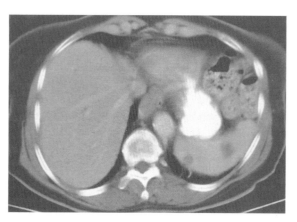

Fig. 9.2. *Mycobacterium tuberculosis* hepatic and splenic abscess. Several hypodense lesions are seen within the spleen and liver

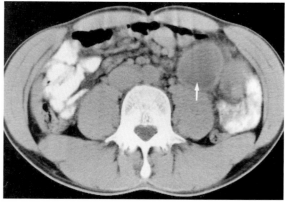

Fig. 9.3. Retroperitoneal lymphadenopathy associated with MAC. This organism was cultured after percutaneous biopsy of the 2-cm lymph node (*arrow*)

9.4.2
Viral Infections

Co-infection with hepatitis B and C viruses, CMV, herpes simplex virus, and Epstein-Barr virus is an important problem in patients with AIDS owing to similar modes of transmission (DIETRICH 1999; VUITTON et al. 1996a). In acute hepatitis, ultrasound may demonstrate hepatomegaly associated with decreased liver echogenicity and prominent portal triads and mural thickening of the gallbladder. CT may show periportal edema, gallbladder wall thickening, and lymphadenopathy in the porta hepatis and hepatomegaly. Hepatitis B and C viruses can cause acute or chronic active hepatitis and ultimately postnecrotic cirrhosis. On cross-sectional imaging, postnecrotic cirrhosis manifests as a nodular hepatic contour, enlargement of the caudate lobe and lateral segment of the left lobe, prominence of the fissures, regenerating nodules, atrophy of the right and quadrate lobes, and perihepatic lymphadenopathy (BARON and GORE 2000). Sonographically, there is increased reflectivity of the fibrous tissue and a concomitant loss of definition of the portal vein walls associated with a generalized coarse, irregular, and heterogeneous hepatic echo architecture.

CMV infection is common in patients with AIDS, seen in up to two-thirds of autopsies. CMV may affect any part of the gastrointestinal tract, generally presenting with ulcers of the esophagus, stomach, and/or colon. Hepatic and pancreatic involvement is observed less frequently. Co-infection with cryptosporidia and *Candida albicans* is common. CMV involves the liver in up to 44% of AIDS patients at autopsy, but generally is clinically silent, unlike biliary, gastrointestinal, or pulmonary infection (PIRATUISUTH et al. 1999). CMV infection may manifest (Fig. 9.4) with multiple echogenic liver lesions sonographically and multiple low-attenuation lesions on CT (VIECO et al. 1990). Hepatic infection by CMV does not significantly alter patient prognosis.

9.4.3
Bacterial Infections

Intravenous drug abusers with AIDS are prone to develop hepatic and splenic septic emboli and abscesses (Fig. 9.5). Usually multiple organisms, most commonly *Staphylococcus aureus,* are cultured from these abscesses.

Peliosis hepatis has been recognized as a bacterial syndrome due to *Rochalimaea henselae* infection in

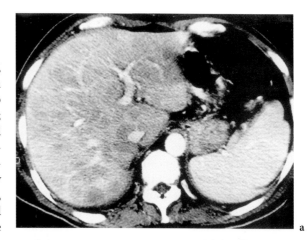

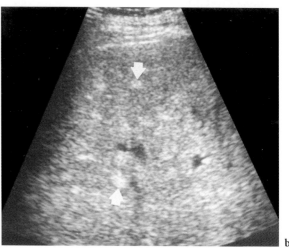

Fig. 9.4a, b. Focal hepatic lesions associated with CMV infection. **a** CT shows multiple hypodense liver masses. **b** These lesions are echogenic (*arrows*) on this transverse sonogram of the liver

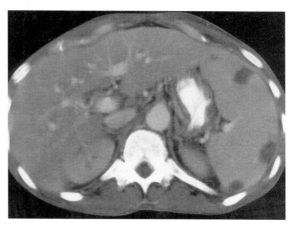

Fig. 9.5. Septic emboli in an intravenous drug abuser with AIDS. The patient has round and wedge-shaped peripheral splenic infarcts and abscesses due to *Staphylococcus aureus*

AIDS patients (MOORE et al. 1995). Histologically, peliosis consists of numerous blood-filled cystic spaces within the hepatic parenchyma without an endothelial lining. There is elevation of serum alkaline phosphatase levels and more modest rises in serum aminotransferase levels. Patients present with cutaneous bacillary angiomatosis as well as fevers, sweats, rigors, and right upper quadrant pain (MOHLE-BOETANI et al. 1996; WYATT and FISHMAN 1993).

The radiologic diagnosis of peliosis hepatis requires a high degree of clinical suspicion because the radiographic and sonographic findings are nonspecific. Sonographically, the tissue texture of the liver is inhomogeneous, with hyperechoic and hypoechoic regions. The CT findings depend upon the size of the vascular cavities. Small cavities are not visible on cross-sectional imaging studies. The blood-filled spaces of larger cavities may appear hypodense early after the intravenous administration of contrast material and become isodense with time. Lesion detection is assisted if there is concomitant hepatic steatosis (GORE et al. 2000).

9.4.4
Fungal Infections

The liver and spleen are often infected in AIDS patients with disseminated fungal infection. These infections share a nonspecific clinical presentation with unexplained fever and hepatosplenomegaly. A nonspecific attenuated granulomatous reaction is seen histologically. Special stains and fungal cultures are generally required for specific diagnosis. Candidiasis can cause hepatic and splenic microabscesses, especially in intravenous drug abusers. These abscesses typically appear as multiple small hypoechoic lesions on sonography or hypodense lesions on CT scans (Fig. 9.6), best seen following intravenous contrast material injection (MURRAY et al. 1995).

9.4.5
Protozoal Infections

The liver is one of the most common extrapulmonary sites of *P. carinii* involvement, occurring in 38% of patients. On liver biopsy, nodules with foamy eosinophilic exudates are seen, often in conjunction with necrosis or hemorrhage, as well as peripheral calcification. Sonography of the liver and spleen (Fig. 9.7a, b) may demonstrate small hypoechoic masses or multiple tiny echogenic foci without shadowing

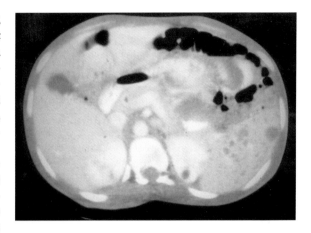

Fig. 9.6. Disseminated candidiasis in a 33-year-old intravenous drug abuser with AIDS. Splenic and renal involvement manifests as multiple small low-attenuation lesions

(BEALE et al. 1995). The echogenic foci are due to calcifications or granulomas (SPONGE et al. 1990). CT scans may demonstrate hypodense lesions or calcifications of the liver and spleen (Fig. 9.7c). Associated findings include punctate calcification of the kidneys, adrenal glands, and lymph nodes (LUBAT et al. 1990). A history of pulmonary *P. carinii* infection, aerosolized pentamidine prophylaxis, and progressive calcification of the liver, spleen, and other organs is suggestive of extrapulmonary *P. carinii* infection.

Calcifications within these lesions do not necessarily signify healed, inactive disease as they do in candidiasis and lymphoma (RADIN et al. 1990). These calcifications were initially believed to be pathognomonic for *P. carinii* infection, but have been described in MAC and CMV infection (BRAY et al. 1992; TOWERS et al. 1991).

9.4.6
Hepatic Steatosis and Cirrhosis

Hepatic steatosis is a common postmortem finding in patients with AIDS (BACH et al. 1992). The pathogenesis of fatty change is complex (FORTGANG et al. 1995) and relates to the effects of circulating cytokines such as tumor necrosis factor, interleukin-1, and interferons. Focal fatty infiltration can mimic other mass lesions. Imaging findings of hepatic steatosis are similar to those in non-AIDS patients. On CT there are diffuse, focal, segmental, or geographic areas of low attenuation in the liver. Sonographically, involved areas show accentuation of echogenic foci resulting from the proliferation of fat-nonfat interfaces. This leads to rapid attenuation of the insonat-

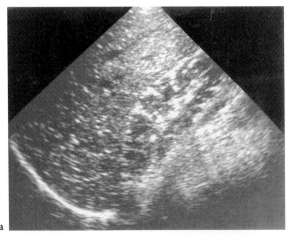

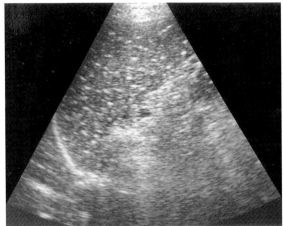

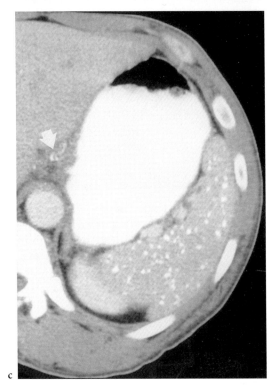

Fig. 9.7a–c. AIDS-related *P. carinii* infection in a 27-year-old man with prior *Pneumocystis* infections who had received prophylactic aerosolized pentamidine. **a** Longitudinal sonogram demonstrates multiple tiny echogenic foci in the liver and right kidney. **b** Multiple tiny echogenic foci are also present in the spleen on this longitudinal scan of the left upper quadrant. **c** Corresponding CT reveals multiple calcifications in the spleen and gastrohepatic ligament (*arrow*). Calcifications are typical of *Pneumocystis* infection and may be present in active and resolved infections

ing ultrasound beam. Magnetic resonance imaging is useful in confidently establishing the presence of focal fatty infiltration (Fig. 9.8).

Multiple hepatic granulomata secondary to infections such as MAC, MTB, cryptococcosis, histoplasmosis, and toxoplasmosis can produce a diffusely echogenic liver as well. Drug toxicity may manifest as hepatic steatosis or as multiple granulomas that also cause an echogenic liver on sonography.

The imaging findings of cirrhosis in AIDS are similar to those seen in patients with hepatitis B and C virus post-necrotic cirrhosis occurring in the absence of AIDS.

9.4.7
Kaposi's Sarcoma

Nearly one-third of patients with cutaneous Kaposi's sarcoma will have hepatic involvement, but this is usually asymptomatic and detected only at postmortem examination (HASAN et al. 1989). The diagnosis is usually made when cutaneous or nodal disease is discovered (Fig. 9.9). Hepatic involvement typically causes only mildly elevated serum alkaline phosphatase levels.

Although specific lesions are rarely identified sonographically, hepatosplenomegaly may be

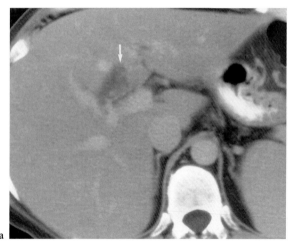

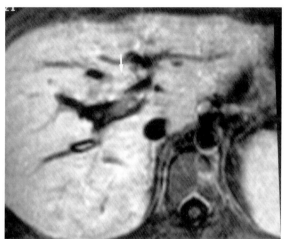

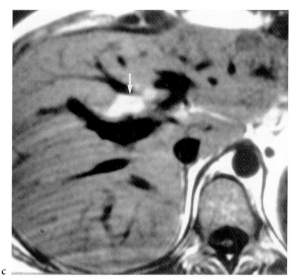

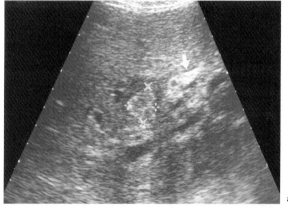

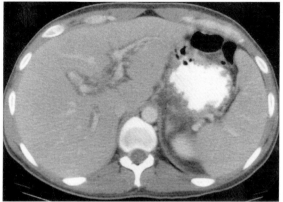

Fig. 9.9a, b. Kaposi's sarcoma: hepatic involvement. **a** Oblique sonogram demonstrates a periportal hyperechoic liver lesion (*calipers*) and echogenic periportal bands (*arrow*). Lymphoma and mycobacterial lesions of the liver tend to be hypoechoic while Kaposi's sarcoma lesions tend to be hyperechoic. **b** Postcontrast CT scan shows low-attenuation periportal changes

Fig. 9.8a–c. A 26-year-old female with AIDS and focal fatty infiltration of the liver. **a** CT demonstrates a hypodense mass (*arrow*). This mass (*arrow*) has a high signal intensity on T1-weighted scan (**b**) which is suppressed on the T1 fat-suppression image (**c**)

present and small hyperechoic periportal and splenic nodules may be visualized, causing increased periportal echogenicity (LUBURICH et al. 1990; VALLS et al. 1991). CT (Fig. 9.10) occasionally demonstrates low-attenuation periportal lesions on noncontrast scans, which subsequently show enhancement on delayed, post-contrast scans (NYBERG and FEDERLE 1987). This finding is nonspecific.

9.4.8
Non-Hodgkin's Lymphoma

Liver involvement in ARL usually occurs in the setting of multiorgan disease (SISKIN et al. 1995). Hepatic lesions usually are asymptomatic although dull right upper quadrant pain or jaundice can occasionally be

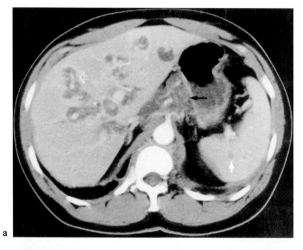

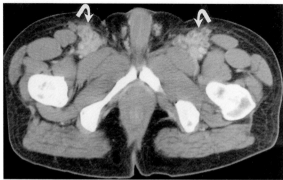

a

b

Fig. 9.10a, b. Kaposi's sarcoma in a 28-year-old man with AIDS. **a** CT scan demonstrates mesenteric and retroperitoneal lymphadenopathy with low-density masses extending into the gastrohepatic ligament (*black arrow*) and portal veins (*white open arrow*). Hypodense splenic lesions (*white arrow*) are also identified. **b** This patient also has enlarged, contrast-enhancing groin lymph nodes characteristic of lymphadenopathy due to Kaposi's sarcoma (*white arrows*)

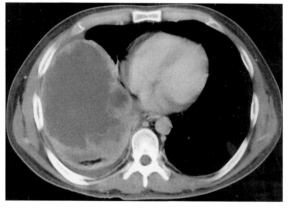

Fig. 9.11. Primary AIDS-related lymphoma in a 45-year-old-man. CT scan shows a large hepatic mass. No extrahepatic disease was identified on other sections

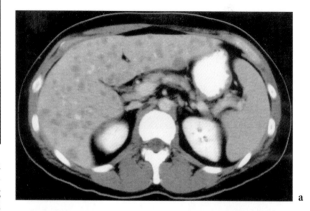

a

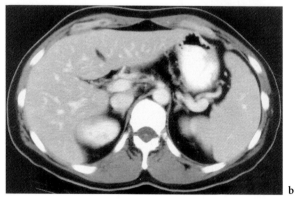

b

Fig. 9.12a, b. A 42-year-old man with AIDS-related non-Hodgkin's lymphoma. **a** Multiple small hypodense liver masses are present. **b** Following chemotherapy, the liver lesions resolved

seen with bulky tumors. Elevations of serum alkaline phosphatase are most sensitive for hepatic involvement, with elevated transaminases and bilirubin identified in advanced disease (SCERPELLA et al. 1996).

On cross-sectional imaging, ARLs present with hepatosplenomegaly and focal lesions (NYBERG et al. 1986). These lesions may vary in size and number, from a large isolated mass (Fig. 9.11) to innumerable tiny lesions (TOWNSEND et al. 1989). Focal lesions can also cause biliary dilatation (TOWNSEND 1991). Focal hepatic lesions (Fig. 9.12) are observed much more commonly on ultrasound (45%) and CT (29%) in ARLs when compared with the 5%–10% incidence of focal abnormalities observed in sporadically occurring lymphoma (RADIN et al. 1993). Focal splenic lesions are observed in 7% of AIDS patients and splenomegaly in 40% of cases (SOYER et al. 1993). Exten-

sive retroperitoneal and/or mesenteric lymphadenopathy (Fig. 9.13) is observed in 56% of ARLs. These nodes usually have soft tissue density, but can occasionally show central necrosis (POMBO et al. 1994).

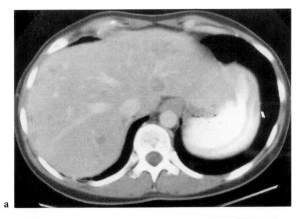

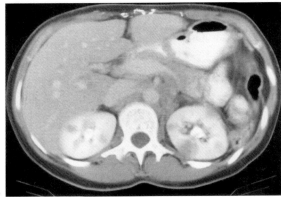

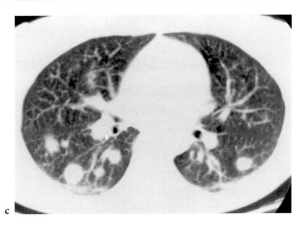

Fig. 9.13a, b. A 33-year-old women with disseminated extra-nodal AIDS-related lymphoma. **a** Multiple low-attenuation liver masses are identified. **b** Low attenuation renal lesions and retroperitoneal lymphadenopathy are also seen. **c** Multiple pulmonary masses are also present. Renal and pulmonary bi-opsies demonstrated non-Hodgkin's lymphoma in this patient

9.4.9
Focal Splenic Lesions

Although splenomegaly is seen in 30%–45% of pa-tients with AIDS, focal lesions are only encountered in 8% of cases (BERNABEU-WITTEL et al. 1999). Most

(86%) focal lesions are due to MTB and typically present as small, multiple hypoechoic, rounded or oval splenic defects on ultrasound (PORCEL-MARTIN et al. 1998). Fine-needle aspiration biopsy of the spleen is usually not needed because other, more accessible lesions are usually present.

Although splenic microabscesses are common in disseminated candidiasis in neutropenic patients, they are uncommon in AIDS patients. Microabscess-es can have a number of sonographic appearances: multiple hypoechoic lesions, a wheel-within-a-wheel pattern, or a bull's eye pattern.

Intravenous drug users may have septic abscess but these are usually larger and more heterogeneous than those seen in MTB infection (Fig. 9.14).

Splenic infarcts may also occur secondary to bac-terial endocarditis. These lesions are usually large, wedge-shaped, hypoechoic, and well-demarcated ar-eas, with the apex directed toward the splenic hilus.

9.5
AIDS-Related Biliary Tract Disease

There are three general categories of biliary tract dis-ease in AIDS patients: acalculous cholecystitis, AIDS cholangiopathy, and non-HIV-associated conditions of the bile ducts (GRENDELL and CELLO 1996). A sub-stantial number of AIDS patients will have common conditions such as gallstones, benign bile duct stric-tures, and even periampullary neoplasms, so it is im-portant to exclude these treatable conditions rather than assume that they are untreatable lesions associ-ated with AIDS (GRENDELL and CELLO 1996).

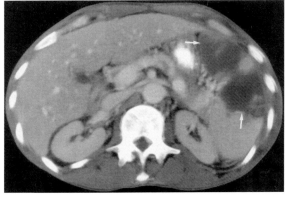

Fig. 9.14. Pyogenic and protozoan abscesses in a 34-year-old febrile man with AIDS and splenic abscesses. CT demon-strates several hypodense splenic lesions (*arrows*). Percuta-neous aspiration revealed *P. carinii*, *Klebsiella*, and *E. coli*

9.5.1
Acalculous Cholecystitis

Acalculous cholecystitis is an uncommon disease in patients with AIDS (VUITTON et al. 1996b). These patients are typically ambulatory, tolerate oral intake, have right upper quadrant pain, have markedly elevated serum alkaline phosphatase and/or mild increase in serum bilirubin, and present with concurrent CMV and/or cryptosporidial infection; they also commonly have HIV-associated sclerosing cholangitis or papillary stenosis (ADOLPH et al. 1992).

Ultrasound typically demonstrates thickening of the gallbladder wall (Fig. 9.15), pericholecystic fluid, and occasionally a sonographic Murphy's sign and intramural air (ROMANO et al. 1988). The patient biliary scintiscan is usually positive as well (QUINN et al. 1993).

Patients with AIDS-related acalculous cholecystitis respond well to cholecystectomy, and histopathology usually shows CMV inclusion bodies in the gallbladder mucosa.

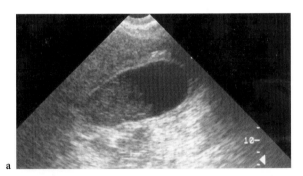

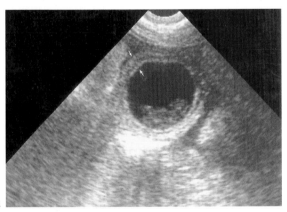

Fig. 9.15a, b. Mural thickening of the gallbladder in an AIDS patient with acalculous cholecystitis and cryptosporidial infection. Sagittal (**a**) and transverse (**b**) sonograms show marked gallbladder wall thickening (*arrows*). There is pericholecystic fluid and sludge within the gallbladder lumen

9.5.2
AIDS-Related Cholangiopathy

Patients with AIDS-related cholangiopathy are typically middle-aged males who have had AIDS for approximately 1 year. There is dramatic elevation of the serum alkaline phosphatase and more modest elevation of the serum transaminase and bilirubin levels (CELLO 1989).

The histopathologic findings include acute and chronic submucosal infiltrates with CMV (21%) and/or cryptosporidial (32%) infection. Some 5% of patients have MAC or microsporidial infiltration. One-year survival is usually less than 20%, although most patients experience relief of biliary-type pain following endoscopic sphincterectomy (CELLO 1989; NASH and COHEN 1997).

Four different patterns of HIV-related cholangiopathy have been reported (CELLO 1989):
1. *Papillary stenosis*, in which there is dilatation of bile ducts and delayed drainage of contrast into the duodenum (28%)
2. *Sclerosing cholangitis*, characterized by focal strictures and dilatations of the intra- and/or extrahepatic bile ducts (12%)
3. Combined *papillary stenosis* and *intra- and/or extrahepatic sclerosing cholangitis* (49%)
4. Long *extrahepatic bile duct strictures* with lengths exceeding 1–2 cm (10%)

Biliary tract infections by several organisms, but especially CMV and cryptosporidia, have been implicated in the development of AIDS-related cholangitis but not directly demonstrated as causative (BENHAMOU et al. 1993). Other associated infections include MAC, microsporidia, and *Isospora* (HEYWORTH 1996). Direct involvement by HIV infection has also been postulated as causative. CMV-associated acalculous cholecystitis has been described, but does not appear to be associated with HIV cholangiopathy, as the two are rarely observed in the same patient. Pathologically, there is inflammation and edema of the gallbladder wall and mucosal ulceration. CMV inclusion bodies characteristically are located near mucosal ulcers (FORBES 1992).

Cryptosporidiosis infection is present in 6% of all AIDS patients and 21% of those with diarrhea (TEXIDOR et al. 1991). The identification of biliary cryptosporidial infection is difficult; currently, there is no effective therapy for the eradication of this organism.

Ultrasound, CT, and endoscopic retrograde cholangiopancreatography are complementary in the diagnosis of AIDS-related cholangiopathy (DASILVA et al. 1993) (Figs. 9.16–9.18). The cholangiographic

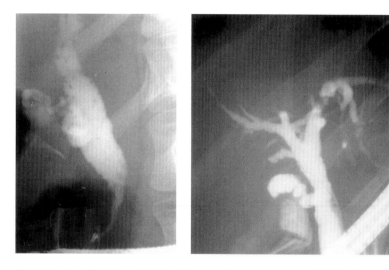

Fig. 9.16a, b. AIDS-related cholangitis secondary to cryptosporidial infection. **a** Cholangiogram shows narrowing of the distal common bile duct and multiple mucosal filing defects. **b** Cholangiogram in a different patient shows irregular beading of the intrahepatic ducts

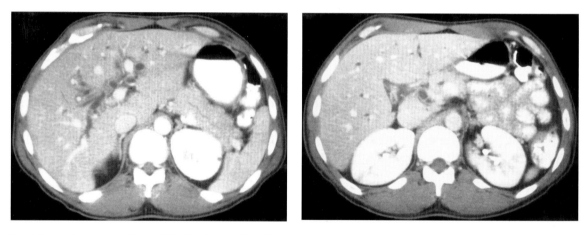

Fig. 9.17a, b. Cryptosporidiosis of the bile ducts and small bowel. **a** CT scan shows dilated intrahepatic ducts. **b** Scan obtained at a lower level reveals mural thickening of the gallbladder and small bowel

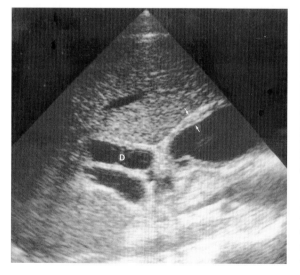

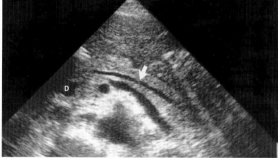

Fig. 9.18a, b. AIDS-induced papillary stenosis due to cryptosporidiosis. **a** Oblique sonogram demonstrates dilatation of the common hepatic duct (*D*) and mural thickening of the gallbladder (*arrows*). **b** Transverse sonogram of the pancreas shows dilatation of the common bile duct (*D*) and pancreatic duct (*arrow*)

features (Fig. 9.16) of AIDS cholangiopathy include common bile duct tapering, beading of the mucosa, irregular dilatation of the extrahepatic biliary system, disproportionately distorted left intrahepatic ducts, irregular focal sacculations and dilations, and focal intraductal debris (FARMAN et al. 1994). In one series, 81% of sonograms and 78% of CT scans were abnormal, showing intra- and extrahepatic bile ducts, irregular focal dilation of intrahepatic segmental ducts, and mural thickening of the common bile duct (CELLO 1989; KIM and CELLO 1999). An echogenic nodule may be seen at the distal end of the common bile duct, representing an edematous papilla of Vater. Gallbladder dilatation and sludge are also commonly found in AIDS patients. On CT, inflammation of the gallbladder or biliary tree is manifested by mural thickening and/or abnormal contrast enhancement (REEDERS et al. 1994) (Fig. 9.17). The cholangiographic signs of beading, pruning, and nodular mural thickening can also be observed (MACCARTY 2000).

9.6
Pancreatic Disease

AIDS-related pancreatic disease is often not recognized during life, although it is commonly detected at autopsy (CAPPELL 1997). AIDS patients are subject to a variety of pancreatic disorders in addition to those seen in the general population: opportunistic infections, drug-induced inflammation, and neoplasms (CAPPELL and HASSAN 1993). Involvement can range from asymptomatic findings detected at autopsy to fulminant pancreatitis leading to death (DASSOPOUBS and EHRENPREIS 1999; PARITHIVEL et al. 1999). Gross pathologic changes vary from a normal pancreas in some infections and tumors to massive necrosis and abscess formation (DUTTA et al. 1997). Special stains for fungi and mycobacteria and detection of viral inclusions are required for diagnosis following biopsy. Generally, the patients are asymptomatic, with the clinical picture dominated by involvement of other organs. CMV, MAC, MTB, *Cryptococcus neoformans*, aspergillosis, and candidiasis are other opportunistic infections that affect the pancreas. Extrapulmonary *P. carinii* rarely involves the pancreas and may be seen as tiny echogenic foci on ultrasound (Fig. 9.19) or calcifications on CT examination. Medications including pentamidine and trimethoprim-sulfamethoxazole, both used to treat *P. carinii* pneumonia, can cause pancreatitis indistin-

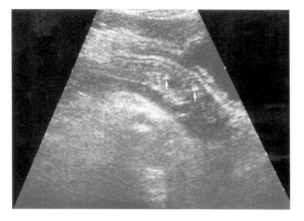

Fig. 9.19. Several echogenic foci (*arrows*) are seen on this transverse pancreatic sonogram in an AIDS patient with disseminated extrapulmonary *P. carinii* infection

guishable from other causes. There is a 7% prevalence of pancreatic neoplasms in AIDS patients at autopsy, most commonly Kaposi's sarcoma and lymphoma (EVRARD et al. 1999). The involvement appears to be subclinical and usually is associated with disseminated disease.

The radiologic features of pancreatitis (Figs. 9.20, 9.21) and pancreatic abscesses in patients with AIDS are similar to those observed in the general population (MILLER et al. 1996). When comparing pancreatic with hepatic parenchymal echogenicity, it should be remembered that the liver is often echogenic in patients with AIDS owing to fatty infiltration, so that the normal pancreas may appear rel-

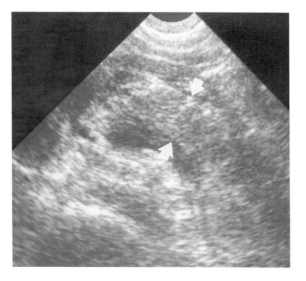

Fig. 9.20. Transverse sonogram shows enlarged hypoechoic pancreas (*arrows*) in an AIDS patient with pentamidine-induced pancreatitis

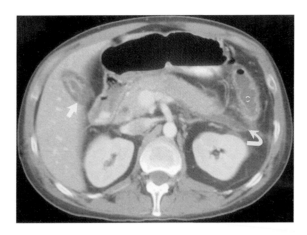

Fig. 9.21. Cytomegalovirus pancreatitis, cholecystitis, and colitis. Inflammatory fluid is present surrounding the pancreatic tail and left anterior interfascial plane (*curved arrow*). Note the mural thickening of the gallbladder (*solid arrow*) and colon (*C*)

atively hypoechoic, simulating pancreatitis. Similarly, the kidney is not always a reliable internal reference: the parenchyma may be hyperechoic due to HIV-associated nephropathy.

9.7 Summary

The hepatic, splenic, biliary tract, and pancreatic manifestations of HIV disease are diverse. Some are unique and specifically attributable to HIV infection, whereas others are coincidental, reflecting the nature and severity of the underlying primary illness. With AIDS patients living longer, solid abdominal visceral involvement is becoming more common, and an understanding of the spectrum of HIV-associated disease is essential for improving patient management (ROSEN et al. 1999).

References

Adolph MD, Bass SN, Lee SK, et al. (1992) Cytomegalovirus acalculous cholecystitis in acquired immunodeficiency virus infection. Am J Med 92:404–411

Alvarez OA, Vanegas F, Maze GL, et al. (2000) Polymicrobial cholangitis and liver abscess in a patient with acquired immunodeficiency syndrome. South Med J 93:232–234

Bach N, Theise ND, Schaffner F (1992) Hepatic histology in the acquired immunodeficiency syndrome. Semin Liver Dis 12:205–212

Baron RL, Gore RM (2000) Diffuse liver disease. In: Gore RM, Levine MS (eds) Textbook of gastrointestinal radiology, 2nd edn. Saunders, Philadelphia, pp 1590–1638

Beale TJ, Wetton CWN, Crofton ME (1995) A sonographic pathological correlation of liver biopsies in patients with AIDS. Clin Radiol 50:761–764

Benhamou Y, Caumes E, Gerosa Y, et al. (1993) AIDS-related cholangiopathy. Dig Dis Sci 38:1113–1118

Bernabeu-Wittel M, Villanueva JL, Pachon J, et al. (1999) Etiology, clinical features and outcome of splenic microabscesses in HIV-infected patients with prolonged fever. Eur J Clin Microbiol Infect Dis 18:324–329

Bray HJ, Lail VJ, Cooperberg PL (1992) Tiny echogenic foci in the liver and kidney in patients with AIDS: not always due to disseminated *Pneumocystis carinii*. AJR 158:81–82

Cappell MS (1997) The pancreas in AIDS. Gastroenterol Clin North Am 26:337–366

Cappel MS, Hassan T (1993) Pancreatic disease in AIDS – a review. J Clin Gastroenterol 17:254–263

Cavert W (1997) Viral infections in human immunodeficiency virus disease. Med Clin North Am 81:411–426

Cello J (1989) Acquired immune deficiency syndrome-related sclerosing cholangitis. Am J Med 86:539–546

Chalasani N, Wilcox CM (1996) Etiology, evaluation, and outcome of jaundice in patients with acquired immunodeficiency syndrome. Hepatology 23:728–733

Chung CJ, Sivit CJ, Rakusan TA, et al. (1994) Hepatobiliary abnormalities on sonography in children with HIV infection. J Ultrasound Med 13:205–210

DaSilva F, Boudghene F, Lecornte I, et al. (1993) Sonography in AIDS-related cholangitis. AJR 160:1205–1207

Dassopoubs T, Ehrenpreis ED (1999) Acute pancreatitis in human immunodeficiency virus-infected patients: a review. Am J Med 107:78–84

DeToma G, Codacci-Pisanelli M, Nicolanti V, et al. (1999) Obstructive biliary symptomatology as the first sign of HIV-infection. J Exp Clin Cancer Res 18:459–462

Dietrich DT (1999) Hepatitis C virus and human immunodeficiency virus: clinical issues in coinfection. Am J Med 107:98–84

Dutta SK, Ting CD, Lai LL (1997) Study of prevalence, severity, etiologic factors associated with acute pancreatitis in patients infected with human immunodeficiency virus. Am J Gastroenterol 92:2044–2045

Evrard S, Van Laethem JL, Urbain D, et al. (1999) Chronic pancreatic alterations in AIDS patients. Pancreas 19:335–338

Farman J, Brunetti J, Baer JW, et al. (1994) AIDS-related cholangiopancreatographic changes. Abdom Imaging 19:417–422

Ferrozzi F, Bova D, Campodonico F, et al. (1995) AIDS-related malignancies: clinicopathologic correlation. Eur Radiol 5:477–485

Forbes A (1992) Acquired immune deficiency syndrome-related sclerosing cholangitis. Eur J Gastroenterol Hepatol 4:455–459

Fortgang IS, Belitsos PC, Chaisson RE, et al.(1995) Hepatomegaly and steatosis in HIV-infected patients receiving nucleoside analog antiretroviral therapy. Am J Gastroenterol 90:1433–1436

French AL, Benator DA, Gordin FN (1997) Nontuberculous mycobacterial infections. Med Clin North Am 81:361–380

Friedman SL (1995) Hepatobiliary infections in AIDS. In: Surwicz C, Owen RS (eds) Gastrointestinal and hepatic infections. Saunders, Philadelphia, pp 391–404

Gore RM, Miller FH, Yaghmai V (1998) Acquired immunodeficiency syndrome (AIDS) of the abdominal organs: imaging features. Semin Ultrasound CT MRI 19:175–189

Gore RM, Baron RL, Marn CS (2000) Vascular disorders of the liver and splanchnic circulation. In: Gore RM, Levine MS (eds) Textbook of gastrointestinal radiology, 2nd edn. Saunders, Philadelphia, pp 1639–1668

Gourevitch MN (1996) The epidemiology of HIV and AIDS. Med Clin North Am 80:1223–1233

Grendell JH, Cello JP (1996) HIV-associated hepatobiliary disease. In: Zakim D, Boyer TD (eds): Hepatology, 3rd edn. Saunders, Philadelphia, pp 1699–1706

Gulati MS, Sarma D, Paul SB (1999) CT appearances in abdominal tuberculosis. A pictorial essay. Clin Imag 23:51–59

Hasan FA, Jeffers U, Welsh SW, et al. (1989) Hepatic involvement as the primary manifestation of Kaposi's sarcoma in the acquired immunodeficiency syndrome. Am J Gastroenterol 84:1449–1451

Havlir DV, Barnes PF (1999) Tuberculosis in patients with human immunodeficiency virus infection. N Engl J Med 340:367–373

Herts BR, Megibow AJ, Birnbaum BA, et al. (1992) High-attenuation lymphadenopathy AIDS patients: significance of findings at CT. Radiology 185:777–781

Heyworth MF (1996) Parasitic diseases in immunocompromised hosts: cryptosporidiosis, isosporiasis, strongyloidiasis. Gastroenterol Clin North Am 25:691–707

Horsburgh CR (1999) The pathophysiology of disseminated Mycobacterium avium complex disease in AIDS. J Infect Dis 179:461–466

Jeffrey RB (1992) Abdominal imaging in the immunocompromised patient. Radiol Clin North Am 30:579–596

Kim LS, Cello JP (1999) Hepatobiliary manifestations of AIDS. In: Schiff ER, Sorrell MF, Maddrey WC (eds) Schiff's diseases of the liver, 8th edn. Lippincott Williams & Williams, Philadelphia, pp 1561–1570

Knollmann FD, Grunewald T, Adler A, et al. (1997) Intestinal disease in acquired immunodeficiency – evaluation by CT. Eur Radiol 7:1419–1429

Keogan MT, Freed KS, Paulson EK, et al. (1999) Imaging-guided percutaneous biopsy of focal splenic lesions: update on safety and effectiveness. AJR 172:933–937

Krown SE (1997) Acquired immunodeficiency syndrome associated Kaposi's sarcoma. Med Clin North Am 81:471–494

Lefkowitch JH (1994) Pathology of AIDS-related liver disease. Dig Dis 12:321–330

Levine AM (1992) AIDS-associated malignant lymphoma. Med Clin North Am 76:253–268

Lubat E, Megibow AJ, Balthazar EJ, et al. (1990) Extrapulmonary Pneumocystis carinii infection in AIDS: CT findings. Radiology 174:157–160

Luburich P, Bru C, Aytiso MC, et al. (1990) Hepatic Kaposi's sarcoma in AIDS: US and CT findings. Radiology 175:172–174

MacCarty RL (2000). Inflammatory disorders of the biliary tract. In: Gore RM, Levine MS (eds) Textbook of gastrointestinal radiology, 2nd edn. Saunders, Philadelphia, pp 1375–1394

Marincili DL, Albelda SM, Williams TM, et al. (1986) Nontuberculous mycobacterial infection in AIDS: clinical, pathologic, and radiographic features. Radiology 160:77–82

Markowitz N, Hansen NI, Hopewell PC, et al. (1997) Incidence of tuberculosis in the United States among HIV infected persons. Ann Intern Med 126:123–132

Miller FH, Gore RM, Nemcek A, Fitzgerald SW (1996) Pancreaticobiliary manifestations of AIDS. AJR 166:1–10

Minamoto GY, Rosenberg AS (1997) Fungal infections in patients with acquired immunodeficiency syndrome. Med Clin North Am 81:381–409

Mohle-Boetani JC, Koeffier JE, Berger TG, et al. (1996) Bacillary angiomatosis and bacillary peliosis in patients infected with human immunodeficiency virus: clinical characteristics in a case-controlled study. Clin Infect Dis 22:794–800

Moore EH, Russell LA, Klein JS, et al. (1995) Bacillary angiomatosis in patients with AIDS: multiorgan imaging finding. Radiology 197:67–72

Murray JG, Patel MD, Lee S, et al. (1995) Microabscesses of the liver and spleen in AIDS: detection with 5-MHz sonography. Radiology 197:723–727

Nash JA, Cohen SA (1997) Gallbladder and biliary tract disease in AIDS. Gastroenterol Clin North Am 26:323–336

Nyberg DA, Federle MP (1987) AIDS-related Kaposi's sarcoma and lymphoma. Semin Roentgenol 22:54–65

Nyberg DA, Jeffrey RB, Federle MP, et al. (1986) AIDS-related lymphomas: evaluation by abdominal CT. Radiology 159:59–63

Pantongrag-Brown L, Nelson AM, Brown AE, et al. (1995) Gastrointestinal manifestations of acquired immunodeficiency syndrome: radiologic-pathologic correlation. Radiographics 15:1155–1178

Parithivel VS, Yoosuf AM, Albu E, et al. (1999) Predictors of the severity of acute pancreatitis in patients with HIV infection or AIDS. Pancreas 19:133–136

Piratuisuth T, Siripaitoon P, Sriplug H, et al. (1999) Findings and benefits of liver biopsies in 46 patients infected with human immunodeficiency virus. J Gastroenterol Hepatol 14:146–149

Poles MA, Lew EA, Dieterich DJ (1997) Diagnosis and treatment of hepatic disease in patients with HIV. Gastroenterol Clin North Am 26:291–322

Pombo F, Rodriguez E, Caruncho NIV, et al. (1994) CT attenuation values and enhancing characteristics of thoracoabdominal lymphomatous adenopathies. J Comput Assist Tomogr 18:59–62

Porcel-Martin A, Rendon-Unceta P, Bascuñana-Quirell A, et al. (1998) Focal splenic lesions in patients with AIDS: sonographic findings. Abdom Imaging 23:196–200

Quinn D, Popock N, Freund J, et al. (1993) Radionuclide hepatobiliary scanning in patients with AIDS-related sclerosing cholangitis. Clin Nucl Med 18:417–422

Radin DR (1991) Intra-abdominal Mycobacterium tuberculosis vs Mycobacterium avium-intracellulare infections in patients with AIDS: distinction based on CT findings. AJR 156:487–491

Radin R (1995) HIV infection: analysis in 259 consecutive patients with abnormal abdominal CT findings. Radiology 197:712–722

Radin DR, Baker EL, Klatt EC, et al. (1990) Visceral and nodal calcification in patients with AIDS-related Pneumocystis carinii infection. AJR 154:27–31

Radin DR, Esplin JA, Levine AM, Ralls PW (1993) AIDS-related non-Hodgkin's lymphoma: abdominal CT findings in 112 patients. AJR 160:1133–1139

Reeders JWA, Bartelsman JFWM, Huibregtse K (1994) AIDS-related manifestations of the bile duct system: a common finding? Abdom Imaging 19:423–424

Romano AJ, vanSonnenberg E, Casola G, et al. (1988) Gallbladder and bile duct abnormalities in AIDS: sonographic findings in eight patients. AJR 150:123–127

Rosen MP, Sher S, Bhorade R, et al. (1999) Screening admission CT scans in patients with AIDS – a randomized trial. Eff Clin Prac 2:101–107

Rubin SA (1997) Tuberculosis and atypical mycobacterial infections in the 1990s. Radiographics 17:1051–1059

Scerpella EG, Villareal AA, Casanova PF, et al. (1996) Primary lymphoma at the liver in AIDS. J Clin Gastroenterol 22:51–53

Schacker T, Collier AC, Hughes J, et al. (1997) Clinical and epidemiologic features of primary HIV infection. Arch Intern Med 125:257–264

Siskin GP, Haller JO, Miller S, et al. (1995) AIDS-related lymphoma: radiologic features in pediatric patients. Radiology 196:63–66

Soriano V, Garcia-Samaniego J, Rodriguez-Rosado R, et al. (1999) Hepatitis C and HIV infections: biological, clinical, and therapeutic implications. J Hepatol 31:119–123

Soyer P, Van Beers B, Teillet-Thidbaud F, et al. (1993) Hodgkin's and non-Hodgkin's hepatic lymphoma: sonographic findings. Abdom Imaging 18:339–343

Sponge AR, Wilson ST, Gopinath N, et al. (1990) Extrapulmonary *Pneumocystis carinii* in a patient with AIDS: sonographic findings. AJR 155:76–78

Straus DJ (1997) Human immunodeficiency virus-associated lymphomas. Med Clin North Am 81:495–510

Suri S, Gupta S, Suri R (1999) Computed tomography in abdominal tuberculosis. Br J Radiol 72:92–98

Telzak EE (1997) Tuberculosis and human immunodeficiency virus. Med Clin North Am 81:345–360

Texidor HS, Godwin TA, Ramirez EA (1991) Cryptosporidiosis of the biliary tract in AIDS. Radiology 180:51–56

Towers MJ, Withers CE, Hamilton PA, et al. (1991) Visceral calcification in patients with AIDS may not always be due to *Pneumocystis carinii*. AJR 156:745–747

Townsend RR (1991) CT of AIDS-related lymphoma. AJR 156:969–974

Townsend RR, Laing FC, Jeffrey RB, et al. (1989) Abdominal lymphoma in AIDS: evaluation with US. Radiology 171:719–724

Tshibwabwa ET, Mwaba P, Boyle-Taylor J, et al. (2000) Four-year study of abdominal ultrasound in 900 Central African adults with AIDS referred for diagnostic imaging. Abdom Imaging 25:290–296

Valls C, Cafias C, Turell LG, et al. (1991) Hepatosplenic AIDS-related Kaposi's sarcoma. Gastrointest Radiol 16:342–344

Vieco PT, Rochon L, Lisona A (1990) Multifocal cytomegalovirus-associated hepatic lesions simulating metastases in AIDS. Radiology 176:123–124

Vuitton D-A, Chossegros P, Bresson-Hadni S, et al. (1996a) HIV infection, the liver and biliary tract. Part I. HBV, HDV, and HCV. Gastroenterol Clin Biol 20:269–280

Vuitton D-A, Chossegros P, Bresson-Hadni S, et al. (1996b) HIV infection, the liver and biliary tract. Part II. Hepatobiliary complications of AIDS. Gastroenterol Clin Biol 20:281–293

Wang C-Y, Snow JL, Su WPD (1996) Lymphoma associated with human immunodeficiency virus infection. Mayo Clin Proc 70:665–672

Wetton CWN, McCarty M, Tomlinson D, et al. (1993) Ultrasound findings in hepatic mycobacterial infections in patients with acquired immunodeficiency syndrome (AIDS). Clin Radiol 47:36–38

Wu CM, Davis F, Fishman EK (1998) Radiologic evaluation of the acute abdomen in the patient with the acquired immunodeficiency syndrome (AIDS): the role of CT scanning. Semin Ultrasound CT MR 19:190–199

Wyatt SH, Fishman EK (1993) Hepatic bacillary angiomatosis in a patient with AIDS. Abdom Imaging 18:336–338

10 Imaging Retroperitoneal Disorders in Patients Infected with HIV

Alec J. Megibow

CONTENTS

10.1 Introduction

The retroperitoneum contains the pancreas, kidneys, adrenal glands, ureters, lymph nodes, and great vessels of the abdomen. Most retroperitoneal abnormalities in AIDS patients are not seen in isolation, but rather in combination with findings in other parts of the abdomen or chest, stressing the importance of pattern recognition in attempting to ascribe etiological significance to any given radiological abnormality. The major focus of this chapter will be on the pattern of disease involvement within the abdomen from the viewpoint of analyzing a retroperitoneal abnormality.

10.2 Choice of Imaging Technique

Retroperitoneal imaging may be performed by computed tomography (CT), ultrasound, or magnetic resonance (MR) imaging. Ancillary examinations such as nuclear medicine studies are employed as a secondary test to further characterize an abnormality found on the "anatomic" studies. The choice of procedure will depend on availability of imaging resources and the specific clinical question.

Although CT is most often used as an initial test in the United States and Europe, ultrasound may be the only imaging technique available. This is especially true in sub-Saharan Africa, where the AIDS epidemic rages. Ultrasound is an effective screening modality for a wide variety of retroperitoneal disorders, and is frequently (or exclusively) employed in patients with renal insufficiency. Abdominal ultrasound for diagnostic purposes in AIDS patients is requested by clinicians for a range of primary clinical indications: abdominal pain, fever of unknown origin, hepatosplenomegaly, lymphadenopathy, and abnormal liver function tests. AIDS patients demonstrate higher frequencies of splenomegaly, hepatomegaly, lymphadenopathy, biliary tract abnormalities, gut wall thickening, and ascites (Tshibwabwa et al. 2000). Yee et al. (1989) found lymphadenopathy to be the single most common ultrasound finding in AIDS patients. A similar large series from Canada demonstrated a high prevalence of hepatosplenomegaly and lymphadenopathy in 889 patients (Smith et al. 1994).

As stated above, when available, most radiologists prefer CT scanning as the primary imaging modality for evaluating the symptomatic human immunodeficiency virus (HIV)-infected patient. Radin categorized the most common abdominal CT findings in 259 HIV-infected patients. Diagnoses were mycobacterial infection, lymphoproliferative disease, Kaposi's sarcoma, fungal infection, hepatocellular disease, extrapulmonary *Pneumocystis carinii* infection, and other disorders. In 30, no diagnosis was obtained. Abnormal findings in descending order of frequency included lymph node enlargement, hepatomegaly, splenomegaly, gastrointestinal mass or wall thickening, and low-attenuation lesions in the liver or spleen. Diagnoses thought to account for CT findings were confirmed or suspected in 247 of the 259 patients (Radin 1995). The easy access to imaging

A.J. Megibow, MD, MPH, FACR
Professor of Radiology, Department of Radiology, NYU School of Medicine, 560 First Avenue, New York, NY 10016, USA

all abdominal compartments has made CT the recommended first-line investigation. Furthermore, CT
allows reproducible quantification for monitoring
response to therapy.

Nuclear medicine scanning with gallium-67 citrate
is useful in the detection of inflammation. The major
use has been in the diagnosis of pulmonary *P. carinii*
infection. Gallium has been shown to be effective in
the abdomen in localizing nodal and extranodal abdominal tuberculosis (ABDEL-DAYEM et al. 1997).

Although MR imaging can be used in abdominal
and retroperitoneal diseases, there has been little documented application of the technology to retroperitoneal AIDS-related diseases. The main use of this technique is in the evaluation of hepatobiliary disease. MR
imaging is useful in assessing the potential vascularity
of a renal mass in a patient with renal insufficiency,
but this is clearly not an AIDS-related application.

10.3
Pancreas

Isolated pancreatic disease is uncommon in the
AIDS patient. Most disease has been recognized at
endoscopic retrograde cholangiopancreatography in
patients who are being evaluated for abnormalities
related to the biliary tree. Biliary disease accounts for
a significantly higher morbidity in these patients.
The symptoms are often mild and may not be clinically apparent (MILLER et al. 1996). Pancreatic abnormalities seen at pancreatography include side
branch alterations, multiple strictures, and diffuse
pancreatic duct dilatation. Pancreatic ductal changes
may occur in the absence of opportunistic infection
(EVRARD et al. 1999).

The pancreas may be involved in mycobacterial
diseases. Tuberculosis has been reported as the cause
of pancreatic abscess (JABER and GLECKMAN 1995).
The spectrum of CT changes in pancreatic tuberculosis includes nonspecific mass lesions, low-attenuation
nodules, and diffuse enlargement (POMBO et al. 1998).
The pancreas may be secondarily involved from adjacent peripancreatic lymph node disease (HULNICK et
al. 1985). These patents will present with a febrile systemic illness, the reported cases stressing that clinical
findings do not indicate pancreatic disease. The diagnosis of tuberculous pancreatic abscess should be
considered when a pancreatic mass is detected in a febrile HIV-infected patient. Other infectious etiologies
can produce pancreatic abscess when they present
with disseminated disease (Fig. 10.1).

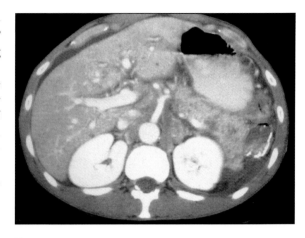

Fig. 10.1. Herpetic abscesses in liver and pancreas. Multiple
low-attenuation lesions are scattered throughout the pancreatic body and tail. Microabscesses are present in the liver. The
patient had disseminated herpes

Fulminant, necrotizing pancreatitis has been observed in patients receiving therapy with 2',3'-
dideoxyinosine (ddI) (ABOULAFIA 1997). Although
the effects of the drug are not precisely known, when
ex vivo dog pancreas is perfused with ddI, there is a
decrease in arterial pressure, reduced oxygen consumption, and a decrease in zymogen granules within acinar cells. These results may explain the higher
incidence of severe necrotizing pancreatitis in individuals receiving the drug (Fig. 10.2) (NORDBACK et
al. 1992).

Pancreatic neoplasms are uncommon in AIDS patients, AIDS-related lymphoma (ARL) being the
most frequent. In a series of 112 patients, a focal pancreatic lymphomatous mass was seen in 5% of cases.
Of these patients, 56% had nodal disease (RADIN et
al. 1993). Focal lymphomatous masses may distort
the pancreatic duct and obstruct the common bile
duct (JONES et al. 1997). Scattered reported cases of
Kaposi's sarcoma resulting in a focal pancreatic
mass have appeared in the literature. In one reported
case, the diagnosis was confirmed by imaging detection of a pancreatic mass with positive identification
of human herpes virus 8 (HHV 8) in the pancreatic
juice (MENGES et al. 1999).

10.4
Kidney

A variety of general and disease specific abnormalities are detected in the kidneys of patients with AIDS
(O'REGAN et al. 1990). Abnormalities may span all

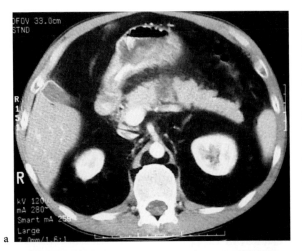

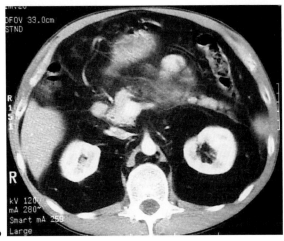

Fig. 10.2. a Necrotizing pancreatitis secondary to ddI. There is an area of central nonperfusion in the body of the pancreas. **b** Necrotizing pancreatitis secondary to ddI therapy. Peripancreatic inflammatory changes are visualized in the root of the small bowel mesentery

Renal cortical calcification in disseminated extrapulmonary *P. carinii* infection was seen for a brief period in the early 1990s. The rapid increase in these cases was ascribed to the widespread use of aerosolized antimicrobial therapy, which was highly successful in controlling pulmonary disease but offered no protection from systemic complications. At CT, these patients present with diffuse punctate calcifications involving a variety of retroperitoneal structures including the adrenal glands, spleen, liver, lymph nodes, and renal cortex. Ultrasound will demonstrate diffuse echogenic foci without shadowing (Fig. 10.3) (BARGMAN et al. 1991; LUBAT et al. 1990; RADIN et al. 1990).

Patients with AIDS who develop renal failure and associated proteinuria will be suspected of having developed AIDS nephropathy. This is a specific lesion seen in HIV-infected patients who have developed AIDS. The disease is histologically characterized as focal segmental glomerulosclerosis, with a variety of tubular abnormalities including epithelial flattening, infolding, and intratubular precipitates (HAMPER et al. 1988). Since most patients have compromised renal function, the diagnosis is most frequently made by ultrasound. The characteristic sonographic feature of AIDS nephropathy is increased cortical echogenicity with variable renal enlargement (Fig. 10.4) (HAMPER et al. 1988; KAY 1992; SCHAFFER et al. 1984).

The introduction of protease inhibitors to the treatment regimen of AIDS patients has significantly improved survival and maintained CD4+ T-lymphocyte counts above 200 per ml^3. The best-studied

manifestations of renal imaging, including: altered cortical echogenicity, renal enlargement, pyelonephritis, lobar nephronia, focal masses (abscess or neoplasm), parenchymal calcifications, hydronephrosis, and infarct (MILLER et al. 1993). When these findings are present in AIDS patients, a different set of etiologic possibilities must be considered to explain the imaging findings.

Abscesses may be due to any one of a variety of infectious agents. There have been several case reports of primary renal aspergillosis presenting with abscesses. Both unilateral and bilateral masses may be present. The authors indicate the rarity with which this infection primarily involves the kidneys and emphasize that the reported cases have all been seen in AIDS patients (MARTINEZ-JABALOYAS et al. 1995).

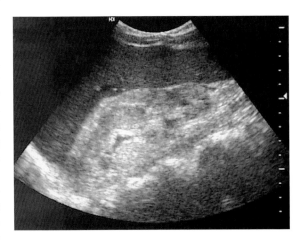

Fig. 10.3. Segmental glomerular sclerosis (AIDS nephropathy). Longitudinal ultrasound image of the right kidney reveals increased echogenicity in the cortex with loss of normal corticomedullary differentiation. The collecting system is unaffected

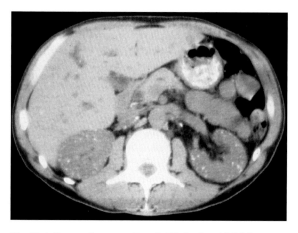

Fig. 10.4. Extrapulmonary *P. carinii* infection. Multiple punctate renal cortical calcifications are present in both kidneys. Diffuse calcifications throughout the liver result in an increased hepatic attenuation despite the scan being performed without contrast enhancement

agent within this class of compounds is indinavir sulfate. The use of these agents is associated with an increased incidence of crystalline nephropathy and uropathy, the estimated prevalence of uropathy being 20% among all who use these drugs. Pure stones are radiolucent on both plain film *and* CT scanning (SCHWARTZ et al. 1999). All patients present with typical features of obstructive uropathy including flank pain and microscopic hematuria. In clinical studies, a mean use time of 11.1 months has been reported. Clinicians recommend that, when clinical symptoms are straightforward, the symptoms should be treated with hydration alone. Medication may be continued during the clinical episode (SCHWARTZ et al. 1999).

In the AIDS patient, renal lymphoma is most frequently seen as a manifestation of disseminated disease; primary renal involvement is rare (EISENBERG et al. 1994). Imaging features of a variety of morphological forms have been described. Histologically, these lymphomas are of the immunoblastic type or small-cell variety. Phenotypically, they are B cell types (TSANG et al. 1993). On CT scanning, renal lymphoma will generally present as a parenchymal mass or masses with a uniform attenuation. Lymphomatous renal involvement may also result in diffuse renal enlargement. In these cases, the normal corticomedullary architecture will be distorted. Nodal involvement, as opposed to disseminated lymphoma, is infrequent in the non-AIDS patient.

10.5
Adrenals

Although adrenal gland pathology is common in AIDS patients, clinically detectable or symptomatic disease is rare. Many patients are discovered to have infections within the adrenal, predominantly with cytomegalovirus (REICHERT et al. 1983). There have been reports of cases of primary adrenal insufficiency in HIV-infected patients (FREDA et al. 1994). Other infections, such as tuberculosis, blastomycosis, histoplasmosis, and extrapulmonary *P. carinii* infection can affect the adrenal gland in these immunosuppressed individuals (LUBAT et al. 1990; RADIN et al. 1990; RADIN 1991a).

Several cases of adrenal stromal tumors, predominantly of smooth muscle origin (leiomyoma and leiomyosarcomas), were reported several years ago. Subsequent cases have shown an increase in these tumors elsewhere within the retroperitoneum. The increasing incidence of these tumors is possibly linked to Epstein-Barr virus (Fig. 10.5).

AIDS-related lymphoma may involve the adrenal gland. This involvement is most frequently seen in the context of disseminated disease (RADIN et al. 1993; BALTHAZAR et al. 1997; TOWNSEND et al. 1989).

10.6
Lymphadenopathy

Lymphadenopathy is a common finding in HIV-infected patients. The detection of lymphadenopathy is problematic because the significance of the finding may be, or more often may not be, correlated with clinical symptoms. As a corollary to this, many patients with AIDS have multiple diagnoses. Because imaging is requested to direct clinical investigation for biopsy and rapid identification of areas highly likely to yield clinically relevant disease, detection of lymphadenopathy may be confounding rather than enlightening.

We have found that lymphadenopathy is best evaluated by applying a pattern approach. The determinants of the pattern include size of individual nodes, distribution within the retroperitoneum and the abdomen, and enhancement characteristics of the nodes themselves. The following discussion will attempt to correlate the above patterns with most likely etiologies of lymph node disease.

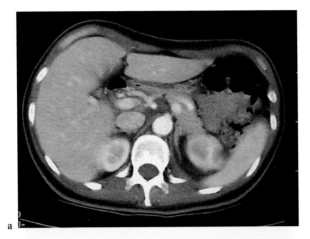

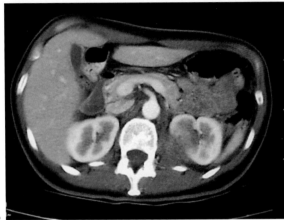

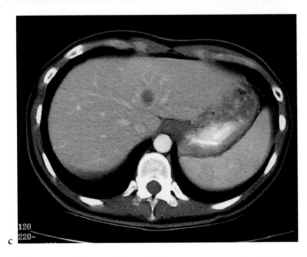

Fig. 10.5a–c. Retroperitoneal leiomyosarcoma. a A soft tissue mass envelops the left adrenal gland. b Same patient as in a. The mass has extended along the left psoas muscle and is invading the left kidney. c A low-attenuation liver metastasis, typical of malignant stromal tumors, is present. The diagnosis of leiomyosarcoma was made at wedge resection of a similar hepatic lesion. The pathologist noted the presence of Epstein-Barr virus in the tumor

10.6.1
Neoplastic Lymphadenopathy

Lymphadenopathy is most frequently associated with neoplasm. In AIDS patients this is almost invariably either Kaposi's sarcoma or lymphoma (RABKIN 1994). Among a group of 25 men with epidemic Kaposi's sarcoma (EKS), 50% of those with lesions in the gastrointestinal tract demonstrated retroperitoneal lymphadenopathy on CT (ROSE et al. 1982). The distribution of lymphadenopathy not specific for EKS. The most likely location of the nodes is within the retroperitoneum and pelvic sidewalls. There is high frequency of inguinal and femoral node involvement, relating to lymphatic drainage from the lower extremities. In many patients, CT will show characteristic "streaky" soft tissue attenuation infiltration in the inguinal fat. This results in obscuration of the borders of the femoral vessels and nodes. The nodes are generally between 2 and 3 cm in size.

On dynamic CT scans, EKS nodes have a distinctive appearance. This can be ascribed to hypervascular hyperplasia of lymph nodes containing interweaving fascicles of spindle cells, extravasated red blood cells, vascular slits, and deposition of hemosiderin (AMAZON and RYWLIN 1988). The results in brightly enhanced nodes on intravenous contrast studies. In a study of the imaging characteristics of lymphadenopathy in 33 AIDS patients, the positive predictive value of hyperattenuating lymphadenopathy for EKS was 79%. These findings were statistically significant at the 95% confidence interval (Fig. 10.6) (HERTS et al. 1992). The lymphadenopathy in the in-

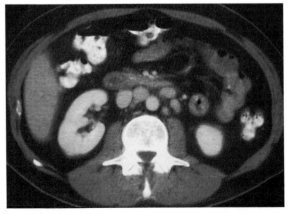

Fig. 10.6. Retroperitoneal adenopathy from EKS. Note that the lymph nodes enhance to a level between that of the inferior vena cava and the aorta

guinal regions is associated with striking infiltration of the surrounding soft tissue, obscuring the margins of the nodes themselves (Fig. 10.7).

AIDS-related lymphomas are often aggressive B cell variants. There is a high predilection for advanced disseminated disease at presentation and a much higher ratio of extranodal to nodal involvement. Radin found lymphadenopathy in 41 of 72 ARL patients with focal abdominal abnormalities on CT scanning (RADIN et al. 1993). When lymphoma is the cause of the adenopathy, the nodes tend to be bulky conglomerate masses measuring >5 cm. The density is close to that of skeletal muscle, without evidence of the enhancement seen in patients with EKS. In our experience, one must be wary of adenopathy in patients with extranodal abdominal AIDS-related lymphomas. When confronted with this finding, we recommend biopsy of an accessible node to assure the clinician that the patient is not harboring a second disease (most frequently mycobacterial). Gallium scanning is also useful in identifying the nodes as lymphomatous. Conversely, if clinical symptomatology and laboratory data do not support infection, one could treat for lymphoma and monitor nodal response.

10.6.2
Non-neoplastic Lymphadenopathy

Lymphadenopathy may be more common in patients with non-neoplastic diseases because of the higher prevalence of these disorders among HIV-infected individuals. Pattern recognition may provide a clue to diagnosis, but most often, tissue or cytological sampling of the affected nodes is necessary to institute timely and appropriate therapy (Fig. 10.8).

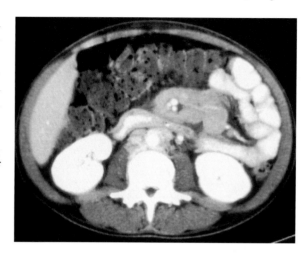

Fig. 10.8. Differentiation of etiology of adenopathy by attenuation. High-attenuation adenopathy surrounds the aorta and inferior vena cava from EKS. Mesenteric adenopathy is less attenuating than the mesenteric vessels it surrounds. This adenopathy was from intra-abdominal *M. tuberculosis*

Mycobacterial disease [*M. tuberculosis* and *M. avium* complex (MAC)] is frequently seen in this population. In an analogous fashion to EKS, MAC was also being recognized as a "new disease" in homosexual men at the beginning of recognition of the epidemic (SOHN et al. 1983). Clinical presentation of fever, diarrhea, and weight loss has been ascribed to other forms of mycobacterial infections. These entities may also present with prominent splenomegaly and lymphadenopathy (GAYNOR et al. 1994).

The imaging findings of lymphadenopathy related to MAC were also recognized in the early AIDS imaging literature (NYBERG et al. 1985). Concurrent reports documented imaging findings in patients with *M. tuberculosis* as well as MAC. The prevalence of *M. tuberculosis* was higher in intravenous drug users with HIV infection as compared to the homosexual population. Although retroperitoneal lymphadenopathy was visualized, peripancreatic and mesenteric locations predominated (HULNICK et al. 1985). While absolute differentiation was impossible, distribution and imaging characteristics of the nodes themselves were thought to have sufficient features to allow a prebiopsy diagnosis. Radin compared abdominal CT scans of 71 patients with AIDS who had proven disseminated infection due to *M. tuberculosis* or *M. avium-intracellulare*. Of the patients with *M. tuberculosis* infection, 93% demonstrated lymphadenopathy, with the majority showing central or diffuse low attenuation. In contrast, patients with lymphadenopathy from MAC demonstrated soft tissue homogeneous adenopathy in the

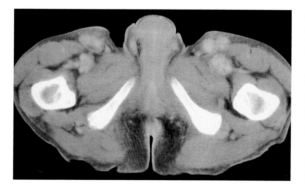

Fig. 10.7. EKS with inguinal infiltration. High-attenuation lymphadenopathy is present in inguinal and femoral lymph nodes. Note the poor definition of the margins of these nodes. This infiltrative pattern is typical in EKS

majority of cases (RADIN 1991b). A more recent study found adenopathy in 10 of 24 patients with MAC, soft tissue attenuation homogeneous lymphadenopathy being present in 80% of cases (Fig. 10.9) (PANTONGRAG-BROWN et al. 1998).

Noninfectious causes of lymphadenopathy may be the result of reactive lymph nodes. These may be seen in patients with so-called AIDS-related complex, ARC or pre-AIDS. The current term is "HIV-infection associated lymphadenopathy." The finding of this adenopathy is correlated with the CD4+ T-lymphocyte count. The nodes are diffusely scattered throughout the retroperitoneum, pelvic sidewalls, and small bowel mesentery. They are uniform in size. Histologically, these nodes will show reactive follicular hyperplasia. If the finding is made by imaging, and the CD4+ count is above 300 cells/mm^3, the assumption that the adenopathy is benign and reactive can be made without biopsy. Many patients also have peripheral adenopathy which can be biopsied if necessary.

Bacillary angiomatosis is a newly recognized entity afflicting AIDS patients. The etiology is a bacteria, *Bartonella henselae* or *B. quintana*. The lesion is characterized by a vascular proliferation within the affected areas. Cutaneous, mediastinal, intra-abdominal, osseous, and nodal lesions are described (HAUGHT et al. 1993; KUNBERGER and MONTALVO 1994). The vascular proliferation results in adenopathy which markedly enhances on contrast CT scanning, as in cases of EKS. Ultrasound may demonstrate high flow on Doppler studies (KUNBERGER and MONTALVO 1994).

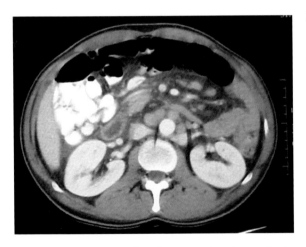

Fig. 10.9. Retroperitoneal and mesenteric adenopathy in MAC. Homogeneous soft tissue adenopathy is present within the para-aortic retroperitoneum, with several enlarged nodes in the small bowel mesentery as well. The homogeneous attenuation and combined retroperitoneal and mesenteric distribution are typical for MAC

10.7 Conclusion

The retroperitoneal diseases rarely occur in the absence of intra-abdominal findings. Although the findings of imaging alone are rarely sufficient to make the specific diagnosis, familiarity with patterns of involvement will often allow a more precise differential diagnosis, which will have the benefit of permitting faster institution of appropriate therapy.

References

Abdel-Dayem HM, Naddaf S, Aziz M, et al. (1997) Sites of tuberculous involvement in patients with AIDS. Autopsy findings and evaluation of gallium imaging. Clin Nucl Med 22:310–314

Aboulafia DM (1997) Acute pancreatitis. A fatal complication of AIDS therapy. J Clin Gastroenterol 25:640–645

Amazon K, Rywlin AM (eds) (1988) Systemic manifestations of Kaposi's sarcoma. Lea & Febiger, Philadelphia

Bach MC, Bagwell SP, Masur H (1986) Utility of gallium imaging in the diagnosis of *Mycobacterium avium-intra-cellulare* infection in patients with the acquired immunodeficiency syndrome. Clin Nucl Med 11:175–177

Balthazar EJ, Noordhoorn M, Megibow AJ, Gordon RB (1997) CT of small-bowel lymphoma in immunocompetent patients and patients with AIDS: comparison of findings. Am J Roentgenol 168:675–680

Bargman JM, Wagner C, Cameron R (1991) Renal cortical nephrocalcinosis: a manifestation of extrapulmonary *Pneumocystis carinii* infection in the acquired immunodeficiency syndrome. Am J Kidney Dis 17:712–715

Eisenberg PJ, Papanicolaou N, Lee MJ, Yoder IC (1994) Diagnostic imaging in the evaluation of renal lymphoma. Leuk Lymphoma 16:37–50

Evrard S, Van Laethem JL, Urbain D, Deviere J, Cremer M (1999) Chronic pancreatic alterations in AIDS patients. Pancreas 19:335–338

Freda PU, Wardlaw SL, Brudney K, Goland RS (1994) Primary adrenal insufficiency in patients with the acquired immunodeficiency syndrome: a report of five cases. J Clin Endocrinol Metab 79:1540–1545

Gaynor CD, Clark RA, Koontz FP, Emler S, Hirschel B, Schlesinger LS (1994) Disseminated *Mycobacterium genavense* infection in two patients with AIDS. Clin Infect Dis 18:455–457

Hamper UM, Goldblum LE, Hutchins GM, et al. (1988) Renal involvement in AIDS: sonographic-pathologic correlation. Am J Roentgenol 150:1321–1325

Haught WH, Steinbach J, Zander DS, Wingo CS (1993) Case report: bacillary angiomatosis with massive visceral lymphadenopathy. Am J Med Sci 306:236–240

Herts BR, Megibow AJ, Birnbaum BA, Kanzer GK, Noz ME (1992) High-attenuation lymphadenopathy in AIDS patients: significance of findings at CT. Radiology 185:777–781

Hulnick DH, Megibow AJ, Naidich DP, Hilton S, Cho KC, Balthazar EJ (1985) Abdominal tuberculosis: CT evaluation. Radiology 157:199–204

Jaber B, Gleckman R (1995) Tuberculous pancreatic abscess as an initial AIDS-defining disorder in a patient infected with the human immunodeficiency virus: case report and review. Clin Infect Dis 20:890–894

Jones WF, Sheikh MY, Mcclave SA (1997) AIDS-related non-Hodgkin's lymphoma of the pancreas. Am J Gastroenterol 92:335–338

Kay CJ (1992) Renal diseases in patients with AIDS: sonographic findings . Am J Roentgenol 159:551–554

Kunberger LE, Montalvo BM (1994) Bacillary angiomatosis in the abdomen: Doppler and CT features. J Comput Assist Tomogr 18:308–309

Lubat E, Megibow AJ, Balthazar EJ, Goldenberg AS, Birnbaum BA, Bosniak MA (1990) Extrapulmonary Pneumocystis carinii infection in AIDS: CT findings. Radiology 174:157–160

Martinez-Jabaloyas J, Osca JM, Ruiz JL, Beamud A, Blanes M, Jimenez-Cruz JF (1995) Renal aspergillosis and AIDS. Eur Urol 27:167–169

Menges M, Pees HW, Aboulafia DM, et al. (1999) Kaposi's sarcoma of the pancreas mimicking pancreatic cancer in an HIV-infected patient.. Int J Pancreatol 26:193–199

Miller FH, Parikh S, Gore RM, Nemcek AA Jr, Fitzgerald SW, Vogelzang RL (1993) Renal manifestations of AIDS. Radiographics 13:587–596

Miller FH, Gore RM, Nemcek AA Jr, Fitzgerald SW (1996) Pancreaticobiliary manifestations of AIDS. Am J Roentgenol 166:1269–1274

Mohle-Boetani JC, Koehler JE, Berger TG, et al. (1996) Bacillary angiomatosis and bacillary peliosis in patients infected with human immunodeficiency virus: clinical characteristics in a case-control study. Clin Infect Dis 22:794–800

Nordback I, Olson J, Chaisson R, Cameron J (1992) Acute effects of a nucleoside analog dideoxyinosine (DDI) on the pancreas. J Surg Res 53:610–614

Nyberg DA, Federle MP, Jeffrey RB, Bottles K, Wofsy CB (1985) Abdominal CT findings of disseminated Mycobacterium avium-intracellulare in AIDS. Am J Roentgenol 145:297–299

Nyberg DA, Jeffrey R Jr, Federle MP, Bottles K, Abrams DI (1986) AIDS-related lymphomas: evaluation by abdominal CT. Radiology 159:59–63

O'Regan S, Russo P, Lapointe N, Rousseau E (1990) AIDS and the urinary tract. J Acquir Immune Defic Syndr 3:244–251

Pantongrag-Brown L, Krebs TL, Daly BD, et al. (1998) Frequency of abdominal CT findings in AIDS patients with M. avium complex bacteraemia. Clin Radiol 53:816–819

Pombo F, Diaz Candamio MJ, Rodriguez E, Pombo S (1998) Pancreatic tuberculosis: CT findings. Abdom Imaging 23:394–397

Rabkin CS (1994) Epidemiology of AIDS-related malignancies. Curr Opin Oncol 6:492–496

Radin DR (1991a) Disseminated histoplasmosis: abdominal CT findings in 16 patients. Am J Roentgenol 157:955–958

Radin DR (1991b) Intraabdominal Mycobacterium tuberculosis vs Mycobacterium avium-intracellulare infections in patients with AIDS: distinction based on CT findings. Am J Roentgenol 156:487–491

Radin R (1995) HIV infection: analysis in 259 consecutive patients with abnormal abdominal CT findings. Radiology 197:712–722

Radin DR, Baker EL, Klatt EC, et al. (1990) Visceral and nodal calcification in patients with AIDS-related Pneumocystis carinii infection. Am J Roentgenol 154:27–31

Radin DR, Esplin JA, Levine AM, Ralls PW (1993) AIDS-related non-Hodgkin's lymphoma: abdominal CT findings in 112 patients. Am J Roentgenol 160:1133–1139

Reichert CM, O'Leary TJ, Levens DL, Simrell CR, Macher AM (1983) Autopsy pathology in the acquired immune deficiency syndrome. Am J Pathol 112:357–382

Rose HS, Balthazar EJ, Megibow AJ, Horowitz L, Laubenstein LJ (1982) Alimentary tract involvement in Kaposi sarcoma: radiographic and endoscopic findings in 25 homosexual men. Am J Roentgenol 139:661–666

Schaffer RM, Schwartz GE, Becker JA, Rao TK, Shih YH (1984) Renal ultrasound in acquired immune deficiency syndrome. Radiology 153:511–513

Schwartz BF, Schenkman N, Armenakas NA, Stoller ML (1999) Imaging characteristics of indinavir calculi. J Urol 161:1085–1087

Smith FJ, Mathieson JR, Cooperberg PL (1994) Abdominal abnormalities in AIDS: detection at US in a large population. Radiology 192:691–695

Sohn CC, Schroff RW, Kliewer KE, Lebel DM, Fligiel S (1983) Disseminated Mycobacterium avium-intracellulare infection in homosexual men with acquired cell-mediated immunodeficiency: a histologic and immunologic study of two cases. Am J Clin Pathol 79:247–252

Sundaram CP, Saltzman B (1999) Urolithiasis associated with protease inhibitors. J Endourol 13:309–312

Townsend RR, Laing FC, Jeffrey R Jr, Bottles K (1989) Abdominal lymphoma in AIDS: evaluation with US. Radiology 171:719–724

Tsang K, Kneafsey P, Gill MJ (1993) Primary lymphoma of the kidney in the acquired immunodeficiency syndrome. Arch Pathol Lab Med 117:541–543

Tshibwabwa ET, Mwaba P, Bogle-Taylor J, Zumla A (2000) Four-year study of abdominal ultrasound in 900 Central African adults with AIDS referred for diagnostic imaging. Abdom Imaging 25:290–296

Yee JM, Raghavendra BN, Horii SC, Ambrosino M (1989) Abdominal sonography in AIDS. A review. J Ultrasound Med 8:705–714

11 Radiologic Evaluation of the Acute Abdomen in AIDS

Karen M. Horton and Elliot K. Fishman

CONTENTS

11.1 Introduction

Many patients with AIDS develop abdominal symptoms, usually related to opportunistic infections or neoplasms. Approximately 4.2% of these patients will require abdominal surgery, often in an emergency setting (Bouillot et al. 1995; LaRaja et al. 1989; Nugent and O'Connell 1986). Radiologic evaluation of AIDS patients with acute abdominal complaints is essential for two main reasons. First, AIDS patients are usually immunosuppressed and thus the classic physical signs and symptoms of peritonitis and sepsis are often absent (Scott-Conner and Fabrega 1996). For instance, many AIDS patients with acute

K.M. Horton, MD
Assistant Professor of Radiology, The Russell H. Morgan Department of Radiology and Radiological Science, Johns Hopkins Medical Institutions, 601. N. Caroline Street, JHOC 3255, Baltimore, MD 21287, USA
E.K. Fishman, MD
Professor of Radiology, The Russell H. Morgan Department of Radiology and Radiological Science, Johns Hopkins Medical Institutions, 601. N. Caroline Street, JHOC 3254, Baltimore, MD 21287, USA

intra-abdominal pathology will have a normal or low white blood cell count, often without a "left shift" (Binderow and Shaked 1991; Bizer et al. 1995; Whitney et al. 1992). Since the physical examination in these patients is often not reliable, radiologic imaging plays a crucial role in the diagnosis of acute abdominal conditions in AIDS patients who present with vague and nonspecific symptoms. Second, patients with AIDS are often debilitated with very poor nutritional status and low albumin (Diettrich et al. 1991). These factors undoubtedly contribute to the high morbidity and mortality rates associated with emergency abdominal operations in patients with AIDS (Bizer et al. 1995; Davidson et al. 1991). Radiologic examinations can help distinguish nonsurgical disorders such as acute colitis or enteritis from those which will require surgical intervention, thus avoiding unnecessary high-risk operations.

This chapter will review the radiologic evaluation and findings of the acute abdomen in patients with AIDS, with an emphasis on the value of computed tomography (CT). Both infectious and neoplastic conditions affecting the gastrointestinal tract, liver, and biliary tract will be discussed and illustrated.

11.2 Radiologic Examinations

Plain radiographs of the abdomen can sometimes be useful as a quick inexpensive initial study in AIDS patients who present with acute abdominal complaints. They may reveal pneumoperitoneum, pneumatosis, or bowel obstruction. However, in most cases the plain film will be normal or will demonstrate a nonspecific bowel gas pattern and further imaging will be necessary.

Barium studies such as the small bowel series or the contrast enema can be helpful in patients with suspected bowel obstruction. These studies may detect the presence and level of obstruction, but typically provide little information regarding the cause of the obstruction, especially if there is extraintestinal disease. Also, barium studies allow visualization of the small bowel and colonic mucosa and can be useful for evaluation of patients in the nonacute setting with nonspecific complaints such as nausea or diarrhea.

Sonography is particularly valuable for imaging the gallbladder and hepatobiliary disease in evaluation of the acute abdomen in patients with AIDS (TAOUREL et al. 1995; WU et al. 1998). Sonography is superior to CT for the evaluation of acalculous cholecystitis and AIDS cholangitis, which are well-described conditions in patients with AIDS (DaSILVA et al. 1993; JEFFREY and SOMMER 1993). Compression-graded sonography is also a reliable technique for the evaluation of suspected appendicitis, especially in children and thin patients (YACOE and JEFFREY 1994). Sonography may be the initial imaging modality of choice when these conditions are suspected. However, ultrasound plays little role in evaluation of the gastrointestinal tract or in patients with vague complaints without localizing signs and symptoms.

Although plain radiographs, barium studies, and sonography each may be useful in evaluation of the acute abdomen, CT remains the diagnostic modality of choice (WU et al. 1998; WYATT and FISHMAN 1994). CT is fast and accurate. On modern spiral scanners, the entire abdomen and pelvis can be imaged in less than a minute. CT is the most sensitive modality for the detection of pneumoperitoneum and pneumatosis and in most cases will be able to determine the cause. CT is also valuable in evaluation of the gastrointestinal tract. CT can detect bowel wall thickening in patients with enteritis and colitis, and in many cases can suggest the correct etiology such as infection vs ischemia vs tumor. CT is both sensitive and specific for the detection of bowel obstruction and for identifying the cause (DANESHMAND et al. 1999; SURI et al. 1999). CT is also excellent for the evaluation of the solid viscera such as the liver, spleen, and pancreas as well as lymph nodes, all of which may be involved in infectious or neoplastic processes.

11.3
Infections

11.3.1
Cytomegalovirus

Cytomegalovirus (CMV) is one of the most common opportunistic infections which occur in patients with AIDS. It can affect any portion of the gastrointestinal tract, although the colon is the most common site of involvement. Patients with CMV colitis can present with crampy abdominal pain and high fever and in cases of colon involvement, severe watery or bloody diarrhea. With colonic involvement, the CT will characteristically demonstrate circumferential wall thickening with inflammatory stranding in the pericolonic fat (Fig. 11.1). Ulcerations may also be identified (BALTHAZAR and MARTINO 1996). The entire colon may be affected, or involvement can be limited to the terminal ileum and right colon (BALTHAZAR and MARTINO 1996; BALTHAZAR et al. 1985a). Segmental involvement of the colon can also occur (MURRAY et al. 1995). Occasionally the colonic wall will demonstrate a target appearance, due to severe submucosal edema with stratification of the bowel wall layers. This target appearance is not specific for CMV colitis, and does occur in other conditions such as ischemia and inflammatory bowel disease. In addition to detecting the colonic pathology in AIDS patients with acute abdominal signs and symptoms, CT is helpful for identifying complications such as ischemia, obstruction, abscess, or perforation.

In patients with CMV enteritis, CT may reveal nonspecific small bowel thickening, usually confined to the distal ileum, although the proximal ileum and jejunum can also be involved (Fig. 11.2). (WALL and JONES 1992). The wall thickening is presumably a result of small vessel vasculitis resulting in hemorrhage and ischemia. Ascites and small nodes may also be present.

CMV can affect the esophagus and stomach, resulting in acute abdominal complaints (BALTHAZAR et al. 1985b). CMV esophagitis is best demonstrated on a

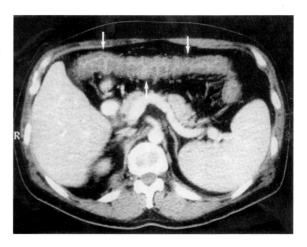

Fig. 11.1. Contrast-enhanced spiral CT demonstrates minimal to moderate diffuse thickening of the transverse colon (*arrows*) in an HIV-positive patient. This is an example of CMV colitis

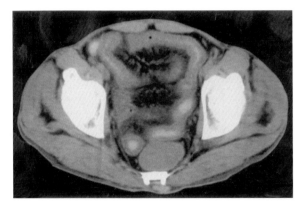

Fig. 11.2. Spiral CT with oral contrast only in a 39-year-old man with HIV and acute abdominal pain demonstrates diffuse thickening of the small bowel. This is an example of CMV enteritis

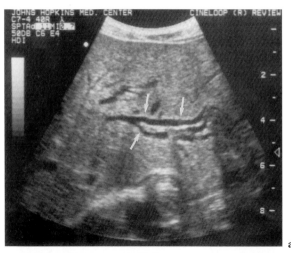

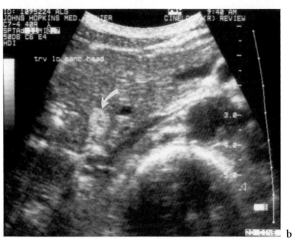

Fig. 11.3a, b. A 35-year-old female with AIDS and right upper quadrant pain. a Ultrasound demonstrates dilatation of the intrahepatic ducts (*arrows*); b in addition there is a small echogenic mass near the ampulla of Vater (*curved arrow*). An echogenic papilla has been described in patients with AIDS cholangitis

contrast esophagogram, which will reveal discrete superficial ulcers, primarily involving the mid and distal esophagus (LEVINE 1989). In severe cases the esophagus may also show fold thickening with only one large flat ulcer. CMV gastritis typically involves the gastroesophageal junction or antrum and results in fold thickening and/or ulcerations (BALTHAZAR et al. 1985b).

CMV as well as *Cryptosporidium* infection can cause cholangitis (BOUCHE et al. 1993). Patients present with right upper quadrant pain and fever, and may be jaundiced. CT may demonstrate intra- and or extrahepatic ductal dilatation, which typically is irregular and simulates the appearance of sclerosing cholangitis (WYATT and FISHMAN 1994). The gallbladder wall may also appear thickened. Ultrasound demonstrates wall thickening of the bile ducts in addition to irregular dilatation. Also, the papilla of Vater can appear echogenic, due to edema (Fig. 11.3) (DASILVA et al. 1993). Endoscopic retrograde cholangiopancreatography can also demonstrate the beading and pruning of the bile ducts, similar to the findings observed in patients with sclerosing cholangitis. Microabscesses can occur in the liver in AIDS patients with ascending cholangitis. These can be detected on ultrasound or CT.

11.3.2
Cryptosporidium

Cryptosporidiosis is a major cause of diarrhea in patients with AIDS and results in significant morbidity. Patients typically present with profuse watery diarrhea and severe abdominal pain. Although ra-

diologic studies are not necessary for diagnosis, they may be the first to suggest the diagnosis in patients presenting with acute abdominal pain. Cryptosporidiosis usually affects the proximal jejunum (Fig. 11.4) although gastric involvement has also been reported. On CT, jejunal wall thickening is characteristic. On barium studies, the proximal jejunum will be dilated with fold thickening. The appearance can resemble sprue. If severe, there may be complete effacement of the jejunal folds, resulting in a "toothpaste" appearance. Gastric involvement is usually characterized by antral narrowing (IRIBARREN et al. 1997). Pneumatosis has been reported as a rare benign complication of intestinal cryptosporidiosis (HERNETH et al. 1998).

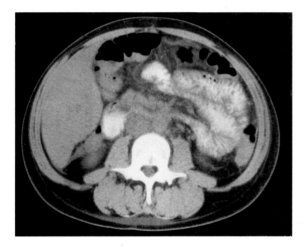

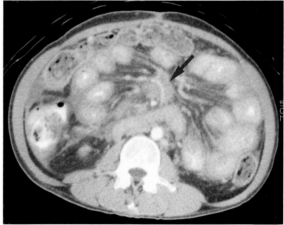

Fig. 11.4. A 29-year-old with AIDS and abdominal pain. CT scan with oral contrast reveals moderate diffuse thickening of the proximal small bowel. This is an example of cryptosporidiosis

Fig. 11.5. Contrast-enhanced spiral CT demonstrates moderate diffuse thickening of the small bowel with stranding in the mesentery and low-density lymphadenopathy (*arrow*). There is also minimal ascites. This is an example of MAI

Cryptosporidiosis can cause cholangitis in patients with AIDS (BOUCHE et al. 1993; DASILVA et al. 1993). The radiologic findings are identical to the cholangitis caused by CMV. In fact, the two organisms are probably coexistent in most patients.

11.3.3
Mycobacterium avium-intracellulare

Mycobacterium avium-intracellulare (MAI) is a very common opportunistic infection in AIDS patients (NYBERG et al. 1985). AIDS patients with abdominal involvement by MAI can present with severe abdominal pain, fever, diarrhea, and weight loss. MAI involvement of the gastrointestinal tract is common. It typically will involve the duodenum and the small bowel (WYATT and FISHMAN 1994). The appearance on barium studies is nonspecific, demonstrating fold thickening and nodularity as well as dilatation. Due to increased intraluminal fluid, there may be segmentation and flocculation of the barium, simulating Whipple's disease. Disseminated infection from MAI has been recognized as a common and severe complication of AIDS. On CT, significant retroperitoneal and mesenteric lymphadenopathy is common, occurring in up to 82%–100% of patients (Fig. 11.5) (NYBERG et al. 1985; RADIN 1995). Typically, the nodes are large and bulky and may demonstrate decreased attenuation due to necrosis. Splenomegaly and hepatomegaly may be present. MAI can also result in small microabscesses in the liver and spleen, which appear as small foci of decreased attenuation on CT (RADIN 1995). On

ultrasound, the small lesions can also be seen and may appear as echogenic or hypoechoic foci. CT or ultrasound can be used as imaging guidance to sample enlarged nodes to confirm the diagnosis of MAI in difficult cases (NYBERG et al. 1985).

11.3.4
Tuberculosis

Patients with AIDS are susceptible to tuberculosis, which is often disseminated. Tuberculosis can affect the gastrointestinal tract, usually resulting from ingestion of contaminated food products or from lymphatic or hematogenous dissemination (HULNICK et al. 1985). Tuberculosis typically involves the distal ileum and cecum, producing wall thickening and occasionally ulcerations (RADIN 1995). This can be demonstrated on barium studies or CT. The radiographic findings of tuberculosis are not specific, as other organisms can affect the ileum and cecum. However, findings such as significant asymmetric thickening of the cecum (predominantly involving the medial wall) or the association of bowel thickening and low-density lymphadenopathy can be suggestive of tuberculosis. Low-density nodes can be seen in up to 89% of patients (Fig. 11.6) (RADIN 1995). In addition to involvement of the gastrointestinal tract, tuberculosis can result in peritonitis (Fig. 11.7). On CT, ascites and soft tissue thickening of the mesentery and omentum can be present in association with lymphadenopathy (HULNICK et al. 1985). The CT appearance can mimic carcinomatosis or perito-

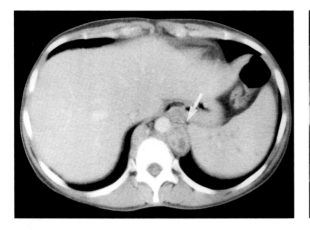

Fig. 11.6. Contrast-enhanced spiral CT of the chest demonstrates extensive low-density lymphadenopathy involving the retrocrural nodes (*arrow*). In addition, smaller density lesions were identified in the spleen. This is an example of tuberculosis

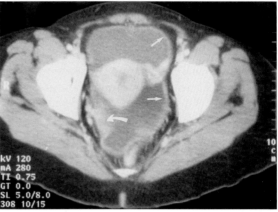

Fig. 11.7. Contrast-enhanced spiral CT demonstrates pelvic ascites with peripheral enhancement (*arrows*) and soft tissue thickening (*curved arrow*). This appearance can be seen in metastatic carcinomatosis from primary tumors such as ovarian cancer. However, laboratory analysis of the fluid demonstrated tuberculosis

neal mesothelioma. Tuberculosis, when disseminated, can also affect the liver and spleen, resulting in small low-density lesions that were found to be present in 73% of patients in one series (Figs. 11.6, 11.8) (RADIN 1995).

11.3.5
Clostridium difficile

Pseudomembranous colitis results from the production of an endotoxin by the overgrowth of *C. difficile* organisms. It is commonly seen in patients treated with antibiotics. Patients can present with severe abdominal pain and may sometimes require surgical resection.

CT findings of pseudomembranous colitis include marked colonic wall thickening, often measuring greater than 1.5 cm in thickness (Fig. 11.9) (FISHMAN et al. 1991; KAWAMOTO et al. 1999b). Other infections which can cause colitis usually do not result in this degree of wall thickening. In addition, patients with pseudomembranous colitis can demonstrate stranding in the pericolic fat that is often much less pronounced than would be expected with the degree of colonic involvement. Ascites has been reported in up to 30% of cases and can help suggest the diagnosis of

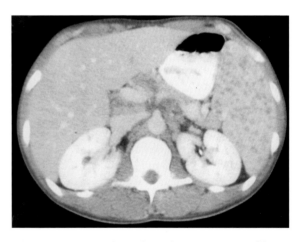

Fig. 11.8. Contrast-enhanced spiral CT in a 31-year-old man with AIDS and abdominal pain demonstrates multiple low-density lesions in the spleen. Biopsy of a retroperitoneal lymph node (not shown) demonstrated tuberculosis

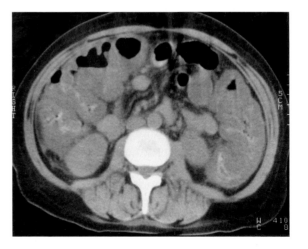

Fig. 11.9. Contrast-enhanced spiral CT demonstrates moderate to marked low-density thickening of the colonic wall. There is also ascites. This is an example of the CT appearance of pseudomembranous colitis occurring in a patient with AIDS

pseudomembranous colitis, although this is not specific (KAWAMOTO et al. 1999a). Although typically thought of as a pancolitis, pseudomembranous colitis can be segmental or even focal, mimicking a soft tissue mass (FISHMAN et al. 1991; KAWAMOTO et al. 1999a). In addition to wall thickening and ascites, the colonic wall may demonstrate enlargement of the haustral folds, which can trap the oral contrast, producing an appearance similar to an accordion. Although this can be suggestive of pseudomembranous colitis, it is neither sensitive nor specific. CT may be the first modality to suggest the diagnosis, which can be confirmed with toxin assays of the stool. In a series of patients with pseudomembranous colitis reported by KAWAMOTO et al. (1999a), CT demonstrated a variety of findings but was unable to predict which patients would require surgical intervention. Surgery is usually considered if there is associated ischemia, pneumatosis, pneumoperitoneum, or significant obstruction. It may also be considered in patients who do not respond to antibiotic therapy.

11.3.6
Other Infections

Amebiasis has also been reported in AIDS patients. In contrast to cryptosporidiosis, amebiasis usually affects the distal small bowel and colon, producing wall thickening and inflammation which can be detected on barium studies or CT scan (WU et al. 1998). In addition, *Giardia* infection can result in abdominal complaints and diarrhea. The radiologic appearance on barium studies and CT can be identical to that of cryptosporidiosis, with proximal small bowel thickening and dilatation.

11.4
Urinary Tract Calculi

Indinavir sulfate is a protease inhibitor which is used in the treatment of HIV infection. This medication is associated with a significant incidence of crystallization and stone formation in the urinary tract. In one study by REITER et al., 105 patients were treated with the drug. The incidence of symptomatic nephrolithiasis during the indinavir treatment was 12.4% (REITER et al. 1999). These patients can present with the usual symptoms of urinary colic, including flank pain and/or nausea and vomiting. Patients may also de-

scribe dysuria, urgency, hematuria, and/or proteinuria. Recently, spiral CT has been used in patients with suspected ureteral calculi to detect radiopaque stones. However, the urinary stones associated with this protease inhibitor are radiolucent and cannot be identified on unenhanced abdominal CT scans (Fig. 11.10) (GENTLE et al. 1997; SCHWARTZ et al. 1999). Secondary signs of obstruction including hydronephrosis and/or perinephric stranding can be detected on CT, although the stones themselves will not be visualized.

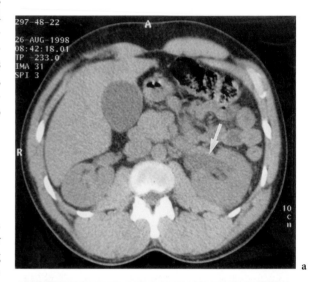

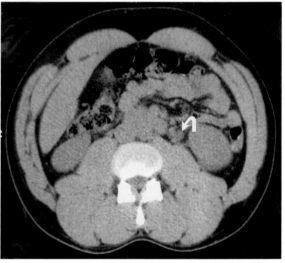

Fig. 11.10a, b. Noncontrast CT with thin collimation was performed in a 22-year-old man with HIV and renal colic. CT demonstrates enlargement of the left kidney with hydronephrosis (*straight arrow*) and hydroureter (*curved arrow*). However, no radiopaque stones were identified. This is an example of ureter obstruction resulting from lucent stones, which form in patients treated with indinavir sulfate

11.5
Pneumatosis

Pneumatosis intestinalis refers to the presence of air within the bowel wall. This can be due to a variety of etiologies; the most worrisome of which is ischemia with bowel ischemia/necrosis. This has been reported in an AIDS patient with necrotizing enterocolitis, and in such cases the patient will be symptomatic. However, a more indolent form of pneumatosis intestinalis has also been described in asymptomatic patients with AIDS in association with various infections including CMV and cryptosporidiosis (GELMAN and BRANDT 1998), and therefore the clinical significance of pneumatosis in AIDS patients is not certain. In a series of six cases of AIDS-associated pneumatosis intestinalis reported by WOOD et al. (1995), five of the patients were managed conservatively without surgical resection. Similarly, in another series of AIDS patients with pneumatosis intestinalis reported by GELMAN and BRANDT (1998), all five patients were managed conservatively. When present, pneumatosis typically involves the right colon or cecum in patients with AIDS. Asymptomatic pneumatosis intestinalis along with free abdominal air has also been described (HEGENER et al. 1998). Therefore, the finding of pneumatosis intestinalis in patients with AIDS should be correlated carefully with the clinical symptoms, as it may indicate bowel necrosis in patients with severe intestinal infections or may simply be an incidental finding which can be treated conservatively in asymptomatic patients (Fig. 11.11).

11.6
Neoplasms

Patients with AIDS are not only predisposed to various infections but are also at risk for certain neoplasms. The two most important neoplasms associated with AIDS are non-Hodgkin's lymphoma and Kaposi's sarcoma. There are several other cancers which appear to have a slighter increased incidence in patients with AIDS, including anal cancer, testicular cancer, and cervical cancer. However, we will limit our discussion to non-Hodgkin's lymphoma and Kaposi's sarcoma.

11.6.1
Non-Hodgkin's Lymphoma

It is estimated that the incidence of intermediate and high-grade B-cell non-Hodgkin's lymphoma in HIV-

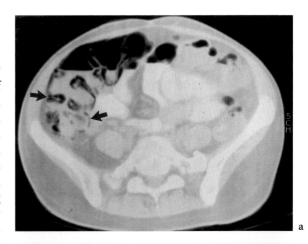

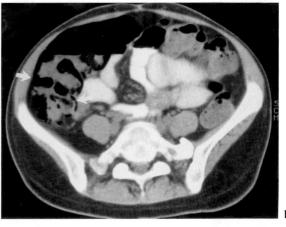

Fig. 11.11a, b. CT of the abdomen with oral contrast only in a 35-year-old female with abdominal pain and AIDS. Pneumatosis involving the cecum is demonstrated (*arrows*) (**a** lung window, **b** soft tissue window). Pneumatosis can be best demonstrated by using lung windows (**a**). The patient was managed conservatively and the pneumatosis resolved over the next 2 weeks. The exact etiology was unclear although the patient had both disseminated MAI and CMV colitis

infected individuals is almost 60 times greater than in the general population (BERAL et al. 1991). These AIDS-related lymphomas tend to be a late manifestation of HIV infection and have unique clinical pathologic features, which are different from classical non-Hodgkin's lymphoma occurring in the general population. In comparison with non-Hodgkin's lymphoma in the general population, lymphomas in patients with AIDS tend to be more aggressive and to display extranodal involvement (BALTHAZAR et al. 1997; ZIEGLER et al. 1984). The central nervous system, bone marrow, and abdomen are the most common sites of involvement. Also, response to treatment is not as good in patients with AIDS as in immunocompetent patients.

AIDS patients with abdominal involvement by non-Hodgkin's lymphoma can present acutely with pain, palpable mass, or gastrointestinal bleeding. Also, lymphoma involving the gastrointestinal tract can cause acute complications such as perforation, obstruction, or intussusception. In these cases, the patients will also present with acute abdominal symptoms, requiring radiologic evaluation. In most cases, CT is considered the imaging modality of choice for detecting, staging, and planning therapy in patients with lymphoma (Figs. 11.12–11.15). CT is sensitive for the detection of bulky abdominal and pelvic lymphadenopathy as well as of lymphoma involving solid organs such as the liver or spleen or gastrointestinal tract (WYATT and FISHMAN 1994). Hepatic or splenic involvement may appear as small

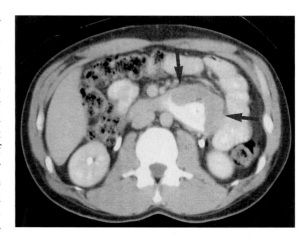

Fig. 11.14. Contrast-enhanced spiral CT demonstrates aneurysmal dilatation of the fourth portion of the duodenum with eccentric wall thickening (*arrows*). Endoscopy and biopsy were performed, revealing Burkitt's lymphoma. The CT appearance is very characteristic of lymphoma resulting in aneurysmal dilatation

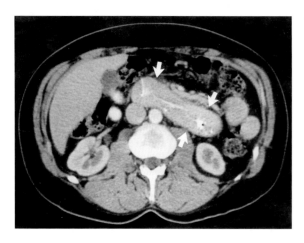

Fig. 11.12. Contrast-enhanced spiral CT demonstrates moderate circumferential thickening along the duodenum (*arrows*), compatible with biopsy-proven small bowel lymphoma

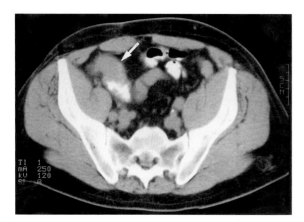

Fig. 11.13. Spiral CT with oral contrast only demonstrates a soft tissue mass involving the terminal ileum (*arrow*). At surgery, a small bowel lymphoma was discovered

low-density masses on CT, which may or may not demonstrate enhancement. Alternatively, lymphoma can appear as a diffuse infiltrative process in the liver or spleen.

Patients with gastrointestinal tract involvement by lymphoma can present with acute abdominal symptoms requiring radiologic evaluation. The stomach is the most common site of involvement (RADIN et al. 1993). The CT appearance of gastric lymphoma can vary from diffuse or segmental wall thickening to a discrete mass with or without ulceration (Fig. 11.16). The CT appearance can resemble adenocarcinoma of the stomach. One differentiating feature is that, despite extensive gastric involvement, lymphoma will very rarely result in gastric outlet obstruction. By contrast, involvement of the stomach by adenocarcinoma will often cause gastric outlet obstruction. Also, in the AIDS population, lymphoma of the stomach is much more common than adenocarcinoma.

The small intestine is the next most likely site of involvement of non-Hodgkin's lymphoma in AIDS patients (RADIN et al. 1993). In a series of 42 consecutive patients with small bowel lymphoma, BALTHAZAR et al. (1997) determined that more than half had AIDS. However, there was no significant difference in the radiologic features of patients with AIDS versus immunocompetent patients. Of the patients with lymphoma and AIDS, 22% demonstrated solid organ involvement such as involvement of the liver, spleen, kidney, or adrenal glands. By contrast, only 10% of the immunocompetent patients with lym-

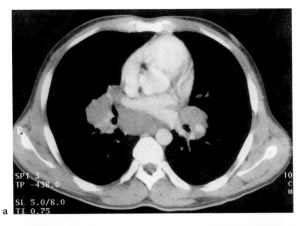

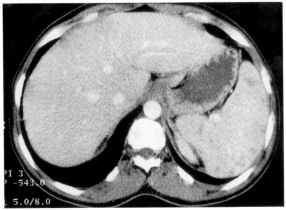

Fig. 11.15a, b. Contrast-enhanced spiral CT in a 29-year-old patient with AIDS and abdominal pain demonstrates multiple low-density lesions in the spleen. In addition, there is significant mediastinal and hilar lymphadenopathy. Bronchoscopy with biopsy demonstrated lymphoma

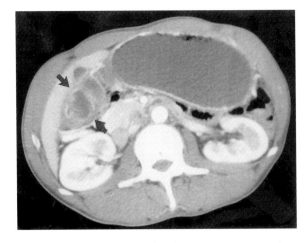

Fig. 11.16. Spiral CT with oral and intravenous contrast in a patient with AIDS and abdominal pain demonstrates distention of the stomach with circumferential thickening of the gastric antrum (*arrow*). At surgery, a gastric lymphoma was discovered

phoma demonstrated solid organ involvement. Two main CT patterns of small bowel involvement were observed (BALTHAZAR et al. 1997). In the first pattern, there were single or multiple segments of circumferential wall thickening which appeared homogeneous in attenuation (1.5–7 cm in thickness). The second pattern of involvement observed was single or multiple cavitary lesions associated with bowel wall thickening. Mesenteric or retroperitoneal lymphadenopathy was demonstrated in 45% of the patients with AIDS, in comparison to 60% of immunocompetent patients (BALTHAZAR et al. 1997). The distribution and pattern of CT presentation were similar for the two groups.

Lymphomas affecting the colon and rectum are uncommon, but have been reported with increased incidence in patients with AIDS (RADIN et al. 1993; WYATT and FISHMAN 1994). Colonic lymphoma can appear as a large polypoid mass or as diffuse thickening. Although the CT appearance of the primary tumor can be similar to that of colon cancer, lymphomas are typically associated with extensive lymphadenopathy.

11.6.2
Kaposi's Sarcoma

Kaposi's sarcoma is the most common AIDS-associated cancer in the United States, although its incidence has decreased from 40% of American men with AIDS in 1981 to less than 20% in 1992 (BIGGAR and RABKIN 1996). This aggressive and frequently fatal variant of Kaposi's sarcoma affects homosexual men with AIDS 20 times as frequently as male patients with AIDS who are not homosexual and have a similar degree of immunosuppression. As with the indolent form of Kaposi's sarcoma, which occurs in non-HIV-infected elderly men, Kaposi's sarcoma in AIDS patients typically involves the skin. However, patients with AIDS who develop Kaposi's sarcoma can show rapid disease progression to include widespread cutaneous involvement as well as involvement of lymph nodes and the gastrointestinal tract. These patients with abdominal involvement may present with acute abdominal symptoms requiring radiologic evaluation. The most common site of gastrointestinal tract involvement is the duodenum, and gastric involvement has also been reported (Fig. 11.17). On upper gastrointestinal tract series, or small bowel series, gastrointestinal tract involvement can appear as small submucosal masses, often with ulcerations. This gives a characteristic target or

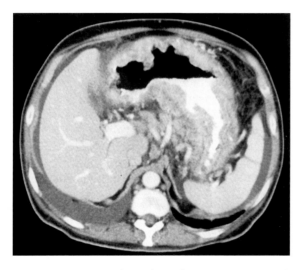

Fig. 11.17. Contrast-enhanced spiral CT in a patient with AIDS demonstrates diffuse thickening of the gastric folds and gastric wall. Endoscopy with biopsy revealed Kaposi's sarcoma

"bull's eye" appearance. Although this appearance is not specific for Kaposi's sarcoma, it is very suggestive in the right population. More extensive involvement of the gastrointestinal tract can appear as fold thickening, plaque, or masses on barium studies. Intestinal perforation has been described as a complication of gastrointestinal Kaposi's sarcoma (YOSHIDA et al. 1997). CT often demonstrates larger masses involving the gastrointestinal tract as well as any associated lymphadenopathy. Hepatic or splenic involvement has also been reported. The radiographic appearance can be similar to that of lymphoma or MAI infection, and biopsy may be required for definitive diagnosis.

Occasionally, the only radiographic finding in patients with Kaposi's sarcoma is lymphadenopathy, simulating lymphoma or MAI infection. One published study by Herts in 1992 suggested that when the lymphadenopathy in AIDS patients has a high attenuation, this is more suggestive of Kaposi's sarcoma than lymphoma or MAI, which often display low-density lymphadenopathy. Typically, in these circumstances, biopsy, with imaging guidance if necessary, will be needed to make the diagnosis (HERTS et al. 1992).

11.7
Conclusions

Radiologic examinations play a valuable role in the evaluation of AIDS patients. Although plain films, barium studies, and sonography all play a defined role in certain patients, CT is considered the modality of choice in patients presenting with acute or nonspecific abdominal complaints. CT allows evaluation of both the gastrointestinal tract and other intra-abdominal organs which are commonly involved in infectious or neoplastic diseases. CT can also help to direct patient management by identifying those patients who require surgical intervention.

References

Balthazar E, Martino J (1996) Giant ulcers in the ileum and colon caused by cytomegalovirus in patients with AIDS. AJR 166:1275–1276

Balthazar E, Megibow A, Fazzini E, et al. (1985a) Cytomegalovirus colitis in AIDS: radiographic findings in 11 patients. Radiology 155:585–589

Balthazar E, Megibow A, Huknick D (1985b) Cytomegalovirus esophagitis and gastritis in AIDS. AJR 144:1201–1204

Balthazar E, Noordhoorn M, Megibow A, et al. (1997) CT of small-bowel lymphoma in immunocompetent patients and patients with AIDS: comparison of findings. AJR 168:675–680

Beral V, Peterman T, Berkelman R, et al. (1991) AIDS-associated non-Hodgkin lymphoma. Lancet 337:805–809

Biggar R, Rabkin C (1996) The epidemiology of AIDS-related neoplasms. Hematol Oncol Clin North Am 10:997–1010

Binderow S, Shaked A (1991) Acute appendicitis in patients with AIDS/HIV infection. Am J Surg 162:9–12

Bizer L, Pettorino R, Ashikari A (1995) Emergency abdominal operations in the patient with acquired immunodeficiency syndrome. J Am Coll Surg 180:205–209

Bouche H, Housset C, Dumont J, et al. (1993) AIDS-related cholangitis: diagnostic features and course in 15 patients. J Hepatol 17:34–39

Bouillot J, Dehni N, Kazatchkine M, et al. (1995) Role of laparoscopic surgery in the management of acute abdomen in the HIV-positive patients. J Laparoendosc Surg 5:101–104

Daneshmand S, Hedley C, Stain S (1999) The utility and reliability of computed tomography scan in the diagnosis of small bowel obstruction. Am Surg 65:922–926

DaSilva F, Boudghene F, Lecomte I, et al. (1993) Sonography in AIDS-related cholangitis: prevalence and cause of an echogenic nodule in the distal end of the common bile duct. AJR 160:1205–1027

Davidson T, Allen-Mersh T, Miles A, et al. (1991) Emergency laparotomy in patients with AIDS. Br J Surg 78:924–926

Diettrich N, Cacioppo J, Kaplan G, et al. (1991) A growing spectrum of surgical disease in patients with human immunodeficiency virus/acquired immunodeficiency syndrome. Experience with 120 cases. Arch Surg 126:860–866

Fishman E, Kavuru M, Jones B, et al. (1991) Pseudomembranous colitis: CT evaluation of 26 cases. Radiology 180:57–60

Gelman S, Brandt L (1998) Pneumatosis intestinalis and AIDS: a case report and review of the literature. Am J Gastroenterol 93:646–650

Gentle D, Stoller, Jarrett T, et al. (1997) Protease inhibitor-induced urolithiasis. Urology 50:508–511

Hegener P, Horst E, Hartman P, et al. (1998) Asymptomatic pneumatosis intestinalis and free abdominal air in a patient with AIDS. Eur J Med Res 12:265–267

Herneth A, Pokieser P, Kettenbach J, et al. (1998) Pneumatosis intestinalis in AIDS-associated chronic intestinal cryptosporidiosis: a benign course in a severe-looking disease. Eur Radiol 8:1499

Herts B, Megibow A, Birnbaum B, et al. (1992) High-attenuation lymphadenopathy in AIDS patients: significance of findings at CT. Radiology 185:777–781

Hulnick D, Megibow A, Naidich D, et al. (1985) Abdominal tuberculosis: CT evaluation. Radiology 157:199–204

Iribarren J, Castiella A, Lobo C, et al. (1997) AIDS-associated cryptosporidiosis with antral narrowing. A new case. J Clin Gastroenterol 25:693–694

Jeffrey R Jr, Sommer F (1993) Follow-up sonography in suspected acalculous cholecystitis: preliminary clinical experience. J Ultrasound Med 12:183–187

Kawamoto S, Horton K, Fishman E (1999a) Pseudomembranous colitis: can CT predict which patients will need surgical intervention? J Comput Assist Tomogr 23:79–85

Kawamoto, S, Horton K, Fishman E (1999b) Pseudomembranous colitis: spectrum of imaging findings with clinical and pathologic correlation. Radiographics 19:887–897

LaRaja R, Rothenberg R, Odom J, et al. (1989) The incidence of intra-abdominal surgery in acquired immunodeficiency syndrome: a statistical review of 904 patients. Surgery 105:175–179

Levine M (1989) Infectious esophagitis. In: Levine M (ed) Radiology of the esophagus, vol I. Saunders, Philadelphia, p 66

Murray J, Evans S, Jeffrey P, et al. (1995) Cytomegalovirus colitis in AIDS: CT features. AJR 165:67–71

Nugent P, O'Connell T (1986) The surgeon's role in treating acquired immunodeficiency syndrome. Arch Surg 121:1117–1120

Nyberg D, Federle M, Jeffrey R, et al. (1985) Abdominal CT findings of disseminated *Mycobacterium avium-intracellulare* in AIDS. AJR 145:297–299

Radin R (1995) HIV infection: analysis in 259 consecutive patients with abnormal abdominal CT findings. Radiology 197:712–722

Radin D, Esplin J, Levine A, et al. (1993) AIDS-related non-Hodgkin's lymphoma: abdominal CT findings in 112 patients. AJR 160:1133–1139

Reiter W, Schon-Pernerstorfer H, Dorfinger K, et al. (1999) Frequency of urolithiasis in individuals seropositive for human immunodeficiency virus treated with indinavir is higher than previously assumed. J Urol 161:1082–1084

Schwartz B, Schenkman N, Armenakas N, et al. (1999) Imaging characteristics of indinavir calculi. J Urol 161:1085–1087

Scott-Conner C, Fabrega A (1996) Gastrointestinal problems in the immunocompromised host. A review for surgeons. Surg Endosc 10:959–964

Suri S, Gupta S, Sudhaker P, et al. (1999) Comparative evaluation of plain films, ultrasound and CT in the diagnosis of intestinal obstruction. Acta Radiol 40:422–428

Taourel P, Pradel J, Fabre J, et al. (1995) Role of CT in the acute nontraumatic abdomen. Semin Ultrasound CT MR 16:151–164

Wall S, Jones B (1992) Gastrointestinal tract in the immunocompromised host: opportunistic infections and other complications. Radiology 185:327–335

Whitney T, Macho J, Russell T, et al. (1992) Appendicitis in acquired immunodeficiency syndrome. Am J Surg 164:467–471

Wood B, Kumar P, Cooper C, et al. (1995) Pneumatosis intestinalis in adults with AIDS: clinical significance and imaging findings. AJR 165:1387–1390

Wu C, Davis F, Fishman E (1998) Radiologic evaluation of the acute abdomen in the patient with acquired immunodeficiency syndrome (AIDS): the role of CT scanning. Semin Ultrasound CT MR 19:190–199

Wyatt S, Fishman E (1994) The acute abdomen in individuals with AIDS. Radiol Clin North Am 32:1023–1043

Yacoe M, Jeffrey R Jr (1994) Sonography of appendicitis and diverticulitis. Radiol Clin North Am 32:899–912

Yoshida E, Chan N, Chan-Yan C, et al. (1997) Perforation of the jejunum secondary to AIDS-related gastrointestinal Kaposi's sarcoma. Can J Gastroenterol 11:38–40

Ziegler J, Beckstead J, Volberding P, et al. (1984) Non-Hodgkin's lymphoma in 90 homosexual men. Relation to generalized lymphadenopathy and the acquired immunodeficiency syndrome. N Engl J Med 311:565–570

12 Musculoskeletal Imaging in AIDS

Jamshid Tehranzadeh and Matthew T. Tran

CONTENTS

12.1
Introduction

Many tiers of immune defenses harmoniously interact to provide a sanctuary against infections. The ability to perceive microorganisms and their products as foreign entities is embodied in lymphocytes, which serve both effector and regulatory functions. Through the elaboration of cytokines and immunoglobulins, lymphocytes recruit nonspecific immune effectors, focus their activity, and modulate the intensity of the immune response. The phylogenically more primitive complement system serves a similar function. Human immunodeficiency virus (HIV) infection is responsible for large numbers of immunocompromised patients worldwide (Rubin and Lotze 1992). Due to the pandemic nature of HIV infection, which encompasses the majority of immu-

J. Tehranzadeh, MD
Professor of Radiology and Orthopaedics, Section Chief of Musculoskeletal Radiology, Department of Radiological Sciences, R140, University of California (Irvine), 101 City Drive, Orange, CA 92868-3298, USA
M.T. Tran, MD
Chief Resident of Radiology, Department of Radiological Sciences, University of California (Irvine), 101 City Drive, Orange, CA 92868-3298, USA

nocompromised patients in the United States and the world, the emphasis of this chapter is on HIV infection.

Although there was an 18% decrease in the incidence of AIDS in 1996–1997 and an 11% decrease in 1997–1998, the number of persons living with AIDS continues to increase. By the end of 1998, there were 297,137 persons living with AIDS, a 10% increase in the United States (Centers for Disease Control 1999).

12.2
Spectrum of Musculoskeletal Involvement in HIV Infection

Musculoskeletal manifestations of HIV infection are not as common as those seen in other parts of the body, including the central nervous system, pulmonary system, and gastrointestinal tract. They tend to occur in advanced stages of HIV infection. The underlying circumstances for the variety of musculoskeletal abnormalities are probably multifactorial. It has been speculated that some of the musculoskeletal abnormalities are related directly to the HIV virus, its components, or circulating immune complexes produced with HIV infection, or to the secondary infections that occur in this patient population.

Different musculoskeletal changes are described in relation to HIV infection. These changes include infection, myopathy, arthritis, and increased prevalence of malignancy. Arthritides include spondylopathic arthropathy, HIV-associated arthritis, painful articular syndrome, and acute symmetric polyarthritis. Malignant diseases with increased prevalence in AIDS patients are Kaposi's sarcoma, non-Hodgkin's lymphoma, and leiomyosarcoma in children. Avascular necrosis, vasculitis, bone marrow changes, and other miscellaneous conditions have been reported in connection with HIV infection (Steinbach et al. 1993; Tehranzadeh and Steinbach 1994). Two specific infections, bacillary angiomatosis and tuberculosis, are discussed.

12.3
Musculoskeletal Infection
in the HIV/AIDS Population

Although opportunistic organisms including *Pneumocystis carinii* and *Toxoplasma gondii* are the most common causes of pulmonary and central nervous system infections in patients with HIV/AIDS, musculoskeletal infection may be caused by common as well as opportunistic agents (MAGID and FISHMAN 1992).

It is of interest that opportunistic infections were not seen at all in a study of 560 HIV-positive patients by SPENCER et al. (1991). *Staphylococcus aureus*, which is the most common cause of musculoskeletal infection in immunocompetent patients (TEHRANZADEH et al. 1992), remains the leading cause of bone and soft tissue infection in HIV-positive patients. A variety of soft tissue and osteoarticular infections and types of inflammation have been reported in AIDS patients. These can be subdivided as follows.

A. Soft tissue infection and inflammation
   1. Cellulitis, lymphedema, and dermatologic disorders
   2. Tenosynovitis
   3. Septic bursitis
   4. Myopathies
B. Osteoarticular infection and inflammation
   1. Osteomyelitis
   2. Arthritis
   3. Spondylitis

12.3.1
Soft Tissue Infection and Inflammation

12.3.1.1
Cellulitis, Lymphedema, and
Dermatologic Disorders

Cellulitis represents inflammation of the skin and subcutaneous tissue and it is usually clinically detectable, particularly in the AIDS patient. Superficial cellulitis and cellulitis associated with deep infection are difficult to distinguish (MAGID and FISHMAN 1992). Owing to its inherent resolution, conventional radiography cannot distinguish the soft tissue and fascial layers, and the early osseous changes cannot be detected (MAGID and FISHMAN 1992). Cellulitis creates inflammation and consequently edema of the subcutaneous fat without a soft tissue mass. For example, BURMAN et al. (1995) observed 11 cases of

Helicobacter cinaedi in HIV-positive homosexual men. Four of these patients developed distinctive cutaneous manifestations of multifocal cellulitis which was preceded by an indolent febrile illness with bacteremia. *Helicobacter cinaedi* (formerly *Campylobacter cinaedi*) was first detected in the fecal flora of homosexual men (BURMAN et al. 1995).

On computed tomographic (CT) examination, cellulitis results in an increase in the density of subcutaneous adipose tissue from 90 to 120 Hounsfield units (HU), attenuation numbers closer to those of soft tissue (MAGID and FISHMAN 1992). On magnetic resonance imaging (MRI), fat normally has a high signal intensity on T1-weighted images and a decreased signal intensity on T2-weighted images. Inflammation and edema cause a decrease in the signal intensity of fat on T1-weighted images and increased signal intensity on T2 (TEHRANZADEH et al. 1992), T2* gradient-echo, and short-tau inversion recovery (STIR) imaging. Cellulitis may spread to involve contiguous structures and lead to myositis, pyomyositis, fasciitis, vascular thrombosis (Fig. 12.1), and lymphedema.

Lymphedema may be primary or secondary to proximal obstruction or destruction of lymphatics and has been described in some patients with AIDS-related lymphoma and Kaposi's sarcoma. The engorged tissues and stagnant lymphatic fluid provide excellent culture media for streptococcal or other secondary infections. A subcutaneous reticular or

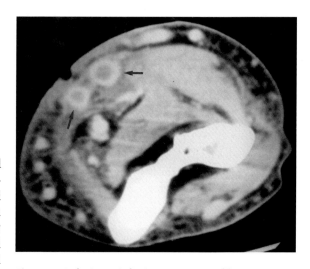

Fig. 12.1. Soft tissue infection. A 40-year-old HIV-positive male with antecubital ulcer. CT scan with intravenous contrast (soft tissue window) shows soft tissue ulcer and edema with brachial artery and vein thrombosis (*arrows*). Note subcutaneous pus collection, inflammation and edema. (From TEHRANZADEH and STEINBACH 1994).

honeycomb pattern can be seen on CT examination. The fibrous septa have the low attenuation of soft tissues (20–30 HU) and are superimposed against a background of residual fatty subcutaneous densities and normal deep muscle layers (MAGID and FISHMAN 1992). On T1-weighted MR images, skin thickening and expansion of subcutaneous tissue with a characteristic honeycomb pattern of low signal intensity streaks may be noted. On STIR images, serpiginous increased signal intensity in the subcutaneous fat is often seen (TEHRANZADEH and STEINBACH 1994).

MRI, CT, and occasionally scintigraphy play an important role in determining the diagnosis and extent of soft tissue infections, myositis, myonecrosis, pyomyositis, fasciitis, and soft tissue abscess. Sequelae such as periostitis and osteomyelitis can also be successfully imaged and evaluated with these modalities (TEHRANZADEH et al. 1992). A noninfectious diagnostic consideration in HIV-infected patients with focal calf pain and swelling is HIV-related "hyperalgesic pseudothrombophlebitis" (ABRAHAMSON et al. 1985; SCHWARTZMAN et al. 1991).

In recent years, newly described dermatologic abnormalities have been described in patients with immunodeficiency syndromes. Eosinophilic folliculitis and pruritic papules of HIV infection are clinically similar lesions that respond to phototherapy. Bacillary angiomatosis (which will be discussed later) may present with skin lesions caused by a pleomorphic gram-negative organism. (These resemble lesions of Kaposi's sarcoma clinically but are curable if treated early with antibiotics). "Toxic strep" syndrome, a scarlatiniform, desquamative eruption associated with hypotension, fever, and multiorgan system dysfunction, is caused by group A streptococcal soft tissue infection. A noninfectious dermatologic abnormality is paraneoplastic pemphigus, a recently characterized autoimmune vesicular eruption that produces painful mucocutaneous ulcerations in patients with an occult neoplasm, such as chronic lymphocytic leukemia or malignant lymphoma (KHORENIAN and LEBWOHL 1995).

12.3.1.2
Tenosynovitis

Pyogenic tenosynovitis may be seen in immunocompromised patients. We observed a 42-year-old HIV-positive female with pyogenic tenosynovitis of the extensor common tendon sheath of the wrist (Fig. 12.2). TOWNSEND et al. (1994) reported a case of *Candida* tenosynovitis in an AIDS patient.

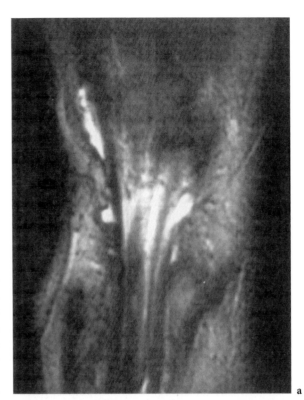

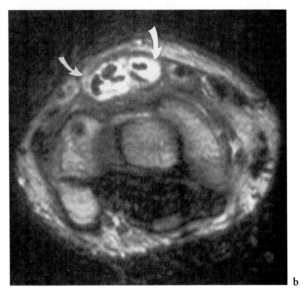

Fig. 12.2a, b. Pyogenic tenosynovitis of extensor sheath of the wrist. A 42-year-old HIV-positive woman with prominent bulging and swelling of the dorsum of the wrist. **a** Coronal T2-weighted posterior section image (3,200/116) of the wrist shows bright signal indicating fluid around the extensor tendons of the wrist. **b** Axial T2-weighted image (4,800/92) of the wrist shows fluid in the extensor common tendon sheath of the wrist (*curved arrows*). (From TEHRANZADEH 1997)

12.3.1.3
Septic Bursitis

Septic bursitis is a well-described entity in immuno-compromised patients (HUGHES et al. 1992; BUSKILA and TENENBAUM 1989), including HIV-infected patients, alcoholics, and those who are on steroids. Infection in the subcutaneous bursae often localizes to the olecranon, prepatellar, and, less frequently, subdeltoid regions. A history of recent trauma and occupational injury or puncture is frequently, although not invariably, present. *S. aureus* is often the etiologic organism involved. Other less frequent agents include *Streptococcus pneumoniae*, *Mycobacterium marinum*, and *Sporothrix schenckii*. Hematogenous causes are uncommon (RESNICK and NIWAYAMA 1988). BUSKILA and TENENBAUM (1989) described two patients with *S. aureus* olecranon bursitis with evidence of HIV infection. ROSCHMANN and BELL (1987) have demonstrated that even though the presenting clinical features of septic bursitis in immunocompetent and immunocompromised patients are similar, immunocompromised patients must be treated with a significantly longer duration of therapy in order to guarantee a successful outcome.

12.3.1.4
Myopathies

Weakness is a common feature of AIDS. It is often assumed to result from a variety of common and uncommon AIDS-related central nervous system complications (BERMAN and JENSEN 1990; BRITTON and MILLER 1984) but other types of muscular change may complicate HIV infection:

a) *Pyomyositis* is caused by bacteria, fungi, and parasites. Viral myositis caused by HIV itself is extremely rare, if it exists at all (Simpson and Bender 1988; Wiley et al. 1989). Pyomyositis (FLECKENSTEIN et al. 1991; WIDROW et al. 1991) or pyogenic infection of muscle is most commonly caused by *S. aureus* (Table 12.1) and usually occurs in the tropics, rarely in the continental United States. Defects of neutrophil function may contribute to the development of the disease in some HIV-infected patients (SCHWARTZMAN et al. 1991) in whom polymorphonuclear leukocytes manifest decreased chemotaxis (RAS et al. 1984a, b). Of 46 cases of HIV-related pyomyositis reported in the literature, 32 (69%) were due to *S. aureus*, three were caused by mycobacterial agents, and three were cryptococcal infections (Table 12.1). Group A ß-hemolytic streptococci have been reported to cause

Table 12.1. Pyomyositis in AIDS patients (review of literature)

Microorganism	No. of cases
Staph. aureus	32
Cryptococcus	3
M. tuberculosis	2
M. avium complex	1
Nocardia asteroides	1
C. freundii	1
Salmonella enteritidis	1
Microsporidia	1
Strep. pyogenes	1
Unknown organism	3
Total	46

a more progressive and malignant pyomyositis (GARDINER et al. 1990).

Other etiologic factors include parasites, viruses, spirochetes, and nutritional imbalances (GARDINER et al. 1990). Antecedent trauma has been reported in 25%–70% of the patients. Myonecrosis initiated by tissue anoxia or trauma, especially when contaminated with foreign material, may lead to pyomyositis and finally muscle abscess. The predominance of nonclostridial myonecrosis in AIDS patients reflects the increasing number of intravenous drug abusers infected with HIV. These patients traumatize their muscles, fail to observe sterile technique, and occasionally have a prolonged state of stupor and immobility, all risk factors for pyomyositis.

Clinical manifestations of pyomyositis have three stages (CHIEDOZI 1979). First pain localizes to one muscle group. There is a woody, hardened area of induration and a low-grade fever. There may be a mild leukocytosis, but needle aspiration will not reveal any pus. In the second stage or so-called suppurative stage, pain, fever, and edema of the affected muscle are noted in 90% of patients. Needle aspiration at this stage reveals thick yellow pus (Fig. 12.3). In the third or "late" stage, patients often appear septic and toxic. A fluctuant abscess may be noted, and the entire muscle may be replaced by pus. This condition may soon be followed by septicemia and death (GARDINER et al. 1990). In the first and second stages of the disease, pyomyositis may be mistaken for a variety of conditions such as cellulitis, muscle tear, hematoma, appendicitis, arthritis, thrombophlebitis, or tumor (GARDINER et al. 1990; CHIEDOZI 1979). MRI and CT have proven to be very useful in imaging and diagnosing this process. Myonecrotic muscle is enlarged and has a decreased attenuation value compatible with soft tissue edema on CT. A localized intramuscular collection of fluid or gas may be seen. Intramuscular gas may reflect clostrid-

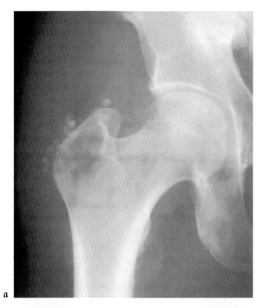

a

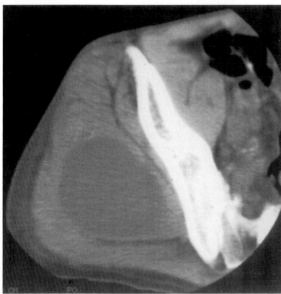

b

Fig. 12.3a, b. Soft tissue abscess. A 40-year-old man presenting with a soft tissue abscess of the right gluteal region. Aspiration revealed *S. aureus*. **a** Plain radiograph of the right hip shows a soft tissue mass with multiple round, small calcific densities in the greater trochanteric region. **b** CT scan (soft tissue window) of the right hemipelvis shows a well-marginated, oval, low-density mass in the gluteal area. (From TEHRANZADEH and STEINBACH 1994)

ial infection (MAGID and FISHMAN 1992). Intravenous contrast material with CT or intravenous gadolinium with MRI differentiates between normal (vascularized) muscle and myonecrotic tissue that does not enhance and may help define the abscess (MAGID and FISHMAN 1992; FLECKENSTEIN et al. 1991).

b) *Polymyositis*, an autoimmune disorder, also occurs in AIDS and may precede the onset of signs and symptoms of AIDS in the HIV-positive patient (TEHRANZADEH and STEINBACH 1994) (Fig. 12.4).

c) *Zidovudine myopathy* is induced by the commonly prescribed antiviral drug, zidovudine (also referred to as azidothymidine or AZT) (BESSEN et al. 1988; DALAKAS et al. 1990). In such cases, histopathology has revealed "ragged red" fibers, indicative of abnormal mitochondria, and paracrystalline inclusions (DALAKAS et al. 1990).

d) *Neurogenic myopathy* (nemaline rod myopathy) (DALAKAS et al. 1987) is a peripheral neuropathy suspected in up to 40% of AIDS patients. This condition may be responsible for the HIV wasting syndrome.

e) *Tumoral infiltration of muscle* due to lymphoma and Kaposi's sarcoma, which may lead to lymphatic obstruction or lymphedema (TEHRANZADEH and STEINBACH 1994), has been described in HIV-infected patients.

f) *Sarcoid myopathy* has only been described in one patient, although neither sarcoidosis nor HIV infection is rare (GRANIERI et al. 1995).

g) *Rhabdomyolysis* has also been reported with HIV infection, and may result from severe muscle infection (CHARIOT et al. 1994) or staphylococcal bacteremia (SESMA et al. 1992).

12.3.2
Osteoarticular Infection and Inflammation

12.3.2.1
Osteomyelitis

Osteomyelitis refers to infection of bone and bone marrow cavity and is relatively uncommon in HIV-positive patients (STEINBACH et al. 1993; FLECKENSTEIN 1994) (Figs. 12.5–12.8). *S. aureus* is the most common cause of osteomyelitis, which is typically acquired hematogenously. In a series of 556 HIV-positive patients, all three reported cases of osteomyelitis were in intravenous drug abusers (MUNOZ-FERNANDEZ et al. 1991). In this series, the involved sites included wrist, tibia, and femoral head. In another series of 560 HIV-positive patients (SPENCER et al. 1991) 12 cases of osteomyelitis were identified. *S. aureus* was the leading cause of infection, followed by salmonella. In another series, two cases of *S. aureus* osteomyelitis, one in the tibia and one in the rib, were noted (STEINBACH et al. 1993). In the same patients, *Nocardia asteroides* was the cause

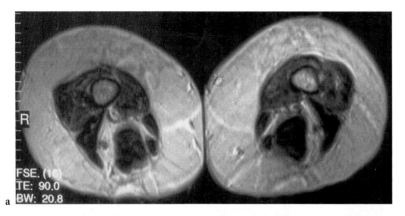

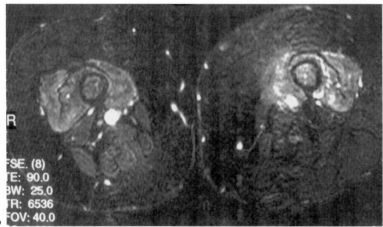

Fig. 12.4a, b. Polymyositis in a 45-year-old HIV-positive female. a Axial FSE T2-weighted image (10,850/90) shows intermediate signal in the vastus medialis, lateralis, and intermedius muscles of the left thigh, more intense than on the right side. b Axial FSE, fat-saturated T2-weighted image (6,536/90) shows bright signal in abnormal vastus medialis, lateralis, and intermedius muscles of the left thigh, again more intense than on the right side

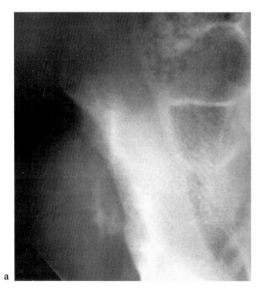

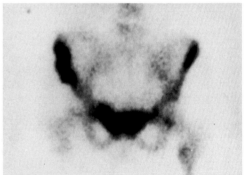

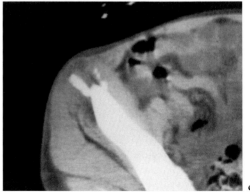

Fig. 12.5a–c. Osteomyelitis of iliac bone. A 28-year-old HIV-positive African-American female with osteomyelitis of right iliac crest and heterotopic calcific changes. a Plain radiograph shows heterotopic ossification with cortical erosion of the right iliac bone. b Bone scan demonstrates increased activity in the right iliac bone. c CT scan of the right iliac bone (soft tissue window) shows heterotopic ossification and cortical erosion of right iliac bone. (From Vanarthos et al. 1992).

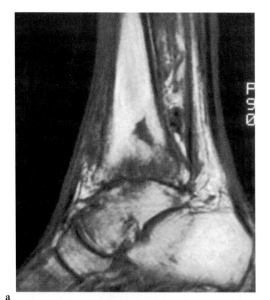

a

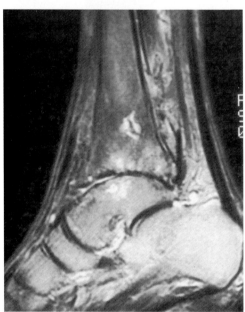

b

Fig. 12.6a, b. Chronic osteomyelitis of the tibia in a 59-year-old HIV-positive man. **a** Sagittal T1-weighted image (600/16) shows subcutaneous edema and inflammation, narrowed ankle joint, and subchondral erosion. Note a focal low signal lesion in the distal tibia. **b** Sagittal T2-weighted image (2,000/102) shows changes similar to those on the T1-weighted image. The focus of osteomyelitis in distal tibia has bright signal with low signal sequestrum in the center

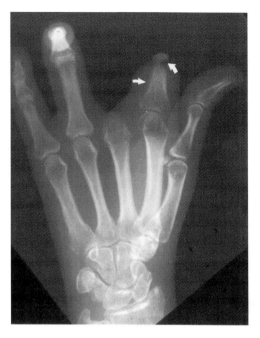

Fig. 12.7. Repeated hand osteomyelitis in a 31-year-old HIV-positive female. The patient had had repeated episodes of osteomyelitis of the hand and had previously undergone amputations of the second and third phalanges. Now there is recurrence of soft tissue and bone infection of the proximal phalanx of the index finger. AP view of the left hand shows osteopenia of the bones, flexion deformity, and previous amputation. Note acute osteomyelitis of the partially amputated proximal phalanx of the index finger with bone erosion (*curved arrow*) and periosteal new bone formation (*arrow*). (From TEHRANZADEH and STEINBACH 1994)

of soft tissue and bone infection in the thoracic cage. *Nocardia* was also the subject of another case (RAY et al. 1994). In a series reported by VANARTHOS et al. (1992), a case of multifocal osteomyelitis with a few skip lesions in the distal tibia was caused by group B streptococcus. Salmonella osteomyelitis was noted in two earlier reports (SPENCER et al. 1991; MASTROIANNI et al. 1992). Isolated cases of bone infection due to gonococcus (WOODS and GERNAAT 1992; ANAYA et al. 1994), cytomegalovirus (BERMAN and JENSEN 1990; FLAITZ et al. 1994), *Candida albicans* (EDELSTEIN and McCABE 1991), invasive aspergillosis (PANTALEO et al. 1993), toxoplasmosis (AL-KASSAB et al. 1995), and disseminated adiaspiromycosis (ECHAVARRIA et al. 1993) have been reported. KASTNER et al. (1994) wrote of an HIV-infected man who presented with symptomatic ulnar osteitis as the initial finding of secondary syphilis, which subsequently led to osteomyelitis and pathologic fracture. The reported cases of osteomyelitis in HIV infection in the literature are probably skewed because esoteric infections are more frequently reported (Table 12.2).

The radiographic appearance of osteomyelitis in AIDS patients is similar to that in the general population. Deep soft tissue swelling, periosteal reaction, and localized osteopenia in long bones are early

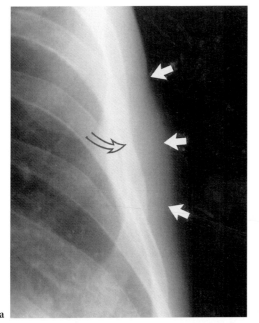

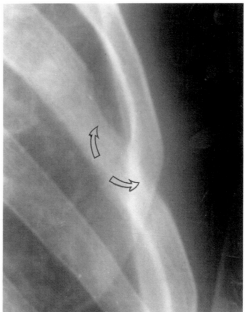

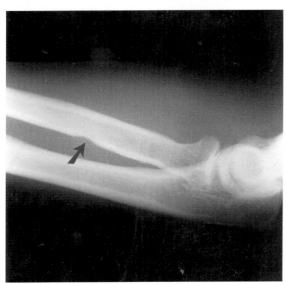

Fig. 12.8a–c. Multifocal osteomyelitis in a 37-year-old HIV-positive female with a history of *Candida* esophagitis and left rib and arm pain. The forearm and rib biopsies showed chronic infection and culture was negative. **a, b** Plain radiographs of the left ribs show soft tissue swelling (*arrows*) and bony erosion (*open arrows*) of the sixth rib with pleural reaction. **c** Lateral radiograph of the left forearm shows erosion of the posterior cortex of proximal radial shaft (*arrow*). (From TEHRANZADEH and STEINBACH 1994)

changes on conventional radiographs. Smaller bones, such as the phalanges and flat bones, may not show periosteal elevation. In these bones, soft tissue changes and cortical erosions are considered early signs. As infection progresses, osteolytic and osteosclerotic changes appear. Triphasic bone scintigraphy and MRI are helpful for early detection of osseous involvement and can differentiate cellulitis and soft tissue changes from osteomyelitis. In addition, these modalities demonstrate the extent of bone marrow infection. Bone scintigraphy, although nonspecific, has the advantage of screening the entire skeleton and is useful for early detection of mul-

tifocal osteomyelitis. MRI is highly sensitive in demonstrating deep soft tissue inflammation and marrow abnormalities. Cortical erosions and marrow sequestrum are better appreciated with CT. CT examination is also advantageous for imaging infection in flat bones of the pelvis and scapula (TEHRANZADEH et al. 1992).

The HIV-infected population is specifically prone to bacillary angiomatosis and mycobacterial infection. These infections will now be discussed separately. Table 12.2 cites 13 cases of osteomyelitis caused by bacillary angiomatosis and nine cases caused by mycobacterial agents.

Table 12.2. Osteomyelitis in HIV infection (review of literature)

Microorganism/disorder	No. of cases
Bacillary angiomatosis	13
Staph. aureus	7
Staph. sanguis	1
M. haemophilum	5
M. tuberculosis	3
M. kansasii	1
Salmonella	2
Cytomegalovirus (CMV)	2
Multifocal strep. group B	1
Torulopsis glabrata	1
Neisseria gonorrhoeae	1
Histoplasma capsulatum	1
Nocardia asteroides	1
Candida albicans	1
Phialophora richardsiae	1
Invasive aspergillosis	1
Disseminated adiaspiromycosis	1
Unknown	3
Total	46

Bacillary angiomatosis. Bacillary angiomatosis results from infection by members of the Rickettsiace-
ae family, *Bartonella (Rochalimaea) henselae* and
Bartonella (Rochalimaea) quintana, which are also
suspected agents for cat-scratch disease and trench
fever, respectively. It occurs predominantly in HIV-
positive patients, although it has been reported in
immunocompetent patients and organ transplant
recipients. It typically produces angiomatous cutaneous lesions but can be accompanied by lesions of
the viscera, lymph nodes, brain, and bone (STEIN-
BACH 1994a; MAJOR and TEHRANZADEH 1997). An
unusual form of osteomyelitis caused by bacillary
angiomatosis has been described in HIV-positive
patients (STEINBACH et al. 1993; BARON et al. 1990)
(Fig. 12.9). The distinct vascular proliferation in the
skin can have several presentations. These include
superficial lesions of the papillary and upper reticular dermis, which present as reddish or flesh-colored
rubbery to firm papules. Sometimes nodules that resemble pyogenic granulomas are seen. These can ulcerate or bleed profusely when traumatized. The lesions are found anywhere, commonly on the upper
trunk and face, and occasionally on the anal, oral, or
gastrointestinal mucosa. Some lesions may be deeper within the subcutaneous tissue. Clinically, fever,
anemia, and elevated erythrocyte sedimentation rate
may be seen (STEINBACH 1994a).

Histologic examination of the lesions of bacillary
angiomatosis demonstrates circumscribed, lobular
aggregates of ectatic capillaries lined with protuber-
ant endothelial cells, surrounded by a mucinousstro-

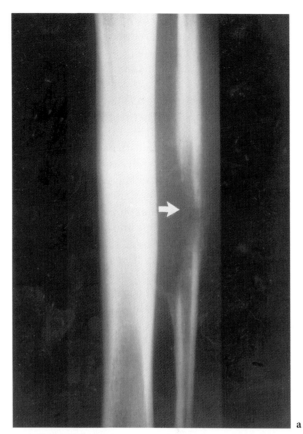

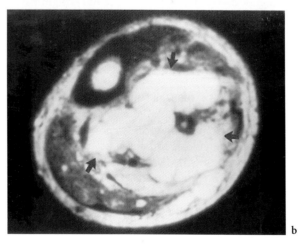

Fig. 12.9a, b. Soft tissue and fibular bacillary angiomatosis. **a**
AP radiograph of tibia/fibula demonstrates an aggressive
destructive lesion which is invading the fibular diaphysis (*arrow*). **b** A corresponding axial T2-weighted image (2,000/80)
also demonstrates a large high signal intensity soft tissue
mass that surrounds the fibula and extends into the anterior
and posterior compartments of the leg (*arrows*). (From
TEHRANZADEH and STEINBACH 1994)

ma, and with a predominantly neutrophilic inflammatory infiltrate. Bacillary forms can be identified in the lesion by Warthin-Starry staining (STEINBACH 1994a). BARON et al. (1990) originally described six patients with osseous lesions among 17 patients with cutaneous bacillary angiomatosis. Since then, seven more cases of osteomyelitis related to bacillary angiomatosis have been reported (STEINBACH et al. 1993; STANDIFORD et al. 1994) (Table 12.2).

The osseous lesions seen with bacillary angiomatosis are lytic and frequently associated with an overlying soft tissue mass and periostitis (Fig. 12.9). Like most active bone lesions, they demonstrate increased uptake on technetium-99m methylene diphosphonate (^{99m}Tc-MDP) bone scans and occasionally are identified by bone scintigraphy in patients without clinical or radiographic findings. Intense contrast enhancement of soft tissue lesions of bacillary angiomatosis has been noted by several authors (HERTS et al. 1991; MOORE et al. 1995). The level of contrast enhancement in bacillary angiomatosis lesions exceeds that of Kaposi's sarcoma (MOORE et al. 1995), a vascular lesion which is very common in AIDS patients and could be confused with bacillary angiomatosis. KOEHLER et al. (1992) has described methods to isolate the infecting bacterium from HIV-infected patients' cutaneous lesions or blood. A dramatic response of bacillary angiomatosis to appropriate antibiotics is characteristic. The organism is sensitive to erythromycin, clarithromycin, and doxycycline, as well as antibiotics directed against mycobacterial disease (MOORE et al. 1995).

Tuberculosis. In 1985, the number of tuberculosis cases began to rise in the United States. Several lines of epidemiologic evidence supported this resurgence of tuberculosis to be related to the HIV epidemic. Patients with HIV infection are at a much higher risk for primary or reactivation tuberculosis. Among HIV-infected individuals with positive tuberculin skin tests, the risk of active tuberculosis is estimated to be 8% per year. The incidence of tuberculosis in patients with AIDS is almost 500 times that in the general population (BARNES et al. 1991; Joint Position Paper of the American Thoracic Society and the Centers for Disease Control 1987; TEHRANZADEH and WONG 1994).

Tuberculosis is often the first indication of immunodeficiency in patients with HIV infection and may precede the diagnosis of AIDS. Clinical presentation reflects the degree of immunosuppression. Patients with tuberculosis who are in the early stage of HIV infection are usually indistinguishable from non-HIV-infected patients. In the later stages of HIV infection, after the diagnosis of AIDS has been established, the clinical presentation of tuberculosis may be more unusual.

It is generally accepted that skeletal tuberculosis occurs mainly by hematogenous spread. Seeding of the skeleton may arise at the time of primary infection of the lung or at a later date, from a quiescent primary site or other extraosseous focus. Skeletal lesions result from implantation of the bacilli in medullary bone. Classically, the vertebral column is most commonly affected. In other bones, metaphyseal involvement is perhaps more common. Hips and knees are the most commonly affected joints. Diagnosis is confirmed by demonstration of tubercle bacilli in smear or culture and may require closed or open biopsy of bone and aspiration of the joint or biopsy of the synovial membrane.

Tuberculous osteomyelitis may affect any bone. The disease may remain in bone or progress to involve adjacent joints. Radiologically, there are foci of osteolysis with varying amounts of eburnation and periostitis. Sequestrum formation is present. The initial appearance is similar to other types of osteomyelitis and even aggressive neoplasm.

Cystic tuberculosis is a special type of tuberculous osteomyelitis affecting the peripheral skeleton of children more frequently than adults. Disseminated lesions of the axial and extra-axial skeleton may be symmetric in distribution and are of variable size without surrounding sclerosis.

Tuberculous dactylitis is also seen more frequently in children than in adults. Soft tissue swelling is usually the initial manifestation. There is mild or exuberant periostitis of the phalanges, metacarpals, or metatarsals. SORIANO and TOR (1992) reported two HIV patients with tuberculous osteomyelitis of the foot. Tuberculous dactylitis may resemble sickle cell dactylitis and luetic dactylitis. Cystic expansion of bone is termed spina ventosa.

Tuberculous spondylitis most commonly affects the thoracic and lumbar spine, especially the first lumbar vertebra. Involvement of the cervical spine and sacrum is uncommon, although involvement of the sacroiliac joint is not rare. In a large series of AIDS patients (MUNOZ-FERNANDEZ et al. 1991), one case of *M. tuberculosis* was noted (Table 12.3). JOHNSON et al. (1990) also reported a patient with HIV infection and tuberculosis with a psoas abscess as well as disseminated *M. avium* and *M. intracellulare* infection. The abscess occurred 18 months after completion of a 12-month course of chemoprophylaxis with isoniazid that was given

Table 12.3. Septic spondylitis in AIDS patients (review of literature)

Microorganism/infection	No. of cases
Staph. aureus	6
M. tuberculosis	2
M. avium-intracellulare	1
Cryptococcus	1
E. coli	1
Pseudomonas	1
Candida tropicalis	1
Candida albicans	1
Nocardia asteroides	1
Aspergillosis	1
Unknown	1
Total	17

because of a positive tuberculin test (JOHNSON et al. 1990). Tuberculosis is a relatively frequent finding in HIV-infected patients and such patients are more likely to develop tuberculosis at extrapulmonary sites (FRANK and FISHMAN 1994; TEHRANZADEH and MESGARZADEH 1994).

HEARY et al. (1994) reviewed 32 patients with spinal infection, 13 of whom were HIV patients. In both HIV-positive and HIV-negative groups, *S. aureus* predominated (72%) as the causative organism. *M. tuberculosis* was the second most common organism. The clinical presentation in both groups was similar, with pain as the most frequent symptom and objective neurologic abnormalities on physical examination in 29 of the 32 patients (91%).

Clinically, there may be spinal cord compression causing paralysis from abscesses, granulation tissue, bone fragments, arachnoiditis, and ischemia of the cord. The clinical presentation and organisms cultured do not differ depending upon whether there is concurrent HIV infection. The ultimate neurologic outcome of patients with spinal infections depends on their neurologic status at the time of treatment and not on their HIV status.

Infection most often begins in the anterior portion of the vertebral body, then spreads to involve the intervertebral disc and neighboring vertebral body. Posterior elements may be initially or predominantly affected in some individuals. (RESNICK and NIWAYAMA 1988; CHAPMAN et al. 1979). There is frequent ligamentous and soft tissue extension from the vertebrae and discs, usually anterolaterally and, rarely, posteriorly into the peridural space. In the lumbar region, a psoas abscess, occasionally containing calcium, may form and may extend into the groin and thigh. Paravertebral abscesses may penetrate the

esophagus, bronchus, mediastinum, liver, kidney, intestine, bladder, rectum, vagina, and aorta.

Radiologically, there is bone destruction involving the anterior vertebral body along with narrowing of the adjacent intervertebral disc and similar bone destruction of the contiguous vertebral body. The end-plates adjacent to the affected intervertebral disc lose their definition and, eventually, progressive vertebral collapse with anterior wedging leads to the characteristic gibbus deformity.

Ultrasound and CT can provide important information in patients with psoas or paraspinal abscesses. SHARIF et al. (1990) reported that MRI permitted prediction of neurologic complications in 93% of patients and diagnosis of the type of infection in 94%. Vertebral intraosseous abscesses, meningeal involvement, subligamentous spread, and paraspinal abscess location were best identified on contrast-enhanced studies. High signal intensities of previously affected vertebrae on T1-weighted images suggested healing and correlated well with symptoms.

Atypical Mycobacterial Infection. With atypical mycobacterial infection, lesions tend to be multiple rather than solitary (Fig. 12.10). The metaphyses and diaphyses of long bones are most commonly affected by discrete lesions which may contain sclerotic margins. Osteoporosis may not be as striking as that seen with tuberculosis. There is a tendency toward the development of abscesses and sinus tracts (TEHRANZADEH and WONG 1994).

Mycobacterium avium-intracellulare complex (MAC) is a group of atypical *Mycobacteria* which are potentially pathogenic and commonly found in the environment. Disseminated disease is the most common form seen in AIDS patients. The diagnosis of disseminated MAC is usually made late in the course of HIV infection, often in conjunction with or after the occurrence of at least one other opportunistic infection (Joint Position Paper of the American Thoracic Society and the Centers for Disease Control 1987). Clinical symptoms that have been attributed to MAC are nonspecific and may include intermittent fever, weight loss, cachexia, and gastrointestinal symptoms ranging from vague abdominal pain to chronic diarrhea and significant malabsorption. MAC has been isolated from bone marrow, lymph nodes, lung, gastrointestinal tract, liver, spleen, urine, and blood. We observed a 12-year-old girl with AIDS and diffuse tuberculous osteomyelitis of the proximal and distal ulna due to MAC (Fig. 12.10).

Mycobacterium haemophilum, an unusual pathogen, has been reported to induce skin infection and

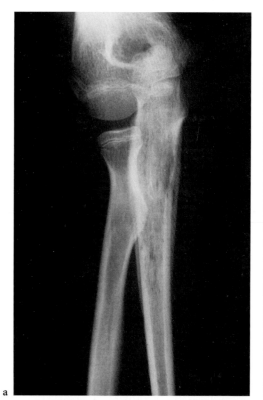

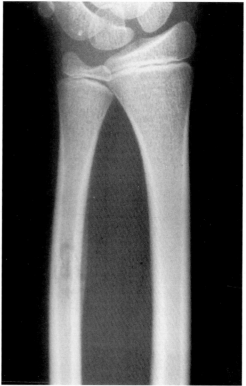

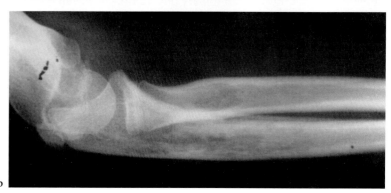

Fig. 12.10a–c. Tuberculous osteomyelitis. Twelve-year-old girl with AIDS and diffuse tuberculous osteomyelitis of the proximal and distal ulna of the right forearm. **a, b** AP and lateral views of the right forearm show permeative lytic lesions of the proximal ulna with diffuse periosteal reaction on the medial and lateral sides. **c** AP view of the distal forearm shows lytic changes of the distal third of the ulnar shaft with periosteal reaction. (From TEHRANZADEH and STEINBACH 1994)

septic arthritis in AIDS patients (KRISTJANSSON et al. 1991; MALES et al. 1987). *M. haemophilum* infection was previously found in patients immunocompromised secondary to renal transplant and Hodgkin's lymphoma. *M. haemophilum* skin lesions begin as painful erythematous nodules and may progress to form abscesses and ulcerate. *M. haemophilum* can also cause tenosynovitis of the knee, ankle, wrist, digit, and tendon sheath. Only one out of five reported cases in a series by GUPTA et al. (1992) responded to antimycobacterial therapy with clinical improvement. This agent is the most common cause of osteomyelitis among atypical mycobacteria in HIV patients.

12.3.2.2
Arthritis

The association of AIDS and arthritis is well documented in the literature, beginning with the first reports of Reiter's syndrome and psoriasis in HIV-infected persons in 1987 (DUVIC et al. 1987; OBERLIN et al. 1987). Up to 78% of patients with AIDS develop rheumatologic manifestations (EUSTACE et al. 1995). Arthritis in HIV-infected persons has a wide spectrum of presentations ranging from mild arthralgias to very severe and disabling joint disorders. The presentation of arthritis may occur during any stage of the HIV disease (WINCHESTER et al. 1987; BERMAN et al. 1988). WINCHESTER et al. (1987) reported a series of 13 HIV-positive patients with arthritis. In their series, two patients had only immunologic abnormalities, six had AIDS-related complex, and five had classic manifestations of AIDS. In a series reported by BERMAN et al. (1988), the majority of patients had full-blown AIDS or an AIDS-associated infection; only one patient was asymptomatic. In the series of ROWE et al. (1989), however, 11 of 36 (31%) patients were not known to be HIV positive when they initially presented with arthritis. This has important implications since the possibility of AIDS must be suspected when any young adult presents with a seronegative arthritis (KEAT and ROWE 1991).

Not only may arthritis be the first manifestation of AIDS, but some data suggest that the onset of arthritis in HIV-positive patients may actually lead to more rapid progression to AIDS (KEAT and ROWE 1991). In the majority of patients, the clinical course of arthritis is variable. Some patients develop a severe arthritis which does not respond well to treatment (WINCHESTER et al. 1987; ROWE et al. 1989), while others have only short-lived joint symptoms which resolve without treatment. Still others present with acute synovitis which responds rapidly to anti-inflammatory medication. Arthritis has also been shown to recur (KEAT and ROWE 1991).

Studies in Tampa, New York, and Cleveland have reported the incidence of inflammatory arthritis in HIV-positive patients to be 16% (BERMAN et al. 1988), 15% (BRANCATO et al. 1989), and 25% (CALABRESE 1989), respectively. The prevalence for Reiter's syndrome was 10% (BERMAN et al. 1988), 4.6% (BRANCATO et al. 1989), and 4.3% (CALABRESE 1989), respectively. A study from London, however, noted a minimum prevalence of inflammatory arthritis in approximately 1% of the HIV-infected population (RYNES et al. 1988), while another study from San Francisco showed that the prevalence of arthritis in AIDS patients was 0.3% (CLARK et al. 1989). It is likely that arthritis is underreported, and clearly more detailed epidemiologic studies need to be performed.

The etiology of arthritis in AIDS patients is unclear. It is known that HIV binds to the membrane glycoprotein, CD4. The CD4 receptor is found predominantly on the T-helper lymphocytes. After binding to the CD4 receptor, the virus quickly enters the cell and kills the T-helper lymphocyte. Some researchers feel that the depletion of T-helper lymphocytes allows immune-regulated arthritides to occur. In further support of this hypothesis, the peripheral blood CD4-positive lymphocyte counts have been found to be reduced in the majority of AIDS patients with arthritis (WINCHESTER et al. 1987; ROWE et al. 1989). Others postulate that HIV may directly cause arthritis (SOLOMON et al. 1991). HIV belongs to the subfamily of viruses called Lentivirinae (lentevirus), and the best-described lentevirus, visna virus, causes chronic arthritis in sheep (NARAYAN and CORK 1985). Another lentevirus, caprine arthritis-encephalitis virus (CAEV), also causes arthritis and has been cultured from joint tissue (NARAYAN and CORK 1985), as has HIV itself (SOLOMON et al. 1991), lending further strength to the argument that HIV may directly cause arthritis. The mere presence of HIV in joint fluid, however, may simply be a manifestation of widespread dissemination of the virus.

Another cause of arthritis in AIDS patients may be infection from an enteric pathogen. Approximately one-third of all HIV-positive patients with Reiter's syndrome have a documented infection with enteric pathogens (usually *Shigella flexneri*, *Salmonella*, *Campylobacter jejuni*, *Yersinia enterocolitica*, and *Yersinia pseudotuberculosis*) (SOLOMON et al. 1991). In another third of patients, infections not traditionally linked to a reactive arthritis, most notably infection by *Mycobacterium avium-intracellulare*, have been documented (WINCHESTER and SOLOMON 1987). Clearly, the pathogenetic mechanisms of AIDS and arthritis need to be further clarified. Perhaps one or a combination of all of these postulated mechanisms may play a role in the development of arthritis.

It is best to divide the arthritides in AIDS patients into five separate groups based on their different clinical presentations and their different responses to treatment. These five groups are: spondyloarthropathic arthritis (Reiter's syndrome, psoriatic arthritis, and undifferentiated spondyloarthropathy), HIV-associated arthritis, painful articular syndrome, acute symmetric polyarthritis, and septic arthritis (SOLOMON et al. 1991).

Spondyloarthropathic arthritis. Spondyloarthropathic arthritis consists of Reiter's syndrome, psoriatic arthritis, and undifferentiated spondyloarthropathy. While Reiter's syndrome and psoriatic arthritis have distinctive clinical features, undifferentiated spondyloarthropathy is a default category for patients who do not meet the criteria for the other two diseases (SOLOMON et al. 1991). They are the most common arthritides to affect AIDS patients, although the exact number of affected HIV-positive and non-HIV-infected patients is controversial. The annual incidence of Reiter's syndrome in the general population has been estimated to be approximately 0.0035% (MICHET et al. 1988); this is similar to the results of NOER (1966), who reported 4 out of 100,000 military personnel with clinically documented Reiter's syndrome. In patients with HIV infection, however, the data vary. BERMAN et al. (1988) reported the prevalence to be in the range of 5%–10%, but CLARK et al. (1989) reported the frequency in the male homosexual population to be 0.3%–0.5% with no statistical difference between the incidence in HIV-positive and HIV-negative individuals. HOCHBERG et al. (1990) also found no change in incidence between these two populations. The studies by CLARK et al. (1989) and HOCHBERG et al. (1990) are, however, viewed as flawed since they relied on questionnaires to retrospectively analyze the data, and none of the patients in their studies were examined by rheumatologists. Thus current opinion favors an increased incidence of Reiter's syndrome in the HIV-infected population.

There is also conflicting evidence regarding the increased incidence of psoriatic arthritis in HIV-positive patients. The prevalence of psoriatic arthritis in the general population is approximately 0.01%–0.14% (ARNETT et al. 1991). WINCHESTER et al. (1988) and BERMAN et al. (1988) reported the incidence of psoriatic arthritis in the HIV-infected population to be 2%–3%. DUVIC et al. (1987), however, found no increased incidence of psoriatic arthritis in their HIV-positive patients. Some of the confusion arises from the use of different criteria to establish the diagnosis. Further epidemiologic studies need to be performed to establish the exact incidence of the spondyloarthropathic arthritides in the HIV population.

The etiology of the spondyloarthropathic arthritides in patients infected with HIV appears to be multifactorial. The HLA-B27 antigen seems to play a central role in the pathogenesis of Reiter's syndrome and is present in approximately 70%–80% of HIV-positive and non-HIV-infected patients who develop the disease (WINCHESTER et al. 1987; BERMAN et al. 1988). Moreover, it is well known that HLA-B27-negative patients who develop reactive arthritis have a less severe arthritis and show fewer extra-articular manifestations of Reiter's syndrome (MONTEAGUDO et al. 1991). HLA-B27 is found in 6%–10% of the normal population (ARNETT et al. 1991); therefore, its presence in an HIV-positive patient strongly indicates the possibility of developing Reiter's syndrome. The HLA-B27 antigen, however, is not linked to the development of psoriatic arthritis or undifferentiated spondyloarthropathy (OBERLIN et al. 1987; WIN-

CHESTER et al. 1987). Some authors argue that Reiter's syndrome may be caused by infection (SOLOMON et al. 1991), although an enteric pathogen as a possible cause has only been detected in 33% of the cases.

It is tempting to speculate that a decrease in circulating CD4-positive lymphocytes may play a role in the development of spondyloarthropathic arthritides in HIV-positive patients. Several studies have shown that while the total white blood cell count is normal, the peripheral CD4-positive lymphocyte counts are reduced in the majority of HIV-positive patients with arthritis (WINCHESTER et al. 1987; ROWE et al. 1989). Perhaps the depletion of CD4-positive lymphocytes permits proliferation of inciting organisms or alters the delicate balance of the immune system, allowing for the development of spondyloarthropathic arthritis.

Reiter's syndrome was the first spondyloarthropathic arthritis to be described in association with HIV infection (WINCHESTER et al. 1987). Since then, several articles describing the correlation have been published. (DUVIC et al. 1987; NARAYAN and CORK 1985). These arthritides have several similar clinical features. The foot and ankle are the most commonly involved sites of inflammation. In the foot, enthesopathy is frequent involving the Achilles tendon, plantar fascia, anterior and posterior tibial tendons, and the extensor tendons (SOLOMON et al. 1991). This can be so painful that it can cause confinement to a wheelchair. Some patients walk on the outer aspects of their feet, producing a wide-based gait known as "AIDS foot" (WINCHESTER et al. 1988) which can simulate the appearance of a peripheral neuropathy (SOLOMON et al. 1991). Multidigit dactylitis also commonly occurs and may simulate the appearance of pedal edema. Knee inflammation is common; however, hip disease is rarely seen (ROSENBERG et al. 1989). Some patients complain of spinal pain and tenderness. In a series from London, 12 of 36 HIV-positive patients complained of spinal pain (ROWE et al. 1989). Six patients had pain in the cervical region and ten patients had pain in the thoracolumbar region. In the upper extremities, dactylitis is typical. Wrist and elbow synovitis is uncommon. Enthesopathy is frequently seen in the upper extremities, usually presenting as lateral or medial epicondylitis, rotator cuff tendinitis, de Quervain's disease, or flexor tendinitis (SOLOMON et al. 1991).

Skin and nail changes often accompany the spondyloarthropathic arthritides in AIDS patients. Although several forms of disease have been described, seborrhea, psoriasis, and onychodystrophy are most commonly seen in this setting. Most patients with psoriasis develop an exacerbation of their skin disease when they develop AIDS (Duvic et al. 1987; Johnson et al. 1985; Major and Tehranzadeh 1997). The psoriasis has also been reported to clear with end-stage AIDS (Duvic et al. 1987). We encountered one HIV-positive patient who developed psoriatic arthritis of the hand and wrist as well as other joints following HIV conversion (Fig. 12.11).

Reactive spondyloarthropathies such as psoriatic arthritis and Reiter's disease have common features and are difficult to differentiate from each other. Psoriatic arthritis commonly shows changes in the hands and wrists; while Reiter's disease has a tendency to affect the lower extremities, specifically the feet and ankles. Enthesopathies are common features of spondyloarthopathies. However, unlike ankylosing spondylitis, which symmetrically affects

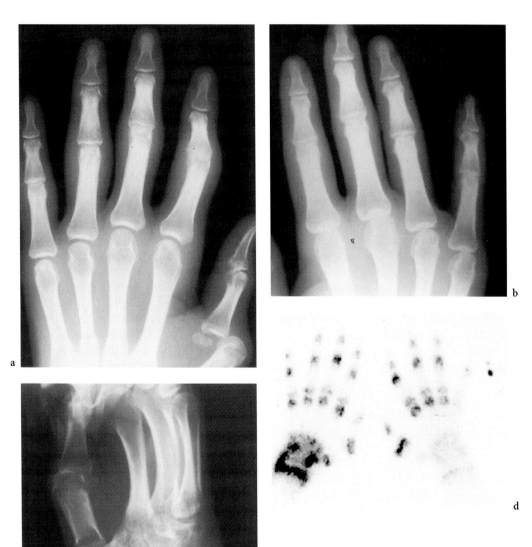

Fig. 12.11a–d. Psoriatic arthritis. A 27-year-old man with AIDS who developed arthritis. **a** AP view of the left hand shows soft tissue swelling at the metacarpophalangeal and proximal interphalangeal joints and dislocation of the first metacarpophalangeal joint. **b** AP view of right hand shows soft tissue swelling of the metacarpophalangeal and proximal interphalangeal joints. **c** Oblique view of the right wrist shows marked ulnar translocation of the carpal bones. **d** AP view of ^{99m}Tc-MDP bone scintigram shows multiple foci of increased activity in the joints of both hands and right wrist, indicating polyarthritis. (From Tehranzadeh and Steinbach 1994)

the sacroiliac joints and is associated with fine syndesmophytes, reactive arthritides create asymmetric sacroiliitis and manifest coarse syndesmophytes and osteophytes. Ankylosing spondylitis shows fine erosions of sacroiliac joints in the form of "serrated edges of a postage stamp" while psoriatic arthritis often creates large erosions at sacroiliac joints. Rheumatoid arthritis shows a tendency for involvement of the proximal interphalangeal and metacarpophalangeal joints of the hands and wrists. Psoriasis may affect any joints in the hands or wrists; however, distal interphalangeal joints are commonly affected. Primary osteoarthritis may cause "seagull wing" osteophytes in distal interphalangeal joints, while a "mouse ear" appearance is typical for psoriatic arthritis. Reactive periosteal reaction and hypertrophic changes are distinguishing features of psoriatic arthritis. "Ray phenomenon" is another classic sign for psoriatic arthritis in hands where all the joints in one ray or several rays, including metacarpophalangeal joints, may be affected.

Although psoriatic arthritis, Reiter's syndrome, and undifferentiated spondyloarthropathy in HIV-positive patients cannot be clinically or radiographically distinguished from each other, there are some important features that are unique to AIDS patients with these arthritides. The arthritis and enthesopathies that occur in AIDS patients are often very severe and less responsive to anti-inflammatory drugs (ARNETT et al. 1991). Usually, psoriatic arthritis or Reiter's syndrome is a mild disease in patients without HIV infection and resolves slowly over 3–12 months (ARNETT 1987). In AIDS patients, however, these arthritides are usually severe and often occur in association with immunodeficiency-related infections. Another important distinguishing feature of patients with HIV-associated spondyloarthropathies is striking muscle atrophy (SOLOMON et al. 1991). The etiology for this is unclear. SOLOMON et al. (1991) speculated that the atrophy may be a result of neuropathy, myopathy, elevated levels of catabolic cytokines, or involuntary splinting of muscles. Physical therapy as well as appropriate splinting of inflamed tendons may help prevent the muscular atrophy (SOLOMON et al. 1991).

It is interesting to note that while there is an increased incidence of spondyloarthropathic arthritis in the HIV population, some rheumatologic conditions improve clinically when a patient is infected with HIV. Systemic lupus erythematosus (SLE) and rheumatoid arthritis (RA) may go into remission in patients with HIV infection (WINCHESTER et al. 1988), and tests for rheumatoid factor and antinuclear antibodies are routinely negative in HIV patients. Why SLE and RA should improve clinically is unclear, although it may be the result of profound immunosuppression. There is a wide range of response to treatment in HIV-positive patients with spondyloarthropathic arthritis. Nonsteroidal anti-inflammatory drugs (NSAIDs) cause moderate to good improvement in some patients (DAVIES et al. 1989) and little improvement in others (WINCHESTER et al. 1987; ROWE et al. 1989). Sulfasalazine and gold benefited two patients (WINCHESTER et al. 1987) but had little effect on others (WITHRINGTON et al. 1987). Intra-articular steroid injections have helped alleviate symptoms (BERMAN et al. 1988; ROWE et al. 1989). Immunosuppressive agents and the use of methotrexate are contraindicated because they may cause worsening of the immunodeficiency (WINCHESTER et al. 1987). More studies using antiviral agents, such as zidovudine, need to be conducted. Finally, it is extremely important that septic arthritis is not mistaken clinically for spondyloarthropathic arthritis. These conditions may be clinically and radiographically similar, so a synovial fluid culture must be performed and broad-spectrum antibiotics administered if septic arthritis is suspected.

HIV-associated arthritis. HIV-associated arthritis was described by RYNES et al. (1988) as a subacute oligoarthritis typically affecting the knees and ankles. It is short in duration, usually lasting 1–6 weeks, but is often characterized by extreme pain. There is usually a good response to nonsteroidal agents, rest, and intra-articular steroids (SOLOMON et al. 1991).

The etiology of this arthritis is unclear; however, many authors favor direct joint infection by HIV. Synovial biopsies have demonstrated only a mild cellular infiltrate, consisting mostly of mononuclear and plasma cells (RYNES et al. 1988). Synovial fluid analysis typically reveals a noninflammatory reaction. HIV has been cultured from the synovial fluid (WITHRINGTON et al. 1987). It is unlikely that this arthritis is related to the spondyloarthropathic arthritides because there is no enthesopathy, the duration of symptoms is shorter, and there is extreme pain and disability. None of the patients with HIV-associated arthritis have had a preceding infection, and none have possessed the HLA-B27 antigen (SOLOMON et al. 1991). The presence of proliferative periostitis (in cases of symmetric rheumatoid-like polyarthritis) should make HIV-associated arthritis a diagnostic consideration (LEE and SARTORIS 1994).

Painful articular syndrome. Painful articular syndrome was described by BERMAN et al. (1988) and RYNES (1991) as an arthralgia in HIV-positive patients consisting of extreme pain of very short duration, typically lasting 2–24 h. The knee joint is most commonly affected; however, the shoulder and elbow can also be involved. Patients usually respond well to NSAIDs. Some patients are confined to a wheelchair because of the extreme pain. HIV infection should be considered when a young patient presents with an intensely painful arthritis, especially if it involves the knee.

Acute symmetric polyarthritis. Acute symmetric polyarthritis was reported by ROSENBERG et al. (1989) as a symmetric polyarthritis involving the hands in four patients. BENTIN et al. (1990) described a similar case. These patients had periarticular osteoporosis, marginal erosions, ulnar deviation, and swan-neck deformities consistent with rheumatoid arthritis, but there were several important distinctions. The disease was acute in all patients, and in two there was marked new bone proliferation, highly unusual for rheumatoid arthritis. Most of the patients were male, and the majority were negative for rheumatoid factor (ROSENBERG et al. 1989). Another patient appeared to respond clinically to zidovudine (BENTIN et al. 1990). The cause of this arthritis is unclear; however, it does not appear to be rheumatoid arthritis, which is rare in the HIV-positive population (FURIE 1991).

Septic arthritis. Septic arthritis is generally seen in HIV-positive patients who are intravenous drug abusers (MUNOZ-FERNANDEZ et al. 1991); the literature is replete with such cases. (STEINBACH et al. 1993; FLECKENSTEIN 1994) (Fig. 12.12). *S. aureus* is the most common cause of this infection (Table 12.4), being seen in 10 of 17 cases of septic arthritis in one series (MUNOZ-FERNANDEZ et al. 1991). *Candida albicans* was the second most common cause of septic arthritis in the same series, accounting for four cases (Table 12.4). All septic arthritis patients in this series were intravenous drug abusers (IVDAs). In another series, three of six cases of septic arthritis were due to *S. aureus*, and one was caused by *Candida albicans* (MONTEAGUDO et al. 1991). Septic arthritis in IVDAs has distinct clinical features, such as a high prevalence in men, young age of affected individuals, and preferential localization to the fibrocartilaginous joints (MUNOZ-FERNANDEZ et al. 1991).

JARZEM et al. (1989) reported seven cases of septic arthritis in HIV-positive hemophiliacs. Septic arthritis in hemophiliacs most commonly involves the knee joint and is caused by *S. aureus* (RAGNI and HANELEY 1989). Septic arthritis is becoming a more

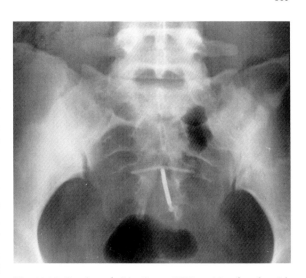

Fig. 12.12. Septic arthritis. Young HIV-positive female with right sacroiliitis. AP view of the pelvis shows cortical indistinctness and sclerosis of the right sacroiliac joint. (From TEHRANZADEH and STEINBACH 1994)

Table 12.4. Septic arthritis in AIDS patients (review of literature)

Microorganism	No. of cases
Staph. aureus	24
Candida albicans	6
M. tuberculosis	5
M. avium complex	6
M. kansasii	5
M. haemophilum	7
M. terrae	1
Salmonella	5
Strep. pneumoniae	3
Neisseria gonorrhoeae	3
Staph. epidermidis	2
Mucormycosis	2
Sporothrix schenckii	2
Haemophilus influenzae	2
Histoplasma capsulatum	2
Pseudomonas	1
Pneumococcus	1
Cryptococcus	1
Yersinia	1
Spir. syphilis (polyarthritis)	1
Chlamydia trachomatis	1
Disseminated *Nocardia asteroides*	1
Campylobacter jejuni	1
Streptococci	1
Gram-negative bacilli	1
Bacteroides melaninogenicus	1
Unknown	9
Total	95

frequent complication of bacterial sepsis in HIV-infected hemophiliacs and a new HIV-associated problem in this group. Thus, a hemophiliac who develops a hemarthrosis associated with fever, poor response to factor treatment, or multiple joint involvement should have joint aspiration and parenteral antibiotic therapy. Although this approach represents a departure from the standard avoidance of joint aspiration in these patients, aggressive management is necessary to avoid joint destruction, disability, and spread to adjacent bones, which can be seen in this patient population (RAGNI and HANELEY 1989; GOLDENBERG and REED 1985). MERCHAN et al. (1992), in another series, described four cases of septic arthritis in HIV-positive hemophiliacs. In three cases, the knee was involved, and in one, the elbow. *Streptococcus pneumoniae* and *S. aureus* were seen in each patient (MERCHAN et al. 1992). COOVELLI et al. (1993) reported three patients with septic arthritis of the sternoclavicular joint. One of these cases was due to *S. aureus* (COOVELLI et al. 1993).

Tuberculous arthritis typically affects large joints and is a monoarticular disease. The majority of joint lesions are secondary to adjacent osteomyelitis. Radiologically, there is a triad of juxta-articular osteoporosis, peripherally located osseous erosions, and gradual narrowing of the interosseous space (Phemister's triad). We have reported two women with HIV infection who had tuberculous arthritis in the ankle and shoulder (TEHRANZADEH and WONG 1994) (Figs. 12.13–12.15).

Three cases of MAC arthritis in AIDS patients have been reported (VINETZ and RICKMAN 1991; BLUMENTHAL et al. 1990). BLUMENTHAL et al. (1990) described a 30-year-old man with AIDS who developed MAC septic arthritis and osteomyelitis of both wrists and feet during the terminal stage of his illness. The patient's clinical course was rapidly progressive and destructive, characteristics usually seen with bacterial septic arthritis. A more indolent arthritis of the left wrist and knee lasting for 1 year has been reported (VINETZ and RICKMAN (1991). There was no bony destruction and the

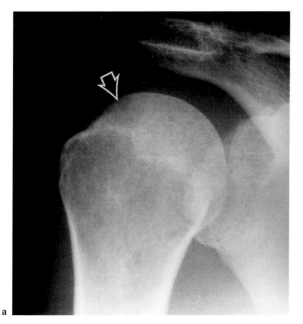

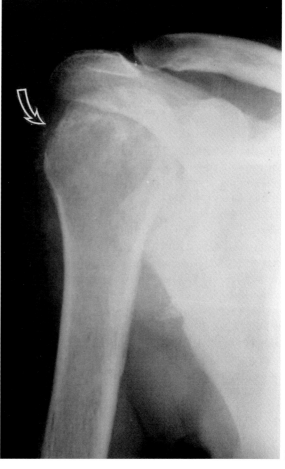

Fig. 12.13a, b. Tuberculous arthritis. A 43-year-old HIV-positive female intravenous drug abuser with tuberculous arthritis of the right shoulder. **a** Initial AP radiograph of the right shoulder shows mild osteopenia and erosion of the cortical margin of the lateral humeral head (*open arrow*). **b** Radiograph of the right shoulder obtained 1 year later shows severe osteoporosis with resorption of the cortical margin of the glenohumeral joint, pathologic nondisplaced fracture with posterior dislocation of the shoulder, extensive soft tissue calcifications (*open arrow*), high-riding humeral head, and atrophy of the rotator cuff. (From TEHRANZADEH and STEINBACH 1994)

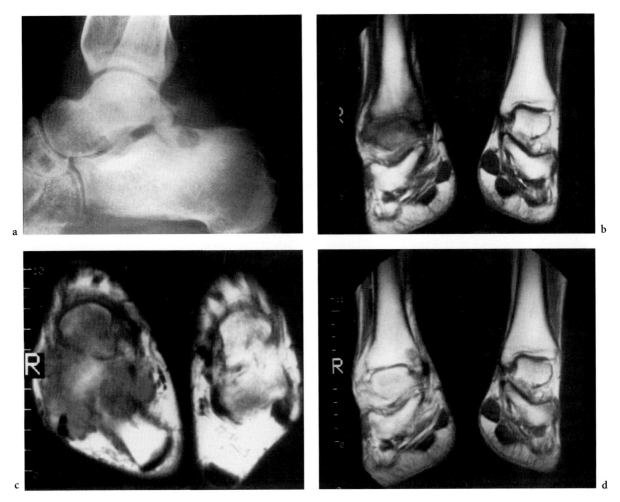

Fig. 12.14a–d. Tuberculous arthritis. 31-year-old HIV-positive female with tuberculous arthritis of the right ankle. **a** Lateral radiograph of the right ankle show osteopenia, loss of cortices of the tibia and talus, narrowed joint spaces, and erosive changes of the talus and calcaneus. Note large joint effusion and soft tissue swelling. **b, c** Coronal and axial T1-weighted images (600/26) show decreased signal intensity of the distal tibia, talus, and calcaneus on the right side, with adjacent soft tissue edema. **d** Coronal T1-weighted image (600/26) with intravenous gadolinium shows enhancement of the inflamed synovium around the ankle joint, with enhancement of the marrow of the distal tibia and talus. Note that the medial malleolus remains relatively low in signal intensity and may be ischemic in relation to other areas. (From TEHRANZADEH and STEINBACH 1994)

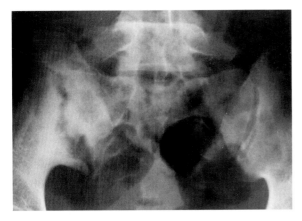

Fig. 12.15. Tuberculous sacroiliitis. Right sacroiliitis in an HIV-positive patient with history of tuberculosis and syphilis AP radiograph of the pelvis shows severe erosive as well as sclerotic changes in the right sacroiliac joint. (From VANARTHOS et al. 1992)

patient was clinically responsive to antimycobacterial therapy. HIRSCH et al. (1996) reported six cases and reviewed nine other cases of HIV-positive patients who developed atypical mycobacterial arthritis with or without osteomyelitis. The organisms include MAC, *M. kansasii*, and *M. haemophilum*.

Other organisms causing septic arthritis include *Sporothrix schenckii* (SOKOLOFF 1990, LIPSTEIN-KRE-SCH et al. 1985), gonococcus in two cases (STRONGIN et al. 1991; MOYLE et al. 1990), and *Haemophilus influenza* (SPACH et al. 1992; HAUGHT et al. 1993).

RADCLIFFE et al. (1991) argue that rheumatic fever ought to be listed along with other recognized causes of arthritis associated with HIV infection. Symptoms are related to a delayed sensitivity immune reaction following group A streptococcal infection. Large joints of the extremities are typically affected in a migratory pattern, in conjunction with fever and often carditis. Radiographic findings are nonspecific, revealing soft tissue swelling without evidence of osseous or cartilaginous destruction; there may be mild osteopenia.

12.3.2.3
Spondylitis in AIDS Patients

Spine infection is relatively common in HIV patients (TEHRANZADEH and MESGARZADEH 1994; STEIN-BACH et al. 1993). Among pyogenic causes, *S. aureus* is implicated most frequently. The disc space is often involved and bony erosion of the adjacent end-plates is generally seen. Often, small or large epidural soft tissue involvement in the form of edema, inflammation, or abscess is noted (Figs. 12.16–12.18; Table 12.3).

PIROFSKI and CASADEVALL (1990) reported a case of an epidural abscess in an HIV-positive patient with a mixed *S. aureus* and cryptococcal infection. In a series by STEINBACH et al. (1993), one of four cases of spondylitis was caused by *Cryptococcus*. In the same series, *E. coli* septicemia in an AIDS patient resulted in septic spondylitis with a large epidural abscess (Table 12.3). The third case of spondylitis was caused by *S. aureus*, and the etiology for the fourth case was unknown. BOIX et al. (1990) reported a case of spine infection with *Candida albicans* and one of our two cases of spondylitis involving the cervical spine with a large anterior epidural abscess was caused by *Candida tropicalis*. Our second case was a 31-year-old intravenous drug abuser with *Pseudomonas* spondylitis. SATHI et al. (1994) reported a case of spinal subdural abscess in an AIDS patient, and Go et al. (1993) described a spinal epidural abscess due to *Aspergillus* in a patient with AIDS. MRI is helpful in imaging spondylitis and discitis. Disc in-

fection is associated with a decreased signal intensity on T1-weighted images, and increasing signal on T2-weighted images. It is often accompanied by paraspinal or epidural inflammation, edema, or abscess formation, and contrast enhancement is usually observed. The vertebral end-plates are also affected (TEHRANZADEH et al. 1992).

12.4
Malignancy

12.4.1
Kaposi's Sarcoma

Kaposi's sarcoma (KS) is the most common neoplasm seen in adults with AIDS, occurring in 14% of patients. (STEINBACH 1994b). The etiology of the tumor is unknown, although ineffective host tumor surveillance, interaction of HIV with transforming viruses, and polyclonal stimulation of B cells and monocytes are believed to contribute. Patients can present with the tumor at any stage of HIV infection. Multifocal involvement of the viscera, skin, and musculoskeletal system may be seen. The lesions may be asymptomatic or painful. The average survival after diagnosis is 14–32 months; KS generally responds poorly to treatment. Osseous lesions of Kaposi's sarcoma have a similar radiographic appearance to certain infections such as bacillary angiomatosis and tuberculosis, as well as lymphoma (STEINBACH 1994b). Bone involvement may manifest on CT as multiple osteolytic lesions in the pelvis, hips, spine, and ribs (WYATT and FISHMAN 1995). These lesions are often associated with periosteal reaction and an overlying soft tissue mass (HO-RUSITZKY et al. 1995). Muscle involvement may show an MRI appearance varying from extensive edema and subcutaneous tissue changes with minimal muscle involvement, to one of extensive muscle involvement with adjacent subcutaneous lesions (LEE and SARTORIS 1994). Even in the presence of bony involvement, bone scintigrams as well as plain radiographs may be negative (HORUSITZKY et al. 1995). MRI has been suggested as the modality of choice in detecting early osseous changes (STEINBACH et al. 1993).

12.4.2
AIDS-Related Lymphoma

AIDS-related non-Hodgkin's lymphoma (NHL) is the second most common tumor found in adults with

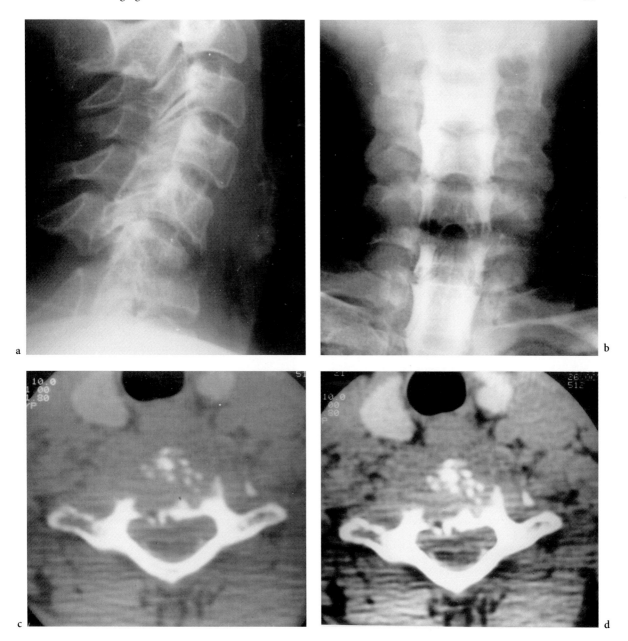

Fig. 12.16a–d. Cervical spondylitis and paravertebral abscess. A 38-year-old HIV-positive female with *Candida tropicalis* spondylitis at C6–7. **a** Lateral radiograph of cervical spine shows destructive changes and collapse of the vertebral bodies of C6 and C7. **b** AP view of cervical myelogram shows epidural defects at C6–7 bilaterally. **c** CT scan (bone window) of cervical spine following myelography at C6–7 shows destructive changes of vertebral end-plates. **d** CT scan (soft tissue window) demonstrates anterior epidural and paravertebral soft tissue mass and inflammation. (From TEHRANZADEH and STEINBACH 1994)

AIDS (Figs. 12.19, 12.20) and the most common tumor found in children with AIDS (LEE and SARTORIS 1994; SISKIN et al. 1995). NHL is approximately 60 times more common in AIDS patients than in the general population (MAJOR and TEHRANZADEH 1997). Lymphoma develops in HIV/AIDS patients at end stages of the disease when the CD4 cell count is very low; its presence signifies a grave prognosis. Though the most

common sites of involvement are the gastrointestinal tract and central nervous system, secondary musculoskeletal involvement is common in NHL, especially in children (LEE and SARTORIS 1994; SISKIN et al. 1995). Patients may present with pain and pathologic fractures; muscle involvement may manifest as painful swelling (SISKIN et al. 1995; CHEVALIER et al. 1993). Bone marrow lesions are found in one-third of pa-

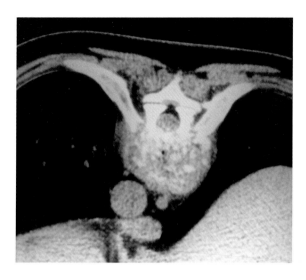

Fig. 12.17. Thoracic spondylitis. A 31-year-old HIV-positive female with history of intravenous drug abuse, with *Pseudomonas* spondylitis. Prone CT scan of thoracic spine (soft tissue window) shows destruction of vertebral endplates at T7–8, discitis, and paravertebral inflammation. (From TEHRANZADEH and STEINBACH 1994)

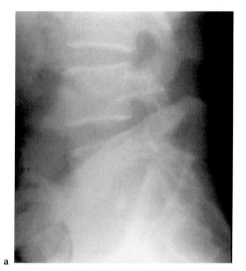

a

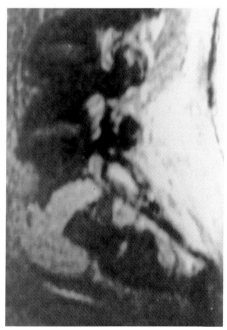

c

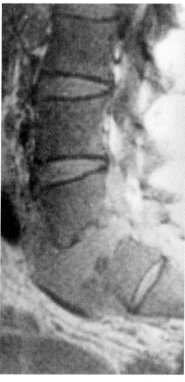

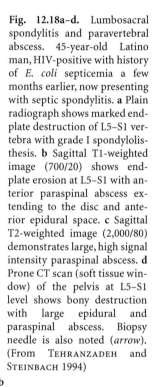

b

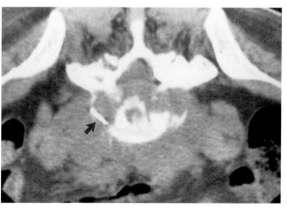

d

Fig. 12.18a–d. Lumbosacral spondylitis and paravertebral abscess. 45-year-old Latino man, HIV-positive with history of *E. coli* septicemia a few months earlier, now presenting with septic spondylitis. a Plain radiograph shows marked endplate destruction of L5–S1 vertebra with grade I spondylolisthesis. b Sagittal T1-weighted image (700/20) shows endplate erosion at L5–S1 with anterior paraspinal abscess extending to the disc and anterior epidural space. c Sagittal T2-weighted image (2,000/80) demonstrates large, high signal intensity paraspinal abscess. d Prone CT scan (soft tissue window) of the pelvis at L5–S1 level shows bony destruction with large epidural and paraspinal abscess. Biopsy needle is also noted (*arrow*). (From TEHRANZADEH and STEINBACH 1994)

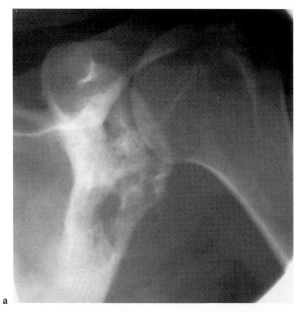

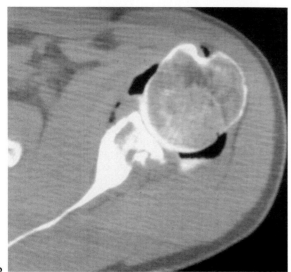

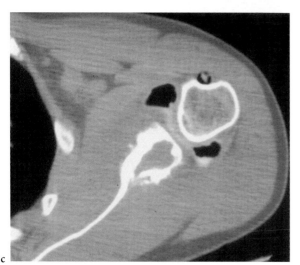

tients with extranodal involvement, whereas in the general population, only 8% suffer from bone lesions (LEE and SARTORIS 1994). The most common site of bone involvement is the lower extremity, as well as the skull, pelvis, and spine; muscle involvement is usually found in the psoas or lower extremity and may clinically mimic pyomyositis or thrombophlebitis (SISKIN et al. 1995; CHEVALIER et al. 1993). Plain radiographs and CT of bone lesions show permeative osteolytic lesions with cortical destruction, sclerosis, an indistinct transition zone, periosteal reaction, pathologic fractures, and an associated soft tissue mass (TEHRANZADEH and BUTLER 1994).

12.5
Miscellaneous

Avascular necrosis (AVN) of bone has been found in patients with AIDS. The reasons for this are varied. An association between antiphospholipid antibodies in HIV-infected individuals and AVN of femoral and humeral heads has been described (WU et al. 1998). BLACKSIN et al. (2000) documented the incidence of AVN in HIV-infected patients and concluded that steroid therapy for the many manifestations of AIDS may be a strong factor in the development of AVN and that HIV infection alone may not cause this phenomenon (BLACKSIN et al. 2000). A vasculitis (Fig. 12.21) seen in HIV/AIDS patients may also be a contributing factor in the development of AVN. Radiographic features of AVN include subchondral fracture and sclerosis with a crescentic radiolucency, flattening of the epiphyseal head, widening of the epiphyseal line, rarefaction of the metaphysis, and preservation of the joint space (TEHRANZADEH and CASSADY 1994) (Figs. 12.22, 12.23). MRI is the best modality for detecting early AVN, with the involved bone showing a low signal intensity band or rings (WYATT and FISHMAN 1995). T2-weighted images manifest a "double line" sign of adjacent low and high signal intensity (WYATT and FISHMAN 1995).

Fig. 12.19a–c. Lymphoma of scapula. A 29-year-old HIV-positive Caucasian male with left shoulder pain. a AP radiograph of the left shoulder shows marked lytic and destructive changes of the glenoid process extending to the body of the scapula with aggressive periosteal reaction and large soft tissue mass. b, c CT scan following shoulder arthrography shows lytic changes of the glenoid process with anterior and posterior soft tissue mass. The articular cartilage remains intact. (From STEINBACH et al. 1993)

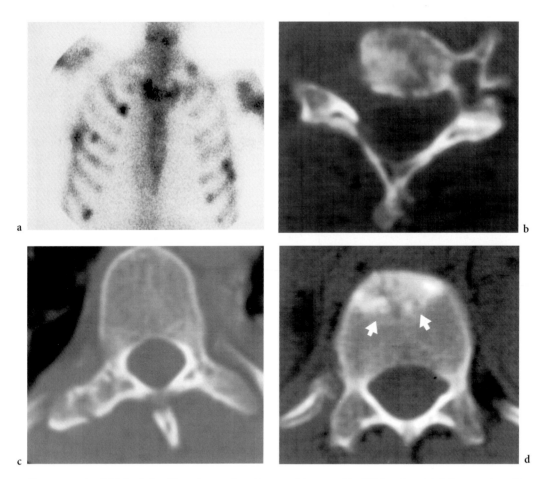

Fig. 12.20a–d. Multiple skeletal lymphomas in a 39-year-old man with AIDS and multiple bone pain. **a** Bone scintigraphy shows multiple foci of increased uptake throughout the thoracic rib cage and both proximal humeri. **b** CT scan of cervical spine (bone window) demonstrates lytic and sclerotic changes of the vertebral body with pathologic fracture. **c** CT scan of thoracic spine (bone window) shows lytic changes with pathologic fracture of the right transverse process with adjacent soft tissue mass. **d** CT scan of thoracic spine (bone window) shows sclerotic involvement, indicating an osteoblastic lesion in the anterior vertebral body (*arrows*). (From TEHRANZADEH and STEINBACH 1994)

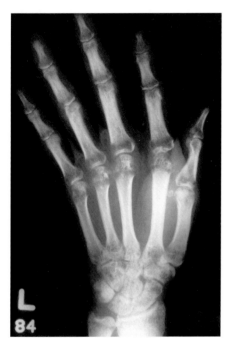

Fig. 12.21. Systemic lupus erythematosus with mixed connective tissue disease in a 38-year-old male AIDS patient. Note acro-osteolysis secondary to vasculitis. (From TEHRANZADEH et al. 1995)

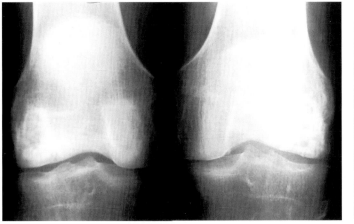
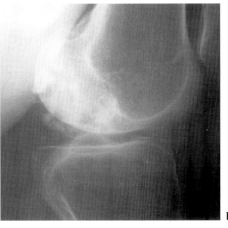

a

b

Fig. 12.22a, b. Osteonecrosis of femoral condyles in a 34-year-old HIV-positive man with meningitis. **a** AP view of bilateral knees shows osteonecrosis of the femoral condyles of both knees. **b** Lateral view of the left knee shows osteonecrosis with subchondral fracture and fragmentation. (From TEHRANZADEH and STEINBACH 1994)

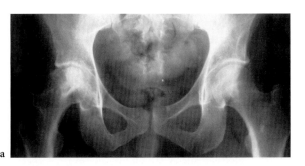

a

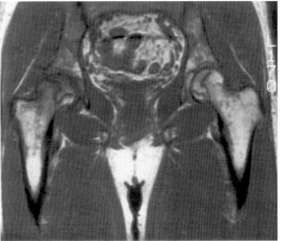

b

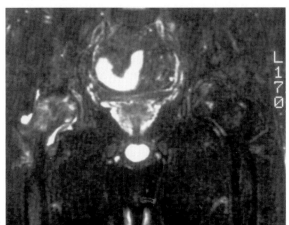

c

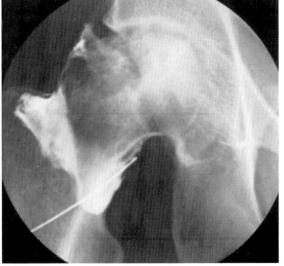

d

Fig. 12.23a–d. AVN of both hips in a 30-year-old man with AIDS. **a** AP radiograph shows sclerosis of both femoral heads and collapse of the superior articular cortex of the right femoral head with joint space narrowing, indicating AVN of the femoral heads with stage IV on the right side and stage II on the left side. **b, c** Coronal T1-weighted image (800/10) and T2-weighted image with fat saturation (4,000/96) show typical changes of AVN on both sides. **d** Palliative right hip arthrograph during injection of Sensorcaine and Depomedrol for pain relief

Hypointense marrow of the vertebral body has been demonstrated on T1- and T2-weighted MR images (LEE and SARTORIS 1994) in AIDS patients. The T2-weighted image does not show increased signal intensity, as it does with pathologic processes, such as infection or lymphoma (MAJOR and TEHRANZADEH 1997). This is probably due to hematopoietic dysfunction in HIV/AIDS patients. HIV may directly infect marrow cells and their precursors, leading to myelosuppression. Other infections, malignancy, and the therapeutic agents used for these conditions may also result in myelosuppression. Ultimately, anemia related to chronic disease may result in an increase in bone marrow iron storage (LEE and SARTORIS 1994; MAJOR and TEHRANZADEH 1997). RUBIES-PRAT et al. (1996) report generalized symmetric increased radionuclide uptake on bone scans to be a common finding in HIV-infected patients who are free of osteoarticular symptoms. They postulate the bone marrow hypercellularity to be responsible for this phenomenon.

Hypertrophic pulmonary osteoarthropathy is found in increased frequency in patients with AIDS and presents as warmth, tenderness, and arthralgias of mid-extremity joints, often relieved by elevation (TEHRANZADEH and CASSADY 1994). The radiographic appearance shows subperiosteal new bone formation, soft tissue thickening, joint effusion, and clubbing of the digits; bone scans reveal increased uptake at areas of new bone formation.

Patients with HIV and severe periodontal disease may progress to necrotizing periodontitis with extensive destruction of bone and soft tissue of the mandible and maxilla (TEHRANZADEH and CASSADY 1994).

Myositis ossificans is characterized by benign, focal heterotopic bone or cartilage formation in the soft tissues, often in association with trauma or nervous system dysfunction (TEHRANZADEH and CASSADY 1994).

Reflex sympathetic dystrophy presents as hyperalgesia, blood flow alterations, changes in sweating, and disturbances in hair and nail growth in an extremity secondary to local autonomic dysfunction. Plain radiographs show severe local osteoporosis (TEHRANZADEH and CASSADY 1994).

Idiopathic Dupuytren's contracture is found with increased frequency in those with AIDS. It appears as a flexion deformity of the metacarpophalangeal joint of the finger secondary to fibrosis and shortening of the palmar fascia (TEHRANZADEH and CASSADY 1994).

12.6 Conclusion

HIV/AIDS patients are prone to different musculoskeletal infections. *S. aureus* is the most common organism. Tuberculosis and atypical mycobacteria are also common. Many HIV patients develop arthritides, especially psoriasis and Reiter's syndrome. Myositis and myopathies manifest in various forms. Malignant neoplasms include Kaposi's sarcoma and lymphoma. Bone marrow changes, avascular necrosis, and miscellaneous conditions have also been described in association with HIV infection.

References

Abrahamson SB, Odagnyk, Grieco AJ, et al. (1985) Hyperalgesic pseudothrombophlebitis, a new syndrome in male homosexuals. Am J Med 78:317–320

al-Kassab AK, Habte-Gabr E, Mueller WF, et al. (1995) Fulminant disseminated toxoplasmosis in an HIV patient. Scand J Infect Dis 27:183–185

Anaya JM, Joseph J, Scopelitis E, et al.(1994) Disseminated gonococcal infection and human immunodeficiency virus (letter). Clin Exp Rheumatol 12:688

Arnett FC (1987) Seronegative spondyloarthropathies. Bull Rheum Dis 37:1–12

Arnett FC, Reveille JD, Duvic M (1991) Psoriasis and psoriatic arthritis associated with human immunodeficiency virus infection. Rheum Dis Clin North Am 17:59–78

Barnes P, Bloch A, Davidson P, et al. (1991) Tuberculosis in patients with human immunodeficiency virus infection. N Engl J Med 324:1644–1650

Baron AL, Steinbach LS, LeBoit PE, et al. (1990) Osteolytic lesions and bacillary angiomatosis in HIV infection: radiologic differentiation from AIDS-related Kaposi sarcoma. Radiology 177:77–81

Bentin J, Feremans W, Pasteels J, et al.(1990) Chronic acquired immunodeficiency syndrome-associated arthritis: a synovial ultrastructural study. Arthritis Rheum 33:268–273

Berman A, Espinoza LR, Diaz JD, et al. (1988) Rheumatic manifestations of human immunodeficiency virus infection. Am J Med 85:59–64

Berman S, Jensen J (1990) Cytomegalovirus-induced osteomyelitis in a patient with the acquired immunodeficiency syndrome. South Med J 83:1231–1232

Bessen L, Greene J, Louie E, et al. (1988) Severe polymyositis-like syndrome associated with zidovudine therapy of AIDS and ARC (letter). N Engl J Med 318:708

Blacksin MF, Kloser PC, Simon J (2000) Avascular necrosis of bone in human immunodeficiency virus infected patients. Clin Imaging 23:314–318

Blumenthal DR, Zucker JR, Hawkins CC (1990) *Mycobacterium avium* complex-induced septic arthritis and osteomyelitis in a patient with the acquired immunodeficiency syndrome (letter). Arthritis Rheum 33:757–758

Boix V, Tovar J, Martin-Hidalgo A (1990) *Candida* spondylodiscitis: chronic illness due to heroin analgesia in an HIV-positive person (letter). J Rheumatol 17:563–565

Brancato L, Itescu S, Skovron ML, et al. (1989) Aspects of the spectrum, prevalence and disease susceptibility determinants of Reiter's syndrome and related disorders associated with HIV infection. Rheumatol Int 9:137–141

Britton C, Miller J (1984) Neurologic complications in the acquired immunodeficiency syndrome (AIDS). Neurol Clin 2:315–339

Burman WI, Cohn DL, Reves RR, et al. (1995) Multifocal cellulitis and monoarticular arthritis as manifestations of *Helicobacter cinaedi* bacteremia. Clin Infect Dis 20:564–570

Buskila D, Tenenbaum J (1989) Septic bursitis in human immunodeficiency virus infection. J Rheumatol 16:1374–1376

Calabrese LH (1989) The rheumatic manifestations of infection with the human immunodeficiency virus. Semin Arthritis Rheum 18:225–239

Centers for Disease Control (1999) HIV/AIDS Surveillance Report – Midyear edn, June 1999. CDC, US Department of Health and Human Services, Atlanta, GA 11:1–21

Chapman M, Murray R, Stoker D (1979) Tuberculosis of the bones and joints. Semin Roentgenol 14:266–282

Chariot P, Ruet E, Authier FJ, et al. (1994) Acute rhabdomyolysis in patients infected by human immunodeficiency virus. Neurology 44:1692–1696

Chevalier X, Amoura Z, Viard J, et al. (1993) Skeletal muscle lymphoma in patients with the acquired immunodeficiency syndrome: a diagnostic challenge. Arthritis Rheum 36:426–427

Chiedozi LC (1979) Pyomyositis: review of 205 cases in 112 patients. Am J Surg 137:255–259

Clark M, Kinsolving M, Cherrihoff D (1989) The prevalence of arthritis in two HIV-infected cohorts. Arthritis Rheum 32:S85

Coovelli M, Lapadula G, Pipitone N, et al. (1993) Isolated sternoclavicular joint arthritis in heroin addicts and/or HIV-positive patients: three cases. Clin Rheumatol 12:422–425

Dalakas M, Pezeshkpour G, Flaherty M (1987) Progressive nemaline (rod) myopathy associated with HIV infection (letter). N Engl J Med 317:1602–1603

Dalakas M, Illa I, Pezeslikpour G, et al. (1990) Mitochondrial myopathy caused by long term zidovudine therapy. N Engl J Med 322:1098–1105

Davies P, Stein M, Latif A, et al. (1989) Acute arthritis in Zimbabwean patients: possible relationship to human immunodeficiency virus infection. J Rheumatol 16:346–348

Duvic M, Johnson TM, Rapini RP, et al. (1987) Acquired immunodeficiency syndrome: associated psoriasis and Reiter's syndrome. Arch Dermatol 123:1622–1632

Echavarria E, Cano EL, Restrepo A (1993) Disseminated adiaspiromycosis in a patient with AIDS. J Med Vet Mycol 31:91–97

Edelstein H, McCabe R (1991) *Candida albicans*, septic arthritis and osteomyelitis of the sternoclavicular joint in a patient with human immunodeficiency virus infection. J Rheumatol 18:110–111

Eustace S, McEnif N, Rastegar J, et al. (1995) Acute HIV polymyositis with complicating myoglobinuric renal failure: CT appearance. J Comput Assist Tomogr 19:321–323

Flaitz CM, Hicks MJ, Nichols CM (1994) Cytomegaloviral. infection of the mandible in acquired immunodeficiency syndrome. J Oral Maxillofac Surg 52:305–308

Fleckenstein JL (1994) Muscular manifestations in the acquired immunodeficiency syndrome (AIDS). In: Tehranzadeh J, Steinback LS (eds) Musculoskeletal manifestations of AIDS. Warren H. Green, St. Louis, pp 84–103

Fleckenstein JL, Burns DK, Murphy FK, et al. (1991) Differential diagnosis of bacterial myositis in AIDS: evaluation with MR imaging. Radiology 179:653–658

Frank I, Fishman N (1994) Epidemiology and clinical manifestations of human immunodeficiency virus infection. Semin Roentgenol 3:230–241

Furie RA (1991) Effects of human immunodeficiency virus infection on the expression of rheumatic illness. Rheum Dis Clin North Am 17:177–187

Gardiner JS, Zank AM, Minnefor AB, et al. (1990) Pyomyositis in an HIV-positive premature infant: case report and review of the literature. J Pediatr Orthop 10:791–793

Gil-Garcia L, Martin-Santos JM, Blanco-Cabero M, et al. (1993) Hypertrophic osteoarthropathy and AIDS (letter). Ann Rheum Dis 52:82–83

Go BM, Ziring DL, Kountz DS (1993) Spinal epidural abscess due to *Aspergillus* sp in a patient with acquired immunodeficiency syndrome. South Med J 86:957–960

Goldenberg DL, Reed JI (1985) Bacterial arthritis. N Engl J Med 312:764–771

Granieri L, Wisnieski JJ, Graham RC, et al. (1995) Sarcoid myopathy in a patient with human immunodeficiency virus infection. South Med J 88:591–595

Gupta I, Kocher J, Miller AJ, et al. (1992) *Mycobacterium haemophilum* osteomyelitis in an AIDS patient. N J Med 89:201–202

Haught WH, Steinbach J, Zander DS, et al. (1993) Case report: bacillary angiomatosis with massive visceral lymphadenopathy. Am J Med Sci 306:236–240

Heary RF, Hunt CD, Krieger AJ, et al. (1994) HIV status does not affect microbiologic spectrum or neurologic outcome in spinal infections. Surg Neurol 42:417–423

Herts BR, Rafii M, Spiegel G (1991) Soft tissue and osseous lesions caused by bacillary angiomatosis: unusual manifestations of cat-scratch fever in patients with AIDS. AJR 157:1249–1251

Hirsch R, Miller SM, Kazi S, et al. (1996) Human immunodeficiency virus-associated atypical mycobacterial skeletal infections. Semin Arthritis Rheum 25:347–356

Hochberg MC, Fox R, Nelson KE, et al. (1990) HIV infection is not associated with Reiter's syndrome: data from the Johns Hopkins Multicenter AIDS Cohort Study. AIDS 4:1149–1151

Horusitzky A, Cariou D, Chicheportiche V (1995) Kaposi's sarcoma involving bone in a patient with AIDS. AIDS 2:206–208

Hughes RA, Row IF, Shanson D, et al. (1992) Septic bone, joint and muscle lesions associated with human immunodeficiency virus infection. Br J Rheumatol 31:381–388

Jarzem P, Tsoukas C, Burke D, et al. (1989) Hemophilia, septic arthritis and human immunodeficiency virus (abstract no. TH.B.P. 7). International Conference on AIDS 5:416

Johnson SC, Stamm CP, Hicks CB (1990) Tuberculous psoas muscle abscess following chemoprophylaxis with isoniazid in a patient with human immunodeficiency virus infection. Rev Infect Dis 12:754–756

Johnson TM, Duvic M, Rapini RP, et al. (1985) AIDS exacerbates psoriasis. N Engl J Med 313:1415

Joint Position Paper of the American Thoracic Society and the Centers for Disease Control (1987) Mycobacterioses and the acquired immunodeficiency syndrome. Am Rev Respir Dis 136:492–496

Kastner RJ, Malone JL, Decker CF (1994) Syphilic osteitis in a patient with secondary syphilis and concurrent human immunodeficiency virus infection. Clin Infect Dis 18:250–252

Keat A, Rowe I (1991) Reiter's syndrome and associated arthritides. Rheum Dis Clin North Am 17:25–42

Khorenian SD, Lebwohl M (1995) New cutaneous manifestations of systemic diseases. Am Fam Physician 51:625–630

Koehler JE, Quinn FD, Berger TG, et al. (1992) Isolation of *Rochalimaea* species from cutaneous and osseous lesions of bacillary angiomatosis (see comments). N Engl J Med 327:1625–1631

Kristjansson M, Bieluch VM, Bveff PD (1991) *Mycobacterium haemophilum* infection in immunocompromised patients: case report and review of the literature. Rev Infect Dis 13:906–910

Lee DJ, Sartoris DJ (1994) Musculoskeletal manifestations of human immunodeficiency virus infection: review of imaging characteristics. Radiol Clin North Am 32:399–411

Lipstein-Kresch E, Isenberg HD, Singer C, et al. (1985) Disseminated *Sporothrix schenckii* infection with arthritis in a patient with acquired immunodeficiency syndrome. J Rheumatol 12:805–808

Magid D, Fishman EK (1992) Musculoskeletal infections in patients with AIDS: CT findings. AJR 158:603–607

Major NM, Tehranzadeh J (1997) Musculoskeletal manifestations of AIDS. Radiol Clin North Am 35:1167–1189

Males BM, West TE, Bartholomew WR (1987) *Mycobacterium haemophilum* infection in a patient with acquired immunodeficiency syndrome. J Clin Microbiol 25:186–190

Mastroianni CM, Vullo V, Delia S (1992) Cranial salmonella abscess with parietal bone osteomyelitis in an HIV-infected patient (letter). AIDS 6:749–750

May T, Rabaud C, Amiel C, et al. (1993) Hypertrophic pulmonary osteoarthropathy associated with granulomatous *Pneumocystis carinii* pneumonia in AIDS. Scand J Infect Dis 25:771–773

Merchan EC, Magallon M, Manso F, et al. (1992) Septic arthritis in HIV-positive haemophiliacs. Four cases and a literature review. Int Orthop 16:302–306

Michet CJ, Machado EB, Ballard DJ, et al. (1988) Epidemiology of Reiter's syndrome in Rochester, Minnesota: 1950–1980. Arthritis Rheum 31:428–431

Monteagudo I, Rivera J, Lopez-Longo J, et al. (1991) AIDS and rheumatic manifestations in patients addicted to drugs: an analysis of 106 cases. J Rheumatol 18:1038–1041

Moore EH, Russell LA, Klein JS, et al. (1995) Bacillary angiomatosis in patients with AIDS: multiorgan imaging findings. Radiology 197:67–72

Moyle G, Barton SE, Midgley J, et al. (1990) Gonococcal arthritis caused by anxotype P in a man with HIV infection. Genitourin Med 66:91–92

Munoz-Fernandez S, Auiralte J, del Arco A, et al. (1991) Osteoarticular infection associated with the human immunodeficiency virus. Clin Exp Rheumatol 9:489–493

Narayan O, Cork LC (1985) Lentiviral infections of sheep and goats: chronic pneumonia leukoencephalomyelitis and arthritis. Rev Infect Dis 7:89–98

Noer HR (1966) An "experimental" epidemic of Reiter's syndrome. JAMA 198:693–698

Oberlin F, Leblonde V, Camus JP (1987) Reactional arthritis in 2 homosexuals with positive HIV serology [in French]. Presse Med 16:355

Pantaleo G, Graziosi C, Demarest JF (1993) HIV infection is active and progressive in lymphoid tissue during the clinically latent stage of disease. Nature 362:355–358

Pirofski L, Casadevall A (1990) Mixed staphylococcal and cryptococcal epidural abscess in a patient with AIDS (letter, comment). Rev Infect Dis 12:964–965

Radcliffe KW, McLean KA, Benbow AG (1991) Acute rheumatic fever in human immunodeficiency virus infection. J Infect 22:187–189

Radin DR, Rosenstein H, Boswell WD, et al. (1984) Burkitt lymphoma in acquired immune deficiency syndrome. J Comput Assist Tomogr 8:173–174

Ragni MV, Haneley EN (1989) Septic arthritis in a hemophiliac patient and infection with human immunodeficiency virus (HIV) (letter). Ann Intern Med 15:110:168–169

Ras GJ, Eftychis HA, Anderson R, et al. (1984a) Mononuclear and polymorphonuclear leukocyte dysfunction in male homosexuals with the acquired immunodeficiency syndrome (AIDS). S Afr Med J 66:806–809

Ras GJ, Anderson R, Lecatsas G, et al. (1984b) Acquired neutrophil dysfunction in male homosexuals with the acquired immunodeficiency syndrome. S Afr Med J 65:873–874

Ray TD, Nimityongskul P, Ramsey KM (1994) Disseminated *Nocardia asteroides* infection presenting as septic arthritis in a patient with AIDS (letter, comment). Clin Infect Dis 18:256–257

Resnick D, Niwayama G (1988) Diagnosis of bone and joint disorders. Saunders, Philadelphia

Roschmann RA, Bell CL (1987) Septic bursitis in immunocompromised patients. Am J Med 83:661–665

Rosenberg ZS, Norman A, Solomon G (1989) Arthritis associated with HIV infection: radiographic manifestations. Radiology 173:171–176

Rowe IF, Forster SM, Seifert MH, et al. (1989) Rheumatological lesion in individuals with human immunodeficiency virus infection. Q J Med 73:1167–1184

Rubies-Prat J, Coll J, del Rio L, et al. (1996) Increased radionuclide uptake on bone scintiscans: a common but not clinically significant finding for human immunodeficiency virus type I-infected patients free of osteoarticular symptoms. Clin Infect Dis 23:170–172

Rubin JT, Lotze MT (1992) Immune function and dysfunction – a primer for the radiologist. Radiol Clin North Am 30:507–523

Rynes RI (1991) Painful rheumatic syndromes associated with human immunodeficiency virus infection. Rheum Dis Clin North Am 17:79–87

Rynes RI, Goldenberg DL, DiGiacomo R, et al. (1988) Acquired immunodeficiency syndrome-associated arthritis. Am J Med 84:810–816

Sathi S, Schwartz M, Cortez S, et al. (1994) Spinal subdural abscess: successful treatment with limited drainage and antibiotics in a patient with AIDS. Surg Neurol 42:424–427

Schwartzman WA, Lambertus MW, Kennedy CA, et al. (1991) Staphylococcal pyomyositis in patient infected by the human immunodeficiency virus. Am J Med 90:595–600

Sesma P, Martinez G, Verdejo C, et al. (1992) Rhabdomyolysis, infection due to the human immunodeficiency virus, and staphylococcal bacteremia (letter). Clin Infect Dis 15:1054

Sharif H, Clark DC, Aabed MY, et al. (1990) Granulomatous spinal infections: MR imaging. Radiology 177:101–107

Simpson D, Bender A (1988) HIV-associated myopathy: analysis of 11 patients. Ann Neurol 24:79–84

Siskin GP, Haller JO, Miller S, et al. (1995) AIDS-related lymphoma: radiologic features in pediatric patients. Radiology 196:63–66

Sokoloff L (1990) A prospective necropsy study of arthritis in acquired immunodeficiency syndrome. Arch Pathol Lab Med 114:1035–1037

Solomon G, Brancato L, Winchester R (1991) An approach to the human immunodeficiency virus-positive patient with a spondyloarthropathic disease. Rheum Dis Clin North Am 17:44–52

Soriano V, Tor J (1992) Multifocal bone tuberculosis in one AIDS patient (letter). Genitourin Med 68:273

Spach DH, Panther LA, Thorning DR, et al. (1992) Intracerebral bacillary angiomatosis in a patient infected with human immunodeficiency virus. Ann Intern Med 116:740–742

Spencer M, Burgener FA, Hampton BA (1991) Osteomyelitis in AIDS patient (abstract). Radiology 181:155–156

Standiford KN, Emery CD, Schiffman RJ (1994) Case report 865. Bacillary angiomatosis. Skeletal Radiol 23:569–571

Stein M, Houston S, Pozniak A, et al. (1993) HIV infection and *Salmonella* septic arthritis. Clin Exp Rheumatol 11:187–189

Steinbach LS (1994a) Bacillary angiomatosis. In: Tehranzadeh J, Steinbach LS (eds) Musculoskeletal manifestations of AIDS. Warren H. Green, St. Louis, pp 44–62

Steinbach LS (1994b) Kaposi sarcoma: skeletal manifestations. In: Tehrandadeh J, Steinbach LS (eds) Musculoskeletal manifestations of AIDS. Warren H. Green, St. Louis, pp 145–155

Steinbach L, Tehranzadeh J, Fleckenstein JL, et al. (1993) Musculoskeletal manifestations of human immunodeficiency virus infection. Radiology 186:833–838

Strongin IS, Kale SA, Raymond MK, et al. (1991) An unusual presentation of gonococcal arthritis in an HIV-positive patient. Ann Rheum Dis 50:572–573

Tehranzadeh J (1997) Musculoskeletal infection in the immunocompromised patient. In: Taveras JM, Ferrucci JT (eds) Radiology: diagnosis - imaging - intervention. Lippincott-Raven, Philadelphia, Chap. 30, pp 1–20

Tehranzadeh J, Butler D (1994) Musculoskeletal lymphoma in AIDS. In: Tehranzadeh J, Steinbach LS (eds) Musculoskeletal manifestations of AIDS. Warren H. Green, St. Louis, pp 123–144

Tehranzadeh J, Cassady C (1994) Miscellaneous musculoskeletal conditions associated with HIV infection. In: Tehranzadeh J, Steinbach LS (eds) Musculoskeletal manifestations of AIDS. Warren H. Green, St. Louis, pp 163–174

Tehranzadeh J, Mesgarzadeh M (1994) Musculoskeletal infection in HIV-positive patients. In: Tehranzadeh J, Steinbach

L (eds) Musculoskeletal manifestations of AIDS. Warren H. Green, St. Louis, pp 3–43

Tehranzadeh J, Steinbach L (1994) Musculoskeletal manifestations of AIDS. Warren H. Green, St. Louis, pp 1–181

Tehranzadeh J, Wong CH (1994) Tuberculosis and other atypical mycobacterial infections in AIDS patients. In: Tehranzadeh J, Steinbach LS (eds) Musculoskeletal manifestations of AIDS. Warren H. Green, St. Louis, pp 63–83

Tehranzadeh J, Wang F, Mesgarzadeh M (1992) Magnetic resonance imaging of osteomyelitis. Crit Rev Diagn Imaging 33:495–534

Tehranzadeh J, Steinbach L, Mesgarzadeh M (1995) Musculoskeletal manifestations of AIDS. Part I. Inflammation, infection, and arthritides. Contemp Diagn Radiol 18:1–5

Townsend DJ, Singer DI, Doyle JR (1994) *Candida* tenosynovitis in an AIDS patient: a case report. J Hand Surg [Am] 19:293–294

Vanarthos W, Ganz WI, Vanarthos JC, et al. (1992) Diagnostic uses of nuclear medicine in AIDS. Radiographics 12:731–749

Vinetz JM, Rickman LS (1991) Chronic arthritis due to *Mycobacterium avium* complex infection in a patient with the acquired immunodeficiency syndrome. Arthritis Rheum 34:1339–1340

Widrow C, Kellie S, Saltzman BR, et al. (1991) Pyomyositis in patients with human immunodeficiency virus: an unusual form of disseminated bacterial infection. Am J Med 91:129–136

Wiley C, Nerenberg M, Cros D, et al. (1989) HTLV-1 polymyositis in a patient also infected with the HIV virus. N Engl J Med 320:992–995

Winchester RW, Solomon G (1987) Reiter's syndrome and acquired immunodeficiency. In: Espinoza L, Goldenberg D, Arnett F, et al. (eds) Infections in rheumatic diseases. Grune and Stratton, Orlando, pp 343–347

Winchester R, Bernstein DH, Fischer HD, et al. (1987) The co-occurrence of Reiter's syndrome and acquired immunodeficiency. Ann Intern Med 106:19–26

Winchester R, Brancato L, Itescu S, et al. (1988) Implications from the occurrence of Reiter's syndrome and related disorders in association with advanced HIV infection. Scand J Rheumatol Suppl 74:89–93

Withrington RH, Cornes P, Harris JRW, et al. (1987) Isolation of human immunodeficiency virus from synovial fluid of a patient with reactive arthritis. Br Med J 294:484

Woods SM, Gernaat HB (1992) Gonococcal osteomyelitis in a Zambian patient with AIDS. Trop Doct 22:47–48

Wu CM, Davis F, Fishman EK (1998) Musculoskeletal complications of the patients with acquired immunodeficiency syndrome (AIDS): CT evaluation. Semin Ultrasound CT MR 19:200–208

Wyatt SH, Fishman EK (1995) CT/MRI of musculoskeletal complications of AIDS. Skeletal Radiol 24:481–488

13 Dermatologic HIV/AIDS-Related Disorders

Hendrik J. Hulsebosch

CONTENTS

13.1
Introduction

From the onset, the human immunodeficiency virus/ acquired immunodeficiency syndrome (HIV/AIDS) epidemic was accompanied by the development of HIV/AIDS dermatology (TSCHACHLER et al. 1996). The gradual deterioration of the immune system resulted in a variety of skin complications that often were a diagnostic challenge for the clinician. Sometimes such complications consisted in well-recognized diseases such as seborrheic dermatitis and asteatosis cutis, but patients also presented with unusual and often severe clinical expressions of skin infections caused by known or new agents, such as herpes simplex, herpes zoster, hairy leukoplakia, bacillary

H.J. HULSEBOSCH, MD
Department of Dermatology, Academic Medical Centre, AO-237, University of Amsterdam, Meibergdreef 9, 1105 AZ Amsterdam, The Netherlands

angiomatosis, cryptococcosis, and histoplasmosis. And there was Kaposi's sarcoma, one of the milestones of the HIV/AIDS epidemic.

With the introduction of highly active antiretroviral therapy (HAART) around 1997, a reverse process started that has changed the dermatologic HIV/ AIDS picture dramatically. Immune restoration, or reconstitution, by HAART has been accompanied by the spontaneous disappearance of skin complications (COSTNER and COCKERELL 1998; HENGGE et al. 2000). However, new phenomena are now being seen, e.g., the development of herpes zoster a few months after the initiation of HAART and the appearance of unsuspected mycobacterial infections (COSTNER and COCKERELL 1998). In addition, there are the side-effects of the antiretroviral drugs, comprising not only drug eruptions but also the fat redistribution syndrome, alopecia, dry skin, cheilitis, paronychia, pruritic skin conditions, and gynecomastia (CARR and COOPER 2000). The influence of longer survival times of patients on the occurrence of skin cancer after a period of immune deficiency is still unknown.

This chapter aims to present an overview of the dermatologic HIV/AIDS-related disorders that occur in the two symptomatic phases of the HIV infection, the primary disease, immediately after HIV has entered the body, and the late stage, when HIV-induced immunodeficiency and AIDS are present. In addition to this, the cutaneous side-effects of HAART will be presented.

13.2
Primary HIV Infection

Primary infection with HIV1 is symptomatic in the majority of cases, with an incubation time of 1–4 weeks and a duration of about 2 weeks. The clinical picture of acute HIV infection varies from influenza-like symptoms to an illness in which the main clinical features are fever ranging from 38° to 40°C, malaise, diarrhea, myalgia, arthralgia, sore throat, headache, lymphadenopathy, and a skin rash. The exanthem consists of maculopapular, roseola-like lesions, sometimes with a central crust, that is typically either disseminated over the upper part of the body or generalized, encompassing the palms and soles (Fig. 13.1). In addition, there is an exanthem with superficial ulcerations. Genital and anal mucosal ulcerations can also be present. During the early stages of primary HIV infection, HIV p24 antigen can be demonstrated in plasma, usually before seroconversion to HIV antibodies takes place. As clinical improvement occurs, so the p24 antigen decreases, while antibody tests become positive after a window phase. As a consequence, sequential testing for HIV antibodies in the serum to document seroconversion can be necessary. The main differential diagnosis of primary HIV infection is secondary syphilis, because of similarities in skin symptoms and the sexual risk behavior in patients' histories (DE JONG et al. 1991).

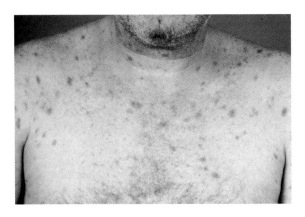

Fig. 13.1. HIV exanthema, part of the primary HIV infection

13.3
Dermatologic Diseases Associated with HIV-Induced Progressive Immunodeficiency

When HIV-induced immunodeficiency develops, finally resulting in AIDS, three groups of HIV-associated skin diseases can be distinguished: infectious dermatoses, skin tumors, and a group of noninfectious, nontumorous skin diseases. Table 13.1 provides an overview. Systematic grouping of HIV-associated dermatologic diseases increases insight and is of practical use when making a (differential) diagnosis.

13.3.1
Infectious Skin Diseases

13.3.1.1
Viral Infections

Viral skin and mucous membrane infections are frequently seen in HIV infection. The clinical picture can be atypical and the course chronic, without the usual spontaneous healing. Besides viral cultures, histopathologic examination, including the use of monoclonal antibodies to detect viruses, may be necessary to make the correct diagnosis.

Herpes simplex virus (HSV) is often the cause of chronic ulcerations, especially in the anogenital region. These ulcerations vary from a small fissure-like chronic defect in the anal rim to large ulcers (Fig. 13.2). Herpes simplex disseminata is another possible presentation, with small ulcerative lesions disseminated over the body. As a matter of routine, every ulcerative lesion in an HIV-infected individual should be cultured for viruses, especially HSV. Acyclovir resistance can be a treatment problem.

Table 13.1. HIV-associated dermatoses

Infectious dermatoses	Tumors	Noninfectious, nontumorous skin diseases
Viral infections	Kaposi's sarcoma	Erythematosquamous dermatoses
Bacterial infections	Lymphomas	Macular and/or papular
Dermatoses	Skin carcinomas	Itchy dermatoses
Fungal infections	Melanoma	Vesiculobullous dermatoses
Protozoan infections		Solitary dermatologic conditions
Infestations		Nail disorders
		Hair disorders
		Pigment disorders
		Oral disorders

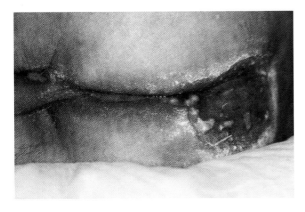

Fig. 13.2. Chronic herpes simplex ulcera in the anal area

Varicella-zoster virus is responsible for herpes zoster, known to be an early clinical sign of developing immunodeficiency. Later on in HIV infection, varicella-zoster disseminata can be observed. Hyperkeratotic varicella-zoster with wart-like lesions is a new entity in the HIV era (Fig. 13.3). Here, too, acyclovir resistance of the virus can be a problem.

Human papilloma virus infections, such as verrucae vulgares, verrucae planae and condylomata acuminata, generally produce familiar clinical pictures, but vary in seriousness and chronicity. Attention should be paid to the oncogenic potential of some of the viral strains with respect to cervical and anal cancer (PALEFSKI 1994) (Fig. 13.4).

Oral hairy leukoplakia was first described in HIV-infected individuals. This new disease of the mucous membranes is caused by the Epstein-Barr virus. The clinical picture consists in linear or sometimes more blotchy white lesions on the lateral sides of the tongue (Fig. 13.5).

Molluscum contagiosum, a harmless self-limiting infection in children, can be opportunistic in HIV-infected patients. The clinical picture varies from the well-known dome-shaped white papules with dull white macules or flat papules, to tumorous and cyst-like lesions (Fig. 13.6). They may be present in large numbers. There is a predilection for the face, especially the beard region.

Cytomegalovirus (CMV) infection of the skin as a primary disease seems to be rare. CMV can be found in histopathologic sections of known dermatoses in HIV-infected patients and is probably secondary to a generalized infection. CMV is sometimes cultured from skin ulcers, especially in the perianal region.

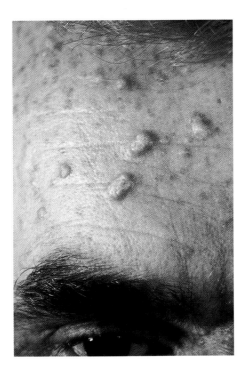

Fig. 13.3. Chronic hyperkeratotic varicella-zoster virus infection

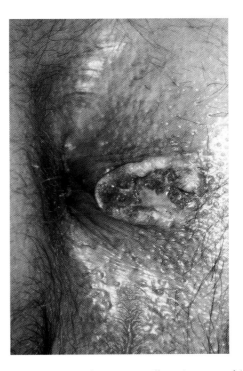

Fig. 13.4. Perianal squamous cell carcinoma resulting from condylomata acuminata

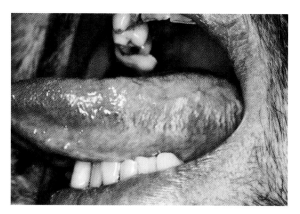

Fig. 13.5. Hairy leukoplakia

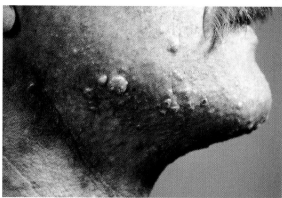

Fig. 13.6. Molluscum contagiosum

13.3.1.2
Bacterial Infections

Bacterial infections of the skin are seen less frequently in HIV-infected patients than viral infections, except in young children, in whom the converse is true.

Pyodermas, caused by *Staphylococcus aureus* and *Streptococcus pyogenes*, can present with unusual clinical pictures. Examples are candidiasis-like intertriginous infections, plaque-like lesions that can be treatment resistant, botryomycosis, and pruritic *Staphylococcus aureus* folliculitis. The last-mentioned is in the differential diagnosis of itch in HIV infection.

Pseudomonas aeruginosa can be the cause of abscesses.

Mycobacterial skin infections, caused by *Mycobacterium tuberculosis* and *Mycobacterium avium-intracellulare* complex, in general are part of systemic disease. They appear as erythematous nodi, skin ulcers, miliary tuberculosis, or lichen scrofulosorum.

Primary syphilis is one of the genital ulcer diseases that play an epidemiologic role in HIV transmission. In the differential diagnosis one should be aware of ulcus molle, lymphogranuloma venereum, donovanosis, and, of course, herpes simplex. Secondary syphilis can present with ulcerative skin lesions, syphilis maligna. In HIV-infected patients the symptomatic stages of syphilis can succeed each other more quickly than is usual; this is especially true for central nervous system involvement, and demands an adequate therapeutic regimen. Syphilis serology can provide unusual results, varying from false-negative to abnormally high titers (ENGELKENS et al. 1991).

Bacillary angiomatosis, initially known as epithelioid angiomatosis and cat-scratch disease in AIDS, is a disease newly recognized in HIV infection and is caused by *Bartonella* (formerly *Rochalimaea*) *henselae* or *B. quintana*. It is characterized

by erythematous, indurated, nodular to tumorous skin lesions, with involvement of internal organs (KOEHLER et al. 1992) (Fig. 13.7).

13.3.1.3
Fungal Infections

Candidiasis of the oral cavity can be an early symptom of HIV infection. When esophageal candidiasis develops, this implies AIDS.

Pityrosporum ovale causes pityriasis versicolor, but more important in HIV-infected patients is pity-

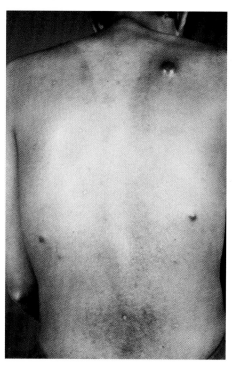

Fig. 13.7. Bacillary angiomatosis; erythematous nodular lesions

rosporal folliculitis, which is in the differential diagnosis of itch.

Fungal infections of the feet, including the nails, are quite common in immunocompetent individuals and will therefore also be frequently seen in HIV-infected individuals. White nails caused by *Trichophyton* species are a special feature in HIV infection. Fungal infections of the groins may show the familiar picture, an elevated border and central healing, but the presentation may be atypical, with erythematosquamous eczematous eruptions.

One should be prepared for rare fungal infections, the most important being cryptococcosis, histoplasmosis, coccidioidomycosis, and sporotrichosis. In general, cryptococcosis and histoplasmosis, presenting with skin lesions, are disseminated infections. The skin lesions vary from papulopustular and plaque-like lesions to molluscum contagiosum- and herpes-like eruptions (Figs. 13.8, 13.9). Making the diagnosis is important with regard to recognition of internal disease, especially involvement of the central nervous system.

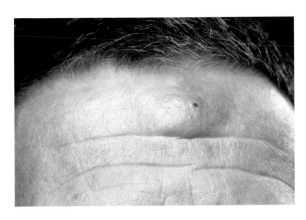

Fig. 13.8. Cryptococcosis; edematous area with central umbilicated ulcer

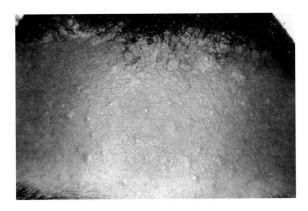

Fig. 13.9. Histoplasmosis; papular eruptions disseminated over the whole body

13.3.1.4
Protozoan Infections

Skin manifestations due to Protozoa in general are part of systemic infection. From the dermatologic point of view, leishmaniasis is prominent; amebiasis, toxoplasmosis, and *Pneumocystis carinii* infection are only occasionally the cause of skin eruptions.

Leishmaniasis may appear as a primary cutaneous infection; however, inconspicuous papular skin lesions may be a symptom of visceral leishmaniasis. Sexual transmission seems possible.

13.3.1.5
Infestations

Sarcoptes scabiei infestation is one of the causes of itch in HIV infection. The clinical picture varies from the usual to Norwegian scabies.

Demodex folliculitis is also in the differential diagnosis of itch in HIV infection.

13.3.2
Tumors

Kaposi's sarcoma is the main skin tumor in HIV infection. The histopathology shows a proliferation of endothelial cells with vessel-like structures and slits containing erythrocytes. In older lesions, a spindle cell component is present, representing transformed endothelial cells. Epidemiologic data give support to a sexually transmissible agent, facilitated by HIV. In 1994, human herpesvirus 8 (HHV8), also called Kaposi sarcoma-associated herpes virus (KSHV), was identified as the probable causative organism (CHANG et al. 1994).

Kaposi's sarcoma of the skin is a polymorphic disease. The "typical" lesion is an oval purple-red nodular lesion with the axis following the lines of cleavage of the skin (Fig. 13.10). But lesions can also be plaque-like, psoriasiform or deep-seated nodules, and on the nose, lupus pernio-like. Obstruction of the lymphatics may cause lymphedema, especially of the legs (Fig. 13.11), of the genitals, and around the eyes. Internal localizations may represent a serious complication. Skin lesions can be treated locally with intralesional diluted vinblastine, radiotherapy, cryosurgery, or infra-red irradiation. When the disease is extensive, systemic chemotherapy can be indicated (LILENBAUM and RATNER 1994).

B cell and T cell lymphomas are also quite common in HIV-infected patients. Skin lesions may be

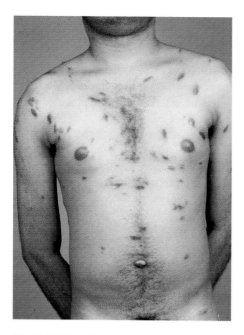

Fig. 13.10. Kaposi's sarcoma

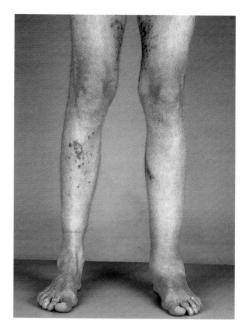

Fig. 13.11. Kaposi's sarcoma on both legs with complicating lymphedema of the left leg

part of the disease and may be the revealing symptom, varying from erythematous nodules to skin ulcers (Figs. 13.12, 13.13).

To date, skin cancers and melanoma have been relatively rare in HIV infection, possibly because the patients are usually young when infected. A longer lifespan induced by HAART may result in an increase in these malignancies.

13.3.3
Noninfectious, Nontumorous Skin Diseases

Noninfectious, nontumorous skin diseases in HIV infection can be subdivided according to clinical characteristics, when necessary in conjunction with histopathologic criteria (Table 13.1). The two main groups are erythematosquamous dermatoses and itchy skin diseases.

13.3.3.1
Erythematosquamous Dermatoses

Seborrheic dermatitis is frequently seen in HIV infection, often as an early skin symptom. Since it is a common disease in non-HIV-infected persons, its presence should not be considered indicative of HIV infection in patients in the HIV risk groups. HIV infection is often accompanied by dry skin, which may develop into asteatotic eczema or even acquired

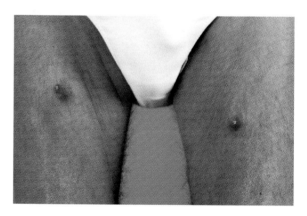

Fig. 13.12. Immunoblastic, non-Hodgkin B-cell AIDS-related lymphoma

ichthyosis. In addition, psoriasis, psoriasiform eruptions, Reiter's disease, pityriasis rosea, pityriasis rubra pilaris, acrodermatitis enteropathica, lichen spinulosus, and Kawasaki syndrome have been described in HIV infection. Drug eruptions are part of the differential diagnosis. Erythroderma may be a complication of the aforementioned diseases.

13.3.3.2
Itchy Skin Diseases

Itch is a frequent complaint in HIV-infected patients, with a multitude of causes. A subdivision into nonfol-

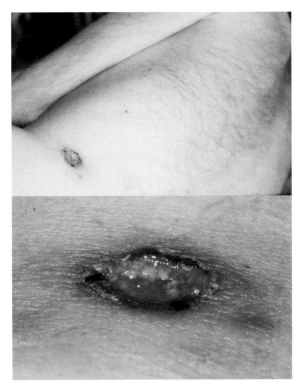

Fig. 13.13. Anaplastic Ki-1-positive T cell lymphoma

licular and follicular itchy skin diseases can be made. The first group includes the prurigo parasitaria-like eruption in HIV infection, the pruritic papular eruption of AIDS, dry skin, seborrheic dermatitis and other eczematous conditions, the hypereosinophilic syndrome, drug eruptions, scabies, prurigo, and pruritus, i.e., itch without perceptible skin disease. In the second group, erythematous papular or papulopustular follicular eruptions occur, including eosinophilic pustular folliculitis in HIV infection (formerly thought to be analogous to Ofuji's disease but, because of a different clinical picture, now distinguished from this entity), pityrosporal folliculitis, *Demodex* folliculitis, itchy *Staphylococcus aureus* folliculitis, itchy folliculitis e.c.i. and itchy folliculitis with a combination of the causes mentioned (HULSEBOSCH 1992).

13.3.3.3
Hair and Nails

HIV/AIDS-associated abnormalities of the hair are thinning, premature greying, and long eye lashes. Nail changes comprise the yellow nail syndrome, zidovudine pigmentation, and, besides the well-known clinical picture of onychomycosis, proximal white subun-

gual onychomycosis that is seen as pathognomonic for HIV infection.

13.3.4
Dermatologic Diseases in Relation to Immunodeficiency

The skin diseases described in this chapter are derived from the HIV literature and may be called HIV associated. This implies that when a patient at risk appears to have one of these diseases, HIV infection may be suspected. But one has to be careful, because most of these skin diseases can also be seen in non-HIV-infected individuals. Only a few skin diseases are AIDS defining. In general, it is impossible to make the diagnosis of HIV infection or AIDS on the basis of skin symptoms alone. Some diseases, however, can be an indication of severe immunodeficiency, represented by low CD4+ lymphocyte counts. Based on investigations in a group of 530 HIV-infected patients with a total of 1,754 dermatovenereal diagnoses who were seen at the Academic Medical Centre in Amsterdam between the beginning of the HIV epidemic and July 1992, it was concluded that herpes simplex ulcera, herpes simplex and varicella-zoster disseminata, hyperkeratotic varicella-zoster, molluscum contagiosum, lymphomas, asteatotic eczema, and acquired ichthyosis are cutaneous signs of severe immunodeficiency. In spite of this, the diagnosis of AIDS, according to the 1987 CDC definition, in general had been made in only about half of the patients with these diseases (HULSEBOSCH 1993).

13.4
Highly Active Antiretroviral Therapy

Highly active antiretroviral therapy (HAART) is a combination of at least three antiretroviral drugs. These belong to three main groups: the nucleoside reverse transcriptase inhibitors (NRTIs), the non-nucleoside reverse transcriptase inhibitors (NNR-TIs), and the protease inhibitors.

As already mentioned in the introduction, HAART has brought about a revolution in HIV/AIDS treatment. With the increase in CD4-positive T lymphocytes and the decrease in the HIV viral load, often to undetectable levels, opportunistic and other infections disappear. This holds true even for many of the dermatologic HIV/AIDS-related dermatoses, including Kaposi's sarcoma (COSTNER and COCKERELL

1998; Hengge et al. 2000). Remission of Kaposi's sarcoma is accompanied by undetectable levels of HHV8 (Dupont et al. 2000; Boivin et al. 2000).

The major toxic effects of the NRTIs, particularly over the medium to long term, are thought to be secondary to inhibition of mitochondrial DNA polymerase gamma, resulting in impaired synthesis of mitochondrial enzymes that generate ATP by oxidative phosphorylation. These side-effects include myopathy, neuropathy, hepatic steatosis and lactic acidemia, pancreatitis, and possibly also peripheral lipoatrophy. Mitochondrial toxicities at the clinical level are generally gradual in onset and disappearance, but they may occur within days of the start of therapy. Another striking feature of these toxicities is their relative tissue-specific and drug-specific nature. Of course, most patients on HAART do not develop mitochondrial toxicity (Carr and Cooper 2000).

13.4.1
Drug Eruptions

Drug hypersensitivity typically manifests as an erythematous, maculopapular, pruritic, and confluent rash, with or without fever. The rash is most prominent on the body and arms and usually begins after 1–3 weeks of therapy. Constitutional features, including fever, rigors, myalgias, and arthralgias, are often prominent and can precede the rash or occur without a rash. Stevens-Johnson syndrome and toxic epidermal necrolysis develop in less than 0.5% of patients. Drug hypersensitivity complicated 3%–20% of all prescriptions in one large series of HIV/AIDS patients. All licensed NRTIs, the NRTI abacavir, and the protease inhibitor amprenavir are common antiretroviral drugs that cause hypersensitivity. Hypersensitivity is rare with the other drugs. In cases of fever, other causes such as infection, malignancy, or immune restoration have to be considered (Carr and Cooper 2000).

13.4.2
Lipodystrophy

The lipodystrophy syndrome, or fat redistribution syndrome, was first described in 1998 in patients on HAART. Its main clinical features are peripheral fat loss from the face, limbs, and buttocks and central fat accumulation within the abdomen, the breasts, and over the dorsocervical area; the so called buffalo hump and also lipomas can occur (Fig. 13.14). The

overall prevalence is about 50% after 12–18 months of therapy. Associated symptoms include hypertriglyceridemia, hypercholesterolemia, insulin resistance, and type II diabetes mellitus. Cardiovascular disease is a matter of concern. The pathogenesis of the syndrome is still unknown (Carr and Cooper 2000; Paparizos et al. 2000; Moreno and Martínez, 2000).

13.4.3
Other Cutaneous Side-effects
of Antiretroviral Drugs

The NRTI zidovudine can cause nail pigmentation, and zalcitabine can cause mouth ulcers. Indinavir seems to be unique among the protease inhibitors in being associated with adverse effects similar to those seen with retinoid therapy, namely alopecia, dry skin, dry lips, and ingrowing nails (Carr and Cooper 2000; García-Silva et al. 2000).

13.4.4
The Immune Restoration
or Immune Reconstitution Syndrome

The restoration of the immune defenses by HAART leads to the disappearance of many HIV/AIDS-com-

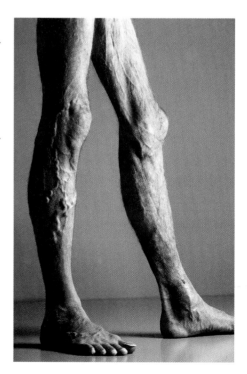

Fig. 13.14. Lipodystrophy; blood vessels become prominent

plicating diseases, but paradoxically some diseases develop or worsen. Examples are herpes zoster developing a few months after initiation of HAART in severely immunocompromised patients, at CD4 cell counts that are comparable to those when they developed herpes zoster earlier in their HIV infection. Eosinophilic folliculitis and inflammatory folliculitis also can be part of the immune restoration syndrome. And a very curious complication is the development of disseminated mycobacterial cutaneous manifestations in patients in whom this infection was previously unsuspected (COSTNER and COCKERELL 1998; DEL GIUDICE et al. 1999) (Fig. 13.15).

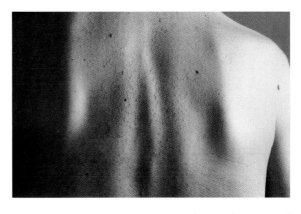

Fig. 13.15. Immune restoration syndrome, disseminated granulomatous papules in a patient on HAART with a history of *Mycobacterium kansasii* infection

13.5
Conclusion

This overview is certainly not complete. For further reading on the dermatologic HIV/AIDS-related disorders, the reader is referred to the book *Skin manifestations of AIDS* (PENNEYS 1995). HIV/AIDS dermatology is still on the move, especially as other side-effects of long-term treatments are still awaited.

References

Boivin G, Gaudreau A, Routy J-P (2000) Evaluation of the human herpesvirus 8 DNA load in blood and Kaposi's sarcoma skin lesions from AIDS patients on highly active antiretroviral therapy. AIDS 14:1907–1910

Bouscarat F, Maubec E, Matheron S, Descamp V (2000) Immune recovery inflammatory folliculitis. AIDS 14:617–618

Carr A, Cooper DA (2000) Adverse effects of antiretroviral therapy. Lancet 356:1423–1430

Chang Y. Cesarman E, Pessin MS, Culpepper J, Moore PS (1994) Identification of herpesvirus-like DNA sequences in AIDS-associated Kaposi's sarcoma. Science 266:1803–1804

Costner M, Cockerell CJ (1998) The changing spectrum of the cutaneous manifestations of HIV disease. Arch Dermatol 134:1290–1292

de Jong M, Hulsebosch HJ, Lange JMA (1991) Clinical and immunological features of primary HIV-1 infection. Genitourin Med 67:367–373

del Giudice P, Durant J, Counillon E, et al. (1999) Mycobacterial cutaneous manifestations: a new sign of immune restorations. Arch Dermatol 135:1129–1130

Dupont C, Vasseur E, Beauchet A, et al., on behalf of CISIH 92 (2000) Long-term efficacy on Kaposi's sarcoma of highly active antiretroviral therapy in a cohort of HIV-positive patients. AIDS 14:987–993

Engelkens HJ, Sluis J van der, Stolz E (1991) Syphilis in the AIDS era. Int J Dermatol 30:254–256

García-Silva J, Almagro M, Juega J, Peña C, López-Calvo S, Pozo J del, Fonseca E (2000) Protease inhibitor-related paronychia, ingrown toenails, desquamative cheilitis and cutaneous xerosis. AIDS 14:1289–1291

Hengge R, Franz B, Goos M (2000) Decline of infectious skin manifestations in the era of highly active antiretroviral therapy. AIDS 14:1069–1070

Hulsebosch HJ. AIDS and itch (1992) J Eur Acad Dermatol 1:311–318. Erratum, legends, figures (1993) J Eur Acad Dermatol 2:62

Hulsebosch HJ (1993) Huidziekten bij HIV-infecties. Thesis, University of Amsterdam

Koehler JE, Quinn FD, Berger TG, et al. (1992) Isolation of *Rochalimaea* species from cutaneous and osseous lesions of bacillary angiomatosis. N Engl J Med 327:1625–1631

Lilenbaum RC, Ratner L (1994) Systemic treatment of Kaposi's sarcoma: current status and future directions. AIDS 8:141–151

Moreno S, Martínez E (2000) Lipodystrophy and long-term therapy with nucleoside reverse transcriptase inhibitors. AIDS 14:905–906

Palefski JM (1994) Anal human papillomavirus infection and anal cancer in HIV-positive individuals: an emerging problem. AIDS 8:283–295

Paparizos VA, Kyriakis KP, Botsis C, Papastamopoulos M, Hadjivassiliou M, Stavrianeas NG (2000) Protease inhibitor therapy-associated lipodystrophy, hypertriglyceridaemia and diabetes mellitus. AIDS 14:903–905

Penneys NS (1995) Skin manifestations of AIDS, 2nd edn. Martin Dunitz, London

Tschachler E, Bergstresser PR, Stingl G (1996) HIV-related diseases. Lancet 348:659–663

14 Pediatric AIDS Imaging

A. Geoffray, M. Spehl, A. Deville

CONTENTS

14.1
Introduction

The presentation of AIDS in children is quite different from that in adults. For example, in children a clinical manifestation of infection or tumor less frequently leads to the diagnosis. In fact, 90% of children with AIDS are now infected by maternofetal transmission and the disease is diagnosed at birth, by biologic tests. There are two presentations in chil-

dren: in the first group, representing 25% of infected individuals, the disease occurs early and is very severe; in the second group, the disease develops later, after an asymptomatic period which can last several years. Manifestations of AIDS in children are generally pulmonary. Gastrointestinal and central nervous system (CNS) infections are much rarer than in adults. Neoplasms are also rarer than in adults but may occur.

14.2
Thoracic Involvement

14.2.1
Lung-Related Diseases

Pulmonary complications occur in almost 80% of children infected with the human immunodeficiency virus (HIV). Lymphocytic interstitial pneumonitis and infections are the main etiologies.

Lymphocytic Interstitial Pneumonitis (LIP). LIP occurs secondary to infiltration of the alveolar and interlobular septa by lymphocytes and plasma cells. It has also been called pulmonary lymphoid hyperplasia. Children with LIP are usually asymptomatic but may present with cough, dyspnea, and hypoxia. Parotidomegaly and peripheral lymphadenopathy are common associated features. Chest radiographs typically show diffuse micronodular opacities (Fig. 14.1) with or without hilar enlargement but at times are nonspecific, with prominent bronchovascular or sometimes localized heterogeneous opacities (Berdon et al. 1993). Diagnosis was previously made by open lung biopsy, but this is rarely performed now. Bronchoalveolar lavage is not specific but large numbers of CD8 lymphocytes are com-

A. Geoffray, MD
Chief of Pediatric Radiology, Fondation Lenval, 57 avenue de la Californie, 06200 Nice, France
M. Spehl, MD
Professor of Radiology, Hopital universitaire Saint Pierre, 322 rue Haute, 1000 Bruxelles, Belgium
A. Deville, MD
Pediatric Oncology, Fondation Lenval, 57 avenue de la Californie, 06200 Nice, France

Most of the figures shown in this chapter were published in *Journal de Radiologie*, 1997; 78:1233–1243, and are reproduced here with the permission of the publisher

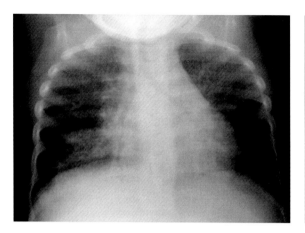

Fig. 14.1. Lymphocytic interstitial pneumonitis. Asymptomatic 5-year-old girl. A chest radiograph demonstrates multiple more or less confluent micronodules and mediastinal lymphadenopathy

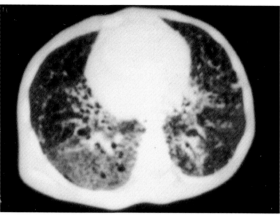

Fig. 14.2. Bronchiectasis. Same child as in Fig. 14.1, 6 years later. A chest CT reveals multiple dilated bronchi coexisting with persistent interstitial disease

monly seen. Computed tomography (CT) is more sensitive to subtle interstitial opacities than chest radiographs (AMBROSINO et al. 1995) but is nonspecific. Radiologic abnormalities may resolve with corticosteroid therapy or even spontaneously. Secondary infections are frequent but children with LIP have a better prognosis than others. With prolonged survival, complications of LIP have appeared. The pathogenesis of bronchiectasis is probably multifactorial. It may be due to LIP itself or secondary to chronic abnormalities of the mucociliary apparatus that result in chronic atelectasis. The role of superimposed infection cannot be excluded. CT is useful in the diagnosis of bronchiectasis (Fig. 14.2), especially in cases of chronic atelectasis. The CD4 T lymphocyte count is less than 100 cells/mm³ in all cases of bronchiectasis (SHEIKH et al. 1997). LIP has also been described in adults (ETTENSOHN et al. 1988).

Pulmonary Infections. In children with HIV, pulmonary infections are very frequent; they represent the most common cause of death in this population (MAROLDA et al. 1991).

Bacterial pneumonia due to common pathogens such as *Streptococcus pneumoniae* or *Haemophilus influenzae* occurs often. Clinical signs are nonspecific. On chest films more extensive disease is seen than in non-HIV-infected children. Frequently multilobar homogeneous opacities are apparent. Hilar or paratracheal lymph node involvement is a common finding. Bronchoalveolar lavage may be required to identify the causal organism(s) so that appropriate antibiotic treatment can be administered.

Pneumocystis carinii pneumonia (PCP) used to be a common finding. Its frequency has decreased significantly in recent years, owing to early detection of HIV status and effective prophylactic therapy. However, PCP may still be the first manifestation of AIDS in children with previously unknown seropositivity. The diagnosis may then occasionally be made in an emergency situation with the child exhibiting respiratory distress. Chest films typically show a diffuse heterogeneous pattern which, with severe disease, will progress to associated focal and eventually diffuse homogeneous alveolar opacities (Fig. 14.3). Complications such as pneumothorax (SCHROEDER et al. 1995), pneumomediastinum, or cavitary or bullous disease may occur (Fig. 14.4). The diagnosis is typically made by identifying organisms on bron-

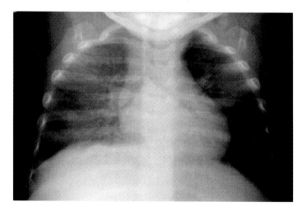

Fig. 14.3. *Pneumocystis carinii* pneumonia. Child with moderate respiratory distress. A chest film demonstrates interstitial disease without adenopathy

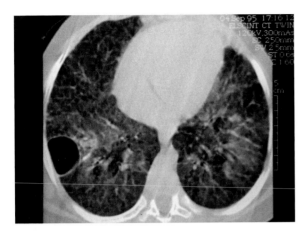

Fig. 14.4. *Pneumocystis carinii* pneumonia. Child with known PCP. CT demonstrates a bulla and bilateral ground-glass and reticular opacities. (Courtesy of Prof. J.P. Montagne, Hopital Trousseau, Paris)

choalveolar lavage; but if the child is too unstable, specific treatment may be initiated even without any laboratory proof. Rapid appearance of diffuse homogeneous opacities may suggest impending death. However, apart from this dramatic presentation, PCP is usually a more chronic disease. Clinical symptoms are nonspecific, as is the radiologic presentation. This is emphasized because PCP should be considered with a variety of chest film abnormalities (SIVIT et al. 1995). The chest film may even be normal in some cases, and in almost one-third of cases, abnormalities are minimal. In about 50% of cases, focal or scattered parenchymal lung abnormalities mimicking bacterial pneumonia may be the initial presentation. Hilar or mediastinal lymphadenopathy is rare in PCP and should suggest another etiology. Pleural effusion is also rare and most likely due to another or coexistent pathogen or neoplasm.

Tuberculosis (TB) is seen with increasing frequency in the HIV population (GOODMAN 1995). It is now the most common opportunistic infection in HIV-infected adults. TB also occurs in HIV-infected children, but the true role of HIV immunosuppression is difficult to assess because these children frequently live in poor economic conditions and in areas with high promiscuity, which are also factors in the development of TB. Clinically the child presents with fever and weakness. Radiographic findings may be nonspecific such as diffuse heterogeneous opacities which mimic other abnormalities, e.g., LIP or PCP (HALLER and GINSBERG 1997). Lobar consolidation or collapse, pleural effusion, and large hilar or paratracheal lymph nodes are more suggestive findings (BERDON et al. 1993). CT may better demon-

strate the abnormalities. Lymph nodes may have low attenuation values secondary to necrosis. This can also be seen with *Mycobacterium avium-intracellulare* complex (MAC) infections in adults but is not typical with other infections or lymphoma (HALLER and COHEN 1993). A miliary pattern may be encountered. Increase in the size of the miliary nodule is very suggestive of TB and distinguishes this entity from LIP. Because of the generally nonspecific radiographic pattern, TB is frequently included in the differential diagnosis and searched for on laboratory analysis. Extrapulmonary TB infection may coexist, especially in the CNS.

The presentation of MAC is similar to that of TB. Diagnosis relies on sputum analysis and cultures.

Other infections are possible: *Varicella or zoster* in the herpesvirus group may lead to interstitial pneumonia. *Cytomegalovirus* (CMV) is frequently encountered in HIV-infected children with pulmonary disease but its role is difficult to assess (AMBROSINO et al. 1992) Other concomitant diseases such as LIP, PCP, or bacterial pneumonia are frequently observed and are more likely responsible for the lung infection. On chest films, diffuse heterogeneous opacities may be suggestive of CMV but are nonspecific. *Toxoplasmosis* is rarely seen in children. *Cryptococcosis* may occur in older children with transfusion-associated HIV infection. Radiologically, peripheral infiltrates or nodules are associated with hilar lymphadenopathy and sometimes pleural effusion. A miliary pattern with hilar lymphadenopathy is also suggestive. Concomitant CNS involvement is frequent. *Aspergillosis* is rare but invasive disease with diffuse opacities and pleural effusion carries a poor prognosis (WRIGHT et al. 1993).

14.2.2
Cardiac Disease

Cardiac disease occurs in 50%–90% of HIV-infected children. The exact cause of cardiac disease is not clear. Direct infection by the virus is possible, but infection by other pathogens such as CMV, *Candida*, bacteria, or even MAC may play a role. Chest films reveal enlargement of the cardiac silhouette (Fig. 14.5). Echocardiography is the best way to evaluate these children. Cardiomyopathy with enlargement of the left and/or right ventricle and low contractility is the most common finding. Cases of myocarditis have been described; the causal agent is still unknown. Pericardial effusion may occur, and be confirmed by echocardiography. It should

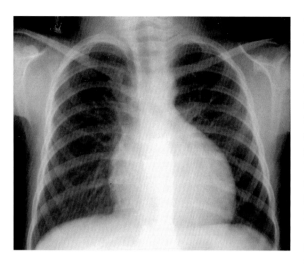

Fig. 14.5. Cardiomyopathy in a 5-year-old girl. A chest film reveals cardiac enlargement

be suspected even with a normal cardiac appearance on chest radiographs, especially if the child is refractory to pulmonary treatment.

14.2.3
Mediastinal Involvement

Lymph nodes are frequently seen and may be associated with several diseases: LIP, bacterial infection, TB, and lymphoma. They are nonspecific although necrotic low-attenuation nodes suggest TB and huge nodes suggest lymphoma.

Thymic involvement is often described as an incidental finding on chest films (Kontny et al. 1997). An anterior multicystic mediastinal mass is a typical appearance on CT. Pathologically, distortion of normal architecture with cystic changes, lymphoid hyperplasia, plasmacytosis, multinucleated giant cells, and HIV particles are found. Spontaneous regression is the rule, so follow-up chest films should be the only recommendation. Thymic volume seems to correlate with preserved immune function in HIV-infected children (Vigano et al. 1999).

14.3
Abdominal Involvement

Abdominal manifestations of AIDS in children are secondary to the HIV infection itself, to other infections (viral, bacterial, opportunistic, mycotic, etc.), or, less frequently, to neoplasm. Every organ may be involved.

14.3.1
Digestive Tract Manifestations

Esophagus. Oral and esophageal infections are most frequently due to *Candida*. Dysphagia and, in younger children, refusal to eat are the more common clinical symptoms. Diagnosis relies mainly on clinical appearance. If further evaluation is required, esophagoscopy seems more indicated than an esophagogram. Radiologic findings include ulcerations, "cobblestone" pattern, and abnormal motility. Esophageal thickening may be seen on US (Fig. 14.6). Other esophageal infections due to herpesvirus or CMV are also common.

Gastrointestinal Infections. Gastrointestinal (GI) infections (Haller and Cohen 1994; Stoane et al.

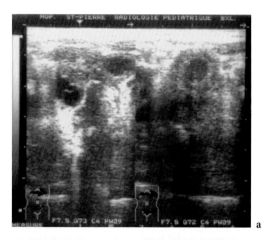

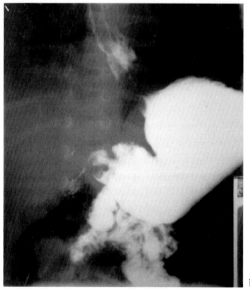

Fig. 14.6. a Esophageal candidiasis. Transverse US under the xyphoid process shows thickening of the esophageal wall. **b** Same child. A barium swallow reveals thickened folds

1996) affect approximately 50% of HIV-infected children. Clinical symptoms are diarrhea, vomiting, anorexia, abdominal pain, malabsorption, and weight loss. Several infectious agents are implicated and diagnosis relies on stool cultures. The diagnosis is usually easy to establish in cases of acute diarrhea, but can be more difficult with chronic diarrhea. The more commonly encountered causal agents are viruses (adenovirus, CMV), bacteria (*Salmonella, Shigella, Campylobacter, Clostridium difficile*, MAC), worms (*Strongyloides*), protozoa (*Cryptosporidium, Giardia, Isospora belli*), and fungi. Diagnosis depends much more on the laboratory results than on radiologic findings. Plain films of the abdomen show nonspecific findings such as bowel dilatation. Pneumatosis has been described in cases of CMV but is also seen with rotavirus or bacterial infection. Ultrasonography (US) may reveal lymphadenopathy, thickened mucosal folds (Fig. 14.7), and free intraabdominal fluid but is not specific for one agent or another. Upper and lower GI contrast studies are also not very specific. *Cryptosporidium* affects the upper intestine and produces fragmentation of barium, thick folds, spasm, and dilatation. CMV occurs in the small intestine and colon, and causes thick folds, ulcerations, spasm, and mucosal nodularity which are well seen on lower GI studies or CT. Severe cases may result in perforation. MAC (PURSNER et al. 2000) affects the distal part of the small intestine with fine nodularity and thick folds. Lesions in the liver, spleen, and nodes (the most common site) have a tumor-like appearance (Fig. 14.8).

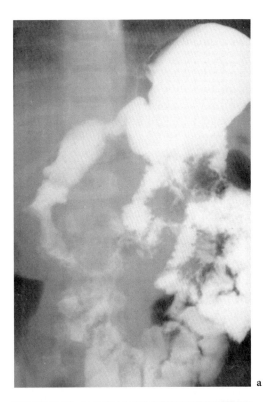

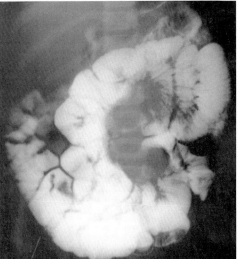

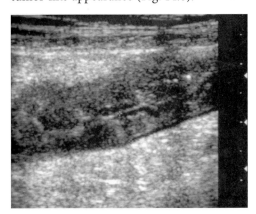

Fig. 14.7. Candidiasis of colon. A 12-year-old girl suffering from abdominal pain and diarrhea. US shows wall thickening of the left colon

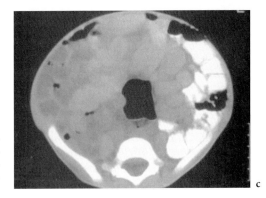

Fig. 14.8. a, b *Mycobacterium avium-intracellulare* complex (MAC). An 8-year-old girl with persistent diarrhea and poor general status. A barium study reveals displacement of bowel loops by extraluminal masses as well as nodular indentation of the duodenal wall. **c** CT scan in the same child reveals multiple juxtaposed nodes due to MAC

14.3.2
Liver and Biliary System

Hepatomegaly. Hepatomegaly is a frequent finding in children with AIDS. It is associated with abnormal hepatic function (HALLER and COHEN 1993) and may be due to hepatitis B or C or occur secondary to infections caused by MAC, TB, *Crypto-coccus*, *Histoplasma*, CMV, cat-scratch bacillus (*Bartonella henselae*), *Toxoplasma*, *Pneumocystis*, or *Microsporidium* (WOOD 1992). US findings are not specific (e.g., hyperechogenicity may be due to steatosis, a common finding). Acute panhepatic infection presents as a hypoechoic liver. Focal, usually hypoechoic lesions, may be encountered with TB, MAC, or PCP. The prognosis of hepatic infections depends on the patient's general condition, being worse when the infection is generalized. A biopsy may be necessary to identify the causal pathogen. Cytolytic or cholestatic hepatitis may also be secondary to drugs. Many hepatic abnormalities are not specific and several etiologies may be acting at the same time, making precise diagnosis difficult.

Tumor infiltration of the liver is usually due to lymphoma, although leiomyomas and leiomyosarcomas have been described and must be considered in the diagnosis of hepatic nodules or masses.

Biliary Complications. Acalculous cholangitis (RUSIN et al. 1992) and cholecystitis present with abdominal pain and fever, sometimes clinical jaundice, and evidence of cholestasis on liver function tests. US reveals enlargement of the intrahepatic and common bile duct. The gallbladder may also be enlarged, with wall thickening. *Cryptosporidium* seems to be a frequent causal agent (TEIXIDOR et al. 1991); CMV has also been incriminated.

14.3.3
Splenic Involvement

Splenomegaly is frequently identified and is usually related to infections. A nodular pattern (Fig. 14.9) is encountered in diseases such as MAC, CMV, cat-scratch disease, or PCP. The nodules of PCP may become calcified (Fig. 14.10). If US is performed with high-frequency transducers, small hypoechoic splenic nodules are often found; these may represent lymphoid infiltration, as in other organs (Fig. 14.11) (GEOFFRAY et al. 1997).

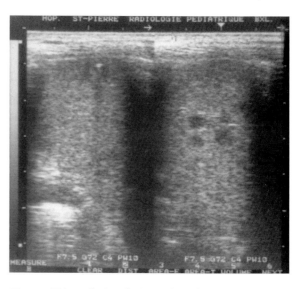

Fig. 14.9. Tuberculosis. Splenic US shows hypoechoic nodules

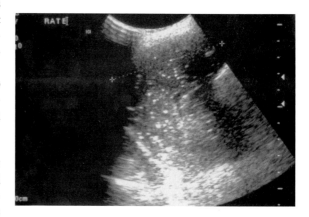

Fig. 14.10. Pneumocystosis. US reveals multiple splenic calcifications

14.3.4
Pancreatic Involvement

Pancreatic abnormalities are frequently found at autopsy of HIV-infected children but are rarely the cause of death (KAHN et al. 1995). Acute pancreatitis is usually due to treatment by 2',3'-dideoxyinosine (DDI) (LEVIN et al. 1997) (Fig. 14.12). Pentamidine has also been incriminated. An enlarged echogenic pancreas can be noted on US. Necrotizing pancreatitis (Fig. 14.13) sometimes occurs with pseudocyst formation; healing usually takes place when drug therapy is suspended. Pancreatitis may arise due to opportunistic infections, such as CMV, *Cryptosporidium*, MAC, or PCP. Tumor involvement of the pancreas is rare.

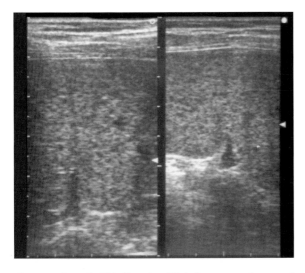

Fig. 14.11. Lymphoid infiltration. High-frequency ultrasound shows multiple hypoechoic micronodules in the spleen

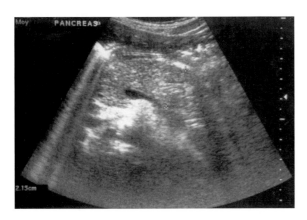

Fig. 14.12. Pancreatitis. A 4-year-old boy treated with DDI, who presented with sudden abdominal pain. US shows pancreatic enlargement secondary to iatrogenic pancreatitis

14.3.5
Retroperitoneal Disease

Kidneys. Renal disease in AIDS is mainly secondary to HIV infection but other infections as well as lymphoma may occur. HIV-associated nephropathy is characterized by the nephrotic syndrome and progressive renal failure (ZILLERUELO and STRAUSS 1995). Pathologically, focal glomerulosclerosis, mesangial hyperplasia, and microcystic dilated tubules are found. US reveals normal-sized dedifferentiated (Fig. 14.14) or enlarged hyperechoic kidneys. On CT, kidneys appear enlarged, mainly at the level of the pyramids. Opportunistic infections that involve the kidneys produce common sonographic findings [e.g., focal hyperechogenicity in bacterial pyelonephritis, pyelocaliceal thickening (WACHSBERG et al. 1995), or even abscesses if the infection is complicated]. Calcifications have been described with PCP or MAC.

There are also complications secondary to treatment. The protease inhibitor indinavir may crystallize in the urine, resulting in obstruction (NOBLE et al. 1998); the stones are radiolucent on plain films.

Simple renal cysts have been described more frequently in HIV-infected children than in normal children (ZINN et al. 1997). Renal masses due to lymphoma or leiomyosarcoma may also be seen (NORTON et al. 1997).

Abdominal lymphadenopathy. Abdominal lymphadenopathy is related to HIV infection, other infections, or neoplasm. Lymphadenopathy due to HIV infection is frequent in the abdomen and in peripheral lymph node areas. US examination with a high-frequency transducer now allows the frequent visualization of small lymph

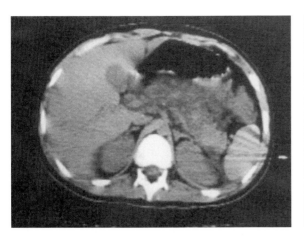

Fig. 14.13. Pancreatitis. CT reveals necrotizing pancreatitis in a 13-year-old boy following DDI treatment

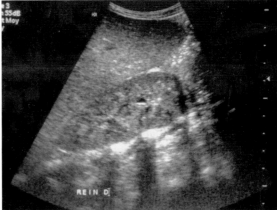

Fig. 14.14. HIV-associated nephropathy. US reveals a dedifferentiated kidney pattern in an HIV-infected child

nodes. The hepatic hilum and celiomesenteric regions are frequently involved with lymphadenopathy related to HIV or to concomitant hepatitis. These nodes do not usually cause symptoms but may occasionally compress the biliary duct, causing acalculous cholecystitis. Lymphadenopathy due to other infections is frequent. One particular and quite typical appearance is encountered with MAC infection, namely multiple, round nodes of intermediate size (Fig. 14.8c) in the iliomesenteric, lumbo-aortic, and iliac regions. These nodes can become large and mimic tumor. On CT, the appearance is suggestive if multiple distinct juxtaposed lymph nodes form a mass which displaces bowel (NYBERG et al. 1985). The node density is usually intermediate; low attenuation values should suggest TB but are also possible with MAC (PURSNER et al. 2000). Differentiation from lymphoma may be suggested if the lymph nodes are confluent and the bowel is infiltrated rather than displaced.

14.4
CNS Disease

Neurologic abnormalities are frequent in children with AIDS. HIV encephalopathy is the most common disorder. Opportunistic infections are rarer than in adults; tumors are usually lymphomas.

14.4.1
HIV Encephalopathy

Clinically, there are two different groups of patients (TARDIEU 1991). The first group includes infants who develop disease early during the first months of life, with severe immunodeficiency and multiple opportunistic infections (NOZYCE et al. 1994). Neurologic symptoms occur during the first year of life; developmental delay, cognitive impairment, and pyramidal signs are the main manifestations. The prognosis of these children is poor, death usually occurring during the early years.

The second group includes older children who remain virtually asymptomatic during the first 2 years. Neurologic symptoms occur later, comprising motor deficits and cognitive abnormalities (as in the first group) or acquired dementia (as in adults). HIV causes encephalitis or leukoencephalopathy. In infants, transfontanellar US may be the first study to reveal atrophy, identified on the basis of ventricular and pericerebral enlargement or basal ganglia calcifica-

tions. CT also demonstrates cerebral atrophy, characterized by ventricular enlargement associated with large pericerebral spaces. These findings are seen in almost all children (90%) when clinical signs are present (KAUFFMAN et al. 1992). Atrophy may also be related to significant weight loss and malnutrition. CT may show focal hypodensities due to abnormality of the white matter [better appreciated on magnetic resonance imaging (MRI)] or calcifications within the basal ganglia (Fig. 14.15) and less frequently in the periventricular frontal white matter. In older children with slowly progressive illness, CT is often normal. MRI should be preferred to CT when analyzing white matter abnormalities. It demonstrates bilateral, symmetric or asymmetric, high signal intensity in the periventricular white matter on proton density, T2-weighted, or FLAIR (fast-fluid attenuated inversion-recovery) images (Fig. 14.16). These areas correspond to demyelination and gliosis.

14.4.2
Opportunistic Infections

Infections of the CNS are infrequently seen in children as compared with adults. In a series of 65 autopsy cases (WROZLEK et al. 1995), they were seen in 14% of the pediatric cases but in 50% of the adult cases. They are probably more frequent in adults owing to

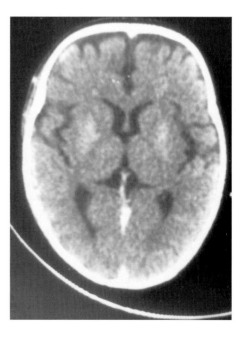

Fig. 14.15. HIV encephalopathy. Subtle calcification of the basal ganglia in a 1-year-old girl is demonstrated on CT

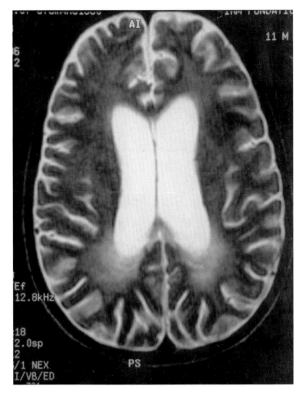

Fig. 14.16. HIV encephalopathy. An 11-year-old boy with recent neurologic symptoms and severe immunodeficiency. MRI reveals high signal intensity of the posterior periventricular white matter

reactivation of a latent pathogen which most children would not have encountered.

Toxoplasmosis, frequently encountered in adults, is rarely seen in children and usually appears in similar fashion to its congenital presentation in immunocompetent children. A few cases of postnatally acquired cerebral toxoplasmosis with brain abscesses, as seen in adults, have, however, been described (TACCONE et al. 1992).

CMV infection is the most frequent cause of secondary CNS infection in children (POST et al. 1986). Pathologically, necrotizing encephalomyelitis with a subependymal and subpial distribution of lesions is observed. On CT or MRI there are findings of atrophy, ventricular enlargement, and periventricular enhancement.

Progressive multifocal leukoencephalopathy due to papovavirus infection is possible, although not as common as in adults. On MRI there is extensive high signal intensity of the white matter, extending to the cortex, including involvement of the U fibers.

Cryptococcosis occurs mainly in children who have become HIV positive through contaminated blood products. Multiple small abscesses, located peripherally near the cortex, with an enhancing ring pattern are seen on CT or MRI. Associated increased meningeal enhancement may also be present. *Aspergillosis* is infrequent but may present as a cerebral abscess with extensive necrosis. *Candidiasis* may affect the brain when the infection is diffuse and severe. *Herpes simplex virus* infection of the CNS is rare. *TB* is of increasing concern in adults and will probably appear in children. *MAC* infection, although common elsewhere in the body, does not often involve the brain. *Bacterial infections* are also rare in the brain and meninges compared with their high frequency in general.

14.4.3
Vasculopathy

Strokes may occur in HIV-infected children secondary to the virus itself, lymphoma, or, rarely, opportunistic infection. Also repeated infections, producing elastases, may alter the elastic lamina of vessels and induce aneurysms (Fig. 14.17) or thrombotic strokes (MORIARTY et al. 1994; PHILIPPET et al. 1994). Hemorrhagic infarcts are another consideration, usually related to thrombocytopenia. HIV-related vasculopathy must be considered in children.

14.5
Other Manifestations

14.5.1
Parotid Gland

Enlargement of the parotid glands secondary to lymphocytic infiltration often occurs concomitantly with peripheral lymphadenopathy and LIP. Lymphoepithelial cysts have also been described. US or CT shows hypertrophy of the gland with multiple hypoechoic or anechoic nodules or cysts (Fig. 14.18).

14.5.2
Musculoskeletal System

Musculoskeletal manifestations of AIDS have been described in adults (STEINBACH et al. 1993) and are also likely to occur in children. Infections such as

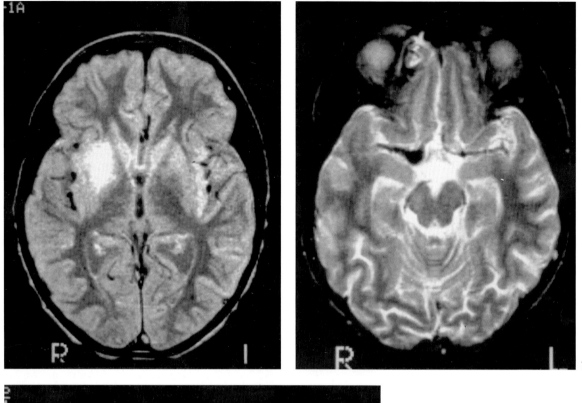

a

b

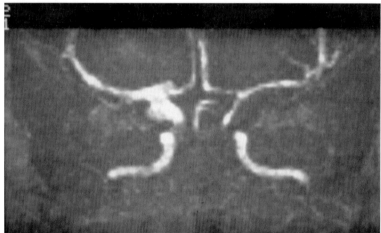

b

Fig. 14.17. a HIV-associated vasculopathy. A 13-year-old girl with severe immunodeficiency and left hemiparesis. MRI demonstrates high signal intensity in the right basal ganglia on a T2-weighted image. b Same child. MRI reveals dilatation of the right sylvian artery on a lower slice. c Same child. MR angiography confirms an aneurysm of the origin of the right sylvian artery. (Courtesy of Prof. Sebag, Hopital Robert Debré, Paris)

osteomyelitis or arthritis due to various pathogens are possible. One particular infection, bacillary angiomatosis due to *Bartonella henselae* or *quintana*, presents with osteolytic lesions associated with periostitis and a soft tissue mass with additional cutaneous or visceral manifestations. It is important to recognize pyomyositis, a multifocal infection of muscles due to *Staphylococcus aureus*, so that appropriate antibiotic therapy can be started. Kaposi's sarcoma and lymphomas may also affect bones and soft tissues.

Polymyositis is characterized by bilaterally symmetric proximal muscle weakness and is associated with creatine phosphokinase elevation. T2-weighted MR images are very useful in demonstrating abnormal increased signal in the involved muscles. Diagnosis relies on biopsy.

14.6
Tumors

For a general discussion of AIDS-related malignancies in children, see HALLER (1997).

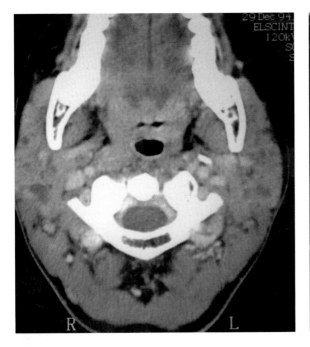

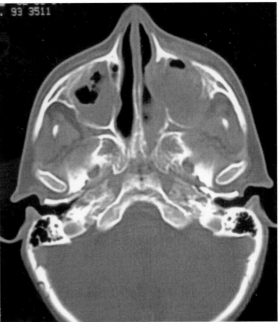

Fig. 14.18. Parotid cysts. CT demonstrates bilateral parotid cysts. (Courtesy of Prof. J.P. Montagne, Hopital Trousseau, Paris)

Fig. 14.19. Lymphoma. An 8-year-old girl with inflammatory periorbital swelling: CT shows maxillary sinus opacity and bone destruction due to B cell lymphoma

14.6.1
Lymphoma

Lymphoma, usually of B cell type, is the most common malignancy in children with AIDS, but is much less common than in adults. Lymphomas may be generalized with multiple sites of involvement or, less frequently, involve only one organ. The majority of children present with manifestations of lymphoid hyperplasia (LIP, lymphadenopathy, hepatosplenomegaly) before developing lymphoma. The role of the Epstein-Barr virus, which stimulates B cell proliferation, has not yet been delineated. Isolated involvement is most frequent in the brain, and lymphomas of the brain were among the first reported (DOUEK et al. 1991).

At presentation, the neoplasm is often unique in appearance. Preferential sites are the basal ganglia, gray-white matter junction, and deep white matter. Tumors can be seen on cranial US if the child is less than 1 year old. CT shows a mass, which is typically hyperdense before contrast injection. Following contrast administration, homogeneous enhancement is observed. Other presentations are also possible, such as a hypodense mass with peripheral enhancement simulating an abscess. MRI shows a mass surrounded by edema, iso- or hypointense signal characteris-

tics on T1-weighted images, hyperintensity on T2-weighted images, and homogeneous or peripheral gadolinium uptake. The diagnosis may be established by lumbar puncture if there is meningeal extension, or at times by stereotactic biopsy. Disseminated lymphomas may also occur with involvement of multiple sites. For example, the facial bones may demonstrate osseous destruction (MUKERJI and HILFER 1993), well imaged on CT (Fig. 14.19). Cervical or peripheral lymph nodes are usually accessible to biopsy, and abdominal organs including the liver, spleen, and kidneys may reveal diffuse infiltration enlarging the organ or solitary or multiple nodules (SISKIN et al. 1995). US shows hypoechoic nodules, which are hypodense on CT (Fig. 14.20). These masses and mesenteric lymphadenopathy have to be differentiated from nodes due to MAC or, more rarely, Kaposi's sarcoma. Thoracic involvement by lymphoma chiefly involves the lymph nodes. Chest radiographs demonstrate mediastinal enlargement; this is, however, usually better appreciated on CT. Pulmonary nodules occasionally occur. Pleural lymphomas are rarely described in children as compared with adults.

Secondary bone lymphoma involves the skull, spine, and pelvis but also long bones, facial bones, and ribs. Lesions are lytic and associated with a soft

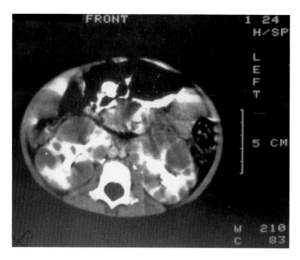

Fig. 14.20. Lymphoma. CT reveals multiple hypodense nodules in both kidneys

tissue mass. Thus, lymphoma should be considered in the differential diagnosis of any mass lesion in HIV-infected children. Hodgkin's lymphoma may also occur but less frequently.

14.6.2
Smooth Muscle Tumors

Leiomyomas and leiomyosarcomas are rare in children (accounting for less than 2% of soft tissue sarcomas) but are seen more frequently in immunodeficient and AIDS children. They may be located in the gastrointestinal tract, tracheobronchial tree, lung, subcutaneous tissue, and liver (MUELLER et al. 1992; LEVIN et al. 1994; TOMA et al. 1997; ROSENFELD et al. 1999). In most instances, the tumor is discovered as an incidental finding at autopsy, having been clinically silent. Radiographically, the mass may be solid or cystic and vascular or avascular on CT. Thus the diagnosis of smooth muscle or spindle cell tumor, although uncommon, must also be considered when a mass is seen in an HIV-infected child.

14.6.3
Kaposi's Sarcoma

Only anecdotal cases have been described but Kaposi's sarcoma may occur in children.

References

Ambrosino MM, Genieser NB, Krasinski K, Greco A, Borkowsky W (1992) Opportunistic infections and tumors in immunocompromised children. Radiol Clin North Am 30:639–658

Ambrosino MM, Roche KJ, Genieser NB, Kaul A, Lawrence RM (1995) Application of thin section low dose chest CT in the management of pediatric AIDS. Pediatr Radiol 25:393–400

Amoroso JK, Miller RW, Laraya-Cuasay, Gaw S, Marone R, Fernkel L, Nosher JL (1992) Bronchiectasis in children with LIP and AIDS. Pediatr Radiol 22:603–607

Berdon WE, Mellins RB, Abramson SJ, Ruzal-Shapiro C (1993) Pediatric HIV infection in its second decade. The changing pattern of lung involvement. Radiol Clin North Am 31:453–463

Douek P, Bertrand Y, Tran-Minh VA, Patet JD, Souillet G, Philippe N (1991) Primary lymphoma of the CNS in an infant with AIDS: imaging findings. AJR 156:1037–1038

Ettensohn D, Mayer KW, Kessimian S, Smith PS (1988) Lymphocytic bronchiolitis associated with HIV infection. Chest 93:201–202

Geoffray A, Spehl M, Chami M, Bosson N, Topet V, Deville A (1997) Imagerie du SIDA chez l'enfant. J Radiol 78:1233–1243

Goodman PC (1995) Tuberculosis and AIDS. Radiol Clin North Am 33:707–716

Haller JO (1997) AIDS-related malignancies in pediatrics. Radiol Clin North Am 35:1517–1538

Haller JO, Cohen HL (1993) Pediatric HIV infection: an imaging update. Pediatr Radiol 24:224–230

Haller JO, Cohen HL (1994) Gastrointestinal manifestations of AIDS in children. AJR 162:387–393

Haller JO, Ginsberg KJ (1997) Tuberculosis in children with acquired immunodeficiency syndrome. Pediatr Radiol 27:186–188

Kahn E, Anderson VM, Greco MA, Magid M (1995) Pancreatic disorders in pediatric AIDS. Hum Pathol 26:765–770

Kauffman WM, Sivit CJ, Fitz CR, Rakusan A, Herzog K, Chandra RS (1992) CT and MR evaluation of intracranial involvement in pediatric HIV infection: a clinical-imaging correlation. AJNR 13:949–957

Kontny HU, Sleasman JW, Kingma DW et al. (1997) Multilocular cysts in children with human immunodeficiency virus infection: clinical and pathological aspects. J Pediatr 131:264–270

Levin TL, Adam HM, van Hoeven KH, Goldman HS (1994) Hepatic spindle cell tumors in HIV positive children. Pediatr Radiol 24:78–79

Levin TL, Berdon WE, Tang HB, Haller JO (1997) Dideoxyinosine-induced pancreatitis in human immunodeficiency virus-infected children. Pediatr Radiol 27:189–191

Marolda J, Paca B, Bonforte RJ, et al. (1991) Pulmonary manifestations of HIV infection in children. Pediatr Pulmonol 10:231–235

Moriarty DM, Haller JO, Loh JP, Fikrig S (1994) Cerebral infarction in pediatric acquired immunodeficiency syndrome. Pediatr Radiol 24:611–612

Mueller BU, Butler KM, Higham MC, et al. (1992) Smooth muscle tumors in children with HIV infection. Pediatr Radiol 90: 460–462

Mukerji PK, Hilfer CL (1993) Burkitt's lymphoma with mandible, intra-abdominal and renal involvement – initial presentation of HIV infection in a 4-year-old child. Pediatr Radiol 23:76–77

Noble CB, Klein LT, Staiman VR, Neu N, Hensle TW, Berdon WE (1998) Ureteral obstruction secondary to indinavir in the pediatric HIV population. Pediatr Radiol 28:627–629

Norton KI, Godine LB, Lempert C (1997) Leiomyosarcoma of the kidney in an HIV-infected child. Pediatr Radiol 27:557–558

Nozyce M, Littelman J, Muenz L, Durako SJ, Fischer ML, Willoughby A (1994) Effect of perinatally acquired HIV infection on neurodevelopment in children during the first two years of life. Pediatrics 94:883–891

Nyberg DA, Federle MP, Jeffrey RB, Bottles K, Wofsy CB (1985) Abdominal CT findings of disseminated *Mycobacterium avium-intracellulare* in AIDS. AJR 145:297–299

Philippet P, Blanche S, Sebag G, Rodesch G, Griscelli C, Tardieu M (1994) Stroke and cerebral infarcts in children infected with human immunodeficiency virus. Arch Pediatr Adoles Med 48:965–970

Post MJ, Hensley GT, Moskowitz LB, Fischl M (1986) Cytomegalic inclusion virus encephalitis in patients with AIDS: CT, clinical and pathological correlation. AJR 146:1229–1234

Pursner M, Haller JO, Berdon WE (2000) Imaging features of *Mycobacterium avium-intracellulare* complex (MAC) in children with AIDS. Pediatr Radiol 30:426–429

Rosenfeld DL, Girgis WS, Underberg-Davis SJ (1999) Bilateral smooth-muscle tumors of the adrenals in a child with AIDS. Pediatr Radiol 29:376–378

Rusin JA, Sivit CJ, Rakusan TA, Chandra RS (1992) AIDS related cholangitis in children: sonographic findings. AJR 159:626–627

Schroeder SA, Beneck D, Dozor AJ (1995) Spontaneous pneumothorax in children with AIDS. Chest 108:1173–1176

Sheikh S, Madijaru K, Steiner P Rao M (1997) Bronchiectasis in pediatric AIDS. Chest 112:1202–1207

Siskin GP, Haller JO, Miller S, Sundaram R (1995) AIDS-related lymphoma: radiologic features in pediatric patients. Radiology 196:63–66

Sivit CJ, Miller CR, Rakusan TA, Ellaune M, Kushner DC (1995) Spectrum of chest radiographic abnormalities in children with AIDS and PCP. Pediatr Radiol 25:389–392

Steinbach LS, Tehranzadeh J, Fleckenstein JL, Vanarthos WJ, Pais MJ (1993) HIV infection: musculoskeletal manifestations. Radiology 186:833–838

Stoane JM, Haller JO, Orentlicher RJ (1996) The gastrointestinal manifestations of AIDS in children. Radiol Clin North Am 34:779–790

Taccone A, Fondelli MP, Ferrea G, Marzoli A (1992) An unusual CT presentation of congenital cerebral toxoplasmosis in an 8 month-old boy with AIDS. Pediatr Radiol 22:68–69

Tardieu M (1991) Encephalopathies au cours des infections par le VIH chez l'enfant. In: Said G, Saimot AG (eds) Manifestations neurologiques et infections rétrovirales. Pradel, Paris, pp 169–182

Teixidor HS, Godwin TA, Ramirez EA (1991) Cryptosporidiosis of the biliary tract in AIDS. Radiology 180:51–56

Toma P, Loy A, Pastorino C, Derchi LE (1997) Leiomyomas of the gallbladder and splenic calcifications in an HIV-infected child. Pediatr Radiol 27:92–94

Vigano A, Vella S, Principi N, et al. (1999) Thymus volume correlates with the progression of vertical HIV infection. AIDS 13:F29–F34.

Wachsberg RH, Obolevich AT, Lasker N (1995) Pelvocalyceal thickening in HIV-associated nephropathy. Abdom Imaging 20:371–375

Wood BP (1992) Children with AIDS; radiographic features. Invest Radiol 27:964–970

Wright M, Fikrig S, Haller JO (1993) Aspergillosis in children with acquired immune deficiency. Pediatr Radiol 23:492–494

Wrozlek MA, Brudlowska J, Kozlowski PB, et al. (1995) Opportunistic infections of the central nervous system in children with HIV infection: report of 9 autopsy cases and review of literature. Clin Neuropathol 14:187–196

Zilleruelo G, Strauss J (1995) HIV nephropathy in children. Pediatr Clin North Am 42:1469–1485

Zinn HL, Rosberger ST, Haller JO, Schlesinger AE (1997) Simple renal cyst in children with AIDS. Pediatr Radiol 27:827–828

15 AIDS in the Tropics

Elizabeth H. Moore and Erik H. L. Gaensler

CONTENTS

E. H. Moore, MD
Department of Radiology, University of California Davis Medical Center, 2616 Stockton Blvd., Sacramento, CA 95817, USA
E. H. L. Gaensler, MD
Department of Radiology, University of California, San Francisco, CA 94143, USA

15.1 Introduction

Almost any discussion of AIDS, verbal or written, generates controversy and strange opinions. The disease has been blamed on the colonial powers, "God's punishment for promiscuity, sexual deviation or intravenous drug usage," "a genetically altered virus pioneered in a military laboratory", abnormal human contact with monkeys or apes in Central Africa, the vaccination programs against smallpox, polio and other infections, or some unknown factor in the border trade between Tanzania and Uganda. Some believe that it is being spread by walking in the footsteps of a sick person. Alternatively, AIDS "does not exist" is "an invention of the western media," is the result of witchcraft, or "is not infectious." Symptoms may be ascribed to diabetes or dysentery rather than

Adapted and modified with permission from Palmer PES, Reeder M (eds) (2001) The imaging of tropical diseases. Springer, Heidelberg Berlin New York

to AIDS. The acceptance of the diagnosis can be fatalistic, "*Acha inuiwe dawa sind*" ("I have no medicine, so let it kill me"), or practical "we have no money" (Chairman of national AIDS committee). Innovative theories regarding AIDS prevention have been suggested: "Women with AIDS should be shot" (a member of parliament), or less final, "anyone with AIDS should be isolated" or banned from school, games, work, and public places or not allowed into the country.

Official responses have often been energetic and occasionally unconventional. At one time it was noted that a Malawian trucker, crossing the border from Mozambique to Zimbabwe, could expect officials to examine his passport, his vehicle's papers, and his genitals. The scientific press is not always more helpful, as is exemplified by a statement in 1986 from the Pasteur Institute in France that "many insects in central Africa are infected with the AIDS virus," to which the Center for Disease Control in the United States replied in 1987, if "mosquitoes are indeed transmitting AIDS, they are being very selective about whom they bite": Only a few percent of AIDS cases are devoid of any identifiable risk factor for transmission.

Researching the literature to establish the incidence of AIDS is equally interesting, particularly looking back over the past 15 years. This illustrates not just the rapid spread of the virus, but the slow process by which people and their governments have come to terms with this epidemic. Many governments denied that there were patients in their countries. Reports, estimates, and authoritative statements abound, and are corrected, amended, and contradicted with great rapidity. The literature is confused and confusing. There is, for example, a report on AIDS in Africa by a medical group from China: however, there are few reports from anyone concerning AIDS in China, and certainly none from an African medical group.

Amidst the plethora of literature on the subject, why a review of AIDS in the tropics? Few doctors anywhere can be unaware of AIDS, yet not all may be aware of how much AIDS varies in its presentations and complications. Most publications on the subject of AIDS have centered around patients in the Western world, often homosexuals or intravenous drug abusers living in urban settings. The vast majority of AIDS patients worldwide do not fit this profile. Over the past 10 years, increasingly numerous reports detailing the presentation of AIDS in the developing countries have appeared, making it clear that the natural history of AIDS differs depending on the microbiologic and nutritional environment, as well as the societal behavior and local customs of the population affected.

In this chapter, the complications of AIDS will be reviewed for various tropical populations. When possible, the reasons for the patterns of illness encountered will be analyzed. In addition, many, if not most of these opportunistic diseases have altogether different clinical and radiologic manifestations when they affect an human immune deficiency virus (HIV)-infected host instead of a normal host. This chapter will emphasize these differences, reviewing the radiographic manifestations of the common opportunistic infections and malignancies as they appear in the AIDS patient. All of this information is needed to produce a geographically and radiologically appropriate differential diagnosis.

In the past, data collection on the frequencies of various complications of AIDS in the tropics has been hampered by the relative lack of diagnostic equipment, laboratories, and sophisticated imaging technology. Even though computed tomography (CT) scanning and magnetic resonance imaging (MRI) are increasingly available in the tropics, few studies are performed on known AIDS patients. A diagnosis of HIV infection frequently ends diagnostic studies and even therapeutic intervention, since scarce resources are assigned instead to patients with potentially curable conditions. The problem of defining complications of AIDS in the tropics has been partially resolved by thorough and carefully performed autopsy studies in the Ivory Coast (LUCAS et al. 1994a).

15.2
Comparative Statistics: the Relative Scope of the Problem

If numbers alone are the trigger for media attention and medical expenditure, then AIDS is unfairly privileged. The estimated incidence figures for many of the diseases described in this book exceed by many times those of AIDS (Table 15.1). Most of these other diseases can be effectively treated or cured if the resources are available, and their incidence is relatively stable; by contrast AIDS is not curable at present and there has been an exponential increase in the numbers affected.

Table 15.1. Worldwide estimates of current infection (2001)

AIDS	34.6 million
Liver and lung flukes	70 million
Malaria	3–500 million (of whom 1 million die every year in Africa)
Schistosomiasis	250 million
Whipworm	360 million
Hookworm	1.25 billion
Amebiasis	600 million
Ascariasis	1.38 billion
Tuberculosis	20+ million

From WHO reports

15.3
Geographic Distribution

Infections by HIV occur worldwide; different subtypes of the virus involve different geographic areas. Currently the highest incidence of AIDS occurs in sub-Saharan Africa, Southeast Asia, and the Caribbean. Even within these broad regions there are major differences; for example, a high rate is found in Haiti, Bermuda, and the Bahamas but a low rate is reported from Cuba. The largest population affected is in Africa, where in some countries 30% of the high-risk population (age 15–50) are infected. Groups such as the military, the elite, diplomats, and businessmen may have even higher rates; 85% of prostitutes in Nairobi are HIV positive. The World Bank and World Health Organization (WHO) in Africa estimate that 25% of the sub-Saharan workforce will die in the next 20 years, that the average life span, which had been increasing to 58–63 years, will fall to 47 years, and that 3 million children will die. Worldwide perhaps 14 million children will be orphaned or be without one parent, and 30% of all neonates will be HIV positive unless education is effective and treatment or prevention becomes available. The social outcome in some countries is already devastating.

15.3.1
Patterns of Spread

The WHO has defined three patterns of spread for the AIDS epidemic. A type 1 pattern, exemplified by the United States and Western Europe, is characterized by disease spread primarily by homosexual behavior and intravenous drug abuse. A type 2 pattern, exemplified by Africa, describes primarily heterosexual spread. It has been estimated that 80% of HIV infections in East Africa are heterosexually transmitted. Homosexuality and drug abuse are rare. A type

2 pattern is also currently seen in the Caribbean and parts of Latin America, although homosexuality and drug abuse are also contributing factors in these areas. A type 3 pattern of spread occurs in areas with recent introduction of HIV by spread from countries with type 1 or type 2 patterns via blood products or sexual contact, often prostitution. The regions thus affected include Eastern Europe, North Africa, the Middle East, and Asia.

Whether AIDS is spread by homosexuals, heterosexuals, bisexuals, intravenous drug users, or transfusion of blood products, it makes little difference to the clinical course of the disease, with some notable exceptions. More important are the individual's general health and hygiene and the bacterial, viral, and parasitic cohabitants of the world in which the patient lives and has lived.

15.3.2
Africa

The first cases of AIDS in black Africans were identified in the 1980s, occurring in young heterosexuals with chronic wasting, opportunistic infections, and/or Kaposi's sarcoma. However, it seems probable that AIDS in Africa has a much longer history. Currently, AIDS is the most common cause of death in many African cities. The highest rates of infection worldwide are in sub-Saharan Africa, particularly Malawi, Zambia, Tanzania, Uganda, Rwanda, Burundi, and Zimbabwe. In sub-Saharan Africa, the trans-Africa highway provides an interesting lesson in social geography. The truck drivers from the coast in Tanzania and Kenya and the prostitutes along the highway form an almost unbroken chain of infection deep into the heart of Africa, from which the epidemic spreads into the countries which are supplied by the trucks. (There is an exactly similar pattern of spread by lorry drivers in India.) In a Tanzanian survey by ATZORI et al. (1993), the level of HIV seroprevalence was directly correlated with the distance between the subject's home village and the nearest main road.

In Africa, the common occurrence of ulcerative venereal diseases, such as chancroid, and the lack of male circumcision increase heterosexual transmission. Condom use is not favored ("no one eats a sweet with the wrapper still on"). Men's dislike of condoms was the major reason for not using them reported by women in a study from Tanzania. In Malawi, with the highest rate of HIV infection in the world, traditional beliefs hold that women require frequent sexual intercourse, the semen acting as a vitamin to restore blood lost during menses (a proposed benefit which would be negated by condom use). Unfortunately, while initiating an educational campaign against AIDS in the new century, the President of one African country forbade mention of condoms.

Contaminated blood products, medical injections with unclean needles, and maternal-fetal spread are also important routes of transmission. Transfusion has contributed an estimated 10%–15% to AIDS transmission in Africa, particularly affecting children with malaria, women with pregnancy-related anemia, trauma victims, and patients with sickle cell disease. Improving standards in blood banking may reverse this trend. Between 5% and 15% of AIDS is perinatally transmitted.

Certain cultural practices may also promote the heterosexual spread of AIDS in Africa. There is a tradition of multiple wives or sexual partners. Networks of concurrent sexual partners, a common situation in sub-Saharan Africa, facilitate transmission. Prostitution is considered more acceptable than in some other parts of the world. Scarification (Fig. 15.1), tattooing, the rites of passage into manhood or womanhood

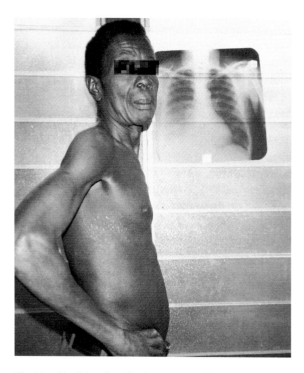

Fig. 15.1. Traditional medical treatment of tuberculous pleurisy by scarification over the right lower chest. The chest film in the background shows a right-sided pleural effusion at the exact site the traditional healer has applied his or her treatment. Such procedures place the individual at risk for transmission of blood-borne diseases, including AIDS

[circumcision, female circumcision (genital mutilation), infibulation], blood letting and blood brotherhood, use of ritual and medicinal enemas given through a dirty reed or horn, and even close head or body shaving, all entail risk of transmission of HIV if, as is almost inevitable, only one instrument is shared by a group.

Heterosexual spread is enhanced by multiple births in rapid succession, with cervicitis, recurrent infection, and scarring. In some societies the surviving spouse after the death of her husband must free the spirit of the deceased by having sex with the nearest relative.

Intensive educational programs have been launched in almost all countries of Africa, with varying success. Knowledge is spreading ("sex is no fun if you are dead" – a high school pupil), but sometimes "knowledge is excellent: behavior is abysmal." However, there is some recent evidence that education may be changing behavior. The first report of decreasing seroprevalence of HIV-l in Ugandan young adults, 13–24 years old, was published in 1995 by MULDER et al. A Ugandan behavioral study published in 1997 by ASIIMWE-OKIROR et al. comparing behavioral patterns in 1989 and 1995 showed increasing condom use, a 2-year delay in the age of first sexual intercourse, and, over the same period, a 40% decline in HIV seroprevalence in women attending antenatal clinics. Similarly, a study of Tanzanian urban factory workers registered a marked decrease in those reporting sex with multiple partners as well as those reporting casual sex partners between 1991 and 1994 (NG'WESHEMI et al. 1996).

Common opportunistic infections and malignancies seen in African AIDS include tuberculosis, bacteremia, cerebral toxoplasmosis, pyogenic pneumonias, cytomegalovirus, Kaposi's sarcoma, and nonspecific enteritis.

15.3.3
Asia

HIV and AIDS rates in Asia vary substantially between countries. Japan demonstrates a very low rate, with the majority of AIDS cases occurring in hemophiliacs infected by blood products produced elsewhere. Homosexuality is rare, as is intravenous drug abuse, and condoms are widely used for contraception. However, some Japanese men participate as customers in the sex trade countries of Asia, such as Thailand, where a high percentage of prostitutes are infected, providing a possible avenue of infection. Korea demonstrates low levels of seropositivity in all groups. Officially reported statistics of AIDS in the People's Republic of China describe extremely low rates, but the reliability of these reports is unknown. The level of knowledge about sexually transmitted diseases appears to be low: in a 1994 survey involving rural Chinese villagers, only 18% had heard of AIDS, and only 25% and 28% respectively had heard of sexually transmitted diseases or condoms (LIAO et al. 1997).

Hong Kong appears to have a type 1 or Western distribution of infections, with the majority in homosexuals and bisexuals. *Pneumocystis carinii* and tuberculosis are common opportunistic infections. Singapore appears to have a relatively low level of HIV infection. In Vietnam, the infected population primarily comprises male intravenous drug abusers and female sex workers (LINDAN et al. 1997). Thailand has experienced three major HIV epidemics, in intravenous drug users, sex workers, and male sexually transmitted disease (STD) patients. Efforts to limit the epidemic have been ineffective. Two-thirds of the intravenous drug abusers in Myanmar (formerly Burma) are thought to carry the virus. The three most common opportunistic infections encountered in the AIDS population in Southeast Asia are extrapulmonary tuberculosis, cryptococcosis, and *Penicillium marneffei*, a fungal pathogen endemic to the region (KOK et al. 1994; SUPPARATPINYO et al. 1994; KAPLAN et al. 1996).

The first cases detected in India by surveillance were in 1986. The Ministry of Health, plagued by budget cuts, is as yet poorly equipped to handle a large number of AIDS patients. An AIDS epidemic is predicted for India primarily because of the large number of prostitutes, many of whom are infected (47% in a sampling from 1997) (MAWAR et al. 1997). Although only 4.4% of respondents to a 1997 Delhi survey had participated in sex outside or before marriage, most positive respondents were males who frequently sought sex with commercial sex workers (KUMAR et al. 1997b). Almost half had never used a condom during extramarital or premarital encounters.

The male to female infection ratio in India is 5:1, with female cases being primarily seen in prostitutes (PAIS 1996). The typical route of infection among males is heterosexual contact with female sex workers, while in women who are not prostitutes, the most common source of infection is their husband (SRIKANTH et al. 1997). Large numbers of blood donors are HIV positive, particularly professional blood donors.

In the study by CHACKO et al. (1995), of 61 AIDS patients in Vellore, India, the most common presenting symptoms included weight loss, fever, and chronic diarrhea. Common secondary infections included

tuberculosis, both pulmonary and/or extrapulmonary, oropharyngeal candidiasis, and cryptococcal meningitis. Kaposi's sarcoma was not seen in any patient. The mean duration from AIDS diagnosis to death was 4.5 months. Tuberculosis and candidiasis are the most common secondary infections. Secondary infections by virulent bacteria are also common, as are cryptococcosis, cryptosporidiosis, and cytomegalovirus. Although *Pneumocystis carinii* pneumonia was not observed in one Indian study (KAUR et al. 1992), in another 9% of patients expired with *P. carinii* as a terminal infection, with a mean CD4 count of 6 cells/mm^3 (GIRI et al. 1995). In a small study of interstitial pneumonia in Mumbai (Bombay), three of five patients were bronchoalveolar lavage or transbronchial biopsy positive for *P. carinii* (BIJUR et al. 1996). Among Indian AIDS patients examined at autopsy for gastrointestinal disease, 71% of those with diarrhea yielded an organism, as compared with 29% of those without diarrhea. The most frequent pathogens were cytomegalovirus, parasites, fungi, and *Mycobacterium tuberculosis* (LANJEWAR et al. 1996).

Screening of a high-risk population at a sexually transmitted disease clinic in Mumbai (Bombay) also revealed a high incidence of HIV-2 infection, usually occurring as a co-infection with HIV-l (PFUTZNER et al. 1992). However, in another study by SARAN and GUPTA (1995) of all seropositives tested for both viruses, 31% were HIV-2 positive only. Thus, India joins the group of HIV-2 epidemic countries, which has included Western Europe, West Africa, Brazil, and the United States.

15.3.4
Cuba and the Caribbean

A large screening study within Cuba has revealed that the overall prevalence of infection in that country is extremely low, with higher rates in visiting foreigners and in homosexuals. Those infected have been isolated to contain the epidemic. Relaxation of the quarantine and increased tourism have been accompanied by increased rates of infection (HANSEN and GROCE 2001).

Other Caribbean countries differ greatly from Cuba. In these countries transmission appears to be primarily homosexual, bisexual, and heterosexual, with a minor contribution of intravenous drug abuse. Bisexuality is generally believed to be common in the Caribbean because homosexuality is not well tolerated; therefore many homosexuals are married with families. Subsequent spread to the general heterosexual population has occurred, and pediatric AIDS has resulted. Further spread of HIV in the community has been promoted by cultural patterns of multiple sexual partners and a propensity for unprotected sex.

A study of 4,000 women attending a prenatal clinic in Port au Prince, Haiti, demonstrated a 9.2% HIV infection rate (Boulos et al. 1998). High rates of infection have also been seen in the English-speaking Caribbean countries such as the Bahamas, Bermuda, and Curaçao.

Co-infection with HTLV-1 may occur, and this appears to speed progression to AIDS and shorten survival.

Histoplasmosis capsulati is endemic in much of the Caribbean, and AIDS patients are at risk for disseminated disease: there are also high rates of tuberculosis.

15.3.5
Central and South America

In Latin America, HIV infection is most common in Brazil and Mexico. Initial infections appeared in homosexual and bisexual males with subsequent spread to the heterosexual community via bisexuals. Intravenous drug abusers contribute to spread in a limited fashion, particularly in Argentina and Brazil. Unlike Africa and Asia, prostitution does not appear to be a major factor. Mexico is an endemic area for coccidioidomycosis, and Central America is an endemic area for histoplasmosis capsulati. Protozoal infections such as toxoplasmosis, cryptosporidiosis, and isosporiasis are common in South America (Kaplan et al. 1996). Fungal and mycobacterial infections are more common in Brazil than *P. carinii* or viral infections (Moreira et al. 1993).

15.3.6
Australia

The patterns of HIV infection is type 1, with initial cases seen in homosexual and bisexual males in urban centers. Subsequent transmission to the heterosexual population has occurred. Education of the public and the prostitute population and increased condom use have diminished the spread of a variety of sexually transmitted diseases including gonorrhea. Unfortunately, participation as sex tourists in Asian countries by Australian males has produced persistent seeding of penicillinase-producing strains of gonorrhea from Southeast Asia, with obvious implications for the importation of HIV (Donovan et al. 1991). Opportunistic infections appear to be similar to those encountered in the United States, with a high prevalence of *P. carinii* infection and a preponderance of atypical

mycobacterial infection as compared with *M. tuberculosis*.

15.4
Clinical Manifestations

HIV infection causes essentially the same immunosuppression in all of its hosts, but the clinical presentation and complications of AIDS in the tropics differ because of preexisting conditions in the host and the host's environment, many of which also contribute to immunosuppression. These include poor hygiene, poor living conditions, preexisting infections (especially parasites), chronic debilitating diseases, nutritional deficiencies, reduced accessibility to diagnosis and treatment, and, possibly but unlikely, unknown factors such as genetic predisposition. This variable background also affects the patterns of spread and the progression from infection to AIDS, as well as the time from the development of AIDS to death.

When AIDS does develop, almost any system may be involved. There may be myocarditis, pericarditis, and endocarditis, and opportunistic infections presenting as oral thrush, esophagitis, gastritis, and colitis. Lymphadenopathy, particularly abdominal, may be nonspecific or tuberculous or from atypical mycobacteriosis. There may be cystitis, pyelonephritis, renal abscesses, nephropathy, and renal insufficiency. HIV-neuropathy causes various neurologic symptoms, such as microcephaly, delayed development, ataxia, seizures, dementia, and coma.

In much of the tropics, tuberculosis and the gastrointestinal manifestations of AIDS predominate. *M. tuberculosis* is the most common significant pathogen, and gastrointestinal disease the most common clinical presentation. Common Western pathogens, such as *P. carinii* and atypical mycobacteria, are rare in many regions, but both groups, tropical and temperate, share other complications such as Kaposi's sarcoma, although not always in the same way.

Children with AIDS have their own diagnostic problems. Many of the clinical signs and symptoms resemble common childhood complaints.

15.5
Clinical Definitions

Clinical criteria to define AIDS have been developed by the WHO for use in sub-Saharan Africa and elsewhere to allow the diagnosis of AIDS without laboratory testing. Clinical definitions vary considerably in different locations depending on the local prevalence of opportunistic diseases and the sophistication of diagnostic procedures available. The sensitivity of the clinical definition developed for sub-Saharan Africa has ranged from about 33% to 65%, with a specificity of 78%–90%.

Relying on clinical criteria alone has certain drawbacks. For example, in Africa, the present system includes persistent cough as one of the minor criteria, and severe weight loss and persistent fever as major criteria, making it difficult to distinguish patients with tuberculosis from those with AIDS. Even in patients known to be HIV positive, the presence of pulmonary tuberculosis and the accompanying symptoms need not indicate progression to AIDS. As another example, a common manifestation of AIDS in Africa is "slim disease," manifested by weight loss, chronic diarrhea, and chronic fever. This was incorporated into one definition of the HIV-related wasting syndrome, but only if not associated with other conditions such as cryptosporidiosis or tuberculosis, which might cause similar findings. However, in many cases, these other diseases are related to HIV and it is often difficult in Africa to exclude such concurrent diseases. It has been suggested that in Africa, the HIV-related wasting syndrome might better be defined as requiring greater than 10% weight loss, chronic diarrhea for at least 30 days, and chronic fever for at least 30 days, whether or not there are concomitant diseases which might be responsible for these findings.

A population study in Tanzania by TODD et al. (1997) showed that the proportion of adult deaths attributable to HIV was 35% overall and 53% in the 20–29 age group. However, the applicable WHO clinical case definition of AIDS was satisfied for only 18% of deaths occurring in HIV-positive patients because many signs and symptoms associated with HIV deaths were nonspecific.

A clinical definition of AIDS has been developed for South America, applicable to developing countries with adequate serologic facilities but without other sophisticated diagnostic procedures. Clinical criteria in South America differ from those used in Africa: diarrhea and weight loss are less common in South American patients, so cachexia was substituted. The South American definition also has the advantage of including symptoms of central nervous system dysfunction. Using a complex scoring system of symptomatology and documented dis-

eases, this system achieves relatively high specificity and sensitivity.

Clinical definitions of AIDS should ideally be equated with a laboratory standard such as a CD4 count of less than 200 cells/mm^3. However, it is unlikely that even tailored clinical definitions can be accurate in locations where there are high endemic rates of diseases which are also HIV associated, such as tuberculosis and Kaposi's sarcoma.

15.6
Children and AIDS

Thirty percent or more of children born to HIV-seropositive mothers will themselves become seropositive, and their AIDS incubation period will be shorter, with clinical signs and symptoms appearing relatively quickly. However, HIV-1 serologic tests in infants must be interpreted with caution because maternal antibodies may persist for as long as 15 months. Thus, if there are no clinical indications of disease, a positive serologic test in an infant under 15 months may not indicate infection and may revert to negative. If the child is antibody positive after age 15 months, he or she is probably infected. When available, viral culture, in vitro production of antibodies, or polymerase chain reaction testing can resolve this dilemma.

Children with AIDS have their own special diagnostic problems. Many of the clinical signs and symptoms of the disease are similar to other common childhood complaints, such as measles (often a severe disease in the tropics), malaria, failure to thrive, chronic cough and fevers, recurrent diarrhea, and respiratory disease. The difficulties are exemplified by pneumonia, which in the developing world is the cause of death of 30% of children under the age of 5 years, even without AIDS. Distinguishing between bacterial pneumonia and tuberculosis and determining which patient might harbor HIV is a major diagnostic challenge, especially where laboratory and imaging facilities are limited or nonexistent. In some regions, Burkitt's lymphoma and acute Kaposi's sarcoma of childhood are endemic and their presence is not AIDS defining.

The most common reasons for hospital admission in Abidjan, Ivory Coast in HIV-positive children were respiratory infection and malnutrition (VETTER et al. 1996). Mortality was 2.4 times higher in HIV-positive children compared with HIV-negative hospitalized children. Most pneumonias in pediatric AIDS are caused by common bacterial pathogens, but if there are severe respiratory signs with any interstitial pneumonia, and a poor response to antibiotics, *P. carinii* pneumonia should be considered, even though it is rare in some countries. On the other hand, lymphocytic interstitial pneumonitis, a persistent interstitial micronodular pulmonary parenchymal pattern, may have minimal respiratory signs.

In an autopsy study, also performed in Abidjan, respiratory infections, *P. carinii* pneumonia, and measles were common causes of death in HIV-positive children as compared with HIV-negative children, while pyogenic meningitis was common in both groups (LUCAS et al. 1996). Surprisingly, in HIV-positive children, tuberculosis, lymphocytic interstitial pneumonitis, and HIV encephalitis were rarely found at autopsy. In a study from Zambia, high HIV rates are found in children with tuberculosis (69%), malnutrition (41%), pneumonia (28%), and diarrhea (24%) (CHINTU et al. 1995). HIV may be responsible for various neurologic symptoms in children, including microcephaly, delayed development, ataxia, seizures, and coma.

15.7
Malaria and Transfusion-Related AIDS

Malaria, particularly infection with *Plasmodium falciparum*, is an immense public health problem in Africa and many other tropical countries, made worse by the increase in drug-resistant strains. Fortunately, concomitant HIV infection does not seem to increase the chances of clinically significant malarial episodes, or change the rate of progression from HIV to AIDS. Indeed, there has even been some evidence that malaria or the chloroquine used to treat malaria may have some effect against HIV (KALYESUBULA et al. 1997). A study from Mama Yemo Hospital in Kinshasa, Zaire, showed no difference in malarial rates in a group of children who had been exposed to HIV in utero, some of whom were HIV positive, some of whom had advanced AIDS, and some of whom were HIV negative or had reverted to the HIV-negative state after birth (COLEBUNDERS et al. 1990). These findings are confirmed by other studies.

However, the severe anemia caused by malaria may necessitate transfusion, which presents a substantial risk for AIDS and other blood-borne diseases. For example, 87% of transfusions in Kinshasa

are performed for malaria and 6% of the blood donors are HIV positive. A study by CHIKWEM et al. (1997) of donated blood in Nigeria revealed that among 364 healthy donors, 14.9% showed hepatitis B, 5.8% HIV-l, 4.1% *Plasmodium falciparum*, and 3.6% *Treponema pallidum*. Worldwide, HIV-positive blood is transfused either because the blood is not properly tested or because blood must be given in an emergency whether or not it has been tested, and testing may be a lengthy process. Needles may be reused without effective sterilization. The risk of transfusion-related AIDS is found over much of the malarial world, compounded in some regions (such as West Africa) by the high prevalence of hemoglobinopathies which also require transfusion.

Falciparum malaria is the most common cause of anemia of pregnancy in sub-Saharan Africa. Malarial parasitemia is highest in the 13th–16th weeks of pregnancy and, for unknown reasons, the rise is most significant in the primigravida patients. It is not, however, the only cause of anemia: parasites, malnutrition, high fertility rates, and chronic ill health all contribute. In Zaire, examination of 2,950 untreated pregnancies revealed that 72% of patients had a moderate anemia (hemoglobin level 7–11 g/dl) and 3.7% of patients had severe anemia (hemoglobin under 7 g/dl) (JACKSON et al. 1991). A 50% mortality is observed when the hematocrit is less than 13% and there is concomitant heart failure. Because the anemia of pregnancy is often treated by transfusion with inadequately screened blood, it is an important cause of AIDS in the maternal and fetal populations.

15.8
Leprosy and AIDS

Although far less common than *Mycobacterium tuberculosis*, *Mycobacterium leprae* is still a significant public health problem in sub-Saharan Africa, India, and other developing countries in Asia, the Middle East, the Caribbean, and Haiti. There has been concern that, due to immunosuppression, HIV may increase susceptibility to leprosy. Data are mixed on this subject. A study in Zambia demonstrated a markedly increased incidence of HIV infection in new leprosy patients as compared with controls (MEERAN 1989), whereas a larger study of leprosy patients in the Ivory Coast, Senegal, and Yemen noted equal HIV positivity rates. In a primate model of leprosy, inoculation led to increased leprosy infection rates in those animals which were SIV positive (GORMUS et al. 1989). It has been postulated (but not proven) that HIV infection may accelerate the development of clinical leprosy; however, active chronic infection with leprosy may accelerate the course of HIV disease due to the preexisting immune response. In Haiti, it was found that although HIV-positive rates in leprosy patients were the same as in the general population, the HIV-positive leprosy patients progressed to symptomatic AIDS more rapidly than would be expected. It also appears that leprosy relapses are more common in HIV-infected individuals.

15.9
Maternal/Fetal AIDS

Maternal-fetal HIV transmission may occur at three stages during the perinatal period: pregnancy, delivery, and nursing. Overall, the rate of perinatal transmission varies from 20% to 60%. Rates of HIV-1 and HIV-2 transmission are similar (PRAZUCK et al. 1995). Intrauterine transmission probably occurs in 20%–30% of HIV-positive mothers, but this rate can be modified if the mother receives antiviral therapy (e.g., zidovudine). Rates of transmission to the fetus are probably higher if the mother becomes infected during her pregnancy and becomes viremic at that time rather than being infected before she becomes pregnant. Transmission during delivery occurs; the risks are unknown but thought to be high. For comparison, 90% of hepatitis B transmissions are known to occur during delivery, and therefore delivery is likely to be a significant risk period for HIV transmission as well. The transmission of AIDS postpartum also occurs, since the virus is found in breast milk. A 15% increase in perinatal HIV transmission has been documented in infants breast fed exclusively, as compared with formula-fed infants (BOBAT et al. 1997). The risk of transmission increases with the number of months of breast feeding. However, without breast feeding, many babies in the tropics will likely be malnourished or develop diarrhea due to poor hygiene. A randomized study by NDUATI et al. (2000) compared breast feeding with formula. The use of breast milk substitutes prevented 44% of infant HIV infections. However, 2-year mortality rates were quite similar: 24% in the breast-feeding arm and 20% in the formula arm. One proposal for utilizing breast milk safely has involved "Pretoria pas-

teurization" of expressed breast milk by submersion in hot water, which would inactivate HIV (JEFFERY and MERCER 2000).

An alternative approach to perinatal infection is the use of single-dose nevirapine to mother and child in the peripartum period, which has demonstrated efficacy in decreasing transmission from mother to child by nearly 50% in a breast-feeding population (GUAY et al. 1999).

In July 1998 the United Nations changed their policy and recommended that women who were HIV-positive should not breast feed their infants. The UN acknowledged that this is a very controversial policy and would be against well-established social customs in many countries. But in 1997 UN-AIDS estimated that 30% (200,000) of the 600,000 children in the world who became HIV infected, acquired their infection from breast feeding. Recent studies have shown that as many as 70% of the women at prenatal clinics may be HIV positive, and 30% or more of women in six African countries were infected. The major problem with the new policy is that 90% of women in developing countries do not know whether or not they are infected and worldwide at least 30% of pregnant women receive no antenatal care.

Women who have symptomatic HIV infections or AIDS have a significantly increased rate of miscarriage, low-birth-weight infants, intrauterine fetal death, and preterm delivery; however, asymptomatic HIV-positive infections have not been associated with increased complications of pregnancy, according to the work of KUMAR et al. (1995). Placental size may be larger in HIV-infected mothers, a nonspecific sign seen in numerous infections.

Although it had been previously believed that a single pregnancy does not adversely affect the course of HIV disease in the mother, a recent controlled study by KUMAR et al. (1997a) from India refutes this. HIV-infected pregnant and nonpregnant women were matched for CD4 counts, age, and parity. The mean survival time was about 19 months for the pregnant women and about 23 months for the nonpregnant women. Many of the infants were delivered preterm, with high infant mortality.

Multiple pregnancies in the HIV-infected mother are thought to speed progression towards clinical AIDS. A possible mechanism for this is the activation of latently infected helper cells by the circulating paternal antigens from the fetus, viral production being stimulated by each successive pregnancy.

15.10
HIV Transmission
and Other Sexually Transmitted Diseases

Key to the understanding of different patterns of spread worldwide are differences in the relative efficiency of heterosexual transmission of AIDS. In the United States, heterosexual contact is relatively inefficient in spreading HIV, with a possibility of conversion estimated at approximately 0.2% with a single sexual contact. In comparison, an infected prostitute in Nairobi may have an HIV transmission rate of 8% with a single sexual contact, rising to 28% if the male was uncircumcised and a genital ulcer was acquired at the same time (TYNDALL et al. 1996).

The rate of heterosexual AIDS transmission is significantly increased if the couple (or one partner) already has an ulcerative sexually transmitted disease. This may affect HIV transmission in one of three ways. First, genital ulcers may increase the infectivity of the donor because of blood or serum from the ulcerated area. Second, open sores may increase the susceptibility of the recipient, both due to nonintact skin or mucosa and also because there may be an increased number of CD4 cells at the ulcer site, making cross-infection easier. Finally, various diseases may be co-factors in any HIV initial infection or progression from increased activation of T4 lymphocytes leading to increased production of HIV-infected cells and viral copies.

The sexually transmitted diseases associated with increased HIV infection include syphilis, chancroid, lymphogranuloma venereum, and herpes simplex. These are all common in most areas in which heterosexual transmission occurs. *Chlamydia trachomatis* is a possible cofactor. Gonorrhea and genital warts, as well as various other nonulcerative sexually transmitted diseases, probably do not increase susceptibility to or transmission of HIV. The incidence of non-AIDS sexually transmitted diseases observed in antenatal clinics in Malawi has been measured by MAHER and HOFFMAN (1995) at 42%, with a 32% HIV positive rate.

Men who have not been circumcised are at increased risk of HIV infection (odds ratio 4.8), with countries in which circumcision is rare closely matching the countries of the "AIDS belt" in Africa. The effect may be due to an increased incidence of ulcerative STDs such as chancroid in uncircumcised males, as well as other factors related to hygiene or a more favorable environment for viral survival and transmission. The relative risk is so striking that some believe circumcision should be considered as

an intervention strategy for AIDS control (TYNDALL et al. 1996). The protective effects of circumcision are most profound when it is performed before the age of 20 (KELLY et al. 1999).

15.11
Complications of AIDS in the Tropics

Many diseases present in the tropics can hasten the development of AIDS, change its clinical course, or attack a host weakened by AIDS. Many of these diseases will have different manifestations than when encountered in the normal host. The clinical presentation and complications of AIDS differ mainly because of preexisting conditions in the host and the host's environment. Some complications of AIDS in the tropics are never seen in Western patients. For example, the protozoan responsible for leishmaniasis has emerged as an AIDS-related pathogen in South America, India, Central Asia, and around the Mediterranean, including North Africa, and penicilliosis is seen exclusively in Southeast Asia.

There is no evidence that amebiasis, malaria, purulent meningitis, schistosomiasis, tetanus, cholera, malignancies (other than Kaposi's sarcoma and lymphoma), and nondisseminated strongyloidiasis are increased in HIV-positive individuals or individuals with AIDS.

As the CD4 count falls, reflecting increasing immunosuppression, the patient will become susceptible to increasingly opportunistic organisms. For instance, thrush may appear when CD4 counts have only fallen to 300–400 cells/mm^3. As long as CD4 lymphocyte counts remain above 200 cells/mm^3, common bacterial pneumonias and *Mycobacterium tuberculosis* predominate. With increasing immunosuppression (CD4 counts less than 200 cells/mm^3), unusual bacterial pathogens and *Pneumocystis carinii* appear. With further declines, disseminated fungal infections and Kaposi's sarcoma are seen. At CD4 counts of below 50 cells/mm^3, lymphoma, cytomegalovirus, and atypical mycobacteria become more likely. Patients in the tropics are likely to die from infections associated with AIDS such as tuberculosis, intestinal parasites, or bacterial pathogens even before a profound level of immunosuppression is reached. This explains why some of the complications of AIDS which are common in more temperate climates are rarely encountered in the tropics. The mean CD4 count of AIDS patients at death in the large autopsy series by LUCAS et al. (1994a) from West Africa was 141 cells/mm^3.

With worsening immunosuppression, some less opportunistic organisms may present with unusual clinical or radiologic features, reflecting the diminished ability of the immune system to control the infection. For example, with CD4 counts below 200/mm^3, the body can no longer mount a granulomatous response: tuberculosis is then less likely to form localized granulomas or cavities and more likely to produce patchy airspace disease or undergo hematogenous dissemination. Similarly, pulmonary cryptococcosis presents as a diffuse pneumonia rather than as well-circumscribed lung nodules.

Categorization of the many pathogens which affect AIDS patients in the tropics is difficult because the majority involve more than one body part or organ system. In the following summary of imaging findings, organisms have been loosely grouped by the region involved. Whenever possible, illustrative radiographs have been obtained from AIDS patients who live in or have recently emigrated from the tropics.

15.12
Organisms Causing Pulmonary Infections

15.12.1
Tuberculosis

The mycobacterial infection most commonly associated with AIDS in the tropics is tuberculosis. The disease is disseminated in most patients and tuberculous meningitis and tuberculous enteritis are common extrapulmonary manifestations (LUCAS et al. 1994a).

Even prior to the onset of the AIDS epidemic, tuberculosis was an extremely common cause of morbidity and mortality in the tropics, with a prevalence of infection much greater than 50%. In the tropics, it is probable that many people are already infected with *M. tuberculosis* before becoming HIV positive, but those with HIV have a greatly increased risk of developing or reactivating tuberculosis as compared with seronegative patients. For example, the study by LEROY et al. (1995) of women in Kigali, Rwanda, demonstrated an 18.2-fold increase in the incidence of active tuberculosis in HIV-positive patients after 4 years of follow-up as compared with HIV-negative controls. As has been confirmed by recent DNA fingerprinting studies, the majority of HIV-associated active tuberculous infections, even those occurring after adequate treatment, are the result of reactivation, although primary infection or reinfection also occurs (GODFREY-FAUSSETT et al. 1994). HIV-infect-

ed tuberculosis patients have a higher incidence of fever, tuberculin skin test anergy, and positive blood cultures than normal hosts.

The interaction between tuberculosis and HIV may have consequences for both epidemics. Cases of tuberculosis have increased twice as fast in countries with high HIV seropositivity as compared to countries with low seropositivity. In very broad terms, about a third of tuberculosis cases can be attributed to HIV. Poor cell-mediated immunity in HIV leads to greater susceptibility to tuberculous infection, and these individuals then transmit the disease to others, further increasing the epidemic. The risk of reactivation of tuberculosis in an AIDS patient over the course of 1 year approximates the risk of reactivation in an HIV-negative patient over a lifetime. The rapid progression to clinical tuberculosis in AIDS patients contributes to the development of resistant strains of tuberculosis. There is increasing evidence that tuberculosis speeds the clinical course of preexisting HIV infection (MURRAY 1997), and recent studies have suggested that treatment for tuberculosis will actually increase CD4+ cell counts in some AIDS patients.

The prevalence of HIV in patients with tuberculosis in sub-Saharan African countries ranges from 20% to 67%; in Mexico it is about 25%, in Central America and South America about 20%–30%. In Central Africa about 40% of HIV-positive autopsies show disseminated tuberculosis. Of those patients dying with "slim disease," 44% had disseminated tuberculosis at autopsy (DE COCK et al. 1992; SERWADDA et al. 1985). Among patients with extrapulmonary tuberculosis, the majority will be HIV positive. Extrapulmonary tuberculosis has been found in 70% of patients with tuberculosis who have CD4 counts of less than 100 cells/mm^3 (DE COCK et al. 1992).

As previously noted, the high incidence of tuberculosis can confuse AIDS statistics. Where only clinical criteria are used for the diagnosis of AIDS, there may be overdiagnosis of AIDS in patients who only have tuberculosis. The same clinical findings may be seen in both, such as weight loss exceeding 10% of body weight, with fever and cough for a month or more. Many patients with untreated tuberculosis, particularly those who are undernourished or in chronic ill health from parasites, will meet the clinical criteria for AIDS without actually having the disease. On the other hand, AIDS patients infected with tuberculosis often have no sputum, negative sputum smears, or negative chest radiographs, making the diagnosis of tuberculosis more difficult.

Extrapulmonary tuberculosis may produce extensive lymphadenopathy in patients with AIDS, often with low-density or hypoechoic necrotic centers seen on CT or ultrasound scanning. It may be impossible to differentiate between tuberculosis and lymphoma, and both may exist together. Tuberculous lymphadenitis in HIV patients (as well as HIV-related lymphadenitis) tends to be bilateral and symmetrical, involving many nodal groups, while tuberculous lymphadenitis in the normal host is usually asymmetrical, focal, and often cervical (BEM 1997). Other extrapulmonary manifestations, such as pleural, pericardial, abdominal, meningeal, and miliary spread, are very common in AIDS patients. Unfortunately, they are also common in undernourished and chronically unwell individuals without AIDS.

In one study, HIV-2 infection appeared to be associated with a lower tuberculosis mortality than HIV-1 infection or dual infection. However, in Abidjan, patients infected with HIV-2 and tuberculosis showed wasting, diarrhea, candidiasis, and lymphadenopathy, similar to patients with HIV-1 (LUCAS et al. 1993). Among those patients presenting with newly diagnosed tuberculosis, 30% were HIV-1 positive, 4% HIV-2 positive, and 9% positive for both strains. It is worthy of note that 25%–30% of these patients with active tuberculosis were PPD (purified protein derivative) negative.

Tuberculosis, provided it is not drug resistant, can be successfully treated even when the patient has AIDS, although a slow response may be expected in advanced HIV infections and the death rate will be much higher in HIV-positive or AIDS patients. Nevertheless, chemoprophylaxis with isoniazid in Zambia resulted in a ninefold decrease in AIDS-related tuberculosis (QUIGLEY et al. 2001). Although there was no change in the mortality statistics within this group, it can be expected that there would have been a decrease in new cases amongst contacts.

Tuberculosis remains an enormous public health problem, and not only in the developing world. There are similar epidemics in eastern Europe and increasing numbers of cases throughout the developed world due to immigration, AIDS, and the emergence of resistant strains. It is estimated that about three million people die of tuberculosis every year, and these figures are probably underestimates.

Imaging Findings. Chest radiographs (see Chap. 7) are not routinely taken in many Third World countries for the diagnosis of tuberculosis except in severely ill patients or if a pneumothorax or pleural effusion is suspected. Thus, the diagnosis of tuberculosis relies mainly on examination of the sputum, but sputum is often scant or absent in the AIDS patient. Conversely, AIDS patients may have acid-fast bacilli (AFB) on sputum smears but a normal chest radiograph. Even if sputum is produced, negative AFB smears do not rule out tuberculosis as the cause of an abnormal chest radiograph. In an African study of AIDS patients, bronchoscopy of AFB smear-negative pneumonias which were unresponsive to penicillin yielded a diagnosis of tuberculosis in 39% of cases (MALIN et al. 1995).

The appearance of tuberculosis (Figs. 15.2–15.7) on chest radiographs has been described in Chap. 7.

Comparison by LONG et al. (1991) of radiographic findings of tuberculosis in Haitians with and without

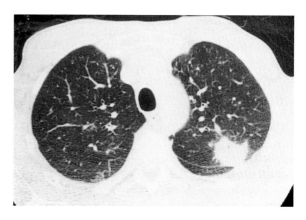

Fig. 15.2. In the earlier stages of AIDS, pulmonary tuberculosis may be similar to that in the non-AIDS patient, with upper lobe nodules or cavities

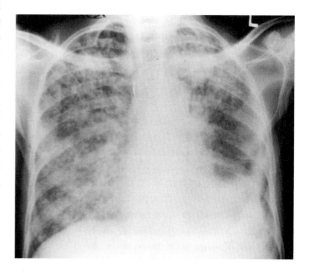

Fig. 15.3. Extensive transbronchial spread of tuberculosis from upper lobe foci

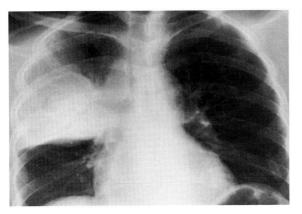

Fig. 15.4. Upper lobe consolidation and massive right paratracheal lymphadenopathy, resembling "primary" tuberculosis

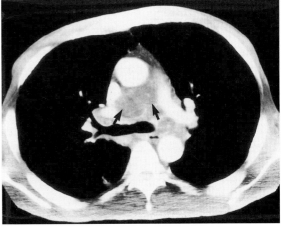

Fig. 15.6. Extensive mediastinal lymphadenopathy with some necrosis *(arrows)*

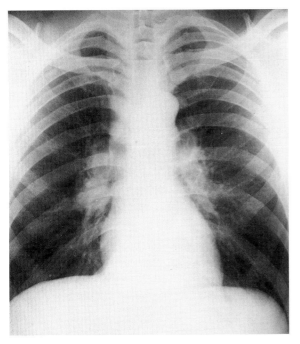

Fig. 15.5. Enlarged hilar and mediastinal lymph nodes may be the only manifestations of tuberculosis in AIDS

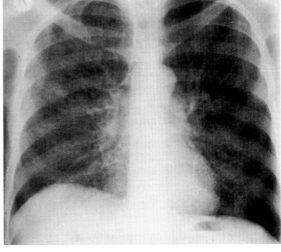

Fig. 15.7. Miliary tuberculosis: innumerable very small nodules resulting either from "primary" or postprimary progressive tuberculosis

HIV or AIDS showed a typical reactivation pattern in 80% of HIV-negative patients, 51% of HIV-positive non-AIDS patients, and 20% of AIDS patients. Similarly, a typical "primary" pattern was seen in 80% of AIDS patients, 30% of HIV-positive non-AIDS patients, and 11% of HIV-negative patients.

Chest radiographic findings in Zambia and Zaire in a study by TSHIBWABWA-TUMBA et al. (1997) confirm that, compared with HIV-negative tuberculosis patients, those who are infected with HIV have a higher incidence of lymphadenopathy (26% vs 13%), pleu-

ral effusions (16% vs 7%), miliary disease (10% vs 5%), interstitial pattern (12% vs 7%), and consolidation (10% vs 3%), but a lower incidence of atelectasis (12% vs 24%) and a much lower incidence of cavitation (33% vs 78%).

AIDS-related tuberculosis is an important cause of empyema. Two-thirds of the empyemas treated in surgical units at a Zambian Hospital were from AIDS-related tuberculosis (DESAI and MUGALA 1992). Pericardial effusions are also common.

15.12.2
Atypical Mycobacteria

Ten strains of atypical mycobacteria cause clinical disease, but *M. avium-intracellulare*, also known as MAC *(Mycobacterium avium* complex), is a particularly common opportunistic organism in AIDS. The atypical mycobacteria are present in the environment worldwide. High rates of infection have been found in Australian AIDS patients, which is not surprising because a high prevalence was noted there before the AIDS epidemic. In Brazil, atypical mycobacterial isolates from bone marrow aspirates are more than twice as common as *Mycobacterium tuberculosis* in AIDS patients with persistent fever, anemia, and leukopenia (BARRETO et al. 1993). In the United States, the atypical mycobacteria are one of the most common manifestations of AIDS, but clinical atypical mycobacterial infections are relatively rare in African AIDS patients. Atypical mycobacterial infections were seen in only 3% of HIV-positive patients, and were not primarily responsible for any death (LUCAS et al. 1994a). Culture of environmental and water supply samples from the United States, Finland, Zaire, and Kenya showed that African samples were less likely to be contaminated with atypical mycobacteria than those from the United States or Finland (VON REYN et al. 1993). Although one study found atypical mycobacteria in 13% of African AIDS patients (PORTEALS et al. 1988), these infections did not appear to be clinically relevant. Similarly, atypical infections are not often encountered in most South America countries, other than Brazil.

In the developed world, most patients do not develop clinically relevant atypical mycobacterial infection until CD4+ counts fall below 100 cells/mm^3, below the mean value at death in the tropics (LUCAS et al. 1993; RIGSBY and CURTIS 1994). However, this would not seem to completely explain the marked disparity in the numbers of cases encountered, so it has been theorized that prior infection with tuberculosis, very common in the African HIV population and elsewhere in the tropics, may produce some class resistance to the development of clinically significant atypical infections. This is contrary to the commonly accepted belief held before AIDS that there is no cross-resistance between *M. tuberculosis* and the atypical mycobacteria.

Imaging Findings. Atypical mycobacterial infection in the AIDS patient is often a disseminated infection, with correspondingly variable radiographic presentations (Figs. 15.8–15.10), as described in Chap. 7. It must be remembered that in spite of the differences

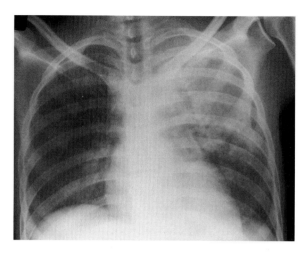

Fig. 15.8. Atypical mycobacterial infection *(Mycobacterium avium* complex): extensive airspace disease in patient with advanced AIDS

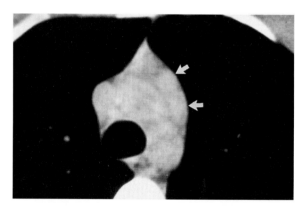

Fig. 15.9. Enlarged lymph nodes *(arrows)* caused by atypical mycobacterial disease are usually of soft tissue density

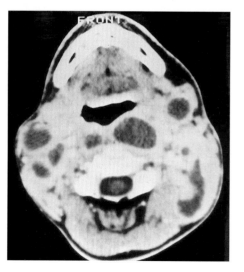

Fig. 15.10. Extensive cervical lymphadenopathy due to *Mycobacterium avium* complex showing the unusual finding of extensive necrosis

in the chest images of HIV-positive and HIV-negative patients, it is not possible to use the imaging findings to make the diagnosis of AIDS. Many HIV-negative patients in the tropics show similar patterns of both *M. tuberculosis* and atypical (MOTT) infections because they are immunocompromised for other reasons.

15.12.3
Pyogenic Infections

Frequently overlooked in discussions of AIDS-related infections are the common organisms which cause pneumonias and other infections in all patients, but for which AIDS patients are at far greater risk. Pyogenic pneumonias were present in 30% and were the primary cause of death in 8% of HIV-positive patients (LUCAS et al. 1994a). The causative organisms were equally divided between gram-positive cocci and gram-negative rods. In a study by GILKS et al. (1996) of sex workers in Nairobi, 79 episodes of invasive pneumococcal disease were seen in 587 HIV-positive women, as opposed to one episode in 132 seronegative women (relative risk 17.8). Occult bacteremia was also seen in this study, a finding not usually encountered in normal adult hosts with pneumococcal pneumonia. HIV-infected patients in Kenya who later developed pneumococcal bacteremia had a significantly lower antibody level towards pneumococcal antigen (pneumolysin) compared with seronegative controls (AMDAHL et al. 1995). Prevention of AIDS-associated pneumococcal disease by means of vaccination has been attempted in Uganda, with poor results (FRENCH et al. 2000).

HIV-positive children with bacterial infections are more likely to exhibit bacteremia, particularly enterobacteremia, and more likely to die if bacteremic [such bacteremia may be due to staphylococci (coagulase negative, followed by *S. aureus*), *Streptococcus pneumoniae*, nontyphoidal *Salmonella*, *E. coli*, *Klebsiella*, and *Rhodococcus equi*].

Bacteremia was present in 16% of HIV + patients, and was responsible for 11% of deaths in the autopsy series of LUCAS et al. (1994a) (Ivory Coast). It was the second most common cause of death after tuberculosis. Etiology of the sepsis, in descending order, included pyelonephritis, pneumonia, enteritis, hepatobiliary disease, and gynecologic infections.

Pyogenic pulmonary, blood, gastrointestinal, renal, sinus, CNS, skin, muscle, soft tissue, and bone and joint infections, as well as endocarditis, are seen with a greater frequency in AIDS patients than in normal hosts.

Imaging Findings. In the AIDS patient, common organisms may have unusual clinical and radiographic presentations (see Chap. 7). *Streptococcus pneumoniae* is very common in the AIDS patient and is more likely to be associated with aggressive spread and multilobar involvement, cavitation, empyema formation, and sepsis than in the normal host.

Pseudomonas bronchopneumonia in the AIDS patient may present with a reticular or reticulonodular pattern, as well as alveolar consolidation. *Staphylococcus aureus*, *Haemophilus influenzae*, and *Streptococcus monocytogenes* are other common pathogens. Nontyphoid strains of *Salmonella* pneumonia may cavitate, form abscesses, or be associated with bacteremia.

Rhodococcus equi pneumonia is characterized by dense pulmonary consolidation with or without cavitation, as well as mediastinal lymphadenopathy and pulmonary nodules (Fig. 15.11). It may be confused with tuberculosis and may be underdiagnosed (GRAY et al. 2000).

Pyogenic infection of the airways is increasingly recognized as a complication of AIDS, causing bronchial wall thickening, impacted bronchioles, and/or bronchiectasis, and primarily involving the lower lobes.

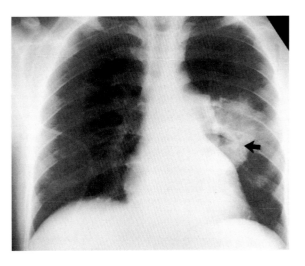

Fig. 15.11. *Rhodococcus equi*, usually encountered in equine foals, can produce mass-like areas of consolidation which may cavitate *(arrow)* in the AIDS patient. (Courtesy of Dr. Charles White)

15.12.4
Bacillary Angiomatosis

Bacillary angiomatosis is a cause of angiomatous skin nodules in AIDS patients, but the infection is not confined to the skin and almost any organ can be involved, particularly at mucocutaneous junctions. The infection is caused by bacilli of the genus *Bartonella*, particularly *B. henselae*, and *B. quintana*, an organism commonly found in cats (24% of cats in Zimbabwe) (KELLY et al. 1996) and also found in fleas and ticks. Clinically the infection presents with fevers, anemia, and angiomatous skin lesions which have an erythematous scale collar. The number of skin lesions seems to reflect the degree of immunosuppression. The individual skin lesions vary considerably but some resemble Kaposi's sarcoma, except that these nodules are painful, while those of Kaposi's sarcoma seldom are.

Bacillary angiomatosis responds rapidly to a variety of antibiotics, but resolution may take many weeks and there may be recurrence when therapy is discontinued. Cases of bacillary angiomatosis have been reported wherever there is AIDS, from the Americas, Africa, Europe, and Asia; however, because the disease is so easily confused with Kaposi's sarcoma, the real incidence is difficult to quantify accurately.

Imaging Findings. Multiorgan involvement is common, with lung nodules, mediastinal lymphadenop- athy, pleural effusions, and ascites (Fig. 15.12) (MOORE et al. 1995). The liver and spleen may be infected and severe hemorrhage can occur. The associated, often pronounced lymphadenopathy and soft tissue masses show dramatic contrast enhancement because the lesions contain well-formed, functional vascular structures (Fig. 15.13).

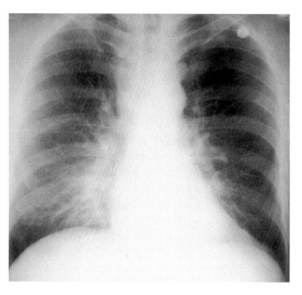

Fig. 15.12. Mediastinal and right hilar lymphadenopathy associated with bacillary angiomatosis

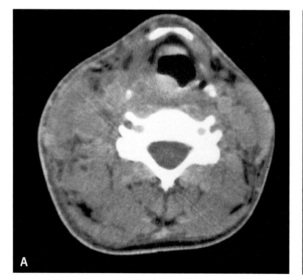
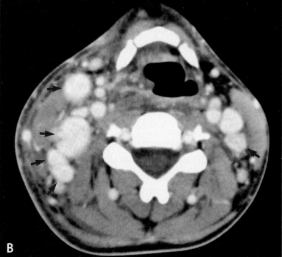

Fig. 15.13A, B. Bacillary angiomatosis. Marked enhancement of lymph nodes of the neck (*arrows*) after contrast injection, equal to the density seen in vascular structures. CT precontrast (**A**) and postcontrast (**B**)

15.12.5
Nocardiosis

A very uncommon manifestation of AIDS in the developed countries, nocardiosis appears to be more common in the tropical world (4% incidence, LUCAS et al. 1994b). The majority of infections are disseminated. Pulmonary disease is most common, followed by cerebral abscesses. Involvement of other organs is rare, but adrenal abscesses have been reported. It is possible that some patients with "smear-negative sputum" for tuberculosis actually have nocardiosis.

Imaging Findings. The manifestations of nocardiosis are protean. The disease may present as multiple nodules which may cavitate, as well as lobar or even diffuse airspace disease, or as a combination thereof. There may be mediastinal lymphadenopathy, pleural effusions, or pleural thickening. Cerebral involvement is most commonly recognized by ring-enhancing abscesses, frequently associated with subependymal nodules and hydrocephalus (LEBLANG et al. 1995).

15.13
Viral Pathogens

15.13.1
Cytomegalovirus

A member of the herpes virus group, cytomegalovirus is present in many HIV-1 patients in both the developed and the nondeveloped world. Immunosuppression leads to reactivation of this common latent infection. However, it has been thought to be an uncommon cause of clinically significant AIDS-related disease in the tropics, perhaps since it is generally seen with CD4+ counts below 50/mm^3. This does not seem to be the case in patients with HIV-2, in whom severe cytomegalovirus infections appear to be more common (LUCAS et al. 1993). Cytomegalovirus is a common isolate from lung and liver at the time of death (JEENA et al. 1996), although the significance of this finding is unclear. Along with P. *carinii*, cytomegalovirus is a common isolate at autopsy in pediatric patients in Chiang Mai, Thailand (BHOOPAT et al. 1994).

Cytomegalovirus infection has an immunomodulating effect, further encouraging the development of superinfections by other organisms in these patients. Thus, it is often part of a multiorganism infection.

The most common manifestation of cytomegalovirus is retinitis, which if untreated may lead to

blindness. Less common manifestations include esophagitis, gastritis, colitis, and pneumonia.

Varicella and herpes simplex are other viral pathogens affecting the lungs and other organs in AIDS.

Imaging Findings. Pulmonary involvement by cytomegalovirus is characterized most commonly by a diffuse reticular or reticulonodular pattern, or ground glass density, and may progress to frank airspace disease (McGUINESS et al. 1994) (see Chap. 7). It may also produce localized masses, usually 1–3 cm in size. Other findings such as pleural effusion or lymphadenopathy are rare. Pulmonary involvement is usually accompanied by clinically significant disease at other sites, such as retinitis, esophagitis, colitis, or cholangitis.

AIDS patients share the same propensity to disseminated varicella infection as other immunocompromised hosts. The appearance in the lungs is similar – a diffuse small nodular pattern (Fig. 15.14).

Herpes simplex pneumonia presents with diffuse airspace disease.

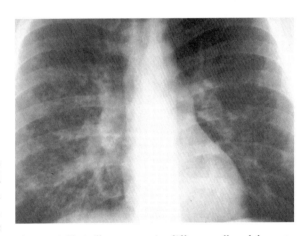

Fig. 15.14. Varicella pneumonia; diffuse small nodular pattern

15.13.2
Pneumocystis carinii

Although P. *carinii* pneumonia is the most common complication of AIDS in the United States and in Western Europe, occurring in 65%–85% of homosexual AIDS patients, it is far less common in Africa and other parts of the world. It may be underestimated because of the lack of availability of diagnostic bronchoscopy, but this does not fully explain the difference. Even within Africa, there is substantial variation. Pneumocystosis is only found in 9% of HIV-positive autopsies (LUCAS et al. 1994a). Numerous other studies from sub-Saharan Africa show that even where there are adequate diagnostic facilities, i.e., bronchoalveolar lavage, transbronchial biopsy, or autopsy, pneumocystosis rates will range between 3% and 22% (the highest value being from Zimbabwe) (McLeod et al. 1990). However, a study by Jeena et al. (1996) of African infants suggests that it is more common than previously thought, occurring in 78% of samples of lungs tested.

Similarly, a recent African study of bronchoscopy isolates in AIDS-related pneumonias unresponsive to penicillin and AFB smear-negative revealed a 33% incidence of pneumocystosis (Malin et al. 1995). In this study, the median CD4 count for these cases was 134/mm^3, while for tuberculosis it was 206/mm^3. Pneumocystosis is uncommon in Haitian AIDS but has been noted to be relatively common among the urban homosexual population in southern Brazil, in Mexico, and in Hong Kong. In a pediatric autopsy study in Thailand, *P. carinii* was a common isolate (Bhoopat et al. 1994).

As has been speculated to explain the situation for atypical mycobacteria, it has been proposed that African AIDS patients die of other, less opportunistic infections prior to onset of the profound immunosuppression required to develop pneumocystosis. It is also possible that P. carinii is a much less prevalent organism. Because of these statistics, prophylactic therapy against pneumocystosis may be of little value in many tropical regions.

Imaging Findings. The early and late manifestations of *P. carinii* infection on chest radiographs (Figs. 15.15–15.19) or CT are described in Chap. 7. Radiographic

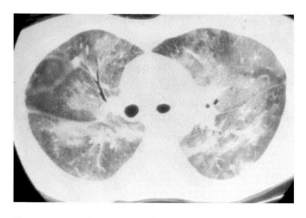

Fig. 15.16. CT of a patient with *P. carinii* pneumonia, clearly demonstrating a diffuse ground glass pattern

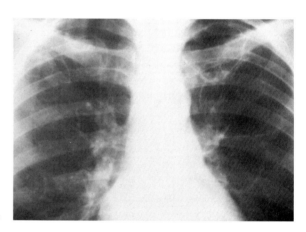

Fig. 15.17. *Pneumocystis carinii* nodules may excavate, creating pneumatoceles, which may trap air and become very large

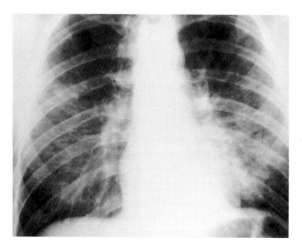

Fig. 15.15. Early *Pneumocystis carinii* pneumonia: interstitial pattern which results in ill-defined borders of the lung vascular markings (*right base*), progressing to ground glass opacities (*left base*)

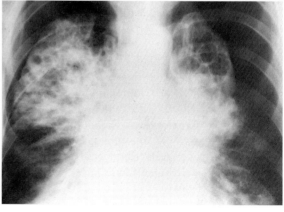

Fig. 15.18. *P. carinii* resulting in numerous peripheral cystic lesions with secondary bilateral pneumothorax. The cystic lesions are best visualized in the periphery of the collapsed left upper lobe

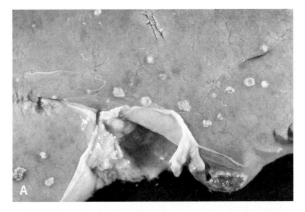

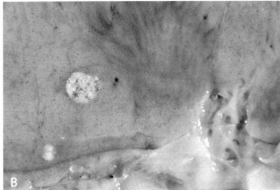

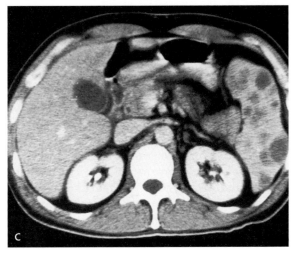

Fig. 15.19A–C. *Pneumocystis carinii.* **A, B** Macroscopically: gray or white nodules are seen in the kidney. **C** CT shows low-density lesions, particularly in the spleen

findings reported in African AIDS have included lobar, multilobar, and diffuse airspace disease. A lobar distribution is rare, and is more likely to be caused by *Streptococcus pneumoniae* or *M. tuberculosis.*

15.14
Fungal Disease and AIDS

15.14.1
Cryptococcosis

Cryptococcus neoformans is an important central nervous system (CNS) pathogen in AIDS. Bird droppings are an extraordinarily rich source of this ubiquitous fungus. Entry into the body is from a pulmonary source; all patients with pulmonary cryptococcosis must be investigated for CNS involvement by examination of the cerebrospinal fluid (CSF). Clinically, meningitis is the commonest presentation, but pseudocysts or cryptococcomas may cause symp-

toms. Primary pulmonary cryptococcosis was found in 13% of AIDS patients with pulmonary disease of unknown etiology: it was best diagnosed by bronchoalveolar lavage because the associated symptoms of cough, weight loss, fever, dyspnea, chest pain, and headache were nonspecific (BATUNGWANAYO et al. 1994a). Treatment of the pulmonary disease appears to prevent the further dissemination of cryptococcal disease.

Imaging Findings (see also Chap. 7). Pulmonary cryptococcosis in the AIDS patient does not form the typical well-circumscribed nodules seen in the normal host who is capable of a healthy granulomatous response; rather, it is usually characterized by diffuse disease. The most common manifestations documented in Rwanda (BATUNGWANAYO et al. 1994a) include a diffuse interstitial infiltrate (76%), an alveolar pattern (19%), mediastinal and/ or hilar lymphadenopathy (11%), nodules (5%), and pleural effusions (5%). A miliary pattern of small nodules may also be seen.

Computed tomography in CNS cryptococcosis is frequently normal but there may be low-density lesions, occasionally showing contrast enhancement, particularly in the basal ganglia. There may occasionally be larger masses, which may enhance.

15.14.2
Histoplasmosis

Histoplasma capsulatum (var. *capsulatum)* occurs in many African and Southeast Asian countries, as well as parts of the United States and Central and South America. Disseminated histoplasmosis is an indicator disease for AIDS. All patients living in or migrating to endemic areas are at risk. Patients tend to be in a relatively advanced stage of the disease, with CD4 counts characteristically under 100 cells/mm^3.

Histoplasmosis had not been considered a significant pathogen in Africa, but cases of disseminated "African" histoplasmosis due to *Histoplasma capsulatum* (var. *duboisii)* in HIV-infected African patients have recently been reported (PILLAY et al. 1997). It was found in 3% of patients who died from AIDS in the Ivory Coast.

Imaging Findings (see also Chap. 7). Focal areas of airspace disease, nodules, and effusions may be seen. Enlarged lymph nodes are seen less often than in the normal host. Disseminated histoplasmosis presents in AIDS as a small nodular pattern on chest radiography similar to any disseminated fungal disease (Fig. 15.20). Histoplasmosis duboisii often affects the skeleton.

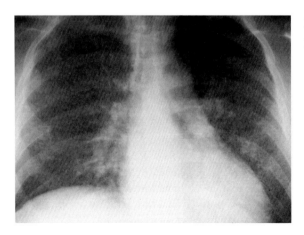

Fig. 15.20. Disseminated histoplasmosis produces a small nodular pattern in the lung, as do most hematogenously disseminated fungal infections. Associated bowel involvement is common in AIDS patients

15.14.3
Penicilliosis

Penicillium marneffei is a fungal infection involving AIDS patients living in or traveling to Southeast Asia. The reservoir for the fungus is the bamboo rat, a root rat living in tunnels in the high plateaus of Southeast Asia, and other rodents. In endemic areas, infection in more frequent in the rainy season than the dry season. It has been known as "Chinese histoplasmosis."

Penicilliosis is the third most common opportunistic infection in HIV disease in parts of Southeast Asia (after extrapulmonary tuberculosis and cryptococcal meningitis). It can clinically resemble tuberculosis, molluscum contagiosum, cryptococcosis, or histoplasmosis. Clinical features include fever, weight loss, hepatosplenomegaly, anemia, skin lesions with central umbilication, lymphadenopathy, pulmonary symptoms, and rarely, gastrointestinal symptoms such as colitis. In AIDS patients, the symptoms are more acute in onset and more intense. The organism can be isolated from skin, blood, bone marrow, and other organs (DUONG 1996). In the study of BHOOPAT et al. (1994) from Thailand, it affected 20% of AIDS patients undergoing autopsy. Treatment with parenteral amphotericin B or itraconazole has been successful.

Imaging Findings. Chest radiographs (see Chap. 7) may show a diffuse reticulonodular, a localized alveolar, a diffuse alveolar, or a localized interstitial pattern. Parenchymal masses, which may cavitate, and enlarged lymph nodes may be seen, though calcification is unusual. There may be pleural or pericardial involvement. Abscesses may also involve the skin, liver, subcutaneous tissues, and lymph nodes. Lytic bone lesions and joint infections may occur.

15.14.4
Aspergillosis

Although a less common pathogen in AIDS than in the neutropenic chemotherapy patient, *Aspergillus* occasionally involves AIDS patients. It was present in 3% of AIDS deaths in the Ivory Coast (LUCAS et al. 1993).

Imaging Findings. The most common radiologic manifestations are thick-walled cavitary lesions and, less commonly, nodules, consolidation, and pleural effusion (see Chap. 7).

15.14.5
Coccidioidomycosis

Endemic to the southwestern United States, Mexico, and portions of Central America, coccidioidomycosis is a substantial risk for AIDS patients residing in or traveling to endemic areas. While usually localized to the lung in the normal host, in AIDS patients dissemination is common.

Imaging Findings. Radiographic manifestations include cavitary masses, localized areas of consolidation, and pleural effusion or empyema. Hematogenous dissemination results in a small nodular pattern, often heralded by pronounced lymphadenopathy. There may be lytic lesions of bone (see Chap. 12).

15.14.6
Candidiasis

Though usually confined to the gastrointestinal tract, *Candida* pneumonias and disseminated candidiasis may occur in AIDS.

Imaging Findings. *Candida* pneumonia produces a nonspecific pattern of airspace disease, often accompanied by pleural effusion. Disseminated candidiasis resembles any hematogenously disseminated fungal infection, producing a small nodular pattern (Fig. 15.21) (see Chap. 7).

15.14.7
Nonspecific Interstitial Pneumonitis

In a large percentage of patients with AIDS and pulmonary symptoms (38%), no cause can be identified even after numerous investigations including open lung biopsy (BATUNGWANAYO et al. 1994b).

Imaging Findings. These patients will demonstrate an interstitial pattern on chest radiograph and nonspecific interstitial pneumonitis on lung biopsy (see Chap. 7). It has been speculated that this may represent the direct effect of HIV on lung tissue.

15.14.8
Lymphocytic Interstitial Pneumonitis

An AIDS-related polyclonal lymphoproliferative disorder known as lymphocytic interstitial pneumonitis

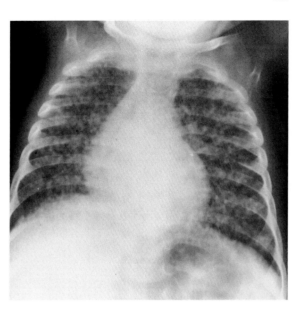

Fig. 15.21. Nine-month-old infant presented with cough and failure to thrive. The chest radiograph demonstrates a diffuse small nodular appearance due to disseminated candidiasis

is particularly common in the pediatric age group (25% of children with AIDS), but it seldom progresses to lymphoma in the AIDS patient The lungs are predominately affected, but it is now known to be a systemic process, with lymphoid infiltrates in many organs. Patients may also seem to have chronic mumps because the salivary glands are often involved.

Imaging Findings. On chest radiographs (see Chap. 7), lymphocytic interstitial pneumonitis appears as an interstitial or reticulonodular pattern, as small nodules (2–4 mm), or as subsegmental consolidation (Fig. 15.22). In some cases, the reticulonodular pattern in the lungs clears as the CD4 counts fall to very low levels, this being considered a poor prognostic sign.

15.14.9
Cardiac Disease in AIDS

Cardiac lesions associated with AIDS include pericardial effusions (often tuberculous, but also viral or fungal), metastases, and cardiomyopathy. In a variety of African studies, the vast majority of patients with tuberculous pericarditis were found to be HIV positive. An AIDS autopsy study from Puerto Rico showed an unexpectedly high rate of cardiac involvement, at 32% (ALTIERI et al. 1994). *Histoplasma capsulatum, Toxoplasma gondii, Mycobacterium tuberculosis,* cytomegalovirus, *Cryptococcus neoformans,*

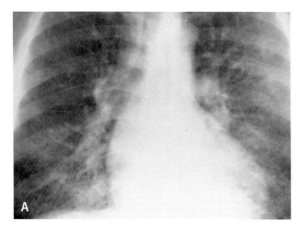

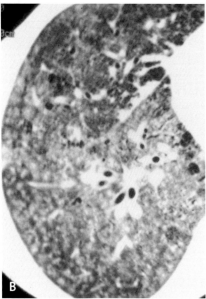

Fig. 15.22A, B. Lymphocytic interstitial pneumonitis. Polyclonal pattern of many small nodules, seen on chest radiograph (**A**) and CT (**B**)

and atypical mycobacteria were all isolated. Nonspecific myocarditis was also identified.

There may be multiple Kaposi's sarcoma nodules affecting the heart and pericardium. The AIDS virus itself may produce a dilated congestive cardiomyopathy in roughly 17% of patients, which may be rapidly progressive; children are often affected.

Imaging Findings. In HIV-related myocarditis, a dilated cardiomyopathy causes increasing cardiac size and, eventually, congestive heart failure. An enlarged cardiac silhouette may also indicate pericardial effusion (Fig. 15.23). In such cases, the classic bag-shaped heart may be seen, with straightening of the left heart border to the level of the transverse portion

of the aorta, the superior extent of the pericardium. Ultrasonography will confirm the diagnosis, because it is very difficult to distinguish cardiomyopathy from pericardial fluid radiographically.

15.15
AIDS-Related Neoplasms

AIDS-related neoplasms may involve the thorax, the abdomen, and other sites.

15.15.1
AIDS-Related Lymphomas

AIDS-related lymphomas are non-Hodgkin's lymphomas: intermediate or high-grade B cell lymphomas, including diffuse large cleaved and noncleaved cell, large cell immunoblastic and small noncleaved cell Burkitt's or non-Burkitt's lymphomas. Over 60% are high-grade lymphomas, especially of the small non-cleaved Burkitt's, non-Burkitt's, or immunoblastic types. These are commonly extranodal; 76% are entirely extranodal, while 98% have some involvement of an extranodal site such as the central nervous system, the bone marrow, the gastrointestinal tract, or mucocutaneous junctions. Twenty percent are primary lymphomas of the brain. Many authors believe that AIDS-related lymphomas are related to the Epstein-Barr virus.

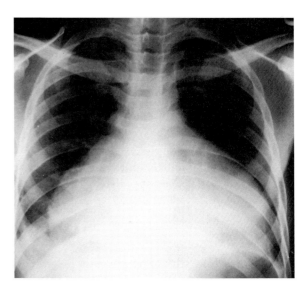

Fig. 15.23. Severe cardiomegaly, due to AIDS-related tuberculosis pericarditis

Lymphoma associated with AIDS usually presents clinically at an advanced stage. It is important that these lymphomas be distinguished from lymphadenopathy due to tuberculosis or other causes. It is also important to separate true lymphoma from the progressive generalized lymphadenopathy which is commonly seen in AIDS. Lucas et al. (1994a) reported that, in Africa, 2.8% of HIV-positive hospital deaths are due to AIDS-related lymphoma (1.6% visceral and 1.2% primary cerebral lymphoma).

About 50% of AIDS patients with lymphoma have had previous (or have concomitant) opportunistic infections. Symptoms of fever and weight loss are frequent. Early diagnosis is of little importance, since the treatment of HIV-related lymphomas is unsatisfactory. The CNS lymphomas have the worst prognosis and are not as radiosensitive as non-HIV-related brain lymphomas: high-grade extracranial lymphomas may show a response to a combination of chemotherapy and radiotherapy. Better results may be seen with large noncleaved cell lymphomas. Compared with lymphomas in the non-HIV patient, complete response is unusual. The mean survival time of patients with AIDS-related lymphomas undergoing chemotherapy is 5.5 months, far less than in other hosts.

Classic pediatric Burkitt's lymphoma is not an AIDS-associated tumor in Africa. Pediatric non-Hodgkin's lymphoma is rare, probably because the children do not survive long enough to develop this malignancy.

Although the incidence of Hodgkin's disease is also increased in the HIV-positive patient group in many settings, this trend was not observed in an African study by Sitas et al. (1997), in which the only cancers to show increased frequency were Kaposi's sarcoma and non-Hodgkin's lymphoma, the latter somewhat less than reported in developed countries.

Imaging Findings. The imaging finding (Figs. 15.24–15.36) of the CNS, chest, and abdomen have been described in Chaps. 5, 7, and 8–11.

15.15.2
Kaposi's Sarcoma

Described in 1872, the hemangiosarcoma of Kaposi has been the subject of much misunderstanding. Two variations have been described, depending on the natural history of the tumor. The "classic" version is a peripheral neoplasm, often presenting as pigmented nodules in the lower limbs, which progresses

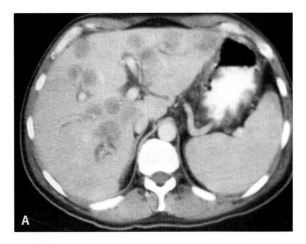

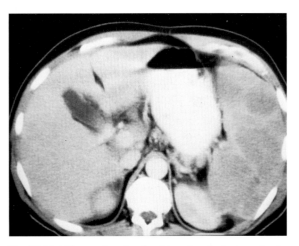

Fig. 15.24. A CT scan of the liver showing multiple low-density lesions due to AIDS-related lymphoma. **B** On ultrasonography these are hypoechoic

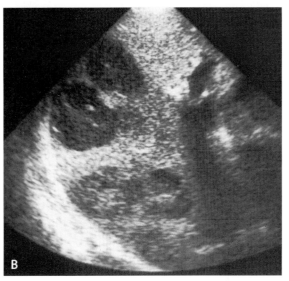

Fig. 15.25. CT scan showing focal low-density lesions due to AIDS-related lymphoma within an enlarged spleen

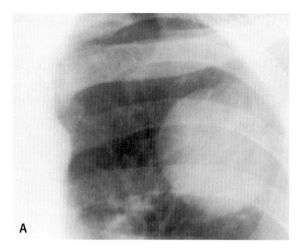

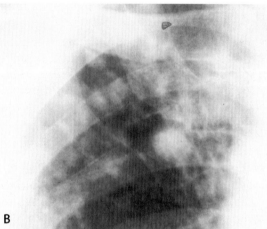

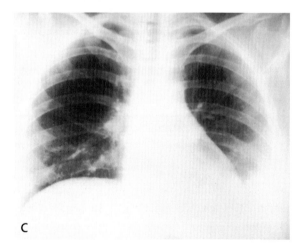

Fig. 15.26A–C. When non-Hodgkin's lymphoma spreads to the lungs there may be discrete round nodules (**A**) or multiple small nodules (**B**). **C** Another common finding is a pleural effusion

slowly in the majority of patients unless there is a change in the status of the patient's immune system. The other version is described in some texts as the "HIV-related generalized aggressive" form. The slow "classic" variety can be transformed into the "aggressive" version by immunosuppression at any age.

Kaposi's sarcoma does not in itself indicate AIDS. In regions such as sub-Saharan Africa, either can exist separately; therefore, HIV serology must be assessed in every patient with Kaposi's sarcoma at any age.

There are regional differences in distribution and aggression. For example, in the United States, unlike most other AIDS complications, Kaposi's sarcoma is concentrated in certain regions: 30% of California and New York homosexuals with AIDS develop Kaposi's sarcoma, whereas in Kansas only 5% of homosexuals with AIDS develop the tumor. Sexual contacts of male homosexuals experience an increased risk of subsequently developing Kaposi's sarcoma. In HIV-negative individuals, it follows a benign course; this is the pattern for 2% of Kaposi's sarcoma in the homosexual population.

Recently a herpes type virus (HHV-8), also called "Kaposi's sarcoma-associated herpes virus" (Kaposi's sarcoma HV), has been found incorporated into the DNA of Kaposi's sarcoma tumor specimens and is now recognized as the cause. Epidemiologically, spread of Kaposi's sarcoma in the homosexual population has been linked to sexual practices involving fecal contact (raising the possibility of spread by other forms of fecal contact). There is a high prevalence of antibodies to Kaposi's sarcoma HV in HIV-infected American homosexual men, but a low prevalence, similar to that in the population at large, in HIV-positive drug users, hemophiliacs, and women. Analysis of tumor lesions from 38 Ugandan Kaposi's sarcoma patients showed that the lesions contained Kaposi's sarcoma HV, and Kaposi's sarcoma HV DNA was also detectable in peripheral blood mononuclear cells (PURVIS et al. 1997). Also noted was the intriguing finding that a high percentage of Kaposi's sarcoma lesions were positive for Epstein-Barr virus sequences. Similar Kaposi's sarcoma HV sequences have been identified in all tested cases of the so-called classic Kaposi's sarcoma, endemic African Kaposi's sarcoma, AIDS-associated epidemic Kaposi's sarcoma, and iatrogenic Kaposi's sarcoma. Examination of serologic evidence of antibodies to Kaposi's sarcoma HV has revealed all patients with African endemic Kaposi's sarcoma to be seropositive. Between 2% and 8% of children are positive, confirming the presence of a nonsexual means of spread (conceivably fecal contact due to poor hygiene practices or perinatal infection). Kaposi's sarcoma HV may, indeed, be a common childhood febrile infection in endemic areas. In Africa and elsewhere, young children may develop Kaposi's sarcoma with minimal skin involvement but with lymphadenopathy, extensive internal organ involvement, and a virulent course.

An additional mystifying statistic is that Kaposi's sarcoma is overwhelmingly a male disease even in the almost exclusively heterosexual population of Africa, and there are few concordant couples even in areas of high incidence. Even in pediatric Kaposi's sarcoma and pre-AIDS era Kaposi's sarcoma, a strong male predominance has been noted, except along the eastern seaboard of South Africa. With the onset of the AIDS epidemic, it has become the most common cancer in African men. However, the male to female ratio has dropped from 19:1 to 1.7:1 (THOMAS 2001).

Kaposi's sarcoma is less common and quite variable in heterosexually transmitted AIDS: it occurs in 8%–18% of heterosexually transmitted AIDS cases in Africa, 30% in Mexico, and 6%–9% in the Caribbean, but in less than 1% of such cases in the United States or India. Patients whose HIV infection is transfusion related rarely develop Kaposi's sarcoma, yet it has developed in patients acquiring HIV via maternal-fetal infection, particularly in the African and Caribbean populations. Kaposi's sarcoma is the most common transplant-associated tumor in Saudi Arabia, but is rare in this setting in Western countries.

It is important to note the clinical variations in Kaposi's sarcoma: although usually characterized by painless deep reddish-purple subcutaneous nodules and similar angiomatous lesions of the mucosae, there may be facial thickening without obvious pigmentation. Kaposi's sarcoma may appear in the gastrointestinal tract or airways without visible skin lesions. Visceral lesions can be solitary or multiple and present as a mass, bleeding, or obstruction. Angiography can demonstrate multiple clinically unsuspected tumors.

It is probable that the development of the aggressive form of Kaposi's sarcoma requires a substantial degree of immunosuppression. In 80% of cases of Kaposi's sarcoma the tumor is the presenting symptom of AIDS. However, particularly in Africa, not every patient with Kaposi's sarcoma has AIDS or is even HIV positive. There is nothing clinically or histologically to distinguish the non-AIDS patient; only serology can do this.

Although chemotherapy produces a clinical response in many patients with endemic African Kaposi's sarcoma, epidemic AIDS-related Kaposi's sarcoma does not respond. Lesions will, however, respond well to local palliative radiotherapy.

Imaging Findings. The CNS, thoracic, abdominal, and musculoskeletal manifestations and imaging findings (Fig. 15.27) have been described in Chaps. 5 and 7–12.

15.16
Organisms Likely to Cause AIDS-Related Diarrhea in the Tropics

The most common presentation of AIDS in Africa is "slim disease," a syndrome characterized by chronic diarrhea and weight loss, leading to severe cachexia. This syndrome affects up to 80% of AIDS patients, and as many as 85% of patients have diarrhea (compared with 50% of Western AIDS patients). However, an autopsy study from West Africa (LUCAS et al. 1994a) indicated that a premortem diagnosis of diarrhea was no more frequent in cachectic patients than in noncachectic patients, and found wasting to be strongly correlated with tuberculosis. Forty-four percent of skeletally wasted cadavers had tuberculosis, compared with 39% of moderately wasted and 23% of nonwasted cadavers. This goes against the conventional wisdom that wasting results from an enteropathy such as that caused by cryptosporidiosis or HIV itself. There is speculation that in some patients, a component of wasting may be related to soluble tumor necrosis factor receptor concentrations (reflecting immune activation and high cytokine activity), rather than being entirely attributable to infections.

The coccidian parasites *Cryptosporidium parvum*, *Isospora belli*, and *Cyclospora*, and the microsporidia are thought to account for at least half of the cases of persistent AIDS-associated diarrhea in the developing world, with contributions from *Mycobacterium avium* complex, other bacteria, and cytomegalovirus.

Cryptosporidiosis and isosporiasis are protozoan diseases (in the same genus as *Toxoplasma gondii*) which affect the epithelial cells of the gastrointestinal tract. In normal hosts, cryptosporidiosis produces transient episodes of diarrhea. In AIDS patients, the diarrhea is far more severe.

Cryptosporidium was the most common pathogen identified in several AIDS diarrhea studies from Africa and Haiti, and is also common in Central and South America. In a study from Brazil, *Cryptosporidium* and *Isospora* were not found in any of the normal hosts examined, but were present in 19% and 10% of AIDS patients respectively (SAUDA et al. 1993). Examina-

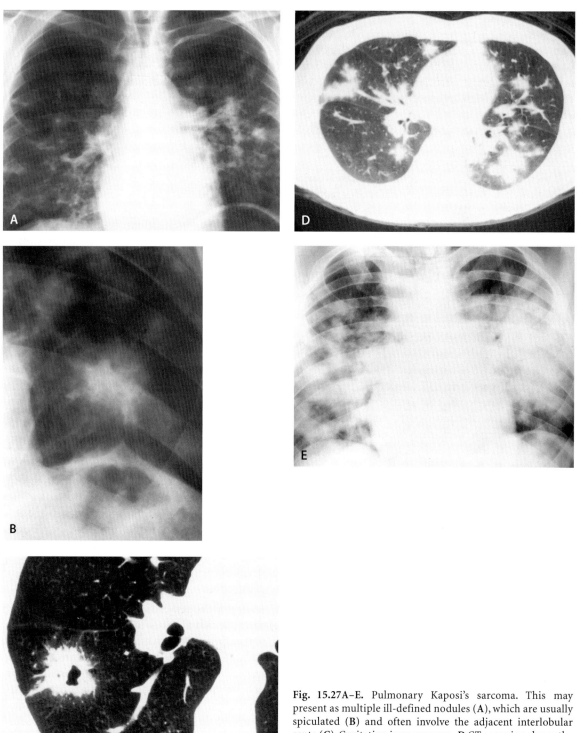

Fig. 15.27A–E. Pulmonary Kaposi's sarcoma. This may present as multiple ill-defined nodules (**A**), which are usually spiculated (**B**) and often involve the adjacent interlobular septa (**C**). Cavitation is uncommon. **D** CT scanning shows the peribronchovascular location. **E** Because the Kaposi's sarcoma nodules are vascular, there may be hemorrhage into the lung, causing airspace disease

tion of the causes of chronic diarrhea in AIDS patients, as compared to the general population in Zambia, showed that *Isospora* occurred in markedly increased numbers in AIDS patients (and was not seen in the general population), and that *Cryptosporidium* was also an important AIDS-related pathogen (HUNTER et al. 1992). *Cryptosporidium* has been documented in 38% of AIDS patients with diarrhea in Mali (PICHARD et al. 1990), and 21% in the Democratic Republic of the Congo (ANANTHA-SUBRAMANIAN et al. 1997). In two Tanzanian studies, cryptosporidiosis and isosporiasis were virtually restricted to HIV-positive individuals with diarrhea (ATZORI et al. 1993; KHUMALO-NGWENYA et al. 1994). Also in Tanzania, a survey of intestinal parasites showed that the prevalence of *Cryptosporidium parvum*, *Isospora belli*, and *Strongyloides stercoralis* was higher in HIV-positive than in HIV-negative patients (and higher in AIDS patients than in HIV-positive patients) (GOMEZ MORALES et al. 1995). *Entamoeba histolytica* and *Ascaris lumbricoides* were more frequent in HIV-negative patients. In a study comparing HIV-positive Zambian diarrhea patients with HIV-negative diarrhea patients, only *Isospora belli* and *Cryptosporidium* were seen exclusively in the HIV-positive group, and an increased incidence of *Entamoeba coli* was also seen (HUNTER et al. 1992). Fecal samples from 108 AIDS patients in southern India revealed that a third of patients with diarrhea were positive for *Cryptosporidium* oocytes (ANANTHASUBRAMANI-AN et al. 1997). In a large Haitian diarrhea study in HIV-positive patients, the most common enteric protozoa included *Cryptosporidium* (30%), *Isospora belli* (12%), *Cyclospora* (11%), *Giardia* (3%), and *Entamoeba histolytica* (1%). Co-infections with *Isospora* and *Cryptosporidium* are seen quite commonly (PAPE et al. 1994).

Cryptosporidia will involve the biliary tract in 10% of AIDS patients. Multisystemic infections involving the respiratory tract, small intestine, biliary tract, and pancreas have occurred. High death rates are seen in the AIDS population because currently there is no effective treatment, although nitazoxanide has recently been shown to be promising. It also shows activity against *Isospora belli*, *Entamoeba histolytica*, *Giardia lamblia*, *Ascaris lumbricoides*, *Enterobius vermicularis*, *Hymenolepis nana*, and *Dicrocoelium dentriticum*.

The ubiquitous microsporidia species *Enterocytozoon bieneusi*, a small protozoan parasite, has been described in 33% of Australian AIDS patients with diarrhea (FIELD et al. 1993). Its contribution to diarrhea in African AIDS patients is probably less significant; it is reported in 2% of patients in Zambia and is not found in patients in Uganda or the Democratic Republic of the Congo.

Cytomegalovirus may produce colitis, with nodular mucosal thickening. Cytomegalovirus infections resulting in diarrhea were identified in only 6% of patients in the Democratic Republic of the Congo and no patients in Uganda and Zambia. However, in India it was found at autopsy in the gastrointestinal tract in 27% of individuals dying from AIDS (LANJEWAR et al. 1996). Intestinal disease due to atypical mycobacteria is also rare in Africa and has not increased in AIDS patients there. Although there is no definitive evidence that AIDS increases the likelihood of infection with *Strongyloides* in the tropics, disseminated strongyloidiasis is much more common in HIV-positive patients (and patients placed on steroids). Dissemination may be associated with the adult respiratory distress syndrome, septic shock, and death. Patients with preexisting colonization by *Strongyloides* appear to have increasing intestinal penetration by the larvae, leading to self-reinfection with increased burdens of juvenile forms. These pass through the lungs and may produce an acute allergic reaction, clinically manifested by asthma, cough, pulmonary infiltrates, and hypoxia. The organisms and surrounding inflammatory reaction may be visible on plain radiographs as a nodular or reticulonodular pattern or on CT scanning as ill-defined nodular densities, about 2–5 mm in size (Fig. 15.28)The patients often present with a combination of gastrointestinal and respiratory symptomatology. This syndrome is frequently accompanied by gram-negative sepsis. The diagnosis may be made by bronchoalveolar lavage and the presence of *Strongyloides* in the intestine, found by examination of the stool for ova and parasites or by duodenal capsule biopsy. Disseminated strongyloidiasis may involve the CNS.

Entamoeba histolytica and *Giardia* appear to be more common in patients with AIDS in the United States than in African and other Third World nations, probably due to increased male homosexual contact. Although unclean water supplies can transmit these diseases, there appears to be no increased risk in AIDS patients in the developing world. Studies from numerous African countries suggest that there is no significant increase in the incidence of extracellular intestinal parasites, such as *Necator americanus* and *Ascaris*, when AIDS patients are compared with controls.

Reports from areas where typhoid and paratyphoid are endemic show that HIV patients may have

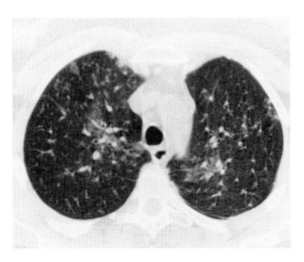

Fig. 15.28. Ill-defined nodules and patchy foci of airspace disease are seen in this patient with asthma: there were *Strongyloides* in both sputum and stool. (Courtesy of Dr. Linda Haramati)

a substantial increase over baseline rates of these diseases. This may reflect the decreased activity of the mononuclear cells in AIDS patients against these organisms. Typhoid and paratyphoid in the AIDS patient are characterized by fulminant diarrhea associated with colitis, and often relapse despite adequate treatment.

Nontyphi salmonellae are also a substantial cause of morbidity in HIV in the tropics, and systemic salmonellosis may be an underdiagnosed cause of death. Of 103 patients in Burundi in hospital for *Salmonella* dysentery, 86 were HIV positive (83%).

Patients with HIV-2 may be more susceptible to bacterial causes of diarrhea than patients with HIV-1 (Ndour et al. 2000).

No etiologic agent can be identified in approximately 20%–40% of the patients in Africa, Haiti, and other parts of the developing world who have both AIDS and chronic diarrhea. This may represent the lack of sophisticated laboratories, but it may also indicate a high incidence of AIDS enteropathy: a chronic diarrhea in AIDS patients for which no identifiable pathogen is found and which possibly results from the direct effect of HIV on the mucosa.

A reasonable guess as to the possible cause can be made on the basis of gastrointestinal symptoms. Dysphagia or odynophagia suggests *Candida*, cytomegalovirus, or herpes simplex esophagitis. Subacute abdominal pain, vomiting, and weight loss raise the possibility of lymphoma or Kaposi's sarcoma. Severe acute abdominal pain suggests pancreatitis or intestinal perforation due to cytomegalovirus.

Right upper quadrant pain suggests hepatic abscess, cholangitis, or cholecystitis. Diarrhea suggests protozoal, parasitic, bacterial, and/or viral disease. Pneumatosis intestinalis should raise the possibility of cryptosporidiosis, rotavirus, cytomegalovirus, *Clostridium difficile*, or *Pseudomonas*.

Many patients with AIDS involving the gastrointestinal tract will have a combination of two or more etiologic factors, such as more than one organism or both infection and malignancy. The documentation of one pathogen or a malignancy does not exclude others. All clinical findings should not be attributed to a single primary diagnosis, particularly in the Third World, where multiple pathologies are not uncommon even in the absence of AIDS.

15.17
Gastrointestinal Disease in AIDS

15.17.1
Esophagus and Stomach (see Chap. 8)

Many AIDS patients experience severe dysphagia or odynophagia, which may be due to a variety of etiologies. Air contrast examination of the esophagus and stomach is important to evaluate focal lesions and the condition of the intervening mucosa.

Esophageal disease may be caused by HIV, resulting in multiple discrete, large shallow ulcers. Esophageal herpes simplex virus infection produces numerous discrete ulcers which may be surrounded by edema and which are separated by normal mucosa, producing a cobblestone appearance on barium swallow (Fig. 15.29). The rectum and anus may also be involved. Cytomegalovirus is another common cause of esophageal ulceration, characteristically producing large, somewhat diamond-shaped ulcers. In the stomach, thickening of mucosal folds and antral stenosis are characteristic findings.

Many of the AIDS patients who complain of dysphagia/odynophagia will have thrush (candidiasis). The condition is widely seen in the tropics. Candidiasis is more common in HIV-1 than in HIV-2 infection (Ndour et al. 2000). Oral thrush is often found in patients with esophageal candidiasis. A barium swallow early in the course of involvement will show small round plaque-like exophytic lesions on the mucosal surface of the esophagus. In more severe cases, the interstices between plaques, mucosal ulcerations, and pseudomembranes produce a "shaggy" appearance.

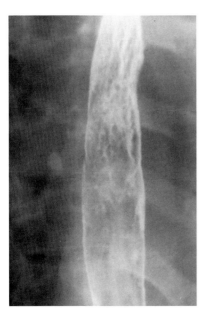

Fig. 15.29. The barium air contrast study of the esophagus of an AIDS patient with herpes simplex esophagitis. There are multiple ulcers separated by areas of normal mucosa

Kaposi's sarcoma may involve the esophagus, stomach, small bowel, or large bowel, originating as flat submucosal lesions but enlarging into polypoid masses often demonstrating central umbilication (target lesion). These lesions may be accompanied by enlarged lymph nodes, which may enhance on contrast injection.

15.17.2
Small Intestine (see Chap. 8)

In the small bowel, *Isospora belli*, *Cryptosporidium*, and microsporidia all produce a similar hypersecretory state, on barium studies causing dilution and fragmentation as well as fold thickening. Isosporiasis may involve the small intestine, the mesenteric and mediastinal lymph nodes, the spleen, and the liver.

Abdominal involvement is common in disseminated histoplasmosis. The gastrointestinal tract will be involved 75% of the time; the terminal ileum and ascending colon are particularly often affected. This involvement is manifested by ulcerations, fold thickening, and marked circumferential bowel wall thickening resembling carcinoma.

The bowel may be involved in tuberculosis, particularly the ileocecal region, which is rich in lymphoid tissue. Ulcers, ulcerating masses, fistulas, stenoses, and wall thickening may be seen, produc-

ing obstruction, bleeding, and perforation. *Mycobacterium avium* complex commonly involves the jejunum as well as the remainder of the small bowel, producing a pattern of irregular thickened folds.

Kaposi's sarcoma involving the small bowel may produce nodular fold thickening, often with the characteristic umbilicated lesions (Fig. 15.30). The lesions are best demonstrated by compression. Cytomegalovirus may also involve the small bowel, particularly the terminal ileum.

15.17.3
Colon and Rectum (see Chap. 8)

Cytomegaloviral colitis is common, often involving the cecum and ascending colon. As in the esophagus, multiple deep or shallow ulcers are produced, often associated with a markedly thickened bowel wall and inflammatory changes in the adjacent fat. Pneumatosis coli or perforation may result. Histoplasmosis may produce fold thickening and apple-core lesions in the ileocecal region. Rectal involvement may be seen in herpes simplex virus infections.

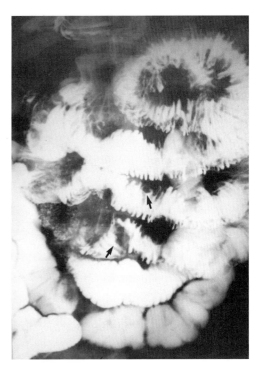

Fig. 15.30. Enteroclysis: multiple nodules in the small intestine in a patient with Kaposi's sarcoma (*arrows*), often associated with thickened mucosal folds. If the nodules ulcerate, they appear as "target" lesions

15.17.4
Liver and Spleen (see Chap. 9)

Liver CT or ultrasonography is frequently abnormal in AIDS patients with hepatic dysfunction. There is often fatty degeneration and the liver may also be the site of bacterial of fungal abscesses (Fig. 15.31) or focal lesions resulting from disseminated cytomegalovirus infection, histoplasmosis, lymphoma, or Kaposi's sarcoma. Focal lesions in the liver or spleen are common in tuberculosis (Fig. 15.32). Bacillary angiomatosis may produce peliosis (multiple blood-filled cystic spaces) of both the liver and the spleen (Fig. 15.33). Disseminated histoplasmosis may produce hepatosplenomegaly, foci of splenic hypoattenuation, adrenal masses, and enlarged lymph nodes, with or without low-density centers. *Pneumocystis carinii* may produce focal low-density liver or spleen lesions which may demonstrate rim calcification. Non-Hodgkin's lymphoma may produce multiple focal lesions in the liver which are low attenuation on CT and hypoechoic on ultrasonography. Hepatomegaly and splenomegaly are both common in AIDS patients. The spleen may be enlarged without invoking a secondary process in addition to AIDS, or it may be involved by lymphoma, Kaposi's sarcoma, or infection. Nonspecific tropical splenomegaly must be excluded.

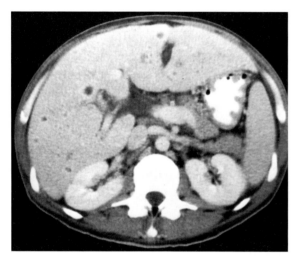

Fig. 15.31. The CT scan of an AIDS patient with multiple cryptococcal abscesses in the liver. There is surrounding enhancement after contrast injection

15.17.5
Biliary System (see Chap. 9)

A wide variety of organisms can cause cholecystitis in AIDS, including microsporidia, *Enterocytozoon bieneusi, Septata intestinalis,* cytomegalovirus, *Cryptosporidium, Pneumocystis carinii,* and *Isospora belli.* AIDS-related cholangitis may produce an echogenic nodule at the distal end of the common bile duct, thought to represent edema of the ampulla of Vater.

AIDS-related cholangiopathy may be due to cryptosporidiosis or cytomegalovirus infection. Patients present with right upper quadrant pain, nausea, vomiting, fever, and cholestasis.

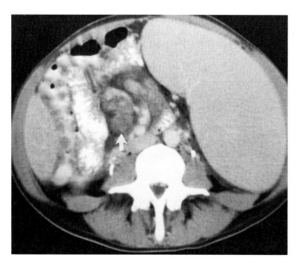

Fig. 15.32. Splenomegaly and lymphadenopathy (*arrow*) due to *Mycobacterium avium* complex

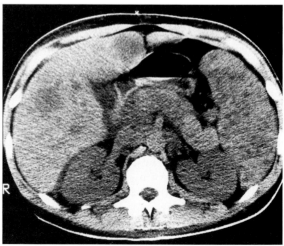

Fig. 15.33. The CT scan of a patient with extensive bacillary angiomatosis, causing peliosis of the liver and spleen. The patient was mistakenly treated for Kaposi's sarcoma, without any benefit, and unfortunately died

On cholangiography, the appearance of AIDS cholangitis is similar to that of sclerosing cholangitis, with diffuse tapered narrowing of the intrahepatic biliary tree. There may be focal stricturing or beading of the biliary tree, focal areas of intrahepatic ductal dilatation, or thickening of the ductal walls or the gallbladder wall. The extrahepatic bile duct may be dilated and thickened but is generally not stenotic. Papillary stenosis may, however, be present, with dilatation to the level of the papilla.

15.17.6
Renal Involvement (see Chap. 10)

HIV itself may produce renal disease characterized by progressive renal failure, proteinuria, and diffuse enlargement of the kidneys which are hyperechoic on ultrasonography. Bacteria, including *Mycobacterium tuberculosis*, and fungi may produce renal abscesses. Non-Hodgkin's lymphoma may develop renal involvement, either by direct extension of adjacent adenopathy or by lymphoma intrinsic to the kidneys.

15.18
AIDS and the Central Nervous System (see Chap. 5)

AIDS produces a variety of neurologic symptoms which may result in the patient being referred for imaging. About 30% of patients will have progressive dementia; CNS presentations also include headache, convulsions, meningeal signs, visual impairment, hemiplegia, focal seizures, and peripheral neuropathy. Meningitis, progressive multifocal leukoencephalopathy, cerebral lymphoma, toxoplasmosis, cryptococcosis, and mycobacterial, mycotic, or bacterial cerebral abscesses are common pathologic conditions in AIDS.

In Africa, focal neurologic findings have been reported in about 10% of HIV-positive adult hospital admissions, and the AIDS dementia complex in 9%–54% (Perriens et al. 1992; Howlett et al. 1989). In the HIV-positive autopsies of Lucas et al. (1994a), 24% died primarily of intracerebral disease, and less than half had normal brains. Cerebral toxoplasmosis was the most common lesion, and this was 12 times more common than primary cerebral lymphoma, with which it can be confused on imaging studies. Tuberculous meningitis was the

second most common intracerebral lesion in this study; other causes of CNS pathology included, in descending order, pyogenic meningitis, cryptococcosis, cytomegaloviral encephalitis, and primary CNS lymphoma. In a study of meningitis in AIDS patients from the South African city of Soweto, tuberculosis was also found to be the most common cause of meningitis, followed by bacterial meningitis (most commonly *Streptococcus pneumoniae*), viral meningitis, and cryptococcal meningitis.

15.18.1
Viral Pathogens

HIV itself is the most common organism to affect the brain in the AIDS patient. Direct HIV encephalopathy causes diffuse brain atrophy with enlargement of the fissures, sulci, and ventricles. White matter atrophy predominates, but subcortical gray matter and cortex can also be affected. Magnetic resonance imaging may show hyperintense signals in the white matter of T2-weighted images.

Cytomegalovirus infection may produce ependymitis (Fig. 15.34).

15.18.2
Toxoplasmosis

Toxoplasma gondii, a parasite often found in cats, is the most common focal brain lesion in AIDS. The majority (about two-thirds) of CNS masses in AIDS patients are due to cerebral toxoplasmosis. This condition is common in AIDS in Africa, representing the third most common cause of death in the HIV-positive autopsy study of Lucas et al. (1994a). It was present in 21% of patients dying with AIDS-defining pathology. CT scanning may aid diagnosis, but even this is not definitive because the appearance of toxoplasmosis and CNS lymphoma may be similar. However, since in the tropics CNS toxoplasmosis is far more common than primary CNS lymphoma, and since the latter is poorly treatable even with sophisticated techniques, focal neurologic manifestations should probably be ascribed to toxoplasmosis. Antimicrobial therapy may be both diagnostic and therapeutic. Improvement is expected within 2 weeks after initiating treatment.

Imaging Findings. The imaging findings (Fig. 15.35) of toxoplasmosis have been described in Chap. 5.

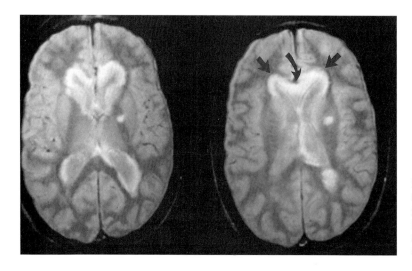

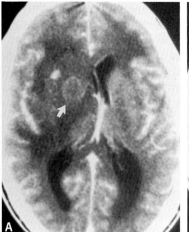
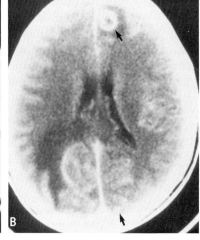

Fig. 15.34. Proton density MR: cerebral CMV infection. There is marked hyperintensity of the ependyma bifrontally (*arrows*). The genu of the corpus callosum has also been affected (*curved arrow*)

Fig. 15.35A, B. Cerebral toxoplasmosis. A A ring-enhancing lesion centered in the right basal ganglia with surrounding edema (*arrow*): this obstructs the foramina of Monro, with resulting hydrocephalus. There is effacement of the sulci. B Multifocal enhancing lesions (*arrows*) are a frequent finding in toxoplasmosis

15.18.3
Cryptococcosis

The third most common process to involve the CNS in AIDS is cryptococcosis, a relatively frequent opportunistic infection in tropical AIDS, found in 5% of the AIDS deaths in an Ivory Coast autopsy study (Lucas et al. 1994a) . CNS disease (meningitis, meningoencephalitis) is most common, followed by lung and skin involvement. Patients with CNS involvement may present with fever, headache, malaise, neck stiffness, nausea, altered mental status, or seizures. Diagnosis is by lumbar puncture with CSF-India ink smears, or, when available, examination for cryptococcal antigen. In a South African study of cryptococcal meningitis, HIV-positive individuals were more likely to suffer neurologic complications and/or death than non-HIV patients.

The site of entry of the organism is the lung. A study from India documented that culture of crypto-

cocci from nonneural sites was more frequent in HIV-positive patients than in normal hosts.

Imaging Findings. Although meningitis is the most common manifestation of cryptococcal infection, it is seldom evident on imaging studies (Fig. 15.36) (see Chap. 5).

15.18.4
CNS Tuberculosis

Tuberculous involvement of the CNS in the tropics most commonly presents as tuberculous meningitis (Fig. 15.37). This may be manifest on CT as infarctions involving the territories supplied by the lenticulostriate arteries (the basal ganglia or frontal lobes) secondary to arteritis of vessels within the basal subarachnoid space) or by meningeal enhancement in the regions of the basal cisterns. Tuberculomas are relatively rare, as are tuberculous cerebral abscesses. Tuberculomas appear as focal lesions which may have central necrosis and which may ring enhance or, in the healing phase, calcify. Tuberculous abscesses resemble other pyogenic brain abscesses.

15.18.5
Syphilis

Many HIV-infected individuals also are seropositive for syphilis. Some authors believe that a more severe

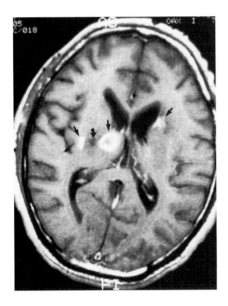

Fig. 15.36. Cryptococcosis: three enhancing cryptococcomas (*arrows*), and a gelatinous pseudocyst (*curved arrow*) in the region of the basal ganglia

clinical presentation and faster development of neurosyphilis may occur in the HIV-positive patient. Syphilis should be considered in any AIDS patient exhibiting unexplained skin or CNS findings. Syphilitic arteritis may be the cause of stroke in this group of patients and appears on arteriography as a vasculitis with focal irregularity of the arterial walls. Syphilitic gummas may appear as focal lesions.

15.18.6
Other Intracranial Infections

In addition to tuberculosis and syphilis, intracranial infections in the HIV patient include *Staphylococcus*, *Streptococcus*, *Salmonella*, *Rhodococcus equi*, *Listeria monocytogenes*, and various fungi (Fig. 15.38). Cerebral involvement by *Nocardia* is most commonly manifested by single or multiple ring-enhancing abscesses, frequently associated with subependymal nodules and hydrocephalus. Bacillary angiomatosis may occasionally involve the brain, producing focal, enhancing lesions (Fig. 15.39).

15.18.7
Progressive Multifocal Leukoencephalopathy

Progressive multifocal leukoencephalopathy is a very rare cause of demyelination and white matter necrosis, beginning in the subcortical white matter in the parietal and occipital lobes and progressing to extensive involvement (see chap. 5). On CT scanning, there are low-density nonenhancing white matter lesions without a mass effect, while on T2-weighted

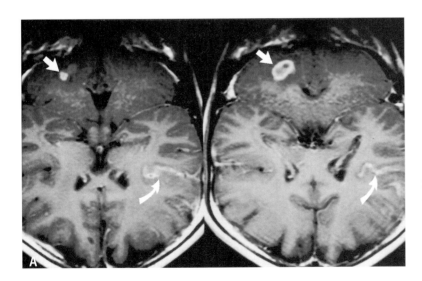

Fig. 15.37. Cerebral tuberculosis. A coronal postgadolinium Tl-weighted image: tuberculoma in the left cerebellar hemisphere (*arrow*) and dense leptomeningeal enhancement in the right sylvian fissure (*curved arrow*) due to tuberculous meningitis

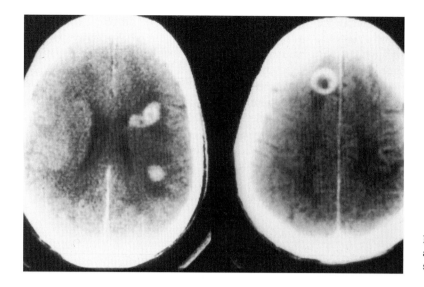

Fig. 15.38. CT: nonspecific appearance of ring-enhancing cerebral abscesses, due to *Candida albicans*

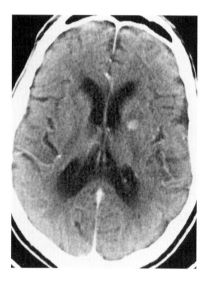

Fig. 15.39. CT: bacillary angiomatosis, showing good contrast enhancement of a lesion of the left basal ganglia

MR images, affected areas show increased signal. The condition is characterized by progressive motor and visual disturbances and is untreatable and rapidly fatal.

Equally important in AIDS, especially in children, is the neurotropic effect of HIV. The encephalopathy may progress slowly or very rapidly. It usually occurs late in the infection but may be the first evidence of HIV, presenting as progressive weakness, mental deterioration, and occasionally seizures (which may occur when there are no discernible focal lesions). CT or MRI will show cerebral atrophy and hydrocephalus. The basal ganglia and periventricular white matter may be mineralized (siderocalcinosis). Necrotizing myelitis has also been observed in the spinal cord (see Chap. 6).

15.18.8
CNS Lymphoma

Primary CNS lymphomas were rare before the AIDS era, and even in AIDS patients, lymphomatous involvement of the CNS may be metastatic. CNS lymphoma (usually B cell, non-Hodgkin's type) is the most common cerebral neoplasm in AIDS, and the second most common mass lesion after toxoplasmosis. Lymphoma is more often a solitary lesion than toxoplasmosis, but since toxoplasmosis is far more common, a solitary toxoplasmoma should be in the differential diagnosis when a single lesion is identified. The presence of ependymal spread or major involvement of the corpus callosum favors lymphoma.

Imaging Findings. The imaging findings (Fig. 15.40) of CNS lymphoma have been described in Chap. 5.

15.19
Bones and Soft Tissues

Patients with AIDS may develop osteomyelitis caused by common organisms such as *Staphylococcus aureus* or *Mycobacterium tuberculosis*, or opportunistic organisms such as *Nocardia*, *Bartonella henselae*, or fungi: these organisms give rise to soft tissue swelling, and later periostitis and lytic lesions develop in bone. Bacillary angiomatosis is another cause of lytic lesions: muscle and soft tissues may also be involved, producing a soft tissue mass which enhances dramatically with contrast (Fig. 15.41). Similar lytic lesions of bone, with associated soft

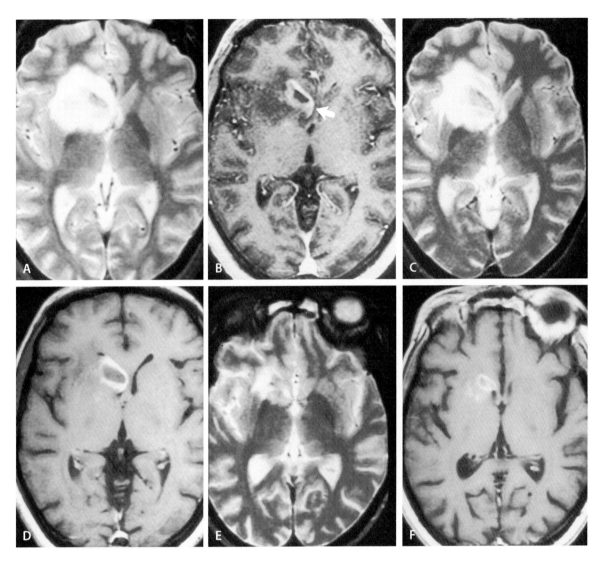

Fig. 15.40A–F. Serial scans of a young male patient with AIDS suffering from seizures. The initial scans (**A, B**) show a hyperintense lesion centered in the right caudate on a T2-weighted image (**A**), with rim enhancement after administration of gadolinium (**B**). The patient was treated presumptively for toxoplasmosis for 3 weeks and the lesion grew (**C, D**) on both T2-weighted (**C**) and enhanced (**D**) images. After these scans and the lack of response to toxoplasmosis therapy, the presumptive diagnosis was changed to lymphoma and radiation therapy was started. Three weeks later (**E, F**), the lesion is much smaller on both T2-weighted (**E**) and gadolinium-enhanced (**F**) images. This strategy averted a biopsy. In retrospect, the ependymal involvement seen on **B** (*arrow*) is very suggestive of lymphoma

tissue abscesses, are also seen in disseminated coccidioidomycosis: in the spine the disc spaces often remain intact (Fig. 15.42). Skeletal tuberculosis is a frequent complication.

Septic arthritis may be due to common bacteria or opportunistic fungi, but also may be due to the HIV, in which case there is characteristically a brief painful reaction involving primarily the knees and ankles. Patients with AIDS also have an increased incidence of the spondyloarthropathies such as Reiter's disease and psoriatic arthritis.

Pyomyositis, occasionally seen in the normal host in tropical regions, is common in AIDS. It characteristically presents with pain in a group of muscles, fever, and leukocytosis. Phlegmonous inflammation progresses to necrosis and abscess formation accompanied by septicemia. *Staphylococcus* is the most common organism, but *Streptococcus*, mycobacteria, *Nocardia*, and *Cryptococcus* are additional sources of muscle infections.

AIDS-related lymphoma may involve bones, particularly in children and often in the leg, causing per-

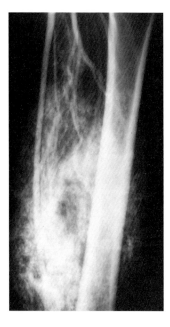

Fig. 15.41. Bacillary angiomatosis: angiography of the upper leg. There is marked contrast enhancement of a large mass in leg muscles

meative destruction. Kaposi's sarcoma involves bone less often, but may cause cortical destruction and periosteal reaction.

An early soft tissue manifestation of HIV infection, often the presenting symptom, is an AIDS-related parotid cyst (lymphoepithelial cyst). When associated with cervical lymphadenopathy, such cysts are extremely suggestive of HIV infection. They probably result from the systemic lymphoid infiltration which affects many organs and which involves periparotid and intraparotid nodes, resulting in obstruction of intranodal ducts (Fig. 15.43). In children the clinical appearance suggests chronic mumps.

In Chap. 12 the different patterns of the musculoskeletal system have been described in more detail.

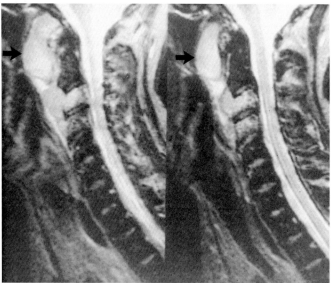

Fig. 15.42. MRI: cervical spine showing osteomyelitis of the C3 and C4 vertebral bodies. The disc spaces are spared, which is suggestive of coccidioidomycosis. There is a large prevertebral abscess (*arrow*)

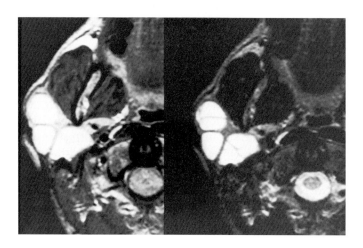

Fig. 15.43. MR proton density (*left*) and T2-weighted (*right*) axial MR images show multiple parotid cysts in an HIV-positive patient

References

Altieri PI, Clement C, Lazala G, et al. (1994) Opportunistic invasion of the heart in Hispanic patients with acquired immunodeficiency syndrome. Am J Trop Med Hyg 51:56–59

Amdahl BM, Rubins JB, Daley CL, et al. (1995) Impaired natural immunity to pneumolysin during human immunodeficiency virus infection in the United States and Africa. Am J Respir Crit Care Med 52:2000–2004

Ananthasubramanian M, Ananthan S, Vennila R, et al. (1997) *Cryptosporidium* in AIDS patients in south India: a laboratory investigation. J Common Dis 29:29–33

Asiimwe-Okiror G, Opio AA, Musinguzi J, et al. (1997) Changes in sexual behaviour and decline in HIV infection among young pregnant women in urban Uganda. AIDS 11:1757–1763

Atzori C, Bruno A, Chichino G, et al. (1993) HIV-1 and parasitic infections in rural Tanzania. Ann Trop Med Parasitol 87:585–593

Barreto JA, Palaci M, Ferrazoli L, et al. (1993) Isolation of *Mycobacterium avium* complex from bone marrow aspirates of AIDS patients in Brazil. J Infect Dis 168:777–779

Batungwanayo J, Taelman H, Bogaerts J, et al. (1994a) Pulmonary cryptococcosis associated with HIV-1 infection in Rwanda: a retrospective study of 37 cases. AIDS 8:1271–1276

Batungwanayo J, Taelman H, Lucas S, et al. (1994b) Pulmonary disease associated with the human immunodeficiency virus in Kigali, Rwanda. A fiberoptic bronchoscopic study of 111 cases of undetermined etiology. Am J Respir Crit Care Med 149:1591–1596

Bem C (1997) Human immunodeficiency virus-positive tuberculous lymphadenitis in Central Africa: clinical presentation of 157 cases. Int J Tuberc Lung Dis 1:215–219

Bhoopat L, Thamprasert K, Chaiwun B, et al. (1994) Histopathologic spectrum of AIDS-associated lesions in Maharaj Nakorn Chiang Mai Hospital. Asian Pac J Allergy Immunol 12:95

Bijur S, Menon L, Deshpande J, et al. (1996) *Pneumocystis carinii* pneumonia in human immunodeficiency virus infected patients in Bombay. Indian J Chest Dis Allied Sci 38:227–233

Bobat R, Moodley D, Coutsoudis A, et al. (1997) Breastfeeding by HIV-1-infected women and outcome in their infants: a cohort study from Durban, South Africa. AIDS 11:1627

Boulos R, Halsey N, Brutus JR, et al. (1988) Risk factors for HIV-1 in pregnant Haitian women. Fourth International Conference on AIDS, Stockholm, Sweden

Chacko S, John TJ, Babu PG, et al. (1995) Clinical profile of AIDS in India: a review of 61 cases. J Assoc Physicians India 43:535–538

Chikwem JO, Mohammed I, Okara GC, et al. (1997) Prevalence of transmissible blood infections among blood donors at the University of Maiduguri Teaching Hospital, Maiduguri, Nigeria. East Afr Med J 74:213–216

Chintu C, Athale UH, Patil PS (1995) Childhood cancers in Zambia before and after the HIV epidemic. Arch Dis Child 73:100

Colebunders R, Bahwe Y, Nekwei W, et al. (1990) Incidence of malaria and efficacy or oral quinine in patients recently infected with HIV in Kinshasa, Zaire. J Infect 21:167–173

De Cock KM, Soro B, Coulibaly IM (1992) Tuberculosis and HIV infection in sub-Saharan Africa. JAMA 268:1581–1587

Desai GA, Mugala DD (1992) Management of empyema thoracis at Lusaka, Zambia. Br J Surg 79:537–538

Donovan B, Bek MD, Pethebridge AM, et al. (1991) Heterosexual gonorrhoea in central Sydney: implications for HIV control. Med J Aust 154:175–180

Duong TA (1996) Infection due to *Penicillium marneffei*, an erneging pathogen: review of 155 reported cases. Clin Infect Dis 23:125–130

Field AS, Hing MC, Miliken ST, et al. (1993) Microsporidia in the small intestine of HIV-infected patients. Med J Aust 158:390–394

French N, Nakiyingi J, Carpenter LM, et al. (2000) 23-Valent pneumococcal polysaccharide vaccine in HIV-1-infected Ugandan adults: double-blind, randomised and placebo controlled trial. Lancet 355:2106–2111

Gilks CF, Ojoo SA, Ojoo JC, et al. (1996) Invasive pneumococcal disease in a cohort of predominantly HIV-1 infected female sex-workers in Nairobi, Kenya [see comments]. Lancet 347:718–723

Giri TK, Pande I, Mishra NM, et al. (1995) Spectrum of clinical and laboratory characteristics of HIV infection in northern India. J Commun Dis 27:131–141

Godfrey-Faussett P, Bithue W, Batchelor B (1994) Recurrence of HIV-related tuberculosis in an endemic area may be due to relapse or reinfection. Tuber Lung Dis 75:199–202

Gomez Morales MA, Atzori C, Ludovisi A, et al. (1995) Opportunistic and non-opportunistic parasites in HIV-positive and negative patients with diarrhoea in Tanzania. Trop Med Parasitol 46:109–114

Gormus BJ, Murphey-Corb M, Martin LN, et al. (1989) Interactions between simian immunodeficiency virus and *Mycobacterium leprae* in experimentally innoculated rhesus monkeys. J Infect Dis 160:405–413

Gray KJ, French N, Lugada E, et al. (2000) *Rhodococcus equi* and HIV-1 infection in Uganda. J Infect 41:227–231

Guay LA, Musoke P, Fleming T, et al. (1999) Intrapartum and neonatal single-dose niviraprine compared with zidovudine for prevention of mother-to-child transmission of HIV-1 in Kampala, Uganda: HIVNET 012 randomised trial. Lancet 354:795–802

Hansen H, Groce NE (2001) From quarantine to condoms: shifting policies and problems of HIV control in Cuba. Med Anthropol 19:259–292

Howlett WP, Nkya WM, Mmuni KA, Missalek WR (1989) Neurological disorders in AIDS and HIV disease in the northern zone of Tanzania. AIDS 3:289–296

Hunter G, Bagshawe AF, Baboo KS, et al. (1992) Intestinal parasites in Zambian patients with AIDS. Trans R Soc Trop Med Hyg 86:543–545

Jackson DJ, Klee EB, Green SD (1991) Severe anemia in pregnancy: a problem of primagravidae in rural Zaire. Trans R Soc Trop Med Hyg 85:829–832

Jeena PM, Coovadia HM, Chrystal V (1996) *Pneumocystis carinii* and cytomegalovirus infections in severely ill, HIV-infected African infants. Ann Trop Paediatr 16:361–368

Jeffery BS, Mercer KG (2000) Pretoria pasturisation: a potential method for the reduction of postnatal mother to child transmission of HIV. J Trop Pediatr 46:219–223

Kalyesubula I, Musoke-Mudido P, Marum L, et al. (1997) Effects of malaria infection in human immunodeficiency virus type 1-infected Ugandan children. Pediatr Infect Dis J 16:876

Kaplan JE, Hu DJ, Holmes KK, et al. (1996) Preventing opportunistic infections in human immunodeficiency virus-infected persons: implications for the developing world. Am J Trop Med Hyg 55:1–11

Kaur A, Babu P, Jacob M, et al. (1992) Clinical and laboratory profile of AIDS in India. J Acquir Immune Defic Syndr 5:883–889

Kelly PJ, Matthewman LA, Hayter D, et al. (1996) *Bartonella (Rochalimaea) henselae* in southern Africa – evidence for infections in domestic cats and implications for veterinarians. J S Afr Vet Assoc 67:182–187

Kelly R, Kiwanuka N, Wawer MJ, et al. (1999) Age of male circumcision and risk of prevalent HIV infection in rural Uganda. AIDS 13:399–405

Khumalo-Ngwenya B, Luo NP, Chintu C, et al. (1994) Gut parasites in HIV-seropositive Zambian adults with diarrhoea. East Afr Med J 71:379–383

Kok I, Veenstra J, Rietra PJ, et al. (1994) Disseminated *Penicillium marneffei* infection as an imported disease in HIV-1 infected patients. Description of two cases and a review of the literature. Neth J Med 44:18–22

Kumar RM, Uduman SA, Khurranna AK (1995) Impact of maternal HIV-1 infection on perinatal outcome. Int J Gynaecol Obstet 49:137–143

Kumar RM, Uduman SA, Khurrana AK (1997a) Impact of pregnancy on maternal AIDS. J Reprod Med 42:429–434

Kumar A, Mehra M, Badhan SK, et al. (1997b) Heterosexual behaviour and condom usage in an urban population of Delhi, India. AIDS Care 9:311–318

Lanjewar DN, Anand BS, Genta R, et al. (1996) Major differences in the spectrum of gastrointestinal infections associated with AIDS in India versus the west: an autopsy study. Clin Infect Dis 23:482–485

LeBlang SD, Whiteman ML, Post MJ, et al. (1995) CNS *Nocardia* in AIDS patients: CT and MRI with pathologic correlation. J Comput Assist Tomogr 19:15–22

Leroy V, Whiteman ML, Post MJ, et al. (1995) Four years of natural history of HIV-1 infection in African women: a prospective cohort study in Kigali (Rwanda), 1988–1993. J Acquir Immune Defic Syndr Hum Retrovirol 9:415–421

Liao S, Choi KH, Zhang K, et al. (1997) Extremely low awareness of AIDS, sexually transmitted diseases and condoms among Dai ethnic villagers in Yunnan province, China. AIDS 11:S27–S34

Lindan CP, Lieu TX, Giang LT, et al. (1997) Rising HIV infection rates in Ho Chi Minh City herald emerging AIDS epidemic in Vietnam. AIDS 11:S5–S13

Long R, Scalcini M, Manfreda J, et al. (1991) Impact of human immunodeficiency virus type 1 on tuberculosis in rural Haiti. Am Rev Respir Dis 143:69–73

Lucas SB, Hounnou A, Peacock C, et al. (1993) The mortality and pathology of HIV infection in a west African city [see comments]. AIDS 7:1569–1579

Lucas SB, Diomande M, Hounnou A, et al. (1994a) HIV-associated lymphoma in Africa: an autopsy study in Cote D'Ivoire. Int J Cancer 59:20–24

Lucas SB, Hounnou A, Peacock C, et al. (1994b) Nocardiosis in HIV-positive patients: an autopsy study in West Africa. Tuber Lung Dis 75:301–307

Lucas SB, Peacock CS, Hounnou A, et al. (1996) Disease in children infected with HIV in Abidjan, Cote d'Ivoire [see comments]. BMJ 312:335–338

Maher D, Hoffman I (1995) Prevalence of genital infections in medical inpatients in Blantyre, Malawi. J Infect 31:77–78

Malin AS, Gwanzura LK, Klein S, et al. (1995) *Pneumocystis carinii* pneumonia in Zimbabwe [see comments]. Lancet 346:1258–1261

Mawar N, Mehendale S, Thilakavathi S, et al. (1997) Awareness and knowledge of AIDS and HIV risk among women attending STD clinics in Pune, India. Indian J Med Res 106:212–222

McGuinness G, Scholes JV, Garay SM, et al. (1994) Cytomegalovirus pneumonitis: spectrum of parenchymal CT findings with pathologic correlation in 21 AIDS patients. Radiology 192:451–459

McLeod DT, Neill P, Gwanzura, Latif AS, et al. (1990) *Pneumocystis carinii* pneumonia in patients with AIDS in Central Africa. Respir Med 84:225–228

Meeran K (1989) Prevalence of HIV infection among patients with leprosy and tuberculosis in rural Zambia. Br Med J 298:364–365

Moore EH, Russell LA, Klein JS, et al. (1995) Bacillary angiomatosis in patients with AIDS: multiorgan imaging findings. Radiology 197:67–72

Moreira ED Jr, Silva N, Brites C, et al. (1993) Characteristics of the acquired immunodeficiency syndrome in Brazil. Am J Trop Med Hyg 48:687–692

Mulder D, Nunn A, Kamali A, et al. (1995) Decreasing HIV-1 seroprevalence in young adults in a rural Ugandan cohort [see comments]. BMJ 311:833–836

Murray JF (1997) Tuberculosis and HIV infection: global perspectives. Respirology 2:209–213

Ndour M, Sow PS, Coll-Seck AM, et al. (2000) AIDS caused by HIV1 and HIV2 infection: are there clinical differences. Results of AIDS surveillance 1986–97 at Fann Hospital in Dakar, Senegal. Trop Med Int Health 5:687–691

Nduati R, Mbori-Ngacha D, Richardson B, et al. (2000) Effect of breastfeeding and formula feeding on transmission of HIV-1: a randomized clinical trial. JAMA 284:956–957

Ng'weshemi JZ, Boerma JT, Pool R, et al. (1996) Changes in male sexual behaviour in response to the AIDS epidemic: evidence from a cohort study in urban Tanzania. AIDS 10:1415–1420

Pais P (1996) HIV and India: looking into the abyss. Trop Med Int Health 1:295–304

Pape JW, Verdier RI, Boncy M, et al. (1994) *Cyclospora* infection in adults infected with HIV: clinical manifestations, treatment, and prophylaxis. Ann Intern Med 121:654–657

Perriens JH, Mussa M, Luabeya MK, et al. (1992) Neurological complications of HIV-1 seropositive internal medicine patients in Kinshasa, Zaire. J Acquir Immune Defic Syndr 5:333–340

Pfutzner A, Dietrich U, von Eichel U, et al. (1992) HIV-1 and HIV-2 infections in a high-risk population in Bombay, India: evidence for the spread of HIV-2 and presence of a divergent HIV-1 subtype. J Acquir Immune Defic Syndr 5:972–977

Pichard E, Doumbo O, Minta D, et al. (1990) Place de la cryptosporidiose au cours des diarrhees chez les adultes hospitalisee a Bamako. Bull Soc Pathol Exot 83:473–478

Pillay T, Pillay DG, Bramdev A (1997) Disseminated histoplasmosis in a human immunodeficiency virus-infected African child. Pediatr Infect Dis J 16:417–418

Porteals F, Taelman H Van den Breen L (1998) Mycobacterial infection in ARC and AIDS patients at the Institute of

Tropical Medicine, Antwerp, Belgium. International Conference on AIDS, Stockholm, Ab. 7533, p 308

Prazuck T, Yameogo JM, Heylinck B, et al. (1995) Mother-to-child transmission of human immunodeficiency virus type 1 and type 2 and dual infection: a cohort study in Banfora, Burkina Faso. Pediatr Infect Dis J 14:940–947

Purvis SF, Katongole-Mbidde E, Johnson JL, et al. (1997) High incidence of Kaposi's sarcoma-associated herpesvirus and Epstein-Barr virus in tumor lesions and peripheral blood mononuclear cells from patients with Kaposi's sarcoma in Uganda. J Infect Dis 175:947–950

Quigley MA, Mwinga A, Hosp M, et al. (2001) Long-term effect of preventive therapy for tuberculosis in a cohort of HIV-infected Zambian adults. AIDS 15:215–222

Rigsby MO, Curtis AM (1994) Pulmonary disease from nontuberculous mycobacteria in patients with human immunodeficiency virus. Chest 106:913–919

Saran R, Gupta AK (1995) HIV-2 and HIV-1/2 seropositivity in Bihar. Indian J Public Health 39:119–120

Sauda FC, Zamarioli LA, Ebner Filho W, et al. (1993) Prevalence of *Cryptosporidium* sp. *Isospora belli* among AIDS patients attending Santos Reference Center for AIDS, Sao Paulo, Brazil. J Parasitol 79:454–456

Serwadda D, Mugerwa RD, Sewankambo NK, et al. (1985) Slim disease: a new disease in Uganda and its association with HTLV III infection. Lancet 2:849–852

Sitas F, Bezwoda WR, Levin V, et al. (1997) Association between human immunodeficiency virus type 1 infection and cancer in the black population of Johannesburg and Soweto, South Africa. Br J Cancer 75:1704–1707

Srikanth P, John TJ, Jeyakumari H, et al. (1997) Epidemiological features of acquired immunodeficiency syndrome in southern India. Indian J Med Res 105:191–197

Supparatpinyo K, Khamwan C, Baosoung V, et al. (1994) Disseminated *Penicillium marneffei* infection in southeast Asia. Lancet 344:110–113

Thomas JO (2001) Acquired immunodeficiency syndrome-associated cancers in sub-Saharan Africa. Semin Oncol 28:198–206

Todd J, Balira R, Grosskurth H, et al. (1997) HIV-associated adult mortality in a rural Tanzanian population. AIDS 11:801–807

Tshibwabwa-Tumba E, Mwinga A, Pobee JO, et al. (1997) Radiological features of pulmonary tuberculosis in 963 HIV-infected adults at three Central African Hospitals. Clin Radiol 52:837–841

Tyndall MW, Ronald AR, Agoki E, et al. (1996) Increased risk of infection with human immunodeficiency virus type 1 among uncircumcised men presenting with genital ulcer disease in Kenya. Clin Infect Dis 23:449–453

U.N./W.H.O. AIDS epidemic update – December 1988. Report of the Joint U.N. Programme on HIV/AIDS. UNAIDS, Geneva, 1998

Vetter KM, Djomand G, Zadi F, et al. (1996) Clinical spectrum of human immunodeficiency virus disease in children in a west African city. Project RETRO-CI. Pediatr Infect Dis J 15:438–442

von Reyn CF, Waddell RD, Eaton T, et al. (1993) Isolation of *Mycobacterium avium* complex from water in the United States, Finland, Zaire, and Kenya. J Clin Microbiol 31:3227–3230

16 AIDS-Related Interventional Procedures

Jeffrey S. Klein and Jeet Sandhu

CONTENTS

16.1
Introduction

Since the initial description of AIDS cases in the early 1980s, over 700,000 patients have been diagnosed with AIDS (Center for Disease Control 1999) in the United States and it remains a leading cause of mortality in younger individuals (Horowitz et al. 1998a, b). Another 100,000 individuals are human immune deficiency virus (HIV) positive but have not yet developed an AIDS index diagnosis. These numbers represent just those who have been tested. An additional 200–300,000 may be seropositive for HIV but are unaware of their infection. HIV/AIDS continues to exact a tremendous toll in both human and economic terms, with a devastating impact on those afflicted. AIDS cases have been documented in every state and U.S. territory, indicative of the pervasive nature of AIDS. Accordingly, it is almost a certainty that a radiologist will encounter an HIV-positive patient during the course of their routine practice.

While the spectrum of radiologic abnormalities

J.S. Klein, MD
Department of Radiology, Fletcher Allen Health Care,
111 Colchester Avenue, Burlington, VT 05401, USA
J. Sandhu, MD
Department of Radiology, University of North Carolina,
CB#7510, Chapel Hill, NC 27599-7510, USA, USA

representing opportunistic infection and malignancy in the AIDS patient has received considerable attention over the past 20 years, the role of image-guided interventions in diagnosis and management of these patients has not been extensively detailed in the radiology literature (Dore et al. 1994). This chapter will review the use of interventional procedures in the HIV-infected individual and review issues relating to the prevention of HIV transmission in the interventional radiology setting.

16.2
Fine-Needle Aspiration Biopsy

As in the general population, the use of image-guided fine-needle aspiration (FNA) biopsy has emerged as a useful diagnostic technique for the definitive characterization of localized intrathoracic and intra-abdominal lesions. In addition, FNA biopsy performed under direct palpation of superficial lesions and lymph nodes with or without imaging guidance has likewise proven useful in the cytologic and microbiologic evaluation of opportunistic disease complicating AIDS. Pathologic findings most commonly seen in biopsy specimens obtained in AIDS patients show a broad spectrum of opportunistic infections and malignancies including mycobacteria, *Pneumocystis carinii*, cytomegalovirus, fungi, Kaposi's sarcoma, non-Hodgkin's lymphoma, and bronchogenic carcinoma (Ioachim 1990; Schofield et al. 1989). A recent report of a series of 655 FNA biopsies in HIV-infected patients found reactive or benign change in 37%, inflammation or specific infection in 30%, and malignancy in 13% (Ellison et al. 1998). Patients with lesions exceeding 2 cm and those with tender lesions or the recent enlargement of lesions were significantly more likely to have specific pathologic findings on FNA.

16.2.1
Head and Neck Lesions

Cervical and axillary lymphadenopathy is an early and common finding in patients with AIDS, and is most often due to follicular hyperplasia. In one series of 113 patients who underwent FNA of palpable lymph nodes on an outpatient basis, 50% had a diagnosis of malignancy or infection, including 20% with non-Hodgkin's lymphoma, 17% with mycobacterial infections, 10% with Kaposi's sarcoma, and 3% with Hodgkin's disease or metastatic carcinoma (BOTTLES et al. 1988). Another series of 65 FNAs in 52 HIV-infected patients with lymphadenopathy showed infection in 17% and malignancy in 11%, with a 25% rate of inadequate sampling that precluded definitive diagnosis (REID et al. 1998). As in the first series, mycobacterial disease was the commonest cause of lymphadenopathy due to infection. In AIDS patients, the presence of unilateral adenopathy or lymph nodes exceeding 3 cm is associated with fine-needle aspirates positive for opportunistic infection (SHAPIRO and PINCUS 1991). FNA diagnosis of cervical tuberculous lymphadenitis by acid-fast staining and culture of aspirated specimens and microscopic detection of caseous necrosis and granulomas is possible in a majority of affected AIDS patients (FINFER et al. 1991).

Additional head and neck lesions in AIDS patients that can be diagnosed by FNA include parotid and salivary gland masses. For example, computed tomography (CT)-detected cystic and solid parotid lesions have been accurately diagnosed by examination of material obtained by FNA (HUANG et al. 1991). In a series of 103 salivary gland lesions in 78 HIV-infected patients, benign lymphoepithelial lesions accounted for 75% of lesions, inflammatory lesions for 14%, and neoplasms for 6% (CHHIENG et al. 1999). In a case report, a patient with hypothyroidism due to *Pneumocystis carinii* infection of the thyroid was diagnosed by FNA (BATTAN et al. 1991).

16.2.2
Chest Biopsy

The thorax is the most common site of opportunistic infection in the AIDS patient (SUSTER et al. 1986). These individuals have increased incidence of infection with *Pneumocystis carinii*, *Mycobacterium tuberculosis* and *avium-intracellulare*, *Aspergillus*, *Coccidioides immitis*, *Histoplasma*, *Cryptococcus*, and pneumonia due to *Streptococcus pneumoniae*, *Haemophilus influenzae*, *Pseudomonas aeruginosa*, *Rhodococcus equi*, *Bartonella henselae*, and cytomegalic inclusion virus. The mainstays in the evaluation of diffuse or focal lung infections have been serologic or skin testing and microscopic or culture exami-

nation of spontaneously produced or induced sputum, bronchoscopic alveolar lavage, transbronchial or Wang needle biopsy, and open (thoracoscopic) biopsy (LUCE and CLEMENT 1989). Analogous to its utility in the mediastinal nodal staging of bronchogenic carcinoma, transbronchial needle aspiration has been shown to be particularly useful in the HIV-infected patient with mediastinal and hilar lymphadenopathy (HARKIN et al. 1998). Although recognized as a useful diagnostic tool in selected immunocompromised patients prior to the AIDS epidemic (CASTELLINO and BLANK 1979), the utility of transthoracic needle biopsy (TNB) has been underpublicized in the setting of AIDS (Fig. 16.1).

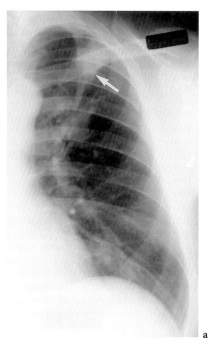

a

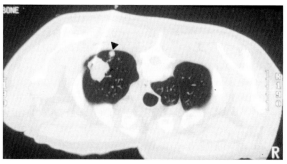

b

Fig. 16.1a, b. Cryptococcosis. **a** Coned down view of the left lung from a frontal radiograph in a 45-year-old male with AIDS demonstrates a left upper lobe nodule (*arrow*). **b** CT scan during needle placement into lateral edge of the large nodule demonstrates a second smaller nodule (*arrowhead*). Stains and cultures of aspirated specimen showed *Cryptococcus neoformans*

Transthoracic needle biopsy for the diagnosis of pulmonary infection in the AIDS patient may be performed with or without direct image guidance. In a series of 45 HIV-infected patients with clinical and radiographic evidence of pulmonary infection, transthoracic needle aspiration with a 25-gauge spinal needle was performed without direct image guidance for localized or diffuse pulmonary infectious disease. None of the patients had a coagulopathy, severe hypoxemia (PaO$_2$ <55 mmHg), bullae, cough, or previous pneumothorax (FALGUERA et al. 1994). For focal disease, the appropriate needle puncture site and depth were estimated from the chest radiographs, while a posterior approach was used for diffuse parenchymal disease. The overall sensitivity of this technique was 62%, with a 93% yield for *Pneumocystis carinii* pneumonia (PCP), 57% for bacterial pneumonia, and 33% for tuberculosis. There were no false-positive results (specificity=100%). Complications were limited to pneumothorax in eight patients (17%), only one of whom required drainage, hemoptysis in two (4%), and persistent pain in three (6%).

Image-guided TNB has been shown to be a safe and effective procedure for the evaluation of focal lung and mediastinal lesions in patients with HIV infection or AIDS. In the largest published study consisting of 32 patients seropositive for HIV (GRUDEN et al. 1993), CT guidance was used for 84% of image-guided biopsies. A coaxial needle system consisting of a 19- or 19.5-gauge outer guide needle and a 20- or 22-gauge inner aspirating or cutting biopsy needle was used to obtain multiple specimens following a single pleural puncture. In 27 (84%) of 32 patients, a specific diagnosis was made on TNB. Importantly, TNB provided a diagnosis in 18 of 21 patients (86%) with negative sputum samples (Fig. 16.2). Similarly, in all seven patients with negative bronchoscopic results, TNB was diagnostic. Infectious agents as a group accounted for the majority of diagnoses (41%) and included bacterial infection in five, fungal infection in 3, localized PCP in two, *Mycobacterium avium* complex in two, and cytomegalovirus in 1. Bronchogenic carcinoma was the most frequent single diagnosis, seen in seven patients (22%). Complications of TNB developed in nine patients (28%) and included pneumothorax in eight (25%) and hemorrhage in two (6%); only two patients required specific treatment of their complications and both recovered within 2 days of the procedure. Fluoroscopically guided TNB in AIDS patients with focal pulmonary lesions has also been described with a similar success rate. In a series of 13 patients undergoing fluoroscopically guided FNA of

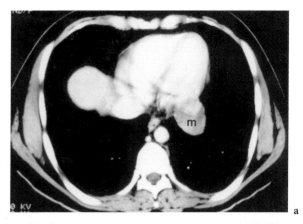

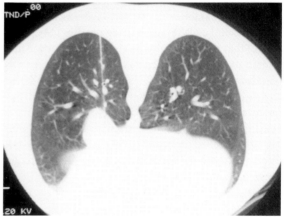

Fig. 16.2a, b. Focal mass-like *Pneumocystis carinii* infection. **a** Contrast-enhanced CT scan at the level of the top of the right hemidiaphragm shows an oval left lower lobe mass (*m*) adjacent to the left ventricle. **b** Prone scan during CT-guided biopsy shows needle tip in mass. Cytology revealed PCP

focal pulmonary lesions, seven of whom had previous negative fiberoptic bronchoscopy, a diagnosis of infection was made in 11 (85%), with only three minor complications (SCOTT and KUHLMAN 1991). While the technique of fluoroscopically guided TNB can provide a diagnosis of PCP in 83% of patients, a high pneumothorax and chest tube insertion rate (44% and 17% respectively) suggests that this technique be reserved for selected patients with diffuse lung disease and negative bronchoscopies prior to subjecting them to open lung biopsy (BATRA et al. 1987). Similar results have been reported for ultrasound-guided FNA of focal pulmonary lesions with or without associated pleural effusion in HIV infection, with one series reporting a diagnostic yield of 80% in 20 HIV-infected patients (HUNG et al. 1999). Another small series of ten HIV-infected patients with solitary pulmonary nodules found that both transthoracic FNA and bronchoscopy with bronchoalveolar lavage and transbronchial needle aspiration had low sensitivity and limited utility in this setting (MARTINEZ-MARCOS et al. 1997).

The technique used for image-guided TNB involves choices of imaging modality, biopsy needles, method of needle placement, and handling of the specimen obtained (KLEIN and ZARKA 2000). CT guidance is used for virtually all mediastinal and hilar lesions and is most useful for small or centrally positioned parenchymal lesions not visualized on orthogonal views of the chest. Recently, the use of CT fluoroscopy, a modality that provides real-time visualization of the needle and lesion, has become more widespread (WHITE et al. 2000). Biopsy needles are generally divided into fine (20–22-gauge) aspirating needles used to obtain cytologic specimens and material for stains and culture, and cutting needles (14- to 20-gauge) that routinely provide core specimens for histologic examination. When expert cytopathology is readily available or material is obtained only for stains and cultures, aspiration biopsy will provide an adequate sample in the majority of cases. Otherwise, specimens obtained using cutting needles with an inner side-notched stylet and outer cutting cannula and a spring-loaded mechanism can be sent for more detailed pathologic examination.

The patient is positioned on the biopsy table to allow the shortest vertical access to the lesion. If the patient is unable to lie comfortably in an optimal position or the lesion is inaccessible from a vertical approach, a nonvertical approach using CT guidance may be necessary. Intravenous analgesia and sedation are administered by a nurse as needed to reduce patient discomfort, but the patient should be able to follow commands to avoid inaccurate needle placement and minimize complications. The chosen needle entry site is marked with an indelible marker and the skin prepared and draped sterilely. Lidocaine is used for local anesthesia to the level of the parietal pleura, and a small skin incision made to ease the entry of the biopsy needle. A single needle technique is utilized for large pleural-based masses where a single aspirate will likely be diagnostic or when multiple passes can be performed without traversing the visceral pleura. For small parenchymal lesions that are difficult to access or when multiple samples are required, a coaxial technique should be used. The coaxial technique involves placement of a thinwalled needle over the superior margin of the rib through the pleura to the edge of the lesion while the patient suspends respiration. Once the proper position of the guide needle has been confirmed, a longer 20- or 22-gauge biopsy needle is placed through the lumen of the guide needle and into the lesion. The coaxial technique allows repeated sampling of the lesion with ei-

ther aspirating or cutting needles, thereby providing multiple cytologic or histologic specimens following a single pleural puncture. An aspirate for cytopathology or microbiologic stains and cultures is obtained with a 20- or 22-gauge needle and attached syringe by piercing the lesion with a rapid repetitive up-and-down and rotatory motion. Specimens for histologic examination are reliably obtained with automated cutting biopsy needles, and in the AIDS patient are most useful in the diagnosis of lymphoma.

Aspirated specimens are expressed onto glass slides for immediate fixation in alcohol. An on-site cytopathologist then performs a fast stain with toluidine blue and examines the slide microscopically. A confident diagnosis of malignancy precludes further needle passes and indicates the biopsy is complete. If additional material is needed for repeat cytologic examination or stains and cultures, repeat aspiration is performed. When inflammatory disease is the primary consideration, as in HIV-infected patients with focal lung lesions, an aspirate is placed in a nonbacteriostatic solution for stains and cultures. If immediate cytopathologic examination is unavailable, several aspirates should be obtained. When a core tissue biopsy is obtained with an automated cutting needle, the specimen is dislodged from the slotted receptacle of the biopsy needle into saline or formalin for later evaluation.

Based on the excellent published results of image-guided TNB in the diagnosis of focal thoracic lesions in AIDS patients, we propose that TNB is the initial diagnostic method of choice in the diagnosis of focal lung lesions. In patients with enlarged mediastinal or hilar lymph nodes, the pertinent imaging studies should be reviewed to determine whether bronchoscopy with transbronchial needle aspiration or transthoracic FNA should be the initial diagnostic procedure. Mediastinoscopy or open biopsy should be reserved for patients with negative results at bronchoscopy or TNB. Patients with diffuse infiltrative lung disease should be evaluated initially with bronchoalveolar lavage and transbronchial biopsy. Those with nondiagnostic bronchoscopic examinations or contraindications to bronchoscopy who do not have respiratory failure should undergo thoracoscopic or open lung biopsy for definitive diagnosis (FITZGERALD et al. 1987; TRACHIOTIS et al. 1992).

16.2.3
Malignancy in AIDS

The diagnosis of non-Hodgkin's lymphoma and Kaposi's sarcoma can be made in the majority of cases by microscopic examination of specimens obtained by needle biopsy. FNA of enlarged lymph nodes detected in a large population of males followed in an AIDS clinic yielded a diagnosis of non-Hodgkin's lymphoma in 20% of patients (BOTTLES et al. 1988). The high frequency of extranodal involvement in non-Hodgkin's lymphoma as detected by CT or ultrasound, particularly thoracic, hepatic, splenic, and omental lesions, can help guide needle sampling for diagnosis (SIDER et al. 1989; TOWNSEND et al. 1989). In a recent report of 12 patients with AIDS-related primary pulmonary lymphoma, five of ten patients who had transthoracic FNA had a definitive diagnosis of high-grade B cell non-Hodgkin's lymphoma and avoided open lung biopsy (RAY et al. 1998). Similarly, an accurate diagnosis of Kaposi's sarcoma from FNA of lymph node, soft tissue, oral, chest, or abdominal masses can be made by the recognition of malignant spindle cells in the aspirated specimen (Fig. 16.3) (HALES et al. 1987). Ultrasound-guided core biopsy of nodal and soft tissue masses for the histologic diagnosis of non-Hodgkin's lymphoma and Kaposi's sarcoma has also been reported (DONALD et al. 1988).

Bronchogenic carcinoma may cause lung and mediastinal masses in the AIDS population (GRUDEN et al. 1993). In HIV-infected patients with lung cancer, the disease behaves in an aggressive manner and is often widespread at the time of diagnosis (Fig. 16.4) (TENHOLDER and JACKSON 1993; WHITE et al. 1995). Image-guided TNB can provide a diagnosis in a majority of affected patients; in one retrospective series, 8 of 13 patients (62%) had a diagnosis by CT-guided TNB (GRUDEN et al. 1995). Adenocarcinoma is the most common cell type; most tumors are poorly differentiated cytologically.

16.3
Treatment of
AIDS-Related Pneumothorax

Cystic or bullous parenchymal lesions have been reported in 7%–34% of AIDS patients with PCP (FEUERSTEIN et al. 1990; SANDHU and GOODMAN 1989). An increased prevalence of premature bullous or cystic disease has also been associated with HIV infection without prior or concurrent PCP and in intravenous drug abusers (GURNEY and BATES 1989; KUHLMAN et al. 1989). The cysts associated with PCP

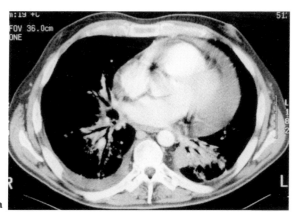

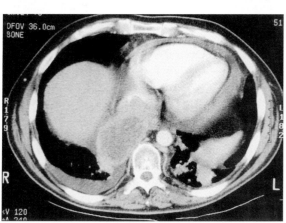

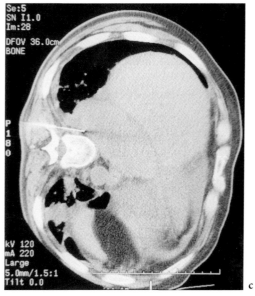

Fig. 16.3a–c. Pulmonary Kaposi's sarcoma. **a** Enhanced CT scan at the level of the left atrium shows thickening of bronchovascular structures and pleural and pericardial effusions. **b** Scan at the level of the interventricular septum shows a large lower lobe mass adjacent to the heart with a thick enhancing wall. Note multiple irregular left basilar lesions. **c** Scan with patient in left decubitus position during biopsy shows the needle at the posterior edge of the mass. Cytologic diagnosis was Kaposi's sarcoma

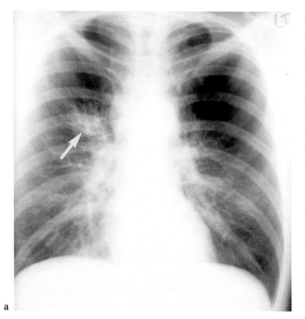

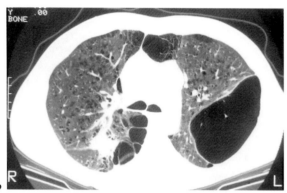

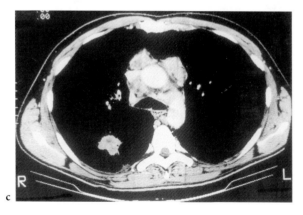

Fig. 16.4a–c. Bronchogenic carcinoma. **a** Frontal chest radiograph shows a spiculated right upper lobe perihilar mass (*arrow*) and enlarged right paratracheal and aortopulmonary window nodes. **b** CT scan at the level of the carina shows a spiculated right upper lobe mass. Note multiple bilateral lung cysts due to prior PCP and centrilobular emphysema. **c** Scan at the same level displayed at lung windows shows bilateral mediastinal lymphadenopathy. CT-guided TNB of the lung mass revealed poorly differentiated adenocarcinoma

are usually multiple and range from 1 to 5 cm in diameter (CHOW et al. 1993). While some have reported an upper zone or apical predilection of the cysts (CHOW et al. 1993; GEREIN et al. 1991), particularly in patients receiving aerosolized pentamidine prophylaxis for PCP, other series show cysts uniformly distributed throughout the lung. These air cysts usually develop during therapy for PCP and resolve or diminish in size within 7–12 months (CHOW et al. 1993; SANDHU and GOODMAN 1989).

The presence of cystic lesions in patients with active or prior PCP accounts for an increased incidence of spontaneous pneumothorax in AIDS (COKER et al. 1993; GOODMAN et al. 1986; MCCLELLAN et al. 1991; SEPKOWITZ et al. 1991). These pneumothoraces may be unilateral or bilateral, simultaneous or sequential, and are frequently recurrent. The mortality from AIDS-related pneumothorax is exceedingly high, with an overall mortality of 54% which increases to 92% for patients with PCP who require mechanical ventilation (BYRNES et al. 1989). Patients with PCP-related pneumothorax have a short survival time, often less than 6 months from initiation of treatment (GEREIN et al. 1991).

The management of AIDS-related pneumothorax has proven to be difficult because of the prolonged air leaks seen in patients with PCP, particularly those receiving systemic corticosteroids (METERSKY et al. 1995). The results of pneumothorax treatment in this population is related more closely to the lung pathology caused by PCP than to the type of treatment employed (GEREIN et al. 1991), yet expedient treatment in this population is particularly important given the occasional need for mechanical ventilation in patients with active PCP. The management of AIDS-related pneumothorax involves (a) treatment of the underlying PCP or other predisposing parenchymal process producing the bronchopleural fistula and (b) evacuation of the pneumothorax and reexpansion of the underlying lung. While small (<10%) stable pneumothoraces in a younger group of AIDS patients with PCP and good lung mechanics can resorb without drainage (MCCLELLAN et al. 1991), the majority of patients require tube drainage for treatment (Fig. 16.5). As with drainage of any moderate or large pleural collection associated with underlying atelectasis that has been present for more than several days, a note of caution is warranted regarding tube drainage of PCP-associated pneumothorax. The rapid evacuation of a large pneumothorax in this setting has resulted in the development of reexpansion edema. Initial attachment of the tube to water seal to allow gradual drainage of pneumothorax is recommended to avoid this complication (LIBRATY 1992).

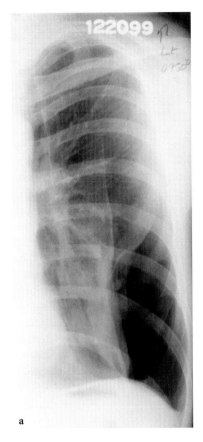

a

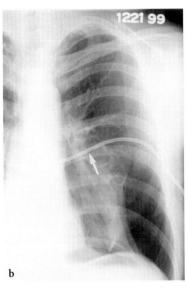

b

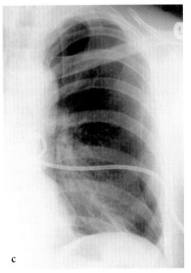

c

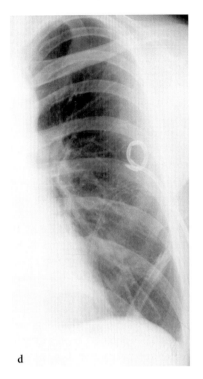

d

Fig. 16.5a–d. Image-guided drainage of PCP-related pneumothorax. **a** Coned-down view of a frontal chest radiograph in a 34-year-old male with AIDS and PCP demonstrates a left pneumothorax. **b** Film obtained on the day following catheter placement (*arrow*) shows persistent but smaller inferolateral pneumothorax. **c** Film obtained 1 month later shows progressive reexpansion of the left lung. **d** Portable film obtained 1 month after catheter placement shows complete reexpansion of the left lung

The ideal treatment of AIDS-related pneumothorax should be safe, should obliterate the bronchopleural fistula while limiting the duration and expense of hospitalization, and should prevent recurrent pneumothorax. Treatment options include pleurodesis via the indwelling tube using a variety of agents such as doxycycline, bleomycin, or talc (HNATIUK et al. 1990; READ et al. 1994; TUNON-DE-LARA et al. 1992), thoracoscopic talc insufflation or cyst stapling and pleurectomy (FEINS 1993; WAIT and DAL NOGARE 1994), and open cyst stapling with pleurectomy and pleural abrasion via a thoracotomy (unilateral disease) or median sternotomy (bilateral disease) (BYRNES et al. 1989; FLEISHER et al. 1988; GEREIN et al. 1991). Although some investigators have reported successful outpatient management of PCP-related pneumothorax using tube drainage attached to underwater suction or a

Heimlich valve (DRIVER et al. 1991; GEREIN et al. 1991), this option does not definitively treat the bronchopleural fistula and appears feasible only in patients with advanced disease with a very limited life expectancy (WALKER and PATE 1993). The results of closed tube drainage and tetracycline/doxycycline pleurodesis have likewise been poor, with a 26% success rate and a mean hospital stay of 18 days (WAIT and DAL NOGARE 1994). For these reasons, several authors have advocated a staged approach to the management of pneumothorax in patients with a reasonable life expectancy. In AIDS patients with lung reexpansion and obliteration of the bronchopleural fistula following tube drainage, chemical pleurodesis with talc or doxycycline should be attempted. Those patients with incomplete lung reexpansion and a persistent air leak beyond 4–8 days of tube placement are candidates for thoracoscopic bleb resection, apical pleurectomy, and pleurodesis (ALBORT et al. 1993; FEINS 1993; FLEISHER et al. 1988). In cases of bilateral disease, sequential thoracoscopy or median sternotomy can be employed.

Pneumothorax drainage in the radiology department using small-gauge catheters is most easily performed under fluoroscopic guidance. CT may be used for loculated collections and for large pneumothoraces which complicate CT-guided chest biopsy or drainage procedures. Several small-gauge catheters are commercially available for percutaneous pneumothorax drainage. These include the Cook pneumothorax catheter (Cook, Bloomington, Ind.), the Sacks catheter (Electro-Catheter, Rahway, N.J.), and the Arrow pneumothorax catheter (Arrow International, Reading, Pa.). A compact, one-piece pneumothorax drainage system available for the treatment of pneumothorax is the Tru-Close Thoracic Vent (UreSil, Skokie, Ill.). This unit is composed of a 12- or 13-French, 10-cm-long catheter connected to a rectangular chamber that contains a self-sealing aspiration port, a red signal diaphragm indicating entry into the pleural space, and a flutter valve. The device also has self-adhesive side flaps that affix the unit to the chest wall.

In most patients, an anterior approach through the second intercostal space in the midclavicular line is used to direct the catheter into the pleural apex. In women, a lateral approach via the third, fourth, or fifth intercostal space in the midaxillary line may be used to avoid traversing the breast. After sterile preparation and draping of the chest wall, 2% lidocaine is administered down over the superior margin of the rib until air is aspirated from the pleural space. After a small skin incision has been made over the rib beneath the interspace to be traversed, the catheter/trocar combination is gradually advanced through the chest wall in a cephalad direction to enter the pleural space over the superior aspect of the rib. Once an intrapleural position has been confirmed by aspirating air through the hollow trocar, the catheter/trocar combination is advanced an additional 1 cm to be certain the catheter tip is intrapleural. The trocar is then steadied and the catheter is advanced over the lung apex under fluoroscopic visualization. To alleviate the pain associated with the catheter contacting the apical parietal pleura, 3 ml of lidocaine can be injected through the catheter once it has reached the pleural apex. The catheter is then affixed to the skin and the pneumothorax is manually aspirated with a large syringe until resistance is encountered. Petroleum gauze is packed around the catheter at the insertion site and an occlusive dressing is applied. The catheter is then attached via an adapter to an underwater seal device with suction or to a flutter (Heimlich) valve.

Patients with indwelling pneumothorax catheters can be managed as inpatients or outpatients. A patient whose lung completely reexpands following pneumothorax evacuation and has no evidence of an air leak is safely managed as an outpatient with a Heimlich valve (KLEIN et al. 1995). Such a patient should return to the hospital in 1 or 2 days for a follow-up chest radiograph. If the lung remains reexpanded, the catheter is removed. Debilitated patients, those with severe lung disease from current or prior PCP, and patients with a persistent air leak precluding complete lung expansion should be hospitalized and placed on suction. These patients should be monitored daily with upright chest radiographs and the water seal chamber of the drainage system should be checked for air leaks. Once the lung has completely reexpanded and there is no evidence of an air leak, the catheter is removed. As discussed above, those patients with prolonged air leaks and incomplete reexpansion of the lung who are candidates for definitive therapy will require a thoracoscopic or open procedure.

Although limited published data are available on the results of AIDS-related pneumothorax drainage which is specifically image guided, successful catheter or tube management of spontaneous or AIDS-related pneumothorax has been reported (DRIVER et al. 1991; GEREIN et al. 1991; MARTIN et al. 1996; MINAMI et al. 1992; WALKER and PATE 1993). Failure of catheter drainage of pneumothorax may be due to kinking of the catheter or occlusion by blood or fibrin, inadvertent withdrawal from the pleural space, or the presence of a large air leak (MARTIN et al. 1996; MINAMI et al. 1992). Chest pain following catheter placement is common and probably results from contact of the catheter with the parietal pleura. Wound infection, chest wall hematoma, hemothorax, and empyema may occur (VAN HENKEL and VAN DE BERGH 1994).

16.4
Management of Pleural Effusion and Empyema

While the pulmonary manifestations of AIDS have been extensively documented, data on the incidence of pleural disease in this population are relatively scarce. Pleural effusion is seen in 14%–27% of AIDS patients, with pulmonary infection accounting for 66%–75% of these cases (JOSEPH et al. 1993; STRAZZELLA and SAFERSTEIN 1991). In patients with documented thoracic empyema, the vast majority develop in injection-drug users and in 91% the empyema is a complication of community-acquired pneumonia (HERNANDEZ BORGE et al. 1999). Noninfectious causes of pleural effusion include hypoalbuminemia, cardiac failure due to AIDS cardiomyopathy, and pleural involvement by Kaposi's sarcoma or non-Hodgkin's lymphoma.

While PCP, fungal infection due to *Cryptococcus*, histoplasmosis, or coccidioidomycosis or mycobacterial infection may rarely present with pleural effusion as the sole manifestation of opportunistic infection in AIDS (MARIUZ et al. 1991; NEWMAN et al. 1987), 94% of patients with infectious effusions have concomitant parenchymal lung disease (STRAZZELLA and SAFIRSTEIN 1991). Despite an increased incidence of bacterial pneumonia due to *Streptococcus pneumoniae* or *Haemophilus influenzae* in this population, the development of complicated parapneumonic effusion and empyema appears to be rare (COKER 1994). An exception seems to be pulmonary tuberculosis in AIDS patients in Africa, which accounted for 19 of 26 cases of concomitant empyema in HIV-infected individuals (DESAI and MUGALA 1992). Empyema complicating pneumonia is a result of polymicrobial infection in approximately 50% of cases. It has been suggested that patients presenting with empyema due to unusual pathogens such as *Salmonella paratyphi* be tested for HIV infection (WOLDAY and SEYOUM 1997).

The management of complicated parapneumonic effusion and empyema in AIDS patients should be similar to that in other patients with infected pleural fluid collections. When physical examination suggests the presence of a parapneumonic effusion, decubitus chest radiographs should be obtained to assess free-flowing or loculated collections. CT or ultrasound are often used as adjuncts to conventional radiographs and accurately characterize the extent of pleural disease and help guide diagnostic thoracentesis and drainage.

Infected pleural collections amenable to image-guided percutaneous catheter drainage include collections in patients with a short duration of symptoms, free-flowing or unilocular effusions, fluid that is easily aspirated by needle, and the absence of a thick pleural peel on CT scans. Imaging guidance is best provided with ultrasound, which is used for free-flowing fluid or collections loculated along the costal pleura (O'MOORE et al. 1987). CT is useful in characterizing complex pleural and parenchymal disease and provides direct visualization of the drainage tract.

A 10- or 12-French catheter provides adequate drainage for serous collections, while collections of purulent or bloody material usually require catheters of 12- to 30-French in diameter to promote the drainage of thick, particulate matter. We have recently started using a 28-French curved tip tube (Thal-Quik, Cook, Bloomington, Ind.) for the drainage of thick infected or bloody pleural fluid collections. A diagnostic 18-gauge trocar needle is placed into the thickest portion of the collection and fluid aspirated. If purulent fluid is aspirated or a gram stain shows microorganisms, a drainage catheter is placed. It is important to note that the nondependent fluid initially aspirated from a loculated pleural collection in a patient who has been supine for a prolonged period may appear serous and noninfected but actually reflects the supernatant of an empyema; therefore the decision to leave a drain in the collection will require microscopic examination of the aspirated fluid or a high clinical suspicion of an empyema. A floppy-tipped guidewire is placed through the needle and into the collection, and the tract is dilated in 2-French increments until the desired diameter is achieved. The drainage catheter is then placed into the dependent portion of the collection (Fig. 16.6) and fluid is manually aspirated until resistance is encountered. For large collections, a single puncture technique may be used, whereby a catheter containing an inner trocar stylet is placed directly into the collection in tandem with the diagnostic needle (KLEIN et al. 1995). The patient is then studied to assess the adequacy of drainage and additional catheters may be placed as necessary. The catheter or tube is then attached to an underwater suction device.

The patient with a pleural catheter or tube is visited daily to maintain catheter patency by flushing the catheter vigorously with saline. The response to drainage is assessed by monitoring fluid output and the patient's temperature and peripheral white blood cell count. Chest radiographs or ultrasound studies are regularly obtained to monitor resolution. The catheter may be removed when output has diminished to <10 ml per day, an improvement in symptoms and signs of infection is noted, and the collection has resolved radiographically. The average duration of catheter drainage is 5–30 days (MERRIAM et al. 1988; HERNANDEZ BORGE et al. 1999).

If pleural drainage is inadequate despite proper catheter placement, a larger diameter catheter or tube may be necessary. New pleural loculations will require additional catheter placement. In patients with collections containing multiple septations or loculations, fibrinolytic therapy with streptokinase

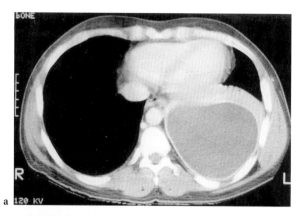

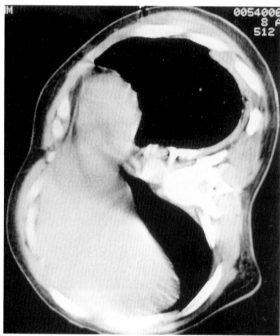

Fig. 16.6a, b. CT-guided empyema drainage. **a** Contrast-enhanced CT scan in a 29-year-old AIDS patient demonstrates a loculated left pleural fluid collection with enhancing pleural layers representing an empyema due to *Streptococcus pneumoniae*. **b** Scan obtained with patient in right lateral decubitus position after CT-guided pleural catheter placement shows complete evacuation of fluid and reexpansion of lung

The success rate of image-guided catheter drainage of infected pleural collections is approximately 80% (SILVERMAN et al. 1988), which compares favorably with the results from placement of large-bore thoracostomy tubes. It should be recognized that while image-guided techniques are often successful at managing infected pleural fluid collections, patients who fail to respond to closed drainage should proceed to thoracoscopy, with open surgical drainage reserved for chronic empyemas with thick pleural peels that require decortication (HORNICK and SMITH 1994). The complications of image-guided pleural drainage are uncommon but include bleeding from intercostal vessel injury, pneumothorax, and lung laceration (KLEIN et al. 1995).

16.5
Drainage of Pericardial Effusion

Pericardial effusion as detected by echocardiography is common in HIV-infected individuals, with a 5%–10% prevalence in the AIDS population and an annual incidence of 11% (CASTELLINO and BLANK 1979; FLEISHER et al. 1988; FREEDBERG et al. 1987). The presence of pericardial effusion in AIDS is associated with a significantly shortened survival (FLEISHER et al. 1988). The etiologies of pericardial effusion include endocarditis, mycobacterial, bacterial, cytomegalovirus, or herpesvirus infection, lymphoma, Kaposi's sarcoma, and myocardial infarction or dysfunction (EISENBERG et al. 1992; FREEDBERG et al. 1987; KARVE et al. 1992; NATHAN et al. 1991; REYNOLDS et al. 1992; STOTKA et al. 1989). While the majority of effusions are small and asymptomatic, large effusions producing pericardial tamponade and requiring emergent pericardiocentesis and surgical intervention have been reported (EISENBERG et al. 1992; KARVE et al. 1992; NATHAN et al. 1991; REYNOLDS et al. 1992; TURCO et al. 1990). Ultrasound-guided pericardiocentesis and drainage can be performed for the emergency treatment of large or symptomatic pericardial collections (Fig. 16.7).

16.6
Lung Abscess Aspiration and Drainage

Bacterial organisms are responsible for 2.5% of severe pulmonary infections in patients with AIDS (MURRAY et al. 1984). In addition to an unusually

or recombinant tissue plasminogen activator (t-PA) may be necessary to enhance drainage. The intrapleural administration of 250,000 units of streptokinase admixed in 100 ml saline or 6 mg of t-PA mixed in 50 cm saline, which is then left dwelling for several hours in the pleural space, can aid in the management of loculated collections and help avoid thoracoscopic or open drainage procedures in selected patients. This technique has been successfully employed in AIDS patients with empyema (MILLER and SEVERN 1995; MOULTON 2000).

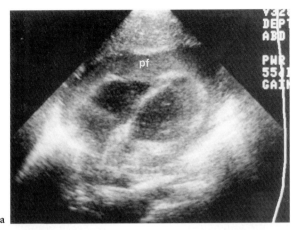

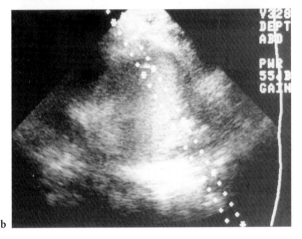

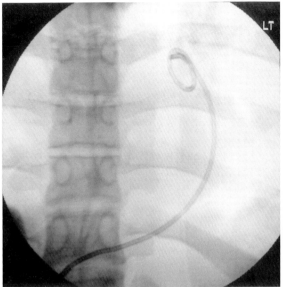

Fig. 16.7a-c. Purulent pericarditis complicating pneumococcal pneumonia and empyema. **a** Transthoracic ultrasound via subxiphoid window shows echogenic pericardial fluid (*pf*) surrounding the cardiac chambers. **b** Scan with needle guide markers shows the anticipated path of the aspiration needle and drainage catheter into the inferior aspect of the pericardial sac. **c** Spot film after placement of a pigtail catheter in the pericardial space; 250 cc of purulent fluid was aspirated

high rate of bacteremia (DALEY 1991), intrathoracic complications of bacterial pneumonia include abscess formation and empyema. While the most common bacterial pathogens are *Streptococcus pneumoniae* and *Haemophilus influenzae*, pneumonia and abscess formation have been described with *Salmonella* (typhoidal and nontyphoidal strains) and *Rhodococcus equi* pulmonary infection (ANKOBIAH and SALEHI 1991; SAMIES et al. 1986; SATUE et al. 1994). In a patient with a cavitating pyogenic infection or lung abscess, image-guided transthoracic needle aspiration and drainage can be performed to obtain material for diagnostic stains and cultures and to promote drainage (Fig. 16.8).

16.7
Abdominal Interventions

In most facets of diagnostic radiology, the patient's underlying HIV status significantly alters the diagnostic possibilities and influences the differential diagnosis for a particular diagnostic finding. However, this principle does not hold true for interventional radiology. There are no unique interventional procedures specifically utilized in the AIDS population. The procedures and interventions performed on AIDS patients are the same as those performed on anyone else. The patient's underlying HIV status may or may not be relevant to the intervention being performed.

For example, a febrile patient with AIDS presented with a cystic hepatic lesion suggestive of an abscess (Fig. 16.9a). While in an HIV-infected patient the causative organisms producing a liver abscess may differ, the treatment remains sonographically guided needle aspiration and lavage (Fig. 16.9b). Since the abscess in this patient was only 3 cm in diameter, a drainage catheter was not placed and aspiration was utilized for diagnostic and therapeutic purposes. The abscess yielded multiple gram-negative enteric organisms from underlying appendicitis and the patient recovered uneventfully with continued antibiotic administration. Another patient presented with renal failure and bilateral hydronephrosis caused by com-

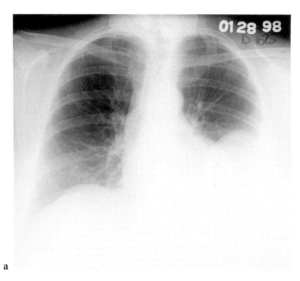

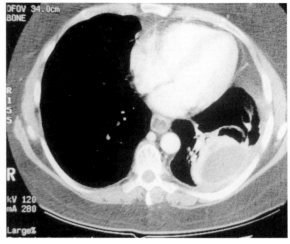

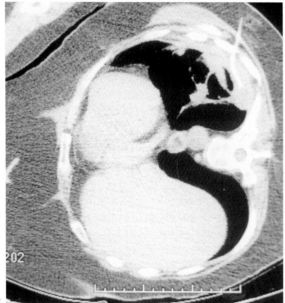

Fig. 16.8a–c. CT-guided lung abscess aspiration and drainage. **a** Frontal chest radiograph in a febrile 31-year-old AIDS patient shows a left lower lobe mass. **b** Contrast-enhanced CT shows a lower lobe fluid collection with adjacent compressed and atelectatic lung and small pleural effusion. **c** Scan with patient in the left decubitus position following catheter placement and aspiration of 35 cc of purulent fluid shows resolution of the collection

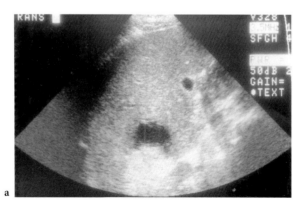

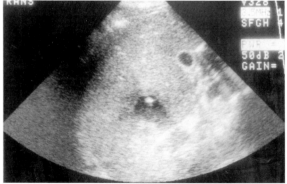

Fig. 16.9a, b. Hepatic abscess. **a** Transverse sonogram of the liver in a patient with AIDS and fever shows a 3-cm right hepatic lobe hypoechoic area. **b** The clinical diagnosis of a hepatic abscess was confirmed via sonographically guided needle aspiration and lavage

pression and obstruction of the ureter by pelvic and retroperitoneal lymphadenopathy (Fig. 16.10). Although the etiology of the obstruction was lymphadenopathy due to non-Hodgkin's lymphoma, the treatment of sonographically guided bilateral nephrostomy tube placement and subsequent internalization of drainage is the same regardless of the cause of ureteral obstruction.

In certain situations, the etiology of the disorder requiring interventional therapy is an opportunistic, neoplastic or infectious process due to the immune suppression of AIDS. However, the procedure employed will be the same as in any non-AIDS patient. For example, intestinal Kaposi's sarcoma or AIDS-related lymphoma may produce gastrointestinal hemorrhage (SHARMA et al. 1992). The treatment algorithm in this situation is to perform routine diagnostic angiography with possible embolotherapy. Similarly, AIDS cholangiopathy is caused by infection from cytomegalovirus, cryptosporidia, or mi-

crosporidia (BENHAMOU et al. 1993). These opportunistic infectious agents then induce multiple stenoses within the intrahepatic bile ducts (Fig. 16.11). In addition to multiple intrahepatic narrowings, AIDS cholangiopathy can cause a focal stenosis at the ampulla (Fig. 16.12a). This narrowing is usually treated with endoscopic papillotomy; metallic stenting of the papillary stenosis via transhepatic biliary drainage can be performed when endoscopic therapy fails (Fig. 16.12b). In patients too unstable to undergo an operative procedure, less invasive interventional techniques may stabilize the patient or preclude the need for surgery. The patient illustrated in Fig. 16.13 had symptoms suggestive of acute cholecystitis and was found on ultrasound to have a markedly thickened gallbladder wall, presumably due to AIDS cholangiopathy as the HIDA scan in this patient was normal. Because of persistent fevers without other identifiable source, percutaneous cholecystostomy was performed to drain the gallbladder.

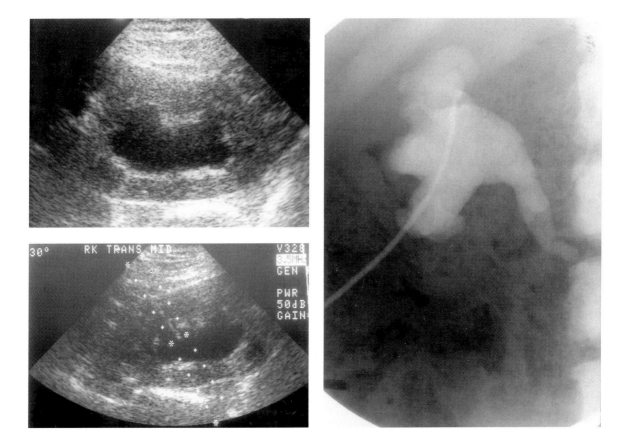

Fig. 16.10a–c. Ureteral obstruction from non-Hodgkin's lymphoma. **a** Longitudinal sonogram of the right kidney shows moderate to severe hydronephrosis. **b** Under sonographic guidance, a needle is advanced through the posterior calyx into the collecting system, allowing a wire to be advanced and a nephrostomy tube placed. **c** Nephrostogram following catheter placement confirms appropriate entry into the collection system and obstruction of the ureter

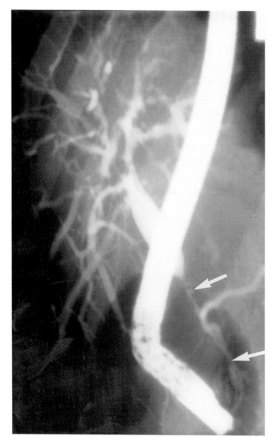

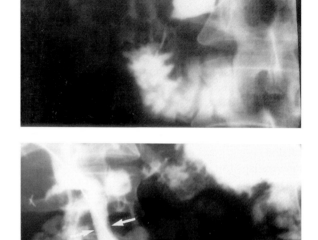

Fig. 16.11. AIDS cholangiopathy treated by percutaneous catheter drainage and stenting of the common bile duct. Spot image from an endoscopic retrograde cholangiopancreaticogram shows multiple intrahepatic strictures with a long segment stricture of the common bile duct (*arrows*), findings compatible with AIDS cholangiopathy

Fig. 16.12a, b. Common bile duct stenosis in AIDS treated with a Wallstent. a High-grade stenosis of the distal common bile duct at the ampulla of Vater indicative of AIDS cholangiopathy. b After endoscopic sphincterotomy failed to improve the patient's symptoms, a percutaneous transhepatic biliary drainage was performed with placement of a woven flexible stainless steel stent (Wallstent) (*arrows*) through the stenotic segment, with relief of obstructive symptoms

16.8
Central Venous Access

One area where interventional radiology plays a significant role in the care and management of the HIV-positive patient is in providing central venous access. Because of requirements for numerous intravenous medications, an HIV-infected patient will often require long-term central venous access. Significant debate persists on the best type of central venous access device (CVAD) to utilize in this patient group. Even before deciding what type of CVAD to place, one has to keep in mind that the infection rate associated with chronic central venous catheterization is higher in the AIDS patient even when compared to patients who are immunocompromised from other etiologies such as organ transplantation or chemotherapy. The differences are especially pronounced

when compared to infection rates for CVAD in immunocompetent patients (SKOUTELIS et al. 1990; DIONIGI et al. 1995).

Central venous access devices can be categorized into those that are inserted through a peripheral vein and those inserted through a central vein such as the subclavian or internal jugular vein. Within each category, the device can be external or totally implanted beneath the skin. Almost all peripheral external devices are non-tunneled and consist predominantly of PICCs (peripherally inserted central catheters) while those inserted through the central veins are usually tunneled and exit external to the skin, such as the Hickman catheter.

Those patients who require short-term access on the order of weeks to several months should receive a PICC line as it is ideally suited for this time period. Often the catheter can be inserted by specially

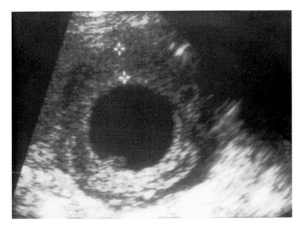

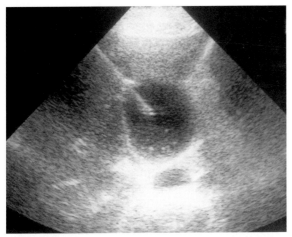

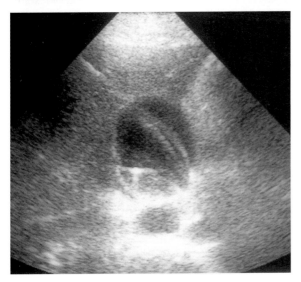

Fig. 16.13a–c. Percutaneous cholecystostomy for acalculous cholecystitis. **a** Transverse sonogram of the gallbladder shows a markedly thickened wall measuring 11 mm. **b** Transverse sonogram from another patient demonstrates a needle being advanced transhepatically into the gallbladder. **c** Once the guidewire is coiled within the gallbladder, a drainage catheter is placed for percutaneous drainage

trained nurses utilizing an antecubital vein for advancement of 3- to 5-French catheters into the central circulation. In those patients in whom a palpable vein is not present, PICC lines can still be inserted via sonographically guided puncture of the deep veins of the upper arm with subsequent advancement of the catheter. When sonographic or venographic guidance is required to gain access to the peripheral deep vein of the upper arm, the PICC line is usually inserted in the interventional suite.

The options for prolonged access greater than 3 months are more limited. The patient can have a peripherally inserted subcutaneous port, a centrally inserted chest port, or a centrally inserted tunneled catheter, all of which can also be placed in the interventional area. Several studies have shown that subcutaneous ports have a much lower infection rate than tunneled catheters (MUSCEDERE et al. 1998; MOORE et al. 1997). Peripheral ports can also function adequately in providing chronic intravenous access in this patient group. Historically, the advantages of peripheral ports were related to significantly decreased number of immediate insertion-related complications such as pneumothorax or puncture of the subclavian artery. There is also a decreased incidence of venous thrombotic complications for peripheral ports when compared to central ports inserted via the subclavian vein. With increasing use of the internal jugular vein as the access site coupled with sonographically guided venipuncture, many of these disadvantages no longer exist. Immediate technical complications are almost nonexistent and symptomatic venous thrombosis is much reduced. Because of the increased incidence of skin breakdown that may occur with intensive use of a peripheral port over a relatively limited septal area, central subcutaneous ports are now preferred. In those patients who have significant body image issues and wish to hide the presence of a port as much as possible, peripheral ports may offer advantages. Otherwise, central subcutaneous ports should be considered as the first-line option for those patients who require long-term intravenous access.

One disadvantage of a subcutaneous port is that access to the system has to be obtained with a sharp special noncoring needle. This increases the risk of occupational exposure to blood-borne pathogens when compared to an external device, where only a Luer lock connection or a needleless system can be utilized to achieve access. If there is concern about accessing ports with needles, this issue should be resolved within each treating unit. From an infection standpoint, subcutaneous chest ports offer the best long-term option. It must be kept in mind that the overall risk of infection from placement of a central venous access in the AIDS population is significantly increased, possibly up to 10 times that in the immunocompetent patient receiving the same type of device. The most critical issue in preventing infections associated with chronic central venous access devices is proper sterile accessing technique and appropriate compliance with site care (SETTLE et al. 1994). If a central venous access device is utilized, every effort should be made to ensure that appropriate site care is administered to further minimize the likelihood of infection.

16.9
Reducing the Risk of Occupational Transmission of HIV in the Interventional Suite

Due to the number of interventional procedures that are performed with the associated used of hollow needles and numerous sharp instruments, the risk of inadvertent transmission of any blood-borne pathogen, including HIV, is significantly higher in interventional radiology than in other areas of radiology. It is thus of paramount importance that extreme care is taken to prevent the transmission of blood-borne pathogens (see also Chap. 17).

As will be discussed in the following sections, the risks of HIV transmission virus from a patient to an operating physician are very low, but every precaution should be taken to further reduce the already remote chance of any accidental viral transmission (WALL et al. 1991). The risk of inadvertent contraction of HIV during an interventional procedure is small; however, once the virus has been acquired, the incidence of progression to AIDS and eventual death is high despite newer and innovative drug therapies. Because of probable fatality and the overwhelming concern and anxiety induced by possibly contracting HIV, the prevention of any occupational transmission of HIV is of the greatest importance. By mid-1999, there had been 191 cases of occupationally acquired HIV infection, of which 136 were probably but not definitely due to occupational exposure and 55 were documented to be due to occupational transmission (Center for Disease Control 1999). The vast majority of these cases were due to percutaneous exposure from needle sticks, but mucocutaneous transmission via inoculation of the mucous membranes or contamination of open skin wounds has occurred. It is estimated that the overall risk of

seroconverting after percutaneous exposure is 0.3% (GERBERDING 1994; HENDERSON et al. 1990). Numerous factors influence the chances of seroconverting, including the route of inoculation as well as the viral load of the patient (HOROWITZ et al. 1998a, b). The use of protease inhibitors, which significantly decrease the patient's viral load, may alter the overall risks of seroconverting after a percutaneous exposure (PALELLA et al. 1998). As a result, the current statistics of seroconversion may actually be lower, but even with this small chance, appropriate precautions should be taken.

While there is a small but real likelihood of HIV seroconversion following exposure to an infected patient's blood or body fluids, one should be even more alarmed by the likelihood of acquiring hepatitis B or C through occupational transmission (LANPHEAR 1994; LANPHEAR et al. 1994; GERBERDING and HENDERSON 1992). The risk of acquiring hepatitis B after an accidental needle stick ranges from 5% to 43%, while the risk of acquiring hepatitis C ranges from 3% to 10% after an accidental needle stick or other percutaneous exposure. Given the infectivity of hepatitis B and C viruses, the health care worker should be more concerned about occupational transmission of hepatitis than HIV (ZUCKERMAN 1995), particularly given the serious health consequences of hepatitis. With hepatitis B, 10% of infected individuals will develop a chronic carrier state, 3.5% will develop chronic persistent hepatitis, 1.5% will develop chronic active hepatitis, and 0.1% will develop acute fulminant hepatitis which is associated with a 70% mortality. With hepatitis C, up to 50% of patients may develop a chronic carrier state, of which 10%–20% will eventually progress to cirrhosis. In addition to the complications of variceal hemorrhage, liver failure, or ascites, a certain percentage will also develop hepatocellular carcinoma. Patients with chronic active hepatitis from hepatitis B may also develop similar problems. In 1991 it was estimated that almost 5,000 health care workers had become infected with hepatitis B from occupational exposure, with 200 deaths attributable to hepatitis B infection. Fortunately, these numbers are decreasing rapidly as a result of the administration of the hepatitis B vaccine. Despite the availability of a suitable vaccine, in 1994 over 1,000 health care workers contracted hepatitis and 22 will die as a consequence of this infection (SHAPIRO 1995). Another 2,200 cases of occupationally acquired hepatitis C infections occur each year among health care workers in the United States (LANPHEAR et al. 1994). Any health care worker who may come into contact with blood or bloody fluid should be vaccinated against hepatitis B to prevent its transmission (GERBERDING and HENDERSON 1992). As there are no immunizations available for HIV or hepatitis C, other measures must be employed to limit occupational exposure to these viruses. Currently, the use of universal precautions as mandated by the Occupational Health and Safety Administration are the most effective means of minimizing occupational exposure to blood-borne pathogens (HERSEY and MARTIN 1994).

Despite the lower infectivity of HIV when compared to hepatitis viruses, it is estimated on the basis of computer modeling that there is still a 0.009%–16% cumulative risk of a practicing interventional radiologist occupationally acquiring HIV infection over a 30-year period (HANSEN and McINTIRE 1996). The overall risk of a health-care worker contracting HIV is related to multiple factors. The three most important factors are (a) the HIV prevalence in the catchment population, (b) the risk of virus transmission after a single exposure to blood or body fluids, and (c) the frequency of occupational blood contact resulting from percutaneous exposure due to needle sticks, lacerations, or mucocutaneous exposure from splashes or glove perforation. These factors along with the number of procedures performed were variables utilized in the computer model to estimate the lifetime risk of occupational exposure to HIV. The practicing radiologist has little if any control over the first two factors but can significantly influence the frequency of blood exposure. The majority of the remainder of the discussion will be devoted to means of reducing blood exposure, and thereby minimizing the likelihood of occupationally contracting blood-borne pathogens.

The prevalence of HIV in the treated clinical population will vary dramatically depending on the demographics of that particular population. Obviously, the higher the incidence of HIV in the clinical population, the higher the chance of being exposed to the patient's blood from a percutaneous injury. Results of a hospital-based seroprevalence study for HIV indicate that approximately 1% of patients hospitalized for non-AIDS-related conditions are HIV positive, with the rate varying from 0.1% to 5.6%, reflecting the significant demographic variations in the patient populations of the hospital (Centers for Disease Control and Prevention 1993). As may be surmised, urban hospitals serving largely indigent inner city populations have much higher rates of HIV positivity when compared to nonurban hospitals. Lest one become too complacent and assume that appropriate precautions are not required because the practice is located in a hospital with an insignificant number of AIDS patients, the results of several other studies are interesting. Another study performed by the Center for Disease Control evaluated the rate of HIV infection among patients presenting to the emergency department in three urban and three suburban areas and found HIV infection rates ranging from 4–9 per 100 patient visits (MARCUS et al. 1993). The HIV status was unknown to the hospital emergency department workers in about 70% of the cases in the inner city hospitals, and this figure varied from 40%–90% in the suburban hospitals. Obviously, the underlying HIV status of a significant number of patients will not be known during the performance of routine procedures. Although the incidence of HIV infection may be low in a particular practice, the corresponding rates of hepatitis B and hepatitis C are likely to be significant enough to warrant protection. A surveillance study of seropositivity for HIV, hepatitis B, and hepatitis C was performed among all surgical patients at Westchester County Medical Center (MONTECALVO et al. 1995). Blood samples were obtained from 1,062 patients undergoing surgical operations and the blood was tested for HIV antibody, hepatitis B surface antigen, and core antibody as well as hepatitis C antibody. It was noted that 1.6% of the surgical patients were HIV positive, 1.4% were hepatitis B positive, and 5.2% were hepatitis C positive. Overall, 8.2% of the patients were at risk for transmitting a blood-borne pathogen. However, when evaluating patients aged 25–44 years, one in six patients was positive for at least one of the three viruses and evaluating for HIV infection alone would have only detected one-quarter of the patients at risk for transmitting a blood-borne pathogen. The results reemphasize the need for adherence to universal precautions to prevent transmission of blood-borne pathogens. Therefore, it would be prudent for any practitioner who is at risk for occupational transmission of blood-borne pathogens to strictly comply with these precautions.

The other significant factor that will determine lifetime seroconversion is the chance of converting with any one single blood exposure. As noted previously, the risk of seroconversion after a needle stick injury is approximately 0.3% (HENDERSON et al. 1990; LANPHEAR 1994). This is the average rate and various factors surrounding the percutaneous injury or mode of blood exposure will influence and determine the true seroconversion rate. Seroconversion can occur after mucous membrane exposure but the incidence is much lower, at only 0.09%, after mucous membrane exposure (IPPOLITO et al. 1993). A study evaluating the risk of the conjunctival exposure or exposure to the buccal mucosa during vascular procedures determined that blood exposure to the eyes or mouth may occur in 7% of the cases, with multiple exposures being common (McWILLIAMS and BLANSHARD 1994). Although it might be assumed that most of the contamination occurs during the initial arterial puncture, the study found that most of the blood exposure occurred later in the procedure. Given the high frequency of exposure to the eyes and mouth, coupled with the risks of transmission of blood-borne pathogen via the conjunctiva or mucosal routes, it is imperative that glasses, goggles, or a face shield, as well as a face mask, as recommended by universal precautions, be worn to prevent transmission of any of the various viruses via this route.

So far, no cases have been reported of seroconversion following simple cutaneous exposure of infected blood to intact skin. Because of this finding, some individuals argue that double gloving is not needed if the skin over the hands is intact. Although this may true, clinically inapparent breakdown in skin integrity may be present and blood exposure in these areas may increase the risk of transmission of blood-borne pathogens. Occult glove perforation occurs in 10% of gloves used in interventional procedures thereby allowing blood to come into contact with skin (HANSEN et al. 1992). The wearer only detected these perforations in 6% of the cases. In addition, there is a 1% rate of preexisting defects or perforations in unused gloves. These two findings suggest that a single pair of gloves is an imperfect barrier against skin contamination. Double gloving will provide a more effective means of preventing skin contamination. The rate of glove perforations significantly increases when they are worn for greater than 2 h and for this reason single gloves, if worn, should be changed after a 2-h procedural time.

Although it can be argued that the use of double gloves results in some minimal loss of manual dexterity, the sensation of decreased manual dexterity is easily overcome with the routine use of double gloving. Double gloving also offers another significant advantage in preventing blood-borne pathogen transmission. If an inadvertent needle stick from a solid suture needle does occur, the use of the second pair of gloves will decrease the volume of blood inoculum by an additional 50% (GERBERDING and SCHECTER 1991; BENNETT and HOWARD 1994; MAST et al. 1993). When a solid needle passes through both layers of the gloves, most of the blood on the surface of the needle appears to be scraped off by the layers of gloves before the needle comes into contact with the skin. Although the results are not as dramatic with hollow-bore needles, as most of the blood is on the inside hollow portion of the needle, there is still a 25% reduction in the volume of blood transferred when a second pair of gloves is used. Despite the effectiveness of the barrier techniques in preventing exposure to blood or body fluids, there is variable compliance with universal precautions and OSHA guidelines in the interventional community (HANSEN et al. 1993b). Given the fact that 87% of the respondents in this survey indicated that they have suffered at least one procedure-related percutaneous injury, it would seem self-evident that use of the routine measures already described will reduce the frequency and extent of percutaneous exposure to blood, thereby reducing the risk of any transmission of blood-borne pathogens. A prospective study of needle stick injuries and blood contacts during interventional procedures found a 3% incidence of cutaneous exposure and parenteral injury in 0.6% of the cases (HANSEN et al. 1993b). Almost all of the cutaneous blood exposure could have been avoided with adherence to proper barrier methods as suggested by universal precautions.

The third significant factor that influences the rate of seroconversion or acquisition of a blood-borne pathogen is the frequency of cutaneous and parenteral exposure. As indicated in the preceding discussion, reducing exposure to cutaneous blood contacts should reduce the incidence of infection, and barrier methods play a critical role in preventing cutaneous exposure. The operating physician has some control over the frequency of needle sticks and lacerations. A greater number of injuries will cumulatively increase parenteral blood exposure and increase the risk of subsequent infection. Adherence to optimal technique and awareness of sharp instruments on the interventional tray and around the patient can minimize the risk of parenteral injury. Papers reviewing means of reducing risk of parenteral injury in the interventional radiology suite (WALL et al. 1991), in the operating room (CHAMBERLAND et al. 1995), and in surgical subspecialty practice (MURR and LEE 1995) are available. The remainder of the article will concentrate on means of reducing parenteral injury in the interventional suite.

Thirty percent of all needle stick injuries are caused by needle recapping (JAGGER et al. 1988). Within interventional radiology, 20% of all percutaneous injuries are from recapping needles (HANSEN et al. 1993a). When recapping a needle, the needle may perforate the side wall of the needle sheath and puncture the operator's finger, or the needle may miss the cap and puncture the individual's finger. By simply not recapping needles, one can eliminate 20%–30% of percutaneous injuries with their attendant risk of blood-borne pathogen transmission. After needle use, the syringe with its needle attached should be discarded in a sharps disposal box. If the needle must be removed, a clamp should be used to remove the needle and dispose of it in the sharps container. If the needle must be recapped for whatever reason, a one-handed technique should be utilized. Any sharp instrument should be discarded after its initial use if at all feasible. If any injury does occur, the chances increase that the injury will be from a clean sterile unused sharp. If the instrument is to be reused, the sharp should be sequestered in a special container on the angiographic tray. Prior to breakdown of the tray, the operating physician should remove and dispose of all sharp objects on the tray to prevent inadvertent needle stick injury to the technologist.

A situation that does not receive sufficient attention in interventional radiology is the use of hollow needles or cannulas with replaceable stylets (WILLIAMS et al. 1991). Replacing the stylet in a needle such as the Chiba or a modified Potts needle is analogous to the situation that occurs when recapping needles. There is a significant opportunity for inadvertent finger puncture and extra attention should be paid when replacing the stylet into these needles.

All glass syringes should be removed from the angiographic tray because of the risk of glass breakage and subsequent laceration or injury to individuals involved in the procedure. Although it may be assumed that plastic syringes cannot cause a percutaneous injury, the use of plastic syringes during hand injection may result in percutaneous injury with sudden breakage of the syringe shaft when performing high-pressure inflations (SANDHU and SCHULTZ 1995). An inflation device or a polycarbonate syringe should be utilized for high-pressure inflations to prevent plastic syringe shaft fracture and subsequent percutaneous injury.

All operators involved in a procedure should be aware of the location of sharp instruments and needles. A no touch means of passing a sharp instrument should be employed to prevent inadvertent injury while passing a sharp instrument from one individual to another. With the no touch pass, the sharp instrument is laid out on the angiographic tray or another stable item and given to the requesting individual. Hand to hand passage of sharp instruments should be avoided.

HIV-positive patients develop conditions that require interventional radiologic attention. The overall risk of seroconverting or acquiring HIV after exposure to a patient's blood is low in general and probably even lower for interventional radiologists. Adherence to appropriate precautions can further reduce this already low risk. Despite all of the concern about HIV transmission, the risk of hepatitis B and hepatitis C are even greater and should encourage an even stricter adherence to universal precautions. Adherence to universal precautions and greater awareness of procedures to minimize occupational injury can significantly reduce the risk of acquiring an infection from blood-borne pathogens. This is not only a theoretical consideration but has proven effective (LOWENFELS et al. 1995).

References

Albort JV, Calleja MA, Canalis EA, Catalan M, Sanchez-Lloret J (1993) Surgical management of spontaneous pneumothorax in patients with AIDS. Ann Thorac Surg 55:808–809

Ankobiah WA, Salehi F (1991) Salmonella lung abscess in a patient with acquired immunodeficiency syndrome. Chest 100:591

Batra P, Wallace JM, Ovenfors CO (1987) Efficacy and complications of transthoracic needle biopsy of lung in patients with *Pneumocystis carinii* pneumonia and AIDS. J Thorac Imag 2:79–80

Battan R, Mariuz P, Raviglione MC, Sabatini MT, Mullen MP, Poretsky L (1991) *Pneumocystis carinii* infection of the thyroid in a hypothyroid patient with AIDS: diagnosis by fine needle aspiration biopsy. J Clin Endocrinol Metab 72: 724–726

Benhamou Y, Caumes E, Gersoa Y, et al. (1993) AIDS-related cholangiopathy: critical analysis of a prospective series of 26 patients. Dig Dis Sci 38:1113–1118

Bennett NT, Howard RJ (1994) Quantity of blood inoculated in a needlestick injury from suture needles. J Am Coll Surg 178:107–110

Bottles K, McPhaul LW, Volberding P (1988) Fine-needle aspiration biopsy of patients with acquired immunodeficiency syndrome (AIDS). Ann Intern Med 108:42–45

Byrnes TA, Brevig JK, Yeoh CB (1989) Pneumothorax in patients with acquired immunodeficiency syndrome. J Thorac Cardiovasc Surg 98:546–550

Castellino RA, Blank N (1979) Etiologic diagnosis of focal pulmonary infection in immunocompromised patients by fluoroscopically guided percutaneous needle aspiration. Radiology 132:563–567

Cegielski JP, Ramiya K, Lallinger GJ, Mtulia IA, Mbaga IM (1990) Pericardial disease and human immunodeficiency virus in Dar es Salaam, Tanzania. Lancet 335:209–212

Center for Disease Control (1999) HIV/AIDS Surveillance Report. 11:5–8

Centers for Disease Control and Prevention (1993) National HIV serosurveillance summary: results through 1992. Atlanta, US Department of Health and Human Services, Public Health Service, Publication HIV/NCID/11–93/036

Chamberland ME, Ciesielski CA, Howard RJ, Fry DE, Bell DM (1995) Occupational risk of infection with human immunodeficiency virus. Surg Clin North Am 75:1057–1070

Chhieng DC, Argosino R, McKenna BJ, Cangiarella JF, Cohen JM (1999) Diag Cytopath 21:260–264

Chow C, Templeton PA, White CS (1993) Lung cysts associated with *Pneumocystis carinii* pneumonia: radiographic characteristics, natural history, and complications. AJR 161:527–531

Coker RJ (1994) Empyema thoracis in AIDS. J R Soc Med 87:65–67

Coker R, Moss F, Peters B, et al. (1993) Pneumothorax in patients with AIDS. Respir Med 87:400–401

Conces DJ, Tarver RD, Gray WC, Pearcy EA (1988) Treatment of pneumothoraces utilizing small caliber chest tubes. Chest 94:55–57

Daley CL (1991) Pyogenic bacterial pneumonia in the acquired immunodeficiency syndrome. J Thorac Imaging 6:36–42

Desai GA, Mugala DD (1992) Management of empyema thoracis at Lusaka, Zambia. Br J Surg 79:537–538

Dionigi P, Cebrelli T, Jemos V, et al. (1995) Use of subcutaneous implantable infusion systems in neoplastic and AIDS patients requiring long-term venous access. Eur J Surg 161:137–142

Donald JJ, Coral A, Shorvon PJ, Lees WR (1988) Ultrasound guided core biopsy in AIDS: experience in six patients. Br Med J 296:606–607

Dore R, Cormalba GP, DiMaggio EM, DiGiulio G, Preda L (1994) Interventional modalities in immunosuppressed patients. Radiol Med 87:77–89

Driver A, Peden J, Adams H, Rumley R (1991) Heimlich valve treatment of *Pneumocystis carinii*-associated pneumothorax. Chest 100:281–282

Eisenberg MJ, Gordon AS, Schiller NB (1992) HIV-associated pericardial effusions. Chest 102:956–958

Ellison E, Lapuerta P, Martin SE (1998) Fine needle aspiration (FNA) in HIV+ patients: results from a series of 655 aspirates. Cytopathology 9:222–229

Falguera M, Nogues A, Ruiz-Gonzalez A, Garcia M, Puig T, Rubio-Caballero M (1994) Transthoracic needle aspiration in the study of pulmonary infections in patients with HIV. Chest 106:697–702

Feins RH (1993) The role of thoracoscopy in the AIDS/immunocompromised patient. Ann Thorac Surg 56:649–650

Feuerstein IM, Archer A, Pluda JM, et al. (1990) Thin-walled cavities, cysts, and pneumothorax in *Pneumocystis carinii* pneumonia. Further observations with histopathologic correlation. Radiology 174:697–702

Finfer M, Perchick A, Burstein DE (1991) Fine needle aspiration biopsy diagnosis of tuberculous lymphadenitis in patients with the acquired immunodeficiency syndrome. Acta Cytol 35:325–332

Fitzgerald W, Bevalacqua FA, Garay SM, Aranda CP (1987) The role of open lung biopsy in patients with the acquired immunodeficiency syndrome. Chest 91:659–661

Fleisher AG, McElvaney G, Lawson L, Gerein AN, Grant D, Tyers GFO (1988) Surgical management of spontaneous pneumothorax in patients with acquired immunodeficiency syndrome. Ann Thorac Surg 45:21–23

Freedberg RS, Gindea AJ, Dieterich DT, Greene JB (1987) Herpes simplex pericarditis in AIDS. N Y State J Med 87:304–306

Gerberding JL (1994) Incidence and prevalence of human immunodeficiency virus, hepatitis B virus, hepatitis C virus, and cytomegalovirus among health care personnel at risk for blood exposure: final report from a longitudinal study. J Infect Dis 170:1410–1417

Gerberding JL, Henderson DK (1992) Management of occupational exposures to bloodborne pathogens: hepatitis B virus, hepatitis C virus, and human immunodeficiency virus. Clin Infect Dis 14:1179–1185

Gerberding JL, Schecter WP (1991) Surgery and AIDS: reducing the risk (editorial). JAMA 265:1572–1573

Gerein A, Brumwell ML, Lawson L, Chan N, Montaner J (1991) Surgical management of pneumothorax in patients with acquired immunodeficiency syndrome. Arch Surg 126:1272–1276

Goodman P, Daley C, Minagi H (1986) Spontaneous pneumothorax in AIDS patients with *Pneumocystis carinii* pneumonia. AJR 147:29–31

Gruden JF, Klein JS, Webb WR (1993) Percutaneous transthoracic needle biopsy in AIDS: analysis in 32 patients. Radiology 189:567–571

Gruden JF, Webb WR, Yao DC, Klein JS, Sandhu JS (1995) Bronchogenic carcinoma in 13 patients infected with the human immunodeficiency virus (HIV): clinical and radiographic findings. J Thorac Imag 10:99–105

Gurney JW, Bates FT (1989) Pulmonary cystic disease: comparison of *Pneumocystis carinii* pneumatoceles and bullous emphysema due to intravenous drug abuse. Radiology 173:27–31

Hales M, Bottles K, Miller T, Donegan E, Ljung BM (1987) Diagnosis of Kaposi's sarcoma by fine-needle aspiration biopsy. Am J Clin Pathol 88:20–25

Hansen ME, McIntire DD (1996) HIV transmission during invasive radiologic procedures: estimate based on computer modeling. AJR 166:263–267

Hansen ME, McIntire DD, Miller GL (1992) Occult glove perforations: frequency during interventional radiologic procedures. AJR 159:131–135

Hansen ME, Miller GL III, Redman HC, McIntire DD (1993a) HIV and interventional radiology: a national survey of physician attitudes and behaviors. JVIR 4:229–236

Hansen ME, Miller GL III, Redman HC, McIntire DD (1993b) Needle-stick injuries and blood contacts during invasive radiologic procedures: frequency and risk factors. AJR 160:1119–1122

Harkin TJ, Ciotoli C, Addrizzo-Harris DJ, et al. (1998) Transbronchial needle aspiration (TBNA) in patients infected with HIV. Am J Respir Crit Care Med 157:1913–1918

Heidenreich PA, Eisenberg MJ, Somelofski CA, et al. (1995) Pericardial effusion in AIDS. Incidence and survival. Circulation 92:3229–3234

Henderson DK, Fahey BJ, Willy M, et al. (1990) Risk for occupational transmission of human immunodeficiency virus type (HIV-1) associated with clinical exposures. Ann Intern Med 113:740–746

Hernandez Borge J, Alfageme Michavilla I, Munoz Mendez J, Campos Rodriguez F, Pena Grinan N, Villagomez Cerrato R (1999) Thoracic empyema in HIV-infected patients: microbiology, management, and outcome. Chest 113:732–738

Hersey JC, Martin LS (1994) Use of infection control guidelines by workers in healthcare facilities to prevent occupational transmission of HBV and HIV: results from a national survey. Infect Control Hosp Epidemiol 15:243–252

Himelman RB, Chung WS, Chernoff DN, Schiller NB, Hollander H (1989) Cardiac manifestations of the human immunodeficiency virus infection: a two dimensional echocardiographic study. J Am Coll Cardiol 13:1030–1036

Hnatiuk OW, Dillard TA, Oster CN (1990) Bleomycin sclerotherapy for bilateral pneumothoraces in a patient with AIDS. Ann Intern Med 113:988–990

Hornick P, Smith PLC (1994) Empyema thoracis in AIDS. J R Soc Med 87:570

Horowitz HW, Telzak EE, Sepkowitz KA, Wormser GP (1998a) Human immunodeficiency virus infection. Part I. Disease-a-Month 44:545–606

Horowitz HW, Telzak EE, Sepkowitz KA, Wormser GP (1998b) Human immunodeficiency virus infection. Part II. Disease-a-Month 44: 679–716

Huang RD, Pearlman S, Friedman WH, Loree T (1991) Benign cystic vs. solid lesions of the parotid gland in HIV patients. Head Neck 13:522–527

Hung CC, Chen MY, Kuo PH, Hsieh SM, Sheng WH, Yang PC (1999) Ultrasound-guided percutaneous transthoracic needle aspiration biopsy for diagnosis of pulmonary lesions in advanced HIV infection. J Formos Med Assoc 98:195–200

Ioachim HL (1990) Biopsy diagnosis in human immunodeficiency virus infection and acquired immunodeficiency syndrome. Arch Pathol Lab Med 114:284–294

Ippolito G, Puro V, De Carli G, et al. (1993) The risk of occupational human immunodeficiency virus infection in health care workers: Italian multicenter study. Arch Intern Med 153:1451–1458

Jagger J, Hunt EH, Brand-Elnaggar J, Pearson RD (1988) Rates of needle-stick injury caused by various devices in a universal hospital. N Engl J Med 319:284–288

Joseph J, Strange C, Sahn SA (1993) Pleural effusions in hospitalized patients with AIDS. Ann Intern Med 118:856–869

Karve MM, Murali MR, Shah HM, Phelps KR (1992) Rapid evolution of cardiac tamponade due to bacterial pericarditis in two patients with HIV-1 infection. Chest 101:1461–1463

Klein JS, Zarka MA (2000) Transthoracic needle biopsy of the chest. Radiol Clin North Am 38:235–266

Klein JS, Schultz S, Heffner JE (1995) Interventional radiology of the chest: image-guided percutaneous drainage of pleural effusions, lung abscess, and pneumothorax. AJR 164:581–588

Kuhlman JE, Knowles MC, Fishman EK, Siegelman SS (1989) Premature bullous disease in AIDS: CT diagnosis. Radiology 173:23–26

Lanphear BP (1994) Trends and patterns in the transmission of bloodborne pathogens to health care workers. Epidemiol Rev 16:437–450

Lanphear BP, Linnemann CC, Cannon CG, et al. (1994) Hepatitis C virus infection in healthcare workers: risk of exposure and infection. Infect Control Hosp Epidemiol 15:745–750

Libraty D (1992) Reexpansion pulmonary edema in AIDS. West J Med 156:657–659

Lowenfels AB, Mehta V, Levi DA, Montecalvo MA, Savino JA, Wormser GP (1995) Reduced frequency of percutaneous injuries in surgeons: 1993 versus 1988. AIDS 9:199–202

Luce JM, Clement MJ (1989) Pulmonary diagnostic evaluation of patients suspected of having an HIV-related disease. Semin Respir Infect 4:93–101

Marcus R, Culver DH, Bell DM, et al. (1993) Risk of human immunodeficiency virus infection among emergency department workers. Am J Med 94:363–370

Mariuz P, Raviglione MC, Gould IA, Mullen MP (1991) Pleural *Pneumocystis carinii* infection. Chest 99:774–776

Martin T, Fontana G, Olak J, Ferguson M (1996) Use of a pleural catheter for the management of simple pneumothorax. Chest 110:1169–1172

Martinez-Marcos FJ, Viciana P, Canas E, Martin-Juan J, Moreno I, Pachon J (1997) Etiology of solitary pulmonary nodules in patients with human immunodeficiency virus infection. Clin Infect Dis 24:908–913

Mast ST, Woolwine JD, Gerberding JL (1993) Efficacy of gloves in reducing blood volumes transferred during simulated needlestick injury. J Infect Dis 168:1589–1592

McClellan M, Miller S, Parsons P, Cohn D (1991) Pneumothorax with *Pneumocystis carinii* pneumonia in AIDS: incidence and clinical characteristics. Chest 100:1224–1228

McWilliams RG, Blanshard KS (1994) The risk of blood splash contamination during angiography. Clin Radiol 49:59–60

Merriam MA, Cronan JJ, Dorfman GS, Lambiase RE, Haas RA (1988) Radiologically guided percutaneous catheter drainage of pleural fluid collections. AJR 151:1113–1116

Metersky M, Colt H, Olson L, Shanks T (1995) AIDS-related spontaneous pneumothorax. Risk factors and treatment. Chest 108:946–951

Miller RF, Severn A (1995) Non surgical treatment of empyema thoracis with intrapleural streptokinase in a patient with AIDS. Genitourin Med 71:259–261

Minami H, Saka H, Senda K, et al. (1992) Small caliber catheter drainage for spontaneous pneumothorax. Am J Med Sci 304:345–347

Montecalvo MA, Lee MS, DePalma H, et al. (1995) Seroprevalence of human immunodeficiency virus-1, hepatitis B virus, and hepatitis C virus in patients having major surgery. Infect Control Hosp Epidemiol 16:627–632

Moore DA, Gazzard BG, Nelson MR (1997) Central venous line infections in AIDS. J Infect 34:35–40

Moulton JS (2000) Image-guided management of complicated pleural fluid collections. Radiol Clin North Am 38:345–374

Murr AH, Lee KC (1995) Universal precautions for the otolaryngologist: techniques and equipment for minimizing exposure risk. ENT J 74: 338–346

Murray JF, Felton CP, Garay SM, et al. (1984) Pulmonary complications of the acquired immunodeficiency syndrome. Report of a National Heart, Lung, and Blood Institute workshop. N Engl J Med 310:1682–1688

Muscedere G, Bennett JD, Lee TY, Mackie I, Vanderburgh L (1998) Complications of radiologically placed central venous ports and Hickman catheters in patients with AIDS. Can Assoc Radiol J 49:84–89

Nathan PE, Arsura EL, Zappi M (1991) Pericarditis with tamponade due to cytomegalovirus in the acquired immunodeficiency syndrome. Chest 99:765–766

Newman TG, Soni A, Acaron S, Huang CT (1987) Pleural cryptococcosis in the acquired immunodeficiency syndrome. Chest 91:459–461

O'Moore PV, Mueller PR, Simeone JF, et al. (1987) Sonographic guidance in diagnostic and therapeutic interventions in the pleural space. AJR 149:1–5

Palella FJ, Delaney KM, Moorman AC, et al. (1998) Declining morbidity and mortality among patients with advanced human immunodeficiency virus infection. N Engl J Med 338:853–860

Ray P, Antoine M, Mary-Krause M, et al. (1998) AIDS-related primary pulmonary lymphoma. Am J Respir Crit Care Med 158:1221–1229

Read CA, Reddy VD, O'Mara TE, Richardson MSA (1994) Doxycycline pleurodesis for pneumothorax in patients with AIDS. Chest 105:823–825

Reid AJ, Miller RF, Kocjan GI (1998) Diagnostic utility of fine needle aspiration (FNA) cytology in HIV-infected patients with lymphadenopathy. Cytopathology 9:230–239

Reynolds MM, Hecht SR, Berger M, Kolokathis A, Horowitz SF (1992) Large pericardial effusion in the acquired immunodeficiency syndrome. Chest 102:1746–1747

Samies JH, Hathaway BN, Echols RM, Veazey JM Jr, Pilon VA (1986) Lung abscess due to *Corynebacterium equi*. Report of the first case in a patient with acquired immunodeficiency syndrome. Am J Med 80:685–688

Sandhu JS, Goodman PC (1989) Pulmonary cysts associated with *Pneumocystis carinii* pneumonia in patients with AIDS. Radiology 173:33–35

Sandhu JS, Schultz SC (1995) Plastic syringe shaft fracture as a risk for percutaneous injury during performance of interventional procedures [letter]. JVIR 6:987–988

Satue JA, Aguado JM, Costa JR, et al. (1994) Pulmonary abscess due to non-typhi *Salmonella* in a patient with AIDS. Clin Infect Dis 19:555–557

Schofield JB, Lindley RP, Harcourt-Webster JN (1989) Biopsy pathology of HIV infection: experience at St. Stephen's Hospital, London. Histopathology 14:277–288

Scott WW Jr, Kuhlman JE (1991) Focal pulmonary lesions in patients with AIDS. Percutaneous transthoracic needle biopsy. Radiology 180:419–421

Sepkowitz K, Telzak E, Gold J, et al. (1991) Pneumothorax in AIDS. Ann Intern Med 114:455–459

Settle JT, Neff-Smith M, Wan GJ (1994) Infections related to venous access devices in patients with AIDS. J Assoc Nurses AIDS Care 5:43–47

Shapiro CN (1995) Occupational risk of infection with hepatitis B and and hepatitis C virus. Surg Clin North Am 75:1047–1056

Shapiro L, Pincus RL (1991) Fine-needle aspiration of diffuse cervical lymphadenopathy in patients with acquired immunodeficiency syndrome. Otolaryngol Head Neck Surg 105:419–421

Sharma VS, Valji K, Bookstein JJ (1992) Gastrointestinal hemorrhage in AIDS: arteriographic diagnosis and transcatheter treatment. Radiology 185:447–451

Sider L, Weiss AJ, Smith MD, VonRoenn JH, Glassroth J (1989) Varied appearance of AIDS-related lymphoma in the chest. Radiology 171:629–632

Silverman SG, Mueller PR, Saini S, et al. (1988) Thoracic empyema: Management with image-guided catheter drainage. Radiology 169:5–9

Skoutelis AT, Murphy RL, MacDonell KB, et al. (1990) Indwelling central venous catheter infections in patients with ac-

quired immune deficiency syndrome. J Acquir Immune Defic Syndr 3:335–342

Stotka JL, Good CB, Downer WR, Kapoor WN (1989) Pericardial effusion and tamponade due to Kaposi's sarcoma in acquired immunodeficiency syndrome. Chest 95:1359–1361

Strazzella WD, Safirstein BH (1991) Pleural effusions in AIDS. N J Med 88:39–41

Suster B, Akerman M, Orenstein M, Wax MR (1986) Pulmonary manifestations of AIDS: review of 106 episodes. Radiology 161:87–93

Tenholder MF, Jackson HD (1993) Bronchogenic carcinoma in patients seropositive for human immunodeficiency virus. Chest 104:1049–1053

Townsend RR, Laing FC, Jeffrey RB Jr, Bottles K (1989) Abdominal lymphoma in AIDS: evaluation with US. Radiology 171:719–724

Trachiotis GD, Hafner GH, Hix WR, Aaron BL (1992) Role of open lung biopsy in diagnosing pulmonary complications of AIDS. Ann Thorac Surg 54:898–901

Tunon-de-Lara JM, Constans J, Vincent MP, Receveur MC, Conri C, Taytard A (1992) Spontaneous pneumothorax associated with *Pneumocystis carinii* pneumonia: successful treatment with talc pleurodesis. Chest 101:1177–1178

Turco M, Seneff M, McGrath B, Hsia J (1990) Cardiac tamponade in the acquired immunodeficiency syndrome. Am Heart J 120:1467–1468

Van Henkel P, Van de Bergh JHAM (1994) Heimlich valve treatment and outpatient management of bilateral spontaneous pneumothorax. Chest 105:1586–1587

Wait MA, Dal Nogare AR (1994) Treatment of AIDS-related spontaneous pneumothorax. A decade of experience. Chest 106:693–696

Walker W, Pate J (1993) AIDS-related bronchopleural fistula. Ann Thorac Surg 55:1048

Wall SD, Olcott EW, Gerberding JL (1991) AIDS risk and risk reduction in the radiology department. AJR 157:911–917

White CS, Haramati LB, Elder KH, Karp J, Belani CP (1995) Carcinoma of the lung in HIV-positive patients: findings on chest radiographs and CT scans. AJR 164:593–597

White CS, Meyer CA, Templeton PA (2000) CT fluoroscopy for thoracic interventional procedures. Radiol Clin North Am 38:303–322

Williams DM, Marx MV, Korobkin M (1991) AIDS risk and risk reduction in the radiology department (commentary). AJR 157:919–921

Wolday D, Seyoum B (1997) Pleural empyema due to *Salmonella paratyphi* in a patient with AIDS. Trop Med Int Health 2:1140–1142

Zuckerman AJ (1995) Occupational exposure to hepatitis B virus and human immunodeficiency virus: a comparative risk analysis. Am J Infect Control 23:286–289

17 HIV Transmission Prevention for Health Care Workers

John R. Mathieson, Eric van Sonnenberg, Jacques W. A. J. Reeders

CONTENTS

17.1 Introduction

The impact of AIDS has included a fundamental reappraisal of methods of disease transmission, and the type of risks posed not only to health care professionals, but also to the public seeking medical care.

In the early days of the epidemic, we did not know what the causative agent was, how it was transmitted, or how to test for the presence of AIDS. Understandably, this stage of ignorance often led to confusion amongst the health care professions (HEILMAN 1991; SHELLEY and HOWARD 1992; BIRD et al. 1991). AIDS patients were regarded with a wide variety of attitudes and prejudices, ranging from a cavalier approach to a state of excessive fear and even hysteria. The latter state of mind prevailed in many institutions early in the epidemic, including a university-affiliated hospital in the same city as one of the authors (J.M.). In this case, the hospital administrators

J.R. MATHIESON, MD
928 Island Road, Victoria BC V8S 2T9, Canada
E. VAN SONNENBERG, MD
Department of Radiology, Dana-Farber Cancer Institute,
44 Binney Street, Boston, MA 02115, USA
J.W.A.J. REEDERS, MD, PhD
Consultant Radiologist, Department of Radiology,
St. Elisabeth Hospital Willemstad, Breedestraat 193 (O),
Curaçao, Netherlands Antilles

publicly refused to allow AIDS patients into their building, fearing transmission of AIDS to their employees.

In this chapter we shall discuss AIDS, its detection, transmission, and prevention, as well as practical safety measures that can be taken so that AIDS patients can be offered the same high standards of compassionate medical care as anyone else, without undue risk to health care workers (HCWs).

We will also briefly discuss the issues surrounding the human immune deficiency virus (HIV)-positive HCW, and subsequent risks to the general public.

17.2 Infection Risks

When an HCW comes into contact with body fluid from an HIV-positive patient, the risk of acquiring the infection depends upon two factors: the type of body fluid and the nature of the contact (FAUCI 1988). Table 17.1 lists the body fluids considered infectious and noninfectious, according to the Centers for Disease Control in Atlanta. In general, the risk of infection parallels the amount of virus present in the fluid. It is now known that body fluids from HIV-positive patients are much less infectious than was feared during the early years of the epidemic. Blood is the most infectious fluid, and even when a needle contaminated with HIV-infected blood accidentally punctures the skin of an HIV-negative person, the risk of infection with HIV is surprisingly low – approximately 0.1%–0.4% (LOWENFELS et al. 1989; MARCUS 1988; WORMSER et al. 1988; HOCHREITER and BARTON 1988; HENDERSON et al. 1990; QUEBBEMAN et al. 1991; IPPOLITO et al. 1993). This is probably due to the relatively low number of virus parti-

This chapter has been modified from Chapter 7 in: Reeders JWAJ, Mathieson Jr (eds) (1998) AIDS imaging. W.B. Saunders, London

cles in HIV-positive patients' blood, compared with other diseases, such as hepatitis B (Centers for Disease Control 1987; GERBERDING et al. 1987). Despite this surprisingly low risk, the tragic fact is that there were at least 32 well-documented cases of HCWs acquiring HIV infection through occupational exposure in the first decade of the epidemic (CHAMBERLAND et al. 1991; ANONYMOUS 1992). Further, it is highly likely that this figure underestimates the actual number of such cases (HAMORY 1983). Since infection with HIV is generally considered universally fatal, every possible precaution must be taken to avoid such accidents (MARCUS 1988; HENDERSON et al. 1990; GERBERDING et al. 1987).

It is also possible, both theoretically and based on case experience, to acquire HIV infection without an actual skin puncture. At least four HCWs have become HIV-positive after mucocutaneous exposure to HIV-positive infected blood (ANONYMOUS 1992). HIV can be transmitted via other body fluids from a mucous membrane or open wounds. Although the risk of such transmission is very low, the additional prognosis of HIV infection makes even a very remote risk unacceptably high (GERBERDING et al. 1990; KELEN et al. 1989; DECKER 1992). It is prudent to recommend strict adherence to the principles of universal precautions. Even though certain fluids are not felt to pose a significant risk unless visibly blood stained (Table 17.1) (Centers for Disease Control 1988), we find it easiest to treat all body fluids (with the exception of sweat and tears) as potentially dangerous.

Table 17.1. Body fluids and risk of HIV transmission

Infectious
  Blood
  Semen
  Vaginal and cervical secretions
  Wound and tissue fluid
  Cerebrospinal fluid
  Amniotic fluid
  Pleural fluid
  Pericardial fluid
  Peritoneal fluid
  Nasal secretions
  Synovial fluid
Noninfectious (unless visibly blood-stained)
  Urine
  Feces
  Saliva
  Sputum
  Vomit
  Sweat
  Tears

17.3 Radiologic Precautions

Early efforts at protecting HCWs from AIDS centered in part on identifying carriers of the disease, so that appropriate protective measures could then be taken by anyone coming into contact with these known AIDS patients. However, this approach has proven futile, for several reasons. The natural history of HIV infection is such that there are significant periods in which an infected individual will be negative to serum testing. Further, many HIV-positive individuals have not been tested, and many are unaware of being at risk for HIV (KELEN et al. 1988). Even when HIV-positive patients are aggressively investigated, there is no clear risk factor identified in a substantial proportion of patients, perhaps as many as 10%. Also, it is impossible to identify potential AIDS patient by their outward physical appearance or behavior (KELEN et al. 1988). Finally, many AIDS patients require treatment on an urgent basis, which may not even allow for an adequate history to be taken, let alone allowing time to obtain results of serologic testing (HOCHREITER and BARTON 1988).

Therefore, most public health recommendations adopt some system of universal precautions, in which blood and other body fluids from all patients are regarded as potentially hazardous. The fact that hepatitis B is also very common in AIDS patients, and is also much more likely to be accidentally transmitted, has served as a useful further motivation to adopt universal precautions (HERSEY and MARTIN 1994). It should be added that while we and others advocate treating all body fluids of every patient as potentially hazardous, there is no doubt that we are even more cautious when we do know we are dealing with an AIDS patient.

The nature of the protective measures required depends upon the nature of the interaction between the patient and the HCW. For example, for casual contact such as routine radiography, ultrasound, or noncontrast computed tomography (CT) and magnetic resonance imaging (MRI), no special precautions are required. For contacts involving intravenous puncture, gloves should be worn, and exquisite care must be taken in the handling of the sharp objects. Needles should never be recapped by hand. All sharp objects should be disposed of immediately after use, using safe point-of-use containers. For radiologists who do not perform interventional procedures, the risk of exposure to HIV is mainly confined to venepuncture for contrast injection. However, radiologists are increasingly asked to perform other more invasive procedures on AIDS patients, and constant vigilance is required to avoid accidental exposure (WALL et al. 1991; WILLIAMS et al. 1988) (see also Chap. 16).

17.3.1
Percutaneous Fine-Needle Aspiration Biopsy

Imaging-guided biopsies are the commonest potential source of accidental infection in most hospital radiology practices, apart from venepuncture. All facets of fine-needle aspiration biopsy (FNAB) procedures must be designed to minimize the possibility of infection. Gloves must be worn routinely. Obviously, gloves help prevent cutaneous contact with body fluids. Also, it has been shown that gloves decrease the volume of blood transferred during accidental needle punctures. "Double gloving" and changing of gloves at intervals during a procedure have been recommended for lengthy procedures in bloody fields. Masks and eye protection should also be worn when there is risk of fluids contacting the face. Masks with attached transparent face shields are available, and we have found these quite convenient to use as they do not impair vision. The use of impermeable gowns, hats, and boots should be considered when appropriate.

Bedside "sharps" disposal containers should be available in every room where biopsies are performed, and must be kept easily accessible to the radiologist. In practice, we find this is the commonest source of procedural errors, as sharps containers are often stored in inconvenient locations, and may have objects piled on top of them, such as papers and charts. Also, standard size sharps disposal containers may be too small for the longer needles and stylets used in radiology departments. Containers must be taller than the longest sharp object used, and must be emptied regularly. Syringes and needles used for local anesthesia should be disposed of immediately after use. Needles must never be recapped by hand, as this is the commonest cause of accidental puncture injuries. If it is necessary to replace a cap on a needle, it must be done without holding the cap by hand. When sharp objects must be reused, such as in angiographic or other interventional procedures, a system of safe storage must be adopted. A film canister is modified with perforations on its top, sized to fit a variety of needles and other sharp objects. Once any sharp object is removed from the patient's body it is immediately inserted into the container, sharp end downwards, and left there until it is needed again. In this way, there are no exposed sharp objects on the equipment tray. Whatever system is used, it must be clearly understood by all personnel and followed without exception.

Although room lighting is kept deliberately low, especially for ultrasound-guided biopsies, there must be sufficient light to see the needle tip and skin puncture marks from local anesthesia. Gauze should always be available to stop any bleeding from the puncture site. Also, gloves and other protective equipment should be available to be worn by any of the attending personnel in the room who may be asked to assist in the procedure. Gloves should be disposed of, and not washed for a second use. It has been shown that "wicking" may occur with wet gloves, with fluids being drawn through very small holes by capillary action. Also, the act of washing gloves is likely to create holes in them.

When biopsies are done for quick stain cytology, the radiologist will pass the needle and syringe containing the biopsy specimen to the cytopathology technologist for immediate plating on slides. It is while the needle is being passed from one person to another that another substantial risk of accidental puncture occurs. Communication between the radiologist and the cytopathology technologist must be clear and explicit, and the needle should be passed with the sharp tip pointing away from the person receiving it. Another solution is to avoid passing the needle from one person to another altogether, by the person performing the biopsy placing the needle and syringe on a table top, and the technologist then picking up the needle from the table. In the hospital of one of the authors (J.M.), more than 10,000 imaging-guided biopsies have been performed since the beginning of the AIDS epidemic, and to our knowledge, only one accidental puncture with a contaminated needle has occurred. In this instance, the radiologist was punctured with the biopsy needle while attempting to pass the needle to the technologist. Although, fortunately, the individual involved remains well and HIV-negative, this accident emphasizes the importance of rigid adherence to universal precautions and safe methods of handling contaminated sharp objects.

Another possible source of accidental contamination occurs when the cytopathology technologist expresses the biopsy specimen from the needle and syringes onto the microscope slides. Sometimes, a plug of material will temporarily occlude the lumen of the needle, and as the plug is dislodged with increasing pressure on the syringe, some material may be sprayed into the air. All personnel in the room should be aware of this potential source of contact. Once the cytopathology technologist has finished plating the material onto the microscope slides, the technologist should directly dispose of the needle and syringes, without passing them to another person.

Consideration must be given to artificial resuscitation procedures, particularly when patients are given narcotic or sedative drugs. Mouth-to-mouth resuscitation is completely abandoned and a variety of respiration devices with one-way valves should be made easily available throughout the department.

17.3.2
Angiography

Angiography is performed for a wide variety of indications in AIDS patients, and is particularly useful in the diagnosis and treatment of bleeding from the gastrointestinal (GI) tract.

Angiography presents the greatest risk for having HIV-infected blood splashed or sprayed onto HCWs, thereby coming into contact with mucous membranes or open wounds. There is an obvious risk of exposure during the act of arterial or venous puncture. Presently, many needle manufacturers are attempting to produce self-contained puncture systems to eliminate or minimize this risk. Additionally, every catheter and wire exchange maneuver presents an opportunity for inadvertent spraying of blood. The use of a sheath with a hemostatic valve helps reduce spraying and splashing of blood. When a needle is being removed over a guide wire, many angiographers are in the habit of wiping the guide wire with gauze that is held in the same hand that is being used to remove the needle. This practice increases the risk of accidental needle puncture, and should be avoided. The puncture needle should be held by its hub while it is being removed from the guide wire, and then the guide wire should be wiped with gauze in a separate motion. Care must be taken when removing a guide wire from a catheter so that the guide wire does not spring loose from the operator's hand, causing it to uncoil and brush against an exposed area of the HCW's body. Particular care must be taken with nitinol wires with hydrophilic coating, as these wires are not only extremely slippery, but can be very springy when coiled excessively. Glass syringes should not be used, owing to the risk of breakage and subsequent injury and contamination.

17.3.3
Other Interventional Procedures

The number of nonangiographic interventional procedures performed in AIDS patients continues to grow rapidly (see Chap. 16). We have performed all manner of interventional procedures on AIDS patients, including abscess draining, nephrostomy, biliary drainage, biliary stone removal, cholecystostomy, gastrostomy, gastrojejunostomy, and chest tube insertion. In many cases, the indications are no different from those in non-AIDS patients. However, there are some special circumstances that apply to AIDS patients. AIDS patients frequently have an abnormal-appearing gallbladder on ultrasound or CT. When a gallbladder wall is thickened, or when pericholecystic fluid is found, the radiologist should personally perform a careful ultrasound examination to see whether these findings are associated with a sonographic Murphy's sign, indicating cholecystitis, either calculous or acalculous. Gallbladder wall thickening is usually not due to acute cholecystitis. However, if the gallbladder is tender as well as thick walled, indicating acute cholecystitis, prompt performance of a percutaneous cholecystostomy can give a dramatic clinical response, and in the case of acalculous cholecystitis, is usually curative.

Pneumothorax is a complication of repetitive pulmonary infections in AIDS patients. We have found that imaging-guided chest tube insertion is very useful under these circumstances and often small (6–8 French) tubes are satisfactory. However, a collapsed lung often may not reexpand quickly in AIDS patients, owing to underlying chronic lung damage. Pleurodesis may be needed. We have also treated AIDS-related pneumothoraces on an outpatient basis, using a one-way Heimlich valve, rather than underwater suction. Patients being considered for outpatient treatment of pneumothoraces must be carefully selected, and must be thoroughly instructed as to how the valve works, as an improperly connected valve could prove disastrous.

We have not found abscesses to be particularly common in AIDS patients, but abscesses can occur in a wide variety of locations. Both typical and atypical tuberculous infections can cause abscesses, often in musculoskeletal sites including psoas, paraspinal, thigh muscles, and feet.

When a liver abscess is found, the primary site of origin in the GI tract must be sought. In particular, we have found infections arising from the colon, appendix, stomach, and distal ileum to cause liver abscesses.

Nutritional support methods bear special mention. AIDS patients are frequently malnourished and, although the reasons are not always straightforward, we have found that AIDS patients can benefit greatly from supplemental nutrition. The radiologist may become involved with transnasal or oral place-ment of feeding tubes into the stomach or duode-num. It may be very difficult for a clinician to place a transnasal tube into the duodenum or jejunum at the bedside. However, for a radiologist skilled in entero-clysis this can be a very simple procedure, particu-larly with the aid of fluoroscopy. When longer term access for supplemental feeding is required, a fluoro-scopically guided percutaneous gastrostomy or gas-trojejunostomy is often the fastest, safest, and least expensive method of achieving external GI tract ac-cess. We have found that a gastrostomy alone is suffi-cient for feeding most AIDS patients, and we reserve gastrojejunostomies for those patients shown to have gastroesophageal reflux after a gastrostomy and for patients with significant neurologic impair-ment. In most cases, we have found that gastrosto-mies can be removed after a few weeks or months, since after patients have gained weight and im-proved their nutritional status, and indeed their gen-eral condition, they can often eat well enough to do without supplemental feeding.

17.4
Accidental Punctures

If an HCW suffers an accidental needle puncture or other exposure to possibly contaminated blood, cer-tain first-aid precautions should be followed imme-diately:

1. Promote active bleeding from the site of puncture or contamination.
2. Wash the site with antiseptic solution, such as 10% povidone iodine.
3. Irrigate the site with normal saline for up to 15 min.

It should also be understood that there are no convincing experimental data to support the above recommendations. However, it is unlikely that this will ever be studied on a randomized, prospective basis, and most authors feel it is sensible to follow these rather elementary measures (FAHEY et al. 1993).

It has also been proposed that the HCW should then begin on a course of zidovudine (AZT). Al-though conclusive data are not yet available, some reports suggest that AZT is beneficial, and some in-stitutions recommend treatment with AZT immedi-ately after exposure (CARDO et al. 1995).

After first-aid measures have been taken, one must then assess the risk of HIV transmission through se-

rologic testing. The source patient from whom the blood or other body fluid was originally obtained must be assessed for HIV infection. If the patient is found or is known to have HIV infection, or if the patient declines serologic testing for HIV, the HCW should be assumed to have been exposed to HIV. Se-rologic testing of the HCW for HIV should be per-formed immediately after the exposure, and if se-ronegative, testing should be repeated at 6 weeks and 3, 6, and 12 months after exposure. If the source pa-tient is seronegative on repeated testing, testing of the HCW can cease. In most centers, testing for hep-atitis B and C is done at the same time.

17.5
AIDS and the Health Care Worker

Until recently, most of the infectious diseases suf-fered by AIDS patients did not pose a substantial risk to HCWs with a normally functioning immune sys-tem. However, since 1990, multidrug-resistant *Myco-bacterium tuberculosis* (MTb) has been found with increasing frequency in AIDS patients, and several cases of transmission to HCWs have been described (DOOLEY et al. 1990). Indeed, in an HIV dental clinic, transmission between two HCWs seems to have oc-curred, one of whom may have acquired the infec-tion from a patient.

The risk of acquiring MTb from an infected per-son depends upon the number of organisms they ex-pel into the air, which in turn depends upon the site of the disease within the patient, and the presence of cough and of cavitary pulmonary disease. CASTRO and DOOLEY (1993) point out that AIDS patients with MTb are no more likely than non-AIDS patients with MTb to transmit the mycobacteria to either ca-sual contacts or to HCWs. However, since MTb is more common in AIDS patients, and given the seri-ous problem posed by the emergence of multidrug-resistant strains, HCWs caring for AIDS patients face a definite risk of acquiring mycobacterial infection. HCWs should be cognizant of these risks, and aware of the importance of identifying patients with tuber-culosis as early as possible, so that appropriate pro-tective measure can be instituted (DI PERRI et al. 1993; CLEVELAND et al. 1995; STROUD et al. 1995).

With the passage of time, the problem of the HIV-positive HCW has received increasing attention.

Difficult practical and ethical issues have been raised of balancing the rights of the HCW to privacy and security of employment, with the rights of the general public to safe medical care (HENDERSON 1990a, b). One highly publicized case of an HIV-positive dentist transmitting HIV to his patients has caused a great deal of alarm and confusion (CIESIELSKI et al. 1992; ANONYMOUS 1993; MISHU and SCHAFFNER 1994). As worrisome and tragic as this case was, it appears to have exaggerated these risks, as the unfortunate patients were probably deliberately infected in this case. However, there have been other cases causing concern and it is difficult to know at the time how this problem should be handled (SCHULMAN et al. 1994).

Certainly, an HIV-positive HCW poses no risk to the patients in the majority of medical circumstances, unless there is a risk of his or her body fluids reaching the patient. This issue has gone beyond theory and conjecture. In one hospital in the United States, the hospital's administrators forced a physician to withdraw from their surgical residency program after he was found to be HIV positive as a result of occupational exposure to the blood of an AIDS patient. He refused the hospital's offer of a position in another medical residency and appealed the court's decision, but the hospital's position was upheld by the appellate court ("Appeals court upholds firing of HIV-positive physician" 1992). The legal and ethical ramifications of this issue are still emerging.

In practical terms, these concerns do not apply to most of the procedures taking place in the radiology department. The possible exceptions would include procedures in which the operator's hands are most likely to be accidentally injured and subsequently come into contact with a patient, such as in procedures which entail the operator's hand being placed in the patient's mouth, e.g., sialography. However, further clarification of the limits that should be placed upon HIV-positive HCWs is needed.

References

Anonymous (1992) Surveillance for occupationally acquired HIV infection – United States, 1981–1992. MMWR Morb Mortal Wkly Rep 1992; 41:823–825

Anonymous (1993) Update: investigations of persons treated by HIV-infected health-care workers – United States. MMWR Morb Mortal Wkly Rep 42:329–331, 337

Appeals court upholds firing of HIV-positive physician (1995) Bull Infect Hosp Epidemiol 16: 492

Bird AG, Gore SM, Leigh-Brown AJ, et al. (1991) Escape from collective denial: HIV transmission during surgery. Br Med J 303:351–352

Cardo DM, Srivastava PU, Ciesielski C, et al. (1995) Case-control of HIV seroconversion in health care workers after percutaneous exposures to HIV-infected blood. Infect Control Hosp Epidemiol 16:536

Castro KG, Dooley SW (1993) Mycobacterium tuberculosis transmission in healthcare settings: is it influenced by coinfection with human immunodeficiency virus? Infect Control Hosp Epidemiol 14:65–66

Centers for Disease Control (1987) Update: human immunodeficiency virus in health-care workers exposed to blood of infected patients. MMWR Morb Mortal Wkly Rep 36:285–289

Centers for Disease Control (1988) Update: universal precautions for prevention of transmission of human immunodeficiency virus, hepatitis B virus, and other bloodborne pathogens in health care settings. MMWR Morb Mortal Wkly Rep 37:377–382, 387–388

Centers for Disease Control and Prevention (1991) Nosocomial transmission of multidrug-resistant tuberculosis among HIV infected persons – Florida and New York, 1988–1991. MMWR Morb Mortal Wkly Rep 40:585–591

Chamberland ME, Conley LJ, Bush TJ, et al. (1991) Health care workers with AIDS. National surveillance update. JAMA 266:3459–3462

Ciesielski CA, Marianos D, Ou CY, et al. (1992) Transmission human immunodeficiency virus a dental practice. Ann Intern Med 116:798–805

Cleveland JL, Kent J, Gooch BF, et al. (1995) Multidrug-resistant Mycobacterium tuberculosis in an HIV dental clinic. Infect Control Hosp Epidemiol 16:7–11

Daley CL, Small PM, Schecter GE, et al. (1992) An outbreak of tuberculosis with accelerated progression among persons infected with the human immunodeficiency virus. N Engl J Med 326:231–235

Decker MD (1992) The OSHA bloodborne hazard standard. Infect Control Hosp Epidemiol 13:407–417

Di Perri G, Cadeo GP. Castelli F et al. (1993) Transmission of HIV-associated tuberculosis to healthcare workers. Infect Control Hosp Epidemiol 14:67–72

Dooley SW Jr, Castro KG, Hutton MD (1990) Centers for Disease Control and Prevention. Guidelines for preventing the transmission of tuberculosis in health-care settings, with special focus on HIV-related issues. MMWR Morb Mortal Wkly Rep 39:1–29

Dooley SW, Villarino ME, Lawrence ME. et al. (1991) Nosocomial transmission of tuberculosis in a hospital unit for HIV-infected patients. JAMA 267:2632–2634

Edlin BH, Tokars JI, Grisco MH, et al. (1992) Nosocomial transmission of multidrug-resistant tuberculosis among hospitalized patients with the acquired immunodeficiency syndrome. N Engl J Med 362:1514–1521

Fahey BJ, Beekmann SE, Schmitt J, et al. (1993) Managing occupational exposures to HIV-1 in the healthcare workplace. Infect Control Hosp Epidemiol 14:405–412

Fauci AS (1988) The human immunodeficiency virus: infectivity and mechanisms of pathogenesis. Science 239:617–622

Fisch MA, Uttanchandani RB, Daikos GL, et al. (1992) An outbreak of tuberculosis caused by multiple-drug-resistant tuberculosis bacilli among patients with HIV infection. Ann Intern Med 117:177–183

Gerberding JL (1990) Current epidemiologic evidence and case reports of occupationally acquired HIV and other bloodborne diseases. Infect Control Hosp Epidemiol 11:558–560

Gerberding JL, Bryant-LeBlanc CE Nelson K, et al. (1987) Risk of transmitting the human immunodeficiency virus, cytomegalovirus, and hepatitis B virus to health care workers exposed to patients with AIDS and AIDS-related conditions. J Infect Dis 1:1–7

Gerberding JL, Littell C, Tarkington A, et al. (1990) Risk of exposure of surgical personnel to patients' blood during surgery at San Francisco General Hospital. N Eng J Med 322:1788–1793

Hamory BH (1983) Underreporting of needlestick injuries in a university hospital. Am J Infect Control 11:174–177

Heilman RS (1991) Doctors and AIDS. Double standard and double jeopardy. RadioGraphics 11:382

Henderson DK (1990a) Zeroing in on the appropriate management of occupational exposures to HIV-1. Infect Control Epidemiol 11:175–177

Henderson DK (1990b) Position paper: the HIV-infected healthcare worker. The Association for Practitioners in Infection Control: The Society of Hospital Epidemiologists of America. Infect Control Hosp Epidemiol 11:647–656

Henderson DK, Fahey BJ, Willy M, et al. (1990) Risk for occupational transmission of human immunodeficiency virus type I (HIV-1) associated with clinical exposures. A prospective evaluation. Ann Intern Med 113:740–746

Hersey JC, Martin LS (1994) Use of infection control guidelines by workers in healthcare facilities to prevent occupational transmission of HBV and HIV: results from a national survey. Infect Control Hosp Epidemiol 15:243–252

Hochreiter MC, Barton LL (1988) Epidermiology of needlestick injury in emergency medical service personnel. J Emerg Med 318:86–90

Ippolito G, Petrosillo N, Puro V, et al. (1993) The risk of occupational HIV infection in health care workers: the Italian multicenter study. Ann Intern Med 153:1451–1458

Kelen GD, Fritz S, Qaqish B, et al. (1988) Unrecognized human immunodeficiency virus infection in emergency department patients. N Engl J Med 318:1645–1650

Kelen GD, DiGiovanna T, Bisson L, et al. (1989) Human immunodeficiency virus infection in emergency department patients. Epidemiology, clinical presentations, and risk to health care workers: the Johns Hopkins experience. JAMA 262:516–522

Lowenfels AB, Wormser G, Jain K (1989) Frequency of puncture injuries in surgeons and estimated risk of HIV infection. Arch Surg 124:1284–1286

Marcus R, CDC Cooperative Needlestick Surveillance Group (1988) Surveillance of health care workers exposed to blood from patients infected with the human immunodeficiency virus. N Engl J Med 319:1118–1123

Mishu B, Schaffner W (1994) HIV transmission from surgeons and dentists to patients: can models predict the risk? Infect Control Hosp Epidemiol 15:114–146

Quebbeman EJ, Telford GL, Hubbard S, et al. (1991) Risk of blood contamination and injury to operating room personnel. Ann Surg 214:614–620

Schulman KA, McDonald RC, Lynn LA, et al. (1994) Screening surgeons for HIV infection: assessment of a potential public health program. Infect Control Hosp Epidemiol 15:146–155

Shelley GA, Howard KJ (1992) A national survey of surgeons' attitudes about patients with human immunodeficiency virus infections and acquired immunodeficiency syndrome. Arch Surg 127:206–212

Stroud LA, Tokars JI, Grieco MH, et al. (1995) Evaluation of infection control measures in preventing the nosocomial transmission of multidrug-resistant *Mycobacterium tuberculosis* in a New York City hospital. Infect Control Hosp Epidemiol 16:141–147

Wall SD, Olcott EW, Gerberding JL (1991) AIDS risk and risk reduction in the radiology department. AJR 157:911–916

Williams DM, Marx V, Korobkin M (1988) AIDS risk and risk reduction in the radiology department. AJR 157:919–921

Wormser GP, Joline C, Sivak SL, Arlin ZA (1988) Human immunodeficiency virus infections: considerations for health care workers. Bull N Y York Acad Med 64:203–215

18 Different Radiologic Patterns in AIDS at a Glance

Jacques W. A. J. Reeders and Phillip C. Goodman

CONTENTS

18.1 Central Nervous System

Organism/ disease	Organ involved	Radiologic abnormality	Extent of disease	Differential diagnosis
Toxo-plasmosis (*Toxoplasma gondii*)	CNS	Encephalitis/leptomeningitis *CT:* Iso/hypodense (82%) lesions with surrounding edema and mass effect; contrast enhancement; well-defined, annular, nodular (rare), subependymal (rare) lesions; calcifications *MR:* Increased signal foci on long TR images with iso/hypointense centers. *Short TR images:* Hypointense/contrast enhancement	• Cerebral hemispheres more frequently affected than cerebellum/ brainstem • Corticomedullary junction • Basal ganglia Other organs involved: • Lymph nodes • GI tract • Respiratory tract	AIDS-related lymphoma

J.W.A.J. Reeders, MD, PhD
Consultant Radiologist, Department of Radiology, St. Elisabeth Hospital Willemstad, Breedestraat 193(O), Curaçao, Netherlands Antilles
P.C. Goodman, MD
Department of Radiology, Duke University Medical Center, P.O. Box 3808, Durham, NC 22710, USA

Organism/ disease	Organ involved	Radiologic abnormality	Extent of disease	Differential diagnosis
AIDS-related lymphoma	CN	*(DDD) CT:* Multiple solid iso- or hypodense masses (less common), hyperdense heterogeneous enhancement (80%); peripheral enhancement due to central necrosis; round, oval, nodular lesions with ringlike enhancement. Linear/nodular subpial and subependymal enhancement *MR:* Hypointense on T1WI; isointense less common; after contrast center remains hypointense; margins enhance in smooth/ringlike appearance. T2WI: variable appearances: increased, isointense or decreased signal intensity to parenchyma. If there is menigeal involvement, this is better visualized on contrast MR than on contrast CT *FDG-PET imaging:* uptake by tumor *Thallium-201 (Tl-201) brain SPECT:* uptake by tumor (not by infection) *MR spectroscopy:* mild to moderate increase in lactate and lipids: markedly evelated choline peak	(Multi)focal lesions: • Basal ganglia • Corpus callosum • Cerebellar vermis • Hemispheric white matter • Periventricular/subependymal Other organs involved: • GI tract • Bone marrow	Toxoplasmosis
Crypto-coccosis *(Cryptococcus neoformans)*	CNS	*CT:* Spherical, well-defined iso/hypodense lesion(s); cryptococcoma, gelatinous pseudocysts *MR:* High signal on long TR images; decreased signal on short TR images; perivascular space dilatation	• Meninges • Basal ganglia • Thalami • Midbrain • Corpus callosum • Cerebral cortex • Posterior fossa Other organs involved: • Respiratory tract • Lymph nodes • Liver/spleen • Bone marrow	Other lesions with CNS mass effect

Organism/ disease	Organ involved	Radiologic abnormality	Extent of disease	Differential diagnosis
Herpes [herpes simplex virus (HSV-1 and HSV-2)]	CNS	*CT:* Necrotizing encephalitis; ventriculitis; necrotizing vasculitis of entire cord/spinal roots; generalized swelling, abnormal density or signal changes in white matter; cortical enhancement (rare) *MR:* Low signal intensity on T1WI, hyperintensity on T2WI. Hemorrhage can be seen (foci of increased signal intensity on T1WI) *SPECT imaging:* Increased perfusion of involved brain areas, even when CT and MR are negative	Diffuse involvement • Frontal/temporal lobes • Brainstem • Cerebellum Other organs involved (mucocutaneous): • Perianal region • Oropharynx • Esophagus	Cytomegalovirus (CMV)
Mycobacteria [*Myco-bacterium tuberculosis, M. avium intracellulare*]	CNS	*CT/MR:* Leptomeningitis; meningeal enhancement of the basal cisterns; granulomata, abscess, calcifications. Infarction and hydrocephalus, usually the communicating type. Parenchymal involvement (less common): ringlike, nodular lesions *Tuberculomas:* *CT:* Ring-enhancing lesions due to central necrosis ("target sign"); central calcifications or punctate enhancement, surrounded by a rim of hypodensity and a rim of enhancement *MR:* Granulomas are isointense on T1WI with a slightly hyperintense rim. Variable signal on T2WI. Usually mass effect and edema surrounding the tuberculoma *MR with contrast:* Intense nodular and/or ringlike enhancement	Solitary/multiple Other organs involved: • Lymph nodes • Liver/spleen • Peritoneum • Bone marrow • GI tract • Respiratory tract • GU tract • Skin (rare) • CVS (rare) • Subarachnoid space • Subdural/epidural space • Corticomedullary junction • Periventricular region • At the side of the perforating end-arteries at the base of the brain	– Toxoplasmosis – AIDS-related lymphoma – Cryptococcosis
		TB abscess *CT:* Hypodense lesion with edema and mass effect; uniform, mostly thin ring enhancement; may occasionally be thick and irregular *MR:* Central pus region and liquefactive necrosis is bright on T2WI; the rim of inflammation is usually iso- to hypointense on T2WI; rim enhancement on TWI after contrast	Mostly solitary	Bacterial
Varicella zoster virus	CNS	Encephalitis, neuritis, myelitis, herpes ophthalmicus CT may be negative while MR may reveal signal abnormalities within brainstem and/or cortical gray matter	Diffuse • Ganglia of cranial nerves (V, VII)	• CMV • Herpes

Organism/ disease	Organ involved	Radiologic abnormality	Extent of disease	Differential diagnosis
Brain atrophy	CNS	*CT/MR:* cortical atrophy; widened sulci	Generalized • Supratentorial (100%) • Infratentorial (70%)	–
Progressive multifocal leuken-cephalopathy Papovavirus (JC virus)	CNS	*CT:* Focal white matter hypodensity without mass effect, usually without enhancement (demyelination); patchy enhancement on occasion *MR:* (More sensitive than CT) T1WI: lesions are hypointense to the parenchyma, sharply circumscribed *Demyelination:* Zones of increased signal on long TR images; decreased signal on short TR images. Lesions against corticomedullary junction, in (deep) gray matter. T2WI: hyperintense signal intensity in periventricular and/or subcortical white matter; lesions: small, but progress to larger areas of involvement. Can be unilateral. No mass effect; rarely enhancement. If enhancement is present: faint and peripheral *MR spectroscopy:* Decreased NAA and Cr, increased CHO	• Asymmetric/multifocal bilateral • Frontal, parietal, occipital region most commonly affected • Corticomedullary junction. • Periventricular subcortical • Posterior fossa (common) • Cervical cord (uncommon) Other organs involved: • Kidneys	• HIV encephalitis • HIV demyelination
Focal white matter hyper-intensities	CNS	*MR:* T1WI/T2WI: zones of perivascular demyelination or dilated perivascular spaces secondary to atrophy: white matter hyperintensity	•Perivascular spaces	–
AIDS-dementia complex	CNS	*CT/MR:* Abnormal in 50%: atrophy/white matter disease *Iodine-123 IMP SPECT:* Multiple focal cortical perfusion abnormalities to be present prior to any evidence of disease on CT/MR *Tc-99m HMPAO:* Regional abnormalities of cerebral blood flow *FDG-PET:* Alternations/decrease in cerebral (subcortical) glucose metabolism	Patchy, diffuse, confluent and homogeneous	–

Organism/ disease	Organ involved	Radiologic abnormality	Extent of disease	Differential diagnosis
Pediatric HIV infections: HIV 1-associated progressive encephalopathy	CNS	*CT/MR:* – Progressive atrophy and ventricular enlargement due to myelin loss or reduced myelin. – White matter hypodensity (infrequent) – Often calcifications in basal ganglia (hypointense on MR), bilaterally or in white matter of frontal lobe – Enhancement within basal ganglia T2WI: hyperintensity in basal ganglia, while CT may be negative *FDG-PET:* Diffuse or focal hypometabolism with subcortical hypermetabolism *MR spectroscopy:* Decreased NAA/Cr ratios in subcortical structures	Patchy, confluent, bilateral	Subacute encephalitis
Pediatric cerebrovascular disease	CNS	HIV-related arteriopathy: *CT/MR:* – Fusiform dilatation of circle of Willis (arteriomegaly) – Ischemia or hemorrhage may be found on contrast CT or as signal voids on T2WI	–	–
Fibrosing sclerosis	CNS	*CT/MR:* Ischemic infarction *MR angiography:* focal areas of vascular stenosis or occlusion	• Basal ganglia • Frontal lobes	–
HIV (subacute) encephalitis	CNS	Nonspecific atrophy with deep white matter changes, without mass effect; microglial nodules undetectable by CT, but rarely seen on MR *CT:* Areas of low attenuation *MR:* – High signal intensity on long TR images – Combined lobal atrophy – Diffuse symmetrical white matter hyperintensity on T2WI	Diffuse, symmetrical • Periventricular • Basal ganglia • Cortex	PML
Acute encephalitis Acute/chronic meningitis	CNS	*Imaging studies* are usually negative; atrophy; white matter lesions less frequently seen on CT; can be seen on serial MR studies.		

Organism/ disease	Organ involved	Radiologic abnormality	Extent of disease	Differential diagnosis
Cytomegalovirus meningoencephalitis	CNS	Calcifications in neonates; microglial nodules predominantly in cortex *CT:* Atrophy: often insensitive! usually normal – White matter hypodensity – Smooth periventricular/subependymal enhancement *MR:* – Ventriculoependymitis; – T2WI: increased signal changes in periventricular white matter *Fat-suppressed MR + Gd-DTPA:* – Thickened and enhancing choroid/retina (CMV retinitis) – less often: subependymal enhancement	Generalized/diffuse Other organs involved: • Respiratory system • Adrenals • GI tract • GU tract • Retina • Biliary tract • Liver/gallbladder • Hematopoietic system	AIDS-related lymphoma
(Acute) syphilitic meningitis	CNS	Meningovascular neurosyphilis *CT:* Often unremarkable • Cerebral atrophy • Small infarcts due to vasculitis *MR:* T2WI: ischemic injuries are bright • Post Gd-DTPA: enhancement in region of subacute infarction • Meningeal enhancement may be present *MR angiography:* Vascular occlusion/narrowing on imaging studies. Gummas appear as mass lesions at the brain surface with nodular/ring enhancement, usually adjacent meningeal enhancement (varogenic edema)	–	–
Nocardiosis (*Nocardia asteroides; Nocardia brasiliensis*)	CNS	Hematogenous spread from pulmonary infection *Chest radiograph:* Cavitary lung infiltrates are common *CT:* Multiple brain abscesses: ring-enhancing lesions, which may be multiple or multiloculated. Meningitis: less common *MR:* Abscess: T1WI: central low signal intensity; T2WI: high signal intensity with a surrounding capsule; extensive edema/mass effect	Multiple/ multiloculated	Other fungal infections: cryptococcosis, histoplasmosis, coccidioidomycosis, blastomycosis

Organism/ disease	Organ involved	Radiologic abnormality	Extent of disease	Differential diagnosis
Bacillary angiomatosis (*Bartonella henselae; Bartonella quintana*)	CNS	*CT/MR:* Intracerebral enhancing lesions, resembling Kaposi's sarcoma	Other organs involved: • Liver, spleen • Coniunctivae • Lymph nodes • Respiratory tract • Skeletal system: Lytic bone lesions in multiple locations	Kaposi's sarcoma
Fungal disease	CNS	• Acute/chronic leptomeningitis/granuloma or abscess • Subacute basilar granulomatous meningitis • Cryptococcomas *CT:* Often unremarkable • Atrophy • Communicating hydrocephalus *MR:* May be negative • Menigeal enhancement on postgadolineum images a) Parenchymal mass lesions (cryptococcomas) b) Dilated Virchow-Robin spaces c) Parenchymal/leptomeningeal nodules d) Mixed pattern *CT:* • Hypodense lesions with solid or ring enhancement • Peripheral small enhancing nodules (granulomas) with punctate calcifications • Small hypodensities without enhancement in basal ganglia • Cysts in basal ganglia ("gelatinous pseudocysts")	• Virchow-Robin spaces in midbrain/basal ganglia • Leptomeninges	• Cryptococcosis • Histoplamosis • Coccidioido- mycosis • Blastomycosis
Mucor- mycosis	CNS	Intracranial abscess and/or infarction	Other organs involved: • Paranasal sinuses	
Aspergillosis	CNS	• Vascular occlusion; hemorrhagic infarction • Focal cerebritis and abscess formation • Hypointense signal on T1WI and T2WI in the paranasal sinuses	Focal	Other fungal infections
Candida albicans	CNS	Meningitis, meningoencephalitis, (micro)abscess, granulomata *CT:* Granulomas: hyperdense nodules with surrounding edema and nodular ring enhancement; iso/hypodense lesions with multiple punctate enhancing nodules on contrast studies *MR:* "Target appearance": central hypointensity on T1WI and surrounding hyperintensity on T2WI		Other fungal infections

DDD, Double-dose delayed; CVS, cardiovascular system; CMV, cytomegalovirus; NAA, *N*-acetylasparate; Cr, creatine; CHO, choline; PML, progressive multifocal leukoencephalopathy

Organism/ disease	Organ involved	Radiologic abnormality	Extent of disease	Differential diagnosis

18.2 Spine and Spinal Cord

Organism/ disease	Organ involved	Radiologic abnormality	Extent of disease	Differential diagnosis
Myelitis	Spine/ spinal cord	*MR:* Early stage: Increase in cord diameter T2WI: diffuse, ill-defined hyperintensity T1WI: poorly defined enhancement on postcontrast T1WI *Later stage* Intramedullary abscess formation: decreased signal intensity on T2WI with well-defined ring enhancement after contrast	• Diffuse • In association with HIV leukoencephalopathy (5%–8%)	Bacterial infections: • *Staphylococcus aureus* • *Streptococcus pneumoniae* • Multiple sclerosis • Lyme's disease • Sarcoidosis of the spine

Myco-bacterium tuberculosis	Spine/ spinal cord	Intramedullary tuberculoma: varied appearance:
		• Noncaseating granulomas:
		  T1WI: hypointense
		  T2WI: hyperintense, homogeneous enhancement
		• Caseating granulomas with solid center:
		  T1WI: hypointense to isointense
		  T2WI: iso- to hypointense with peripheral enhancement after contrast
		• Caseating granulomas with liquid center:
		  T1WI: hypointense
		  T2WI: hyperintense and peripheral enhancement
			10% may have brain lesions	–

Viral infections	Spine/ spinal cord	Vacuolar myelopathy *MR:* T2WI: abnormal intra medullary hyperintensity in the posterior and lateral columns of the cord, surrounding gray matter without cord enlargement or contrast enhancement	Associated with brain lesions Mid/lower thoracic spine	–
Cytomegalo-virus Herpes simplex virus (HSV-1/ HSV-2)	Spine/ spinal cord	Myeloradiculitis Polyradiculomyelitis *CT/MR:* Often unremarkable; thickening of conus and cauda equina. Postcontrast: strong enhancement of the pia lining the cord, conus medullaris, nerve roots and leptomeningis of the cord. In case of necrotizing myelitis: *MR:* T2WI: hyperintense intramedullary lesions with contrast enhancement *Nonenhanced T1WI, myelography and CT myelography are usually normal*	–	–

Organism/ disease	Organ involved	Radiologic abnormality	Extent of disease	Differential diagnosis
Toxoplasmosis (*Toxoplasma gondii*)	Spine/ spinal cord	*MR:* (see CNS) Focal enlargement of the spinal cord with increased T2 signal and homogeneous contrast enhancement	Coexists with brain lesions	AIDS-related lymphoma
Arachnoiditis (leptomeningitis) • Neoplastic • Inflammatory: tuberculosis	Spine/ spinal cord	*MR:* T1WI: indistinct or absent cord outline due to increase in signal intensity of surrounding CSF. T2WI (heavily T2W FSE with fat suppression): CSF loculations and adhesions: • In the cervical and thoracic regions with obliteration of the arachnoidal space • In lumbar region: nerve root fusion seen as irregularly thickened clumped nerve roots. Peripheral adherence of nerve roots to the thecal sac ("featureless or empty sac"). Contrast enhancement in lumbar arachnoiditis: 3 patterns: • Smooth linear layer of enhancement outlining the surface of the cord and nerve roots • Nodular pattern with discrete foci of enhancement, seen along the surface of the cord and nerve roots • Diffuse thick intradural enhancement which completely fills the subarachnoid space	–	• AIDS-related lymphoma • Tethered cord
Discitis/ osteomyelitis	Spine/ spinal cord	Disc space narrowing with osteolytic destruction of the adjacent vertebral endplates. *MR:* • T2WI: hyperintense discs adjacent vertebral marrow: T1WI: hypointense and T2WI hyperintense *Postcontrast MR:* Peripheral diffuse enhancement of the disc space and enhancement of the adjacent vertebral end plates. Paraspinal abscess	–	• *Staphylococcus aureus* • *Mycobacterium* (MAI, MTb)
AIDS-related lymphoma	Spine/ spinal cord	*MR:* • T2WI: enlarged cord with intramedullary iso- to hyperintensity • T1WI: hypointensity; patchy enhancement after contrast administration	• Epidural • Leptomeningeal • Intramedullary Other organs involved: • Skeletal system	–

MAI, Mycobacterium intracellulare; MTb, Mycobacterium Tuberculosis

Organism/ disease	Organ involved	Radiologic abnormality	Extent of disease	Differential diagnosis

18.3 Cardiovascular System

Organism/ disease	Organ involved	Radiologic abnormality	Extent of disease	Differential diagnosis
Pericardial effusion	CVS	Occurs in 10%–15% of HIV infection *Echocardiography:* Diastolic compression of the R atrium; echo-free/echo-poor space between parietal pericardium and epicardium; pericardial tamponade	Pericardium/ epicardium	Mycobacterium, tuberculosis, MAI, CMV, Coxsackie virus, herpes simplex, *Cryptococcus, neoformans, Salmonella typhymurium, Nocardia asteroides, Listeria monocytogenes, Toxoplasma gondii,* Kaposi's sarcoma, AIDS-related lymphoma
Myocarditis, cardio-myopathy/ ventricular dysfunction	CVS	Myocarditis (50%) and dilated myocardiopathy (20%) Endocarditis Pericarditis/pericardial effusion Left ventricular enlargement *Chest radiograph:* Dilated cardiomyopathy with enlarged cardiac silhouette with/without pulmonary venous congestion/edema; cardiac decompensation *Echocardiography:* Four chamber enlargement with right/left ventricle hypokinesia. Abnormal septum position/motion. Marked pulmonary hypertension: both diastolic and systolic flattening of ventricular septum in response to markedly abnormal transeptal pressure gradient	Myocardium Endocardium Pericardium	*Mycobacterium tuberculosis,* MAI, CMV, Coxsackie virus, Epstein-Barr virus, herpex simplex, *Toxoplasma gondii, Pneumocystis carinii, Candida albicans, Cryptococcus neoformans, Aspergillus fumigatus, Staphylococcus aureus, Nocardia asteroides, Streptococcus pneumoniae,* Kaposi's sarcoma, AIDS-related lymphoma
HIV-associated pulmonary hyper-tension	CVS	*Chest radiograph:* central pulmonary arteries are enlarged; marked decreased in caliber peripherally: right ventricular enlargement	–	PCP

CVS, Cardiovascular system; CMV, cytomegalovirus; MAI, Mycobacterium aviumintracellulare

Organism/ disease	Organ involved	Radiologic abnormality	Extent of disease	Differential diagnosis

18.4 Respiratory System

Organism/ disease	Organ involved	Radiologic abnormality	Extent of disease	Differential diagnosis
Pneumocystis carinii pneumonia	Chest	Normal chest radiograph: 10% *Chest radiograph:* *Early disease:* Bilateral symmetric perihilar/or basal fine reticulonodular pattern without pleural effusion *Advanced disease:* Diffuse homogeneous alveolar opacities *Late disease:* Asymmetrically scattered alveolar consolidation (mosaic pattern); reticular pattern; thickening of interlobular/interlobar interstitial tissue *Disseminated disease:* In patients with prophylactic aerosolized penta-midine therapy; enlarged lymph nodes; liver/spleen punctate calcifications or areas of low attenuation Less common: • Miliary/coarse interstitial pattern • Thin-walled air containing cystic lesions (multiple, confluent) • Pneumatoceles: 10%–34% unilateral or less frequently bilateral • Pneumothorax (1%–6%) Atypical pattern: Air space disease; cavitary nodules, hilar/mediastinal lymphadenopathy; pleural effusions (0%–2%) *High-resolution CT:* Symmetric ground-glass appearance with a geographic distribution; pneumatoceles; interstitial pattern; sparing of lung periphery Complications: unilateral or less frequently bilateral pneumothorax	Diffuse; upper or lower zone predominance, sometimes focal Bilateral, often symmetric, multilobar Other organs involved: • Liver/spleen • Lymph nodes	Other opportunistic infections: tuberculosis, fungal infections, toxoplasmosis, HSV, Kaposi's sarcoma, CMV
Staphylococcus aureus	Chest	*Chest radiograph/CT:* Bilateral focal parenchymal opacities (wedge-shaped) with a peripheral predominance. Development of cavitations; Pleural effusions/cardiomegaly uncommon	Bilateral/focal	Other bacterial infections
Toxo-plasmosis (*Toxoplasma gondii*)	Chest	*Chest radiograph/CT:* Predominantly coarse, nodular opacities and reticulonodular opacities; confluent consolidations; pleural effusions, occasionally lymphadenopathy (not typical)	Bilateral Other organs involved: • CNS • GI tract (rare)	• PCP • Tuberculosis • Fungal infections

Organism/ disease	Organ involved	Radiologic abnormality	Extent of disease	Differential diagnosis
Cytomegalo-virus	Chest	*Chest radiograph:* pneumonia: reticular or reticulonodular opacities; areas of consolidation; tiny nodules or symmetrically scattered alveolar opacities with preference for central lower regions; peribronchial thickening *CT:* Bronchiectasis; "tree in bud" pattern of branching; small centrilobular nodules; ground glass attenuation; reticular opacities, nodules, masses; pneumothorax; pneumomediastinum	Bilateral Other organs involved: • Adrenals • GI tract(oropharynx) • CNS • Retina • Biliary tract • Liver/gallbladder	• PCP
Herpes simplex virus (HSV-1, HSV-2)	Chest	*Chest radiograph/CT:* Bilateral interstitial pattern; scattered focal alveolar abnormalities;pleural effusion: rare; lymphadenopathy: rare	–	• PCP • CMV
Varicella zoster virus	Chest	*Chest radiograph/CT:* Bilateral, scattered, round, nodular alveolar opacities with tendency to coalesce; pleural effusions: rare; lymphadenopathy: rare	–	• PCP • CMV
Pyogenic infections	Chest	*Chest radiograph/CT:* Diffuse heterogeneous or lobar consolidation; pleural effusions; empyema; peripheral nodules/nodular infiltrates with a basalar predomi-nance; cavitation does occur (*Staphylococcus aureus, Rhodococcus equi,* and anaerobes); multiple lung abscesses may occur; intrathoracic lymphadenopathy: uncommon; may be present in *Rhodococcus* infection	Diffuse Unilateral/bilateral	• *Haemophilus influenzae* • *Streptococcus pneumoniae* • *Nocardia asteroides* • *Legionella pneumomae* • *Corynebacterium equi (Rhodo-coccus)*
Strongyloides stercoralis	Chest	*Chest radiograph:* May be normal miliary nodules or reticular opacities are seen. Scattered alveolar opacities and lobar consolidations may be present in patient with the hyperinfection syndrome; alveolar opacities and ARDS may develop	• bilateral	PCP
Bacillary angimatosis (*Bartonella henselae; Bartonella quintana*)	Chest	Pulmonary bacillary angiomatosis *Bronchoscopy:* Violaceous endobronchial lesions, mimicking Kaposi's sarcoma *Chest radiograph:* Parenchymal nodules most common; pleural effusions; lymphadenopathy; chest wall masses *CT:* Lymphadenopathy and chest wall masses which enhance greatly on contrast CT	Other organs involved: • Skin • Lymph nodes • Liver/spleen • Ophthalmus, conjuntivae (rare) • Skeletal system	Kaposi's sarcoma

Organism/ disease	Organ involved	Radiologic abnormality	Extent of disease	Differential diagnosis
Pasteurella multocida	Chest	*Chest radiograph:* Focal areas of consolidation which may be complicated by cavitation and pleural effusion	Other organs involved: • Soft tissue	Other opportunistic infections
Bordetella	Chest	*Chest radiograph:* Interstitial infiltrates, focal areas of consolidations, occasionally cavitation	bilateral	Other opportunistic infections
Tuberculosis (*M. tuberculosis*)	Chest	Radiographic appearance of tuberculosis varies with the CD4 cell count Normal chest radiograph: 5% *Primary form (60%)* *Early disease:* >200 cells/mm³: typical pattern of post primary (reactivation) tuberculosis; cavitary infiltrates and consolidation usually in the apical and posterior segments of the upper lobes and /or superior segments lower lobes. Cavitation occurs. Lymphadenopathy: infrequent *Advanced disease:* <200 cells/mm³: Diffuse coarse, nodular, reticulonodular pattern. Cavitation occurs infrequently. Lymphadenopathy is often present, uni- or bilateral. *Third form (15%):* Miliary pattern: diffuse fine nodular pattern; focal alveolar opacities in mid/lower lung; hilar and/or mediastinal lymphadenopathy *CT:* Tuberculous lymphadenopathy: enlarged nodes with central low attenuation (necrosis) and peripheral ring enhancement on contrast CT; <50 cells/mm³: disseminated tuberculosis with miliary infiltrates; pleural effusions; increasing lymphadenopathy	Localized or diffuse; Unilateral or bilateral Other organs involved: • GI tract (esophagus) • Liver/spleen • Lymph nodes • GU tract • Bones • Adrenals	• PCP • Atypical mycobacterial infections • *M. gordonae* • *M. fortuitum* • *M. xenopi* • *M. kansasii* • Fungal infections • AIDS-related lymphoma
Mycobacterium avium complex	Chest	Normal chest radiograph: 20% *Chest radiograph/CT:* • Diffuse, bilateral, reticulonodular opacities or nodules, with or without cavities • Preference for the superior lobes; focal or diffuse alveolar disease: parenchymal consolidation miliary pattern: less common; hilar and/or mediastinal lymphadenopathy; pleural effusions	Disseminated, focal or bilateral Other organs involved: • Lymph nodes • Liver/spleen • Peritoneum • Bone marrow • GI tract • GU tract • CNS (rare) • Skin (rare) • CVS (rare)	Tuberculosis

Organism/ disease	Organ involved	Radiologic abnormality	Extent of disease	Differential diagnosis
Penicillium marneffei	Chest	*Chest radiograph/CT:* Scattered reticulonodular or alveolar opacities and/or intrathoracic lymphadenopathy (80%); single nodule/mass with/without cavitation or focal segmental consolidation (less frequent); pleural effusion; miliary pattern	Solitary/multiple lesions, bilateral, diffuse Other organs involved: • CNS • Lymph nodes • Liver/spleen • Bone marrow	• Toxoplasmosis • PCP • Tuberculosis
Nocardiosis (*Nocardia asteroides; Nocardia brasiliensis*)	Chest	*Chest radiograph/CT:* • Large areas of segmental consolidations, involving several lobes • Diffuse interstitial pattern or solitary defined mass often, with cavitation; pleural or pericardial effusion may occur	Unilateral/focal Other organs involved: • CNS • Skin and soft tissue infections	• Other opportunistic infections • Tuberculosis
Histo-plasmosis (*Histoplasma capsulatum*)	Chest	*Chest radiograph/CT:* Normal in 50% • Diffuse heterogeneous opacities • Diffuse small lung parenchymal nodules • Linear irregular and airspace opacities less common • Miliary pattern; focal infiltrates • Hilar/mediastinal lymphadenopathy (uncommon) • Pleural effusions (uncommon)	Disseminated More diffuse than focal Other organs involved: • Bone marrow	Other opportunistic infections
Coccidio-idomycosis (*Coccidioides immitis*)	Chest	*Chest radiograph/CT:* Normal in 70% • Reticulonodular lung parenchymal opacities • Focal alveolar opacities • Discrete nodules • Hilar lymphadenopathy • Pulmonary thin-walled cavity and pleural effusion occur	Diffuse Other organs involved: • Meninges • Skin	Other opportunistic infections
Aspergillosis (*Aspergillus fumigatus*)	Chest	*Chest radiograph/CT:* • Ill-defined pleural based nodules or masses • Areas of consolidation • Multiple thick-walled cavities ("air crescent sign") in upper lobe less common: • Pleural effusions (uncommon) • Lymphadenopathy (uncommon)	Diffuse systemic dissemination (35%)	• Other opportunistic infections • Tuberculosis
Blasto-mycosis	Chest	*Chest radiograph/CT:* • Focal airspace opacities or masses • Diffuse nodular opacities • Cavitation • Lymphadenopathy and pleural effusions: less common	Disseminated disease	–

Organism/ disease	Organ involved	Radiologic abnormality	Extent of disease	Differential diagnosis
Kaposi's sarcoma	Chest	*Chest radiograph:* *Early disease:* • Diffuse, bilateral, poorly defined, reticulonodular opacities (1–2 cm) in a perihilar distribution • Coarsening bronchovascular bundles and peribronchial cuffing • Bilateral scattered mostly round opacities, whose delineation varies in definition • Parenchymal abnormalities coarser in nature than those in PCP *Advanced disease:* • Lobar consolidation; Kerley B lines • Pleural effusions, mostly bilateral, often in large amounts (<40%) • Intrathoracic lymphadenopathy (30%) *CT:* • Ill-defined nodules; • areas of consolidation along a predominantly bronchovascular distribution; peribronchovascular thickening, radiating from the perihilar region • Subpleural nodules • Ground-glass attenuation adjacent to nodules/ masses (hemorrhage) • Interlobular septal thickening (38%)	Bilateral Unilateral (<10%) Other organs involved: • Mucocutaneous • Sternum • Ribs • Thoracic spine • GI tract • Liver/spleen • Lymph nodes Pulmonary Kaposi's sarcoma is preceded in 95% by mucous membrane/skin lesions	• PCP • CMV • NHL • Typical/ atypical mycobacterial infections • Fungal infections
AIDS-related lymphoma (B cell or T cell lymphoma)	Chest	Intrathoracic involvement: 10%–50% *Chest radiograph/CT:* • Lung parenchymal consolidation • Unilateral or bilateral solitary or multiple masses and nodules, which may rapidly progress • Pleural effusion/masses (60%); air bronchogram; chest wall invasion • Axillary/hilar/mediastinal lymphadenopathy (50%) • Less frequent: interstitial infiltrates; alveolar opacities; pericardial effusion/masses; myocardial involvement	Unilateral or bilateral; solitary or multiple lesions Other organs involved: • CNS • GI tract • Liver, spleen • Pancreas • Retroperitoneum	• Typical/ atypical mycobacterial infections • PCP • Fungal infections
Lymphocytic interstitial pneumonia	Chest	Normal chest radiograph: 50% *Chest radiograph:* Nonspecific findings: • Fine to coarse reticular/ reticulonodular interstitial opacities, • Scattered alveolar/ground-glass opacities • Pleural effusion: unusual • No intrathoracic lymphadenopathy *CT:* Small nodules are the predominant findings; peribronchovascular in distribution; areas of ground-glass opacities	Diffuse, bilateral Most frequent in children	• Other opportunistic infections • PCP

Organism/ disease	Organ involved	Radiologic abnormality	Extent of disease	Differential diagnosis
Lung cancer	Chest	*Chest radiograph:* Peripheral or central nodule or mass; pleural effusion *CT:* Lung mass, extending to the pleura	–	–

HSV, Herpes simplex virus; CMV, cytomegalovirus; PCP, *Pneumocystis carinii pneumonia;* ARDS, adult respiratory distress syndrome; CVS, cardiovascular system; NHL, non-Hodgkin's lymphoma

18.5 Luminal Gastrointestinal Tract

Organism/ disease	Organ involved	Radiologic abnormality	Extent of disease	Differential diagnosis
Candida (Candida albicans)	Oropharynx/ esophagus	*Endoscopy/barium studies:* Oral thrush *Mild disease:* • Edematous folds • Minimal mucosal plaques, covering a friable erythematous mucosa • Coarse filling defects, oriented along the long axis of the esophagus • Ulcerations *Moderate disease:* • Diffuse mucosal plaques; fine longitudinal ulcerations *Severe/advanced disease:* • Fold thickening • Abnormal motility • Diffuse deep ulcerations (longitudinal); "cobblestone" appearance (submucosal edema) • Extensive diffuse or focally clustered plaques ("shaggy esophagus"); barium trapping within plaques and pseudomembranes in conjunction with deep ulceration and mucosal sloughing *Endstage of disease:* Polypoid lesions; strictures; mucosal "bridging"	Focal or confluent Other organs involved: • Skin • Respiratory tract • CNS	Herpes simplex virus
Herpes simplex virus (HSV-1, HSV-2)	Oropharnx/ esophagus	*Endoscopy/barium studies:* *Mild disease:* • Multiple, scattered, diamond/stellate-shaped shallow ulcers, separated by normal mucosa; lucent halo of edema *Advanced disease:* • Diffuse nodularity/ulcerations with "cobblestoning"; inflammatory exudates • Irregular esophageal contour similar to CMV	Focal or diffuse Other organs involved: • Mucocutaneous • Perianal region	• *Candida* • CMV

Organism/ disease	Organ involved	Radiologic abnormality	Extent of disease	Differential diagnosis
Cytomegalo-virus	Esophagus/ stomach	CMV gastritis *Endoscopy/esophagogram:* Diffuse granular mucosa, due to clustered superficial erosions and/or aphthous ulcers; irregular thickening of mucosal folds; shallow, poorly defined, diamond-shaped ulcers, irregular thickening of mucosal folds; nodular wall thickening; tiny ulcers; granularity of mucosa; narrowing of lumen with limited distensibility with attenuation	Distal esophagus with extension into esophagogastricjunction Predilection: antrum Other organs involved: • Adrenals • Respiratory tract • CNS • Retina • Biliary tract • Liver/gallbladder Focal or diffuse: common	• Idiopathic • HIV • Herpes • *Candida* • *Cryptosporidium*
	Small intestine	*Barium studies* Mild dilatation: edematous submucosal nodules (0.25–0.75cm); separation of loops; shallow or deep, round or serpiginous ulceration of various size/depth *Late stage:* narrowing of lumen; fistula, pneumatosis intestinalis	Segmental or diffuse Predilection: terminal ileum	*Cryptosporidium*
	Colon/ano-rectum	*Mild disease:* *Barium studies:* Diffuse mucosal granularity; cecal spasm; irregular thickening of mucosal folds (edema); superficial or deep punctate or linear ulcerations; aphthous ulcers *CT:* Low-density edematous bowel wall; marked mucosal/serosal enhancement *Severe/advanced disease:* *Barium studies:* Large ulcers; skip lesions; areas of mass effect (granulation tissue/submucosal hemorrhage); nodular filling defects (pseudomembranes) *CT:* Increased density in bowel wall (hemorrhage); thickening of bowel wall *Late-stage disease:* Barium studies *CT:* Narrowing of the lumen	Segmental or diffuse Common predilection: • Ascending colon/ cecum/terminal ileum • Sometimes entire colon	

Organism/ disease	Organ involved	Radiologic abnormality	Extent of disease	Differential diagnosis
Idiopathic HIV	Esophagus/ anorectum	*Barium studies:* Giant (2 cm) well-defined flat/shallow ulceration, surrounded by thin rim of edema with surrounding normal mucosa	Usually solitary; can be multiple Predilection: lower esophagus	• CMV • HSV • Mycobacterial infection
	Small intestine	*Barium studies/CT:* "Idiopathic AIDS enteropathy"; nonspecific mild small bowel wall thickening		
Crypto-sporidiosis *(Cryptosporidium)*	Small intestine	*Barium studies:* Mild small bowel dilatation; hypersecretion; "sprue-like appearance" *CT:* Small bowel wall thickening/ dilatation small bowel/increased intraluminal fluids; no associated mesenteric lymphadenopathy	Diffuse Predilection: proximal bowel Other organs involved: • Duodenum • Colon • Biliary tract • Respiratory tract	Other opportunistic infections: • Giardiasis • Isospora belli
Mycobacterium avium-intracellulare complex	Esophagus	*Esophagogram:* Focal extrinsic mass impression; longitudinal deep ulcerations; sinus tract to the mediastinum/ esophago-trachial fistulae; traction diverticula; strictures in chronic disease; fistula formation	Focal Predilection: middle third of the esophagus, duodenum, small bowel Other organs involved: • Lymph nodes • Liver/spleen • Peritoneum • Bone marrow • Respiratory tract • GU tract • CNS (rare) • Skin (rare) • CVS (rare)	• Idiopathic • HIV • CMV • M. tuberculosis
	Stomach/ duodenal bulb	*Barium studies:* Ulceration; hypertrophic fibrotic encasement; bulky gastric mass extending into mesentery. Thickening of mucosal folds; aphthous ulcers, outlet obstruction	Segmental Hepatosplenomegaly common	• Crohn's disease
	Small intestine	*Barium studies/CT:* Mild dilatation with irregular fold thickening; separation/displacement of bowel loops due to low attenuation necrotic lymphadenopathy; spasm, irregularity; fine nodularity; mild hypertension with segmental/ flocculation of barium; appendiceal mass?; "pseudo-Whipple's" disease *CT:* Large mesenteric and retroperitoneal low-attenuation necrotic lymphadenopathy; marked hepatosplenomegaly	Segmental Predilection • Ileocecal area • Jejunoileum Microabscesses in liver/ spleen are an uncommon finding	Other opportunistic infections: • PCP • Giardiasis • Isospora belli • CMV

Organism/ disease	Organ involved	Radiologic abnormality	Extent of disease	Differential diagnosis
Kaposi's sarcoma	Colon	*Barium studies:* Circumferential thickening of cecal wall and terminal ileum; fistula formation *CT:* Regional low-attenuation necrotic lymphadenopathy	Segmental Predilection: ileocecal region Diffuse Other organs involved • Respiratory tract • Lymph nodes • Liver/spleen • CVS • GU tract • Skin	Opportunistic infections • Crohn's disease • AIDS-related lymphoma • MAC • Multiple polyps • Hematogenous metastasis
	Oropharynx/ esophagus/ stomach/ duodenum/ small bowel/ colon/ anorectum	*Barium studies:* *Early disease:* Flat lesions, not demonstrated on barium studies; granularity of mucosa *Advanced disease:* Irregular thickening of mucosal folds; discrete sharp mucosal nodules (6 mm–3 cm) with or without central umbilication (bull's eye/target appearance); normal intervening mucosa; nodular wall thickening or small bowel; sometimes large, bulky polypoid, segmental masses; narrowing of lumen *CT:* High-attenuation lymphadenopathy complications: intestinal perforation		
AIDS-related lymphoma	Stomach/ small intestine/colon/ anorectum	*Barium studies:* Diffuse wall thickening mesenteric polypoid lesions simulating adenocarcinoma; loss of mucosal pattern; irregular fold thickening; discrete Penetrating ulcers; Narrowing of lumen *CT:* Extraluminal extent of enteric lymphomas; abundant retroperitoneal or mesenteric lymphadenopathy. Acute complications: Perforation, obstruction, intussuseption	Other organs involved: • CNS • Bone marrow • Abdominal viscera: kidney (hydronephrosis due to obstructing lymphnodes) • Anorectum/colon • Nonspecific hepatosplenomegaly may be present	• Kaposi's sarcoma • Mycobacterium tuberculosis

HSV, Herpes simplex virus; CMV, cytomegalovirus; PCP, Pneumocystis carinii pneumonia; CVS, cardiovascular system; MAC, Mycobacterium avium-intracellulare complex

Organism/ disease	Organ involved	Radiologic abnormality	Extent of disease	Differential diagnosis

18.6 Liver/Spleen/Biliary tract

Pneumocystis (Pneumocystis carinii)	Liver/spleen	*US:* Numerous nodules (liver/spleen/kidneys) Usually hypoechoic >2 cm, multiple tiny echogenic foci without shadowing *CT:* Calcifications (liver/spleen), usually hypodensity nodules, <2 cm in both liver and spleen	Focal Other organs involved: • CNS • Bone marrow • Respiratory tract • GU tract • Adrenal glands • Retina • Thyroid • Parathyroid glands • Gallbladder • Pancreas	• *Candida albicans* • *Aspergillus fumigatus* • MAC • Cytomegalo virus • *Mycobacterium tuberculosis* • Bacillary angiomatosis • Fungal infections • Kaposi's sarcoma • AIDS-related lymphoma • Smooth muscle tumor
Bacillary angiomatosis (peliosis) (*Bartonella henselae)*	Liver/spleen	*US:* Nonspecific! Heterogeneous liver with hyper- and hypoechoic regions *CT:* Hypodense with isodense lesions after attenuation	Rare • Associated with chronic diseases (malignancies, tuberculosis etc.) Other organs involved: • Respiratory tract • Mediastinum • CNS (rare) • Ophtalmic (rare) • Skeletal system	• Mycobacterium tuberculosis • MAC • PCP • Fungal infections • Kaposi's sarcoma • AIDS-related lymphoma • Smooth muscle tumor
Fungal infections	Liver/spleen	*US/CT:* Multiple small hypoechoic/hypodense nodules <2 cm (liver/spleen); hepatosplenomegaly	Diffuse Other organs involved: • Respiratory tract • Bone marrow • GI tract • CNS • Lymph nodes • Liver/spleen	• *Mycobacterium tuberculosis* • MAC • Bacillary angiomatosis • PCP • Kaposi's sarcoma • AIDS-related lymphoma • *Histoplasma capsulatum* • *Coccidioides immitis* • *Cryptococcus neoformans* • *Candida albicans*

Organism/ disease	Organ involved	Radiologic abnormality	Extent of disease	Differential diagnosis
Cytomegalovirus	Liver/spleen	*US/CT:* Multiple focal small echogenic/hypoechoic/low-attenuation lesions	Focal or diffuse Other organs involved: • Luminal GI tract • Adrenals • Respiratory tract • CNS • Retina • Pancreas	Other opportunistic infections
	Biliary tract	*ERCP:* AIDS-related cholangiopathy; sclerosing cholangitis; irregular dilatation of the CBD; decreased arborization of intrahepatic ducts; irregular/ "brush border" of biliary mucosa; multiple vesicular filling defects; thickened duct wall of intra/ extrahepatic bile ducts; papillary stenosis; acalculous cholecystitis; extrahepatic bile duct strictures (1–2 cm)	Segmental/diffuse	• *Microsporidium* • *Cryptosporidium* • MAC • *Isospora belli* • *Primary sclerosing cholangitis*
Mycobacterium avium-intracellulare complex	Liver/spleen	*US:* Multiple tiny echogenic foci in liver/spleen and kidneys *CT:* Hypoechoic/hypodense nodules <2 cm; hepatosplenomegaly; porta hepatis and pancreatic lymphadenopathy	Diffuse/focal Other organs involved • Lymph nodes • Peritoneum • Bone marrow • GI tract • Respiratory tract • GU tract (kidneys) • CNS (rare) • Skin (rare) • CVS (rare)	• *Mycobacterium tuberculosis* • Bacillary angiomatosis • *P. carinii* (extrapulmonary) • Fungal infections • Kaposi's sarcoma • AIDS-related lymphoma
Mycobacterium tuberculosis	Liver/spleen	*US/CT:* Hypoechoic/hypodense nodules <2 cm; hepatosplenomegaly; often enlarged retroperitoneal and mesenteric lymph nodes with central necrosis (low-density nodes); concomitant segmental ileocecal thickening	Diffuse/multifocal Other organs involved: • Respiratory tract • Lymph nodes • GU tract • Adrenals • Pancreas • Bone marrow • GI tract • CNS • Soft tissue	• MAC • Bacillary angiomatosis • *P. carinii* • Fungal infections • AIDS-related lymphoma
Kaposi's sarcoma	Liver/spleen Bile duct Gallbladder	*US:* Small (5–12 mm) hyperechoic periportal nodules in liver/spleen Increased periportal echogenicity *CT:* Low-attenuation periportal lesions which enhance on delayed postcontrast scans ("prominent portal triads"); hypodense nodules <2 cm (liver/spleen); hepatosplenomegaly	Other organs involved: • Skin • Chest • GI tract • Lymph nodes • Pancreas • CVS • GU tract (kidneys)	• *Mycobacterium tuberculosis* • MAC • Bacillary angiomatosis • *P. carinii* • Fungal infections • AIDS-related lymphoma • Metastatic disease • Hemangiomas

Organism/ disease	Organ involved	Radiologic abnormality	Extent of disease	Differential diagnosis

AIDS-related lymphoma	Liver/ spleen/ bile duct/ gallbladder	Three patterns:
		1. Large infiltrating masses:
		  US: hypoechoic, homogeneous
		  CT: hypodense with homogeneous attenuation
		2. Multiple focal nodules:
		  US: hypoechoic
		  CT: low density; variable size, 1–5 cm or larger
		3. Diffuse infiltrating "peritoneal lympho-matosis":
		  US: hypoechoic
		  CT: hypodense; mimics fluid, also with ascites
		
		In all 3 patterns:
		Extensive retroperitoneal and/or mesenteric lymphadenopathy
		
		CT: soft tissue density with low central attenuation due to central necrosis
			Other organs involved:
			• Respiratory tract
			• CNS
			• Retroperitoneum (pancreas)
			• CVS
			• Luminal GI tract
				• *Mycobacterium tuberculosis*
				• MAC
				• Bacillary angiomatosis
				• *P. carinii*
				• Fungal infections
				• Kaposi's sarcoma
				• Smooth muscle tumor

PCP, Pneumocystis carinii pneumonia; CVS, cardiovascular system; MAC, Mycobacterium avium-intracellulare complex

18.7 Retroperitoneum

Myco-bacterium tuberculosis	Pancreas/ adrenals	*CT:* Nonspecific mass lesions: low-attenuation nodules; diffuse enlargement; retroperitoneal lymphadenopathy with central or diffuse low attenuation; peripancreatic/small bowel mesenteric, retroperitoneal/pelvic sidewalls; Fulminant necrotizing pancreatitis in patient receiving therapy with ddI	• Pancreatic lymph nodes • Liver/spleen	Other myco-bacterial infections
Myco-bacterium avium-intra-cellulare complex	Kidneys	*CT:* Hepatosplenomegaly; diffuse jejunal wall thickening; soft tissue density homogeneous lymph nodes; mesangial proliferative glomeronephritis	Other organs involved: • Lymph nodes • Bone marrow • GI tract • Respiratory tract • Retroperitoneum • CNS • Skin • CVS	• *P. carinii* (extra-pulmonary) • *Mycobacterium tuberculosis* • Fungal infections • Kaposi's sarcoma • AIDS-related lymphoma
AIDS-related lymphoma	Pancreas/ adrenals	*US:* Hypoechoic masses; lymphadenopathy *CT:* Lymphomatous low-attenuation masses; nodal disease; distortion of pancreatic duct; obstruction of CBD; hydronephrosis due to retroperitoneal obstructing lymphadenopathy; bulky conglomerate masses >5 cm; density is close to skeletal muscle without enhancement *Ga-67 citrate* is useful in identifying nodes as ARL lymph nodes	Disseminated disease	Kaposi's sarcoma

Organism/ disease	Organ involved	Radiologic abnormality	Extent of disease	Differential diagnosis
Kaposi's sarcoma	Pancreas/ kidneys	*CT:* Focal pancreatic/kidney mass; retroperitoneal lymphadenopathy (2–3 cm); "streaky" soft tissue attenuation; infiltrations in the inguinal fat; KS nodes have a distinctive appearance on dynamic CT; brightly enhanced nodes on contrast CT	Associated with lymphadenopathy/skin manifestations	AIDS-related lymphoma
Aspergillus fumigatus	Kidneys	*CT:* abscesses	Uni/bilateral	–
Extra-pulmonary *P. carinii*	Kidneys	Renal cortical calcification: *US:* diffuse echogenic foci without shadowing; hepatosplenic involvement *CT:* diffuse punctate calcifications involving a variety of retroperitoneal structures; low-attenuation lesions AIDS nephropathy: focal segmental glomerulosclerosis *US:* increased cortical echogenicity with variable renal enlargement *CT:* hyperdense medulla; enlarged kidneys	Diffuse Other organs involved: • Adrenals • Liver/spleen • Lymph nodes	–
Cytomegalovirus	Kidneys/ adrenals	Focal and segmental glomerulosclerosis; adrenal stromal tumors (leiomyoma, leiomyosarcoma)	–	–
Blastomycosis/histoplasmosis	Adrenals/ kidneys	Acute postinfection glomerulonephritis	–	–
Bacillary angiomatosis (*Bartonella henselae*)	Retroperitoneum	*US:* high flow on Doppler studies *CT:* retroperitoneal lymphadenopathy	Other organs involved: • Skin • Mediastinum • Abdomen • Skeletal system • Lymph nodes	Kaposi's sarcoma
Candida albicans	Kidneys	Focal renal lesions (membranoproliferative glomerulonephritis)	Liver/spleen	–

CBD, Common bile duct; ARL, AIDS-related lymphoma; CVS, cardiovascular system; KS, Kaposi's sarcoma

Organism/ disease	Organ involved	Radiologic abnormality	Extent of disease	Differential diagnosis

18.8 Musculoskeletal System

Organism/ disease	Organ involved	Radiologic abnormality	Extent of disease	Differential diagnosis
Cellulitis	Skin	*Conventional radiology:* Cannot distinguish soft tissue/fascial layers; early osseous changes cannot be detected *CT:* Increase in density of subcutaneous adipose tissue (90–120 HU) *MR:* Decrease in signal intensity of fat on T1WI; increased signal intensity on T2WI, T2 gradient echo and STIR-imaging	May spread to involve contiguous structures and lead to (pyo) myositis, fasciitis, vascular thrombosis, and lymphedema	–
Lymphedema (*Strepto- coccus/* secondary infections)	Subcuta- neous layers	*CT:* Subcutaneous reticular or "honeycomb" pattern fibrous septa: low-attenuation (20–30 HU) *MR:* T1WI: skin thickening; expansion of subcutaneous tissue with a characteristic "honeycomb" pattern of low signal intensity streaks *STIR:* Serpiginous increased signal intensity in subcutaneous fat	–	–
Dermatologic disorders (*Helicobacter cinaedi, Streptococcus pneumoniae,* secondary infections)	Skin	Eosinophilic folliculitis; pruritic papules; bacillary angiomatosis; paraneoplastic pemphigus	–	Kaposi's sarcoma
Tenosynovitis (*candida albicans*)	Tendons sheath	US/CT: edema of tendon sheat; tenosynoritis	–	–
Septic bursitis	Bursa	US/CT: edema of bursa; bursitis	• Olecranon • Prepatellar • Subdeltoid region	• *Staphylococcus aureus* • *Streptococcus pneumoniae* • *Mycobacterium marinum* • *Sporothrix schenkii*
Myopathy	Muscular system	*CT/MR:* Myonecrotic muscle: enlarged, decreased attenuation; localized intramuscular collection of fluid or gas may be seen; *contrast CT/MR* may differentiate between normal and myonecrotic tissue	Localized/diffuse	• Bacterial infections (*Staphylococcus aureus*) • Fungal infections • Parasitic infections

Organism/ disease	Organ involved	Radiologic abnormality	Extent of disease	Differential diagnosis
Osteomyelitis	Skeletal system	*Conventional radiography* • Periosteal reaction • Soft tissue swelling • Cortical erosions As infection progresses: osteolytic + osteosclerotic changes *Bone scintigraphy/MR* are helpful for early detection of osseous involvement and to demonstrate the extent of bone marrow infection	Localized	• *Staphylococcus aureus* • *Nocardia asteroides* • *Salmonella typhimurium* • *Gonococcus* • CMV • *Candida albicans* • *Aspergillus fumigatus* • *Toxoplasma gondii* • Spiromycosis
Bacillary angiomatosis (*Bartonella henselae, Bartonella quintana*)	Skin	Angiomatous cutaneous lesions *Conventional radiography:* Osteolytic lesions with overlying soft tissue mass: periostitis *Tc-99m scintigraphy:* Increased uptake *CT/MR:* Intense contrast enhancement of soft tissue lesions	• Liver/spleen • Lymph nodes • Respiratory tract • Skeletal system • Skin • Conjunctivae	–
Tuberculosis (*Mycobacterium tuberculosis; Mycobacterium avium-intra-cellulare*)	Skeletal system	Tuberculous osteomyelitis: vertebral column/cervical spine • Focal osteolysis with varying amounts of eburnation and periostitis • Sequestrum formation Tuberculous spondylitis of thoracic/lumbar spines *Conventional radiography:* Osteonecrosis; bone destruction involving the anterior vertebral body, narrowing of adjacent intervertebral disc; similar bone destruction of the contiguous vertebral body; progressive vertebral collapse with anterior wedging ("gibbus deformity") *US/CT:* Psoas/paraspinal abscess *Contrast MR:* Vertebral intraosseous abscess; meningeal involvement; subligamentous spread; paraspinal abscess	Other organs involved: • Respiratory tract • Metaphyseal involvement of bones: hips/knee • Sacral bones	*Staphylococcus aureus*

Organism/ disease	Organ involved	Radiologic abnormality	Extent of disease	Differential diagnosis
Atypical mycobacterial infection (*Mycobacterium avium-intracellulare complex*)	Mcta/dia-physes of long bones	*Conventional radiography:* • Discrete osteolytic lesions which have sclerotic margins (osteomyelitis) • Osteoporosis • Abscesses/sinus tracts/sarcoma	Multiple rather than solitary Other organs involved: • Bone marrow • Lymph nodes • Respiratory tract • GI tract • Liver/spleen • GU tract • Blood • Skin	• Tuberculosis • Extrapulmonary *P. carinii* • Fungal infections • Kaposi's sarcoma • AIDS-related lymphoma
Mycobacterium haemophilum	Tendon sheats	Tenosynovitis	• Knee • Ankle • Hip • Digits	–
Arthritis	Synovial joints	• Spondyloarthropathic arthritis (Reiter's syndrome) • HIV-associated arthritis; painful articular syndrome • Acute symmetric polyarthritis • Septic arthritis: common features, difficult to differentiate from each other • Tuberculous arthritis may affect large joints: monoarticular *Conventional radiography:* Phemister's triad: • Juxtra-articular osteoporosis • Peripherally located osseous erosions • Gradual narrowing of interosseous space	• Foot • Ankle • Knee • Hip • Multidigital dactylitis • Ankle • Shoulder	• Enteric pathogens • *Staphyloccocus aureus* • *Candida albicans* • *Streptococcus pneumoniae* • MAC • *M. kansasii* • *Mycobacterium haemophilum*
Avascular necrosis	Skeletal system	*Conventional radiography:* Subchondral fracture; sclerosis with crescentic radiolucency; flattening of epiphyseal head; widening of epiphyseal line; rarefaction of metaphysis; preservation of joint space *MR:* Low signal intensity band or rings of involved bone T2WI: "double line" sign of adjacent low/high signal intensity	Local	–
Hypertrophic pulmonary osteoarthropathy	Skeletal system	*Conventional radiography:* Subperiosteal new bone formation; soft tissue thickening; joint effusion; clubbing of digits *Bone scintigraphy:* Increased uptake at areas of new bone formation	Local	–

Organism/ disease	Organ involved	Radiologic abnormality	Extent of disease	Differential diagnosis
Spondylitis	Intervertebral (disc) space	*Conventional radiography:* Bony erosions of adjacent end-plates Narrowing of disc space *MR:* T1WI: decreased signal intensity of the discs T2WI: increasing signal intensity; paraspinal/epidural inflammation; edema, abscess formation with contrast ehancement; vertebral end-plates are also affected	Localized	• *Staphylococcus aureus* • *Cryptococcus neoformans* • *Candida albicans* • *Candida tropicalis* • *Pseudomonas aeruginosa*
Kaposi's sarcoma (KS)	Musculo skeletal system	*Plain radiographs* may be negative *Scintigraphy* may be negative *CT:* Multiple osteolytic lesions in pelvis, hips, spine, ribs, associated with periosteal reaction and overlying soft tissue mass *MR:* Extensive edema and subcuteneous tissue changes with minimal muscle involvement; extensive muscle involvement with adjacent subcutaneous lesions	Multifocal involvement Other organs involved: • Mucocutaneous • Sternum • Ribs • Thoracic spine • GI tract • Liver/spleen • Lymph nodes	• Bacillary angiomatosis • Tuberculosis • AIDS-related lymphoma
AIDS-related lymphoma	Musculo-skeletal system	*Conventional radiography/CT:* Permeative osteolytic lesions with cortical destruction; sclerosis and indistinct transition zone; periosteal reaction; pathologic fractures and associated soft tissue mass *MR:* T2WI: hyperintense signal mass	• Lower extremities • Skull • Pelvis • Spine • GI tract • CNS	Kaposi's sarcoma

CMV, Cytomegalovirus; MAC, Mycobacterium avium-intracellulare complex STIR; short tau inversion recovery

18.9 Different Radiologic Patterns on Chest Radiographs in AIDS

Observations	Incidence	Differential Diagnosis
Bronchial or bronchiolar wall thickening	Common	Pyogenic infections Mycobacterial infections (MTb, MAC) Kaposi's sarcoma
	Uncommon/absent	ARL Viral infections Fungal infections LIP, PCP

Observations	Incidence	Differential Diagnosis
Bronchiectasis	Common	Mycobacterial infections (MTb, MAC) Pyogenic infections
	Uncommon/absent	Fungal infections, PCP Kaposi's sarcoma ARL Viral infections LIP
Endoluminal polyp/mass	Uncommon	Mycobacterial infections (MTb, MAC) Fungal infections Kaposi's sarcoma ARL (rare)
	Absent	Pyogenic infections, PCP, viral infections LIP
Intrathoracic (mediastinal/hilar) lymph-adenopathy	Common	Mycobacterial infections (MTb, MAC) Fungal infections ARL
	Uncommon/absent	Kaposi's sarcoma PCP Viral infections Bacterial infections
Pleural effusions (isolated)	Common	Kaposi's sarcoma ARL Bacterial infections PCP
	Uncommon/absent	Viral infections Mycobacterial infections (MTb, MAC) Fungal infections LIP
Thick-walled cavities	Common	Fungal infections (*Aspergillus, cryptococcus*) Mycobacterial infections (MTb, depending on CD4 cell count, MAC) Rhodococcus Septic emboli
	Uncommon/absent	PCP Viral infections Kaposi's sarcma LIP ARL
Thin-walled cavities	Common	PCP

Observations	Incidence	Differential Diagnosis
Solitary (paren-chymal) nodules	Common	Kaposi's sarcoma (peribronchovascular and subpleural) ARL Fungal infections *(Aspergillus, cryptococcus)* *Nocardia* Myobacterial infections (MTb, MAC) Septic emboli Bronchogenic carcinoma
	Uncommon	CMV
Multiple (miliary) nodules	Uncommon	PCP CMV Tuberculosis Fungal infections PCP
Homo-geneous consolidation	Common	Bacterial infections Fungal infections
	Uncommon/absent	Mycobacterial infections (MTb, MAC) PCP Viral Kaposi's sarcoma ARL
Ground-glass attenuation (CT)	Common	PCP Pyogenic infections Viral infections (CMV) Kaposi's sarcoma Bacterial infections LIP
Reticular/reticulo-nodular pattern	Common	PCP Viral infections (CMV) Kaposi's sarcoma (coarse) ARL LIP
Ascites	Uncommon	*P. carinii* (extrapulmonary) ARL *Mycobacterium tuberculosis* Atypical mycobacterium Kaposi's sarcoma Bacillary angiomatosis

MTb, Mycobacterium tuberculosis; MAC, Maycobacterium avium-intracellulare complex; ARL, AIDS-related lymphoma; LIP, lymphocytic interstitial pneumonia; PCP, Pneumocystis carinii pneumonia; CMV, cytomegalovirus

18.10 Pathogens and Neoplasms in AIDS: Cytologic Methods

This table is adapted (and modified) from CHAN NH (1998) AIDS imaging; a practical clinical approach, Chap 6. SAUNDERS, London

Infections	Organ involved	Diagnostic method	Cytogenic staining	Pathologic characteristics
Viral infections				
Cytomegalovirus	Adrenals Respiratory tract GI tract CNS Retina	Bronchoalveolar lavage Smears FNA biopsies Transbronchial biopsies Open lung biopsies	PAP, H&E, Giemsa stain Monoclonal antibodies for immunochemistry In situ hybridization	Endothelial cells or histiocytic clusters; Enlarged large violaceous to dark red intranuclear inclusion bodies, surrounded by thin halo
Herpes simplex virus (HSV-1, HSV-2) Herpes zoster virus	Mucocutaneous Perianal region Oropharyngeal region Esophageal region	Sputum Bronchial brushing/washing (BAL) Smears from skin, oral mucosa, esophagus and remaining GI tract FNA biopsies	PAP, H&E, Giemsa stain Monoclonal antibodies for immunochemistry In situ hybridization	Vesicles/ulcerations: small esophilic, intranuclear, inclusion bodies
Bacterial infections				
Mycobacterium tuberculosis *Mycobacterium avium-intracellulare* complex	Lymph nodes Liver/spleen Bone marrow GI tract Respiratory tract CNS (rare) Skin (rare) CVS (rare)	Smears FNA specimen of the lymph nodes or other mass lesions Bone marrow biopsy/aspiration Bronchoscopy specimen Endoscopic biopsy	H&E stain Ziehl-Neelsen stain Kinynon stain Rhodamine-auramine stain DNA probes PAS/GMS/Giemsa stain Metaminamine stain Diff Quik	Multiple noncaseating granulomas within lobular parenchyma and portal tracts of the liver; acid fast microorganisms in cytoplasm of macrophages; single cells, small clusters, or large groups of histiocytes that are filled with small rods; inflammatory infiltrates usually absent
Pneumocystis carinii	Respiratory tract Liver/spleen GU tract	Induction and collection of sputum FNA biopsy of mass lesions for extra-pulmonary disease Bronchial brushing/washing BAL via fiberoptic bronchoscopy FNA biopsy Sputum Smears	PAP stain: specific H&E stain: specific GMS stain Giemsa or toluidine blue stain Autofluorescence Methylene blue stain	Acellular, granular foamy alveolar casts

Infections	Organ involved	Diagnostic method	Cytogenic staining	Pathologic characteristics

Parasitic infections

Infections	Organ involved	Diagnostic method	Cytogenic staining	Pathologic characteristics
Toxoplasma gondii	CNS Respiratory tract Lymph nodes	Open biopsy of enlarged regional lymph nodes FNA or tissue biopsy of intracranial mass BAL Smears	Giemsa stain H&E stain PAP/PAS stain GMS stain Monoclonal antibodies with immunoperoxidase stain Cannot be cultured; morphologic identification is crucial	*Toxoplasma* cysts three morphologic forms: • tachyzoites (acute infection: 3–7 mm × 2–4 mm tear drop, crescent shape; groups or aggregates within membrane, round cytoplasmic vacuoles; oval or rounded) • Bradyzoites (chronic infection): rounded, packed tightly into cysts (30–100 mm) • Oocysts: contain up to eight sporozoites
Cryptosporidium	GI tract Biliary tract Respiratory tract	–	Ziehl-Neelsen stain	Acid-fast micro-organisims (2–6 μm)
Microsporidium/ Isospora belli	GI tract (small bowel) Lymph nodes			Electron microscope examination

Fungal infections

Infections	Organ involved	Diagnostic method	Cytogenic staining	Pathologic characteristics
Candida albicans	Skin Oral cavity Esophagus Respiratory tract	Endoscopy specimen Bronchoscopy specimen	PAP/PAS stain GMS stain Culture Tissue immunohistochemistry or DNA probes not necessary	Invading fungi surrounded by granulocytes; buds and pseudohyphae without branching or true septations
Histoplasmosis (*Histoplasma capsulatum*)	CNS Respiratory tract Liver/spleen Adrenals Kidney	FNA biopsy of mass lesions BAL Peripheral blood smears	PAP/PAS stain Giemsa stain GMS stain Bone marrow culture Tissue immunohisto chemistry or DNA probe not necessary	–
Cryptococcosis (*Cryptococcus neoformans*)	CNS Lymph nodes Liver/spleen Bone marrow	Lumbar puncture (CSF) FNA specimen of a mass lesion Skin biopsy	PAP stain PAS stain GMS or mucicarmine stain India ink stain (CSF)	Epitheloid, multinucleated giant cells with organisms in their cytoplasm; small, sometimes teardrop-shaped budding yeasts with a diameter of 4–7 μm. Cells have prominent capsules
Coccidioidomy-cosis	Respiratory tract CNS	BAL Transbronchial biopsy	PAP stain PAS stain GMS or mucicarmine stain India ink stain (CSF)	

Infections	Organ involved	Diagnostic method	Cytogenic staining	Pathologic characteristics

Neoplasms

Infections	Organ involved	Diagnostic method	Cytogenic staining	Pathologic characteristics
Kaposi's sarcoma	Skin Mucous membrane Bronchial tree Oropharynx GI tract Lymph nodes Liver CVS GU tract (kidneys)	Endoscopy Biopsy	FNA biopsies Cytology plays no role in diagnosis	Five patterns are recognized: early, nodular, aggressive cutaneous, lymphadenopathic, and systemic generalized Kaposi's sarcoma *Histology:* Early angiomatous spindle cell, inflammatory, mixed and pleomorphic variant *Early lesions:* Small red nodules: 1–2 mm, later macular plaque-like lesions; slight to moderate cytonuclear pleomorphism with mitoses. Tumor cells show erythrophagocytosis, perivascular growth. Reactive proliferation of endothelial cells; irregularly dilated vascular spaces coated with swollen endothelial cells, similar to HHV-8
AIDS-related lymphoma	Respiratory tract GI tract CNS Pleura Pericardium Peritoneal cavity	FNA biopsy of mass lesions Smears	H&E stain Diff Quik Ziehl-Neelsen stain Giemsa stain Gram stain AFB	Pleomorphic population of lymphocytes, plasma cells and macrophages in a clear background, without granulomas or necrosis. Mixed cellularity. Histology: • Centroblastic cells • Lymphoblastic cells • Immunoblastic cells

FNA, Fine-needle aspiration; PAP, Papanicolaou stain; H&E, hematoxylin and eosin stain; GMS, Grocott's methenamine silver stain; PAS, periodic acid-Schiff stain; CSF, cerebrospinal fluid; AFB, acid-fast bacilli; BAL, bronchoalveolar lavage; CVS, cardiovascular system

Subject Index

List of Contributors

J. BEDFORD, MD
Assistant Director of River Valley HIV Services
of Western Massachusetts
15 Hospital Drive, Suite 403
Holyoke, MA 01040
USA

J.W. BERLIN, MD
Department of Diagnostic Radiology
Evanston Northwestern Healthcare
2650 Ridge Ave.
Evanston, IL 60201
USA

M.R. CANNINGA-VAN DIJK, MD
Department of Pathology
H04.312, University Medical Center
PO Box 85500
3508 GA Utrecht
The Netherlands

A. DEVILLE, MD
Pediatric Oncology, Fondation Lenval
57 avenue de la Californie
06200 Nice
France

E.K. FISHMAN, MD
Professor of Radiology
The Russell H. Morgan Department of Radiology
and Radiological Science
Johns Hopkins Medical Institutions
601. N. Caroline Street, JHOC 3254
Baltimore, MD 21287
USA

E.H.L. GAENSLER, MD
Department of Radiology
University of California
San Francisco, CA 94143
USA

A. GEOFFRAY, MD
Chief of Pediatric Radiology
Fondation Lenval
57 avenue de la Californie
06200 Nice
France

P.C. GOODMAN, MD
Department of Radiology
Duke University Medical Center
P.O. Box 3808
Durham, NC 22710
USA

R.M. GORE, MD
Department of Diagnostic Radiology
Evanston Northwestern Healthcare
2650 Ridge Ave.
Evanston, IL 60201
USA

L.B. HARAMATI, MD
Department of Radiology
Albert Einstein College of Medicine
and Montefiore Medical Center
111 East 210th Street
Bronx, New York 10467
USA

C.B. HICKS, MD
Associate Clinical Professor of Medicine
Division of Infectious Diseases
Duke University Medical Center
Box 3360
Durham, NC 27710
USA

A.J. HOLZ, MD
Department of Radiology
University of Miami School of Medicine
1115 NW 14th Street
Miami, FL 33136
USA

K.M. HORTON, MD
Assistant Professor of Radiology
The Russell H. Morgan Department of Radiology
and Radiological Science
Johns Hopkins Medical Institutions
601. N. Caroline Street, JHOC 3255
Baltimore, MD 21287
USA

H.J. HULSEBOSCH, MD
Department of Dermatology
Academic Medical Centre, AO-237
University of Amsterdam
Meibergdreef 9
1105 AZ Amsterdam
The Netherlands

E.R. JENNY-AVITAL, MD
Department of Medicine, Division of Infectious Diseases
Albert Einstein College of Medicine
Jacobi Medical Center
1400 Pelham Parkway South
Bronx, New York 10461
USA

J.S. Klein, MD
Department of Radiology
Fletcher Allen Health Care
111 Colchester Avenue
Burlington, VT 05401
USA

P.P. Maeder, MD
Department of Radiology
University Hospital, CHUV
1011 Lausanne
Switzerland

J.R. Mathieson, MD
928 Island Road
Victoria BC V8S 2T9
Canada

A.J. Megibow, MD, MPH, FACR
Professor of Radiology
Department of Radiology, NYU School of Medicine
560 First Avenue
New York, NY 10016
USA

R.A. Meuli, MD
Department of Radiology, University Hospital, CHUV
1011 Lausanne
Switzerland

F.H. Miller, MD
Department of Radiology
Northwestern Memorial Hospital
Northwestern University Medical School
676 St. Clair
Chicago, IL 60611
USA

E.H. Moore, MD
Department of Radiology
University of California Davis Medical Center
2616 Stockton Blvd.
Sacramento, CA 95817
USA

G.M. Newmark, MD
Department of Diagnostic Radiology
Evanston Northwestern Healthcare
2650 Ridge Ave.
Evanston, IL 60201
USA

J.W.A.J. Reeders, MD, PhD
Consultant (Interventional) Radiologist
Department of Radiology
St. Elisabeth Hospital Willemstad
Breedestraat 193 (O)
Curaçao
Netherlands Antilles

G.S. Reiter, MD, FACP
Medical Director Holyoke Hospital
Director of River Valley HIV Services
of Western Massachusetts
575 Beech St.
Holyoke, MA 01040
USA

J. Sandhu, MD
Department of Radiology
University of North Carolina, CB#7510
Chapel Hill, NC 27599-7510
USA

M. Spehl, MD
Professor of Radiology
Hopital universitaire Saint Pierre
322 rue Haute
1000 Bruxelles
Belgium

J. Tehranzadeh, MD
Professor of Radiology and Orthopaedics
Section Chief of Musculoskeletal Radiology
Department of Radiological Sciences, R140
University of California (Irvine)
101 City Drive
Orange, CA 92868-3298
USA

M.T. Tran, MD
Chief Resident of Radiology
Department of Radiological Sciences
University of California (Irvine)
101 City Drive
Orange, CA 92868-3298
USA

J.G. Van den Tweel, MD, PhD
Department of Pathology
H04.312, University Medical Center
PO Box 85500
3508 GA Utrecht
The Netherlands

E. van Sonnenberg, MD
Department of Radiology
Dana-Farber Cancer Institute
44 Binney Street
Boston, MA 02115
USA

M.L. Hansman Whiteman, MD
Department of Radiology
University of Miami School of Medicine
1115 NW 14th Street
Miami, FL 33136
USA

V. Yaghmai, MD
Department of Diagnostic Radiology
Evanston Northwestern Healthcare
2650 Ridge Ave.
Evanston, IL 60201
USA

J. Yee, MD
Chief of CT and GI Radiology
VA Medical Center/UCSF
4150 Clement Street
San Francisco, CA 94121
USA

MEDICAL RADIOLOGY
Diagnostic Imaging and Radiation Oncology

Titles in the series already published

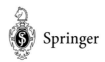

Springer

MEDICAL RADIOLOGY
Diagnostic Imaging and Radiation Oncology

Titles in the series already published

RADIATION ONCOLOGY

Lung Cancer
Edited by C.W. Scarantino

Innovations in Radiation Oncology
Edited by H. R. Withers
and L. J. Peters

**Radiation Therapy of Head
and Neck Cancer**
Edited by G.E. Laramore

**Gastrointestinal Cancer – Radiation
Therapy**
Edited by R.R. Dobelbower, Jr.

**Radiation Exposure and
Occupational Risks**
Edited by E. Scherer, C. Streffer,
and K.-R. Trott

**Radiation Therapy of Benign
Diseases - A Clinical Guide**
S.E. Order and S. S. Donaldson

**Interventional Radiation Therapy
Techniques - Brachytherapy**
Edited by R. Sauer

Radiopathology of Organs and Tissues
Edited by E. Scherer,
C. Streffer, and K.-R. Trott

**Concomitant Continuous Infusion
Chemotherapy and Radiation**
Edited by M. Rotman
and C. J. Rosenthal

**Intraoperative Radiotherapy –
Clinical Experiences and Results**
Edited by F. A. Calvo,
M. Santos, and L.W. Brady

**Radiotherapy of Intraocular
and Orbital Tumors**
Edited by W. E. Alberti
and R. H. Sagerman

**Interstitial and Intracavitary
Thermoradiotherapy**
Edited by M. H. Seegenschmiedt
and R. Sauer

**Non-Disseminated Breast Cancer
Controversial Issues
in Management**
Edited by G. H. Fletcher
and S.H. Levitt

**Current Topics in Clinical Radiobiology
of Tumors**
Edited by H.-P. Beck-Bornholdt

**Practical Approaches to Cancer Invasion
and Metastases**
A Compendium of Radiation
Oncologists' Responses to 40 Histories
Edited by A. R. Kagan with the
Assistance of R. J. Steckel

**Radiation Therapy
in Pediatric Oncology**
Edited by J. R. Cassady

Radiation Therapy Physics
Edited by A. R. Smith

Late Sequelae in Oncology
Edited by J. Dunst and R. Sauer

Mediastinal Tumors. Update 1995
Edited by D. E. Wood
and C. R. Thomas, Jr.

**Thermoradiotherapy
and Thermochemotherapy**

Volume 1:
Biology, Physiology, and Physics

Volume 2:
Clinical Applications
Edited by M.H. Seegenschmiedt,
P. Fessenden, and C.C. Vernon

**Carcinoma of the Prostate
Innovations in Management**
Edited by Z. Petrovich,
L. Baert, and L.W. Brady

**Radiation Oncology
of Gynecological Cancers**
Edited by H.W. Vahrson

**Carcinoma of the Bladder
Innovations in Management**
Edited by Z. Petrovich,
L. Baert, and L.W. Brady

**Blood Perfusion and Microenvironment
of Human Tumors**
Implications for Clinical
Radiooncology
Edited by M. Molls and P. Vaupel

**Radiation Therapy of Benign Diseases.
A Clinical Guide**
2nd Revised Edition
S. E. Order and S. S. Donaldson

**Carcinoma of the Kidney and Testis, and
Rare Urologic Malignancies**
Innovations in Management
Edited by Z. Petrovich,
L. Baert, and L.W. Brady

**Progress and Perspectives in the Treat-
ment of Lung Cancer**
Edited by P. Van Houtte, J. Klastersky,
and P. Rocmans

**Combined Modality Therapy of
Central Nervous System Tumors**
Edited by Z. Petrovich, L. W. Brady,
M. L. Apuzzo, and M. Bamberg

Age-Related Macular Degeneration
Current Treatment Concepts
Edited by W. A. Alberti, G. Richard, and
R. H. Sagerman

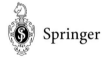

Springer